The APRN's Complete Guide to Prescribing Drug Therapy

2017

Mari J. Wirfs, PhD, MN, RN, ANP-BC, FNP-BC, CNE, is a nationally certified adult nurse practitioner (ANCC since 1997) and family nurse practitioner (AANP since 1998) and certified nurse educator (NLN since 2008). Her career spans 45 years in collegiate undergraduate and graduate nursing education and clinical practice in critical care, pediatrics, psychiatric–mental health nursing, and advanced practice primary care nursing. Her PhD is in higher education administration and leadership. During her academic career, she has achieved the rank of professor with tenure in two university systems. Currently she is adjunct professor in the New Orleans Baptist Theological Seminary Graduate School where she teaches neuropsychology and psychopharmacology in the Guidance and Counseling Program. She is a frequent guest lecturer on a variety of advanced practice topics to professional groups and general health care topics to community groups.

Dr. Wirfs has completed, published, and presented six quantitative research studies focusing on academic leadership, nursing education, and clinical practice issues, including one for the Army Medical Department conducted during her 8 years reserve service in the Army Nurse Corps. Dr. Wirfs has co-authored family primary care certification review books and study materials, authored the *Clinical Guide to Pharmacotherapeutics for the Primary Care Provider* (1999–2014), and now *The APRN's Complete Guide to Prescribing Drug Therapy 2017.*

Dr. Wirfs has been inducted into several honor societies and is a long-time member of the National Organization for Nurse Practitioner Faculties (NONPF), serving as clinical preceptor for several nurse practitioner programs. Since 2002, Dr. Wirfs has served as clinical director and primary care provider at the NOBTS Family Health Care Clinic, serving faculty, staff, students, and their families. She is also a founding member of the medical staff in part-time practice at Baptist Community Health Services, established post-Katrina in the New Orleans Lower Ninth Ward.

The APRN's Complete Guide to Prescribing Drug Therapy

2017

Mari J. Wirfs, PhD, MN, RN, ANP-BC, FNP-BC, CNE

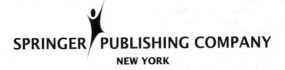

SPRINGER PUBLISHING COMPANY
NEW YORK

Springer Publishing Company, LLC
11 West 42nd Street
New York, NY 10036
www.springerpub.com

Acquisitions Editor: Margaret Zuccarini
Composition: Exeter Premedia Services Private LTD.

ISBN: 978-0-8261-6666-1
e-book ISBN: 978-0-8261-6667-8

16 17 18 19 / 5 4 3 2 1

This book is a quick reference for health care providers practicing in primary care settings. The information has been extrapolated from a variety of professional sources and is presented in condensed and summary form. It is not intended to replace or substitute for complete and current manufacturer prescribing information, current research, or knowledge and experience of the user. For complete prescribing information, including toxicities, drug interactions, contraindications, and precautions, the reader is directed to the manufacturer's package insert and the published literature. The inclusion of a particular brand name neither implies nor suggests that the author or publisher advises or recommends the use of that particular product or considers it superior to similar products available by other brand names. Neither the author nor the publisher makes any warranty, expressed or implied, with respect to the information, including any errors or omissions, herein.

Library of Congress Cataloging-in-Publication Data
Names: Wirfs, Mari J., author.
Title: The APRN's complete guide to prescribing drug therapy 2017 / Mari J.
   Wirfs.
Description: New York, NY : Springer Publishing Company, LLC, [2017]
Identifiers: LCCN 2016013691| ISBN 9780826166661 | ISBN 9780826166678 (e-book)
Subjects: | MESH: Drug Therapy—nursing | Advanced Practice Nursing—methods
   | Handbooks
Classification: LCC RM301 | NLM WY 49 | DDC 615.1—dc23
LC record available at https://lccn.loc.gov/2016013691

Special discounts on bulk quantities of our books are available to corporations, professional associations, pharmaceutical companies, health care organizations, and other qualifying groups. If you are interested in a custom book, including chapters from more than one of our titles, we can provide that service as well.

For details, please contact:
Special Sales Department, Springer Publishing Company, LLC
11 West 42nd Street, 15thFloor, New York, NY 10036-8002
Phone: 877-687-7476 or 212-431-4370; Fax: 212-941-7842
E-mail: sales@springerpub.com

Printed in the United States of America by Edwards Brothers Malloy.

CONTENTS

SECTION I: DRUG THERAPY BY CLINICAL DIAGNOSIS

SECTION II: APPENDICES

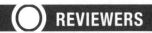

REVIEWERS

Kelley M. Anderson, PhD, FNP
Assistant Professor of Nursing, Georgetown University School of Nursing & Health Studies, Washington, DC

Kathleen Bradbury-Golas, DNP, RN, FNP-C, ACNS-BC
Associate Clinical Professor, Drexel University, Philadelphia, Pennsylvania
Family Nurse Practitioner, Virtua Medical Group, Hammonton and Linwood, New Jersey

Lori Brien, MS, ACNP-BC
Instructor, AG-ACNP Program, Georgetown University School of Nursing & Health Studies, Washington, DC

Jill C. Cash, MSN, APN
Nurse Practitioner, Logan Primary Care, West Frankfort, Illinois

Catherine M. Concert, DNP, RN, FNP-BC, AOCNP, NE-BC, CNL, CGRN
Nurse Practitioner—Radiation Oncology, Laura and Isaac Perlmutter Cancer Center, New York University Langone Medical Center; Clinical Assistant Professor, Pace University Lienhard School of Nursing, New York, New York

Aileen Fitzpatrick, DNP, RN, FNP-BC
Clinical Assistant Professor, Pace University Lienhard School of Nursing, New York, New York

Tracy P. George, DNP, APRN-BC, CNE
Assistant Professor of Nursing, Amy V. Cockroft Fellow 2016–2017, Francis Marion University, Florence, South Carolina

Norma Stephens Hannigan, DNP, MPH, FNP-BC, DCC, FAANP
Clinical Professor of Nursing, Coordinator, Accelerated Second Degree (A2D) Program/Sophomore Honors Program, Hunter College, CUNY Hunter-Bellevue School of Nursing, New York, New York

Ella T. Heitzler, PhD, WHNP-BC, FNP-BC, RNC-OB
Assistant Professor, Georgetown University School of Nursing and Health Studies, Washington, DC

Melissa H. King, DNP, FNP-BC, ENP-BC
Director of Advanced Practice Providers, Director of TelEmergency,
Department of Emergency Medicine, University of Mississippi Medical Center,
Jackson, Mississippi

Michael Watson, DNP, APRN, FNP-BC
Lead Family Nurse Practitioner, Wadley Regional Medical Center, Emergency
Department, Texarkana, Texas

*	single-scored tablet
**	cross-scored tablet
(II), (III), (IV), (V)	Drug Enforcement Agency (DEA) controlled substance schedule
(A), (B), (C), (D), (X)	Federal Drug Agency (FDA) pregnancy category
ABSSSI	acute bacterial skin and skin structure infection
ac	before meal
ACEI	angiotensin converting enzyme inhibitor
ALT	liver enzyme; alanine transaminase (ALT)
AM	antemeridiem, morning
APAP	acetaminophen
AST	liver enzyme, aspartate transaminase
Amp	ampule
Apo-B	apolipoprotein b
ARB	angiotensin receptor blocker
ART	antiretroviral treatment
ASE	adverse side effect
AVB	atrioventricular heart block
bid	bis in die, twice-a-day
BP	blood pressure
CAD	coronary artery disease
calib applicator	calibrated applicator
cap	capsule
CAP	community acquired pneumonia
CCB	calcium channel blocker
CFC	chlorofluorocarbon, inhaler propellant
chew tab	chewable tablet

Child-Pugh A	mild liver disease/dysfunction
Child-Pugh B	moderate liver disease/dysfunction
Child-Pugh C	severe liver disease/dysfunction
CHF	congestive heart failure
CKD	chronic kidney disease
clnsr	cleanser
conc	concentrate, concentration
conj estra	conjugated estrogen
COPD	chronic obstructive pulmonary disease
cplt	caplet
Cr	creatinine
CrCl	creatinine clearance measured in mL/min
CRI	chronic renal insufficiency
CRF	chronic renal failure
crm	cream
CVD	cardiovascular disease
DDAVP	desmopressin acetate
dL	deciliter
DM	diabetes mellitis
DMARDs	disease modifying anti-rheumatoid drugs
DVT	deep vein thrombosis
ent-coat	enteric-coated
EDTA	edatate calcium disodium
EE	ethinyl estradiol
eGFR	estimated glomerular filtration tate
EKG	electrocardiogram
EIA	exercise-induced asthma
EIAED	enzyme-inducing antiepileptic drug
EIB	exercise-induced bronchospasm

elix	elixer
emol, emol crm	emollient, emollient cream
ESA	erythropoiesis stimulating agent
ESR	erythrocyte sedimentation rate
ESRD	end stage renal disease
est	estradiol
EX, ext-rel	extended-release
g	gram
(G)	generic, generic availability
GABHS	group a beta-hemolytic streptococcus
GAD	generalized anxiety disorder
GI	gastrointestinal
gtt, gtts	drop, drops
GU	genitourinary
H_2O_2	hydrogen peroxide
HAART	highly active antiretroviral treatment
HCT	hematocrit
HCTZ	hydrochlorothiazide
HAV	hepatitis A virus
HBV	hepatitis C virus
HCV	hepatitis C virus
HDL, HDL-C	high density lipoprotein cholesterol
HFA	hydrofluoroalkane (inhaler propellent phasing in)
Hgb	hemoglobin
HgbA1c	hemoglobin A1c, the standard POC diagnostic test for diabetes
hgc	hard-gel capsule
HPV	human papilloma virus
HR	heart rate in beats per minute
HRT	hormone replacement therapy

HS	hour of sleep, bedtime
IBS-C	irritable bowel syndrome with constipation
IBS-D	irritable bowel syndrome with diarrhea
ID	intradermal
IM	intramuscular
immed-rel	immediate-release
inhal	inhalation
inj	injection
IU	international unit
IUD	intrauterine device
IV	intravenous
JRA	juvenile rheumatoid arthritis
K+	potassium
kg	kilogram
L	liter, 1000 ml
LAA	long-acting anticholinergic
LABA	long-actine beta agonist
LAR	long-acting release
LDL, LDL-C	low density lipoprotein cholesterol
LFTs	liver function tests
Liq	liquid
lotn	lotion
LR	lactated ringers IV solution
MAOI	monoamine oxidase inhibitor
mcg	microgram
MDD	major depressive disorder
MDI	metered dose inhaler
mfr	manufacturer
mg	milligram

mg/dL	milligrams per deciliter
mg/kg/day	milligram per kilogram per day
ml, mL	milliliter
MRSA	methicillin-resistant staphylococcus aureus
MS	multiple sclerosis
MTX	methotrexate
Na+	sodium
NaCl	sodium chloride
NaHCO3	sodium bicarbonate
NMDA	n-methyl-d-aspartate receptor antagonist
NNRTI	nonnucleoside reverse transcriptase inhibitor
NOH	neurogenic orthostatic hypotension
non-HDL-C	non-high density lipoprotein cholesterol
norgest	norgestimate
nPEP	non-occupational post-exposure prophylaxis
NR	not rated, pregnancy category not ssigned
NRTI	nucleoside reverse transcriptase inhibitor
NS	nasal spray; normal saline
NSAID	nonsteroidal anti-inflammatory drug
OA	osteoarthritis
OCD	obsessive compulsive disorder
OCP	oral contraceptive pill
ODT	orally-disintegrating tablet
Oint	ointment
ophth	ophthalmic, pertaining to the eye
orally-disint	orally-disintegrating
OTC	over-the-counter
Otic	pertaining to the ear
oz	ounce, 30 ml

pc	after meals
PBA	pseudobulbar affect
PCOS	polycystic ovarian syndrome; Stein-Leventhal Disease
Pediatric	newborn to ≤18 years-of-age
PD	Parkinson's disease
PDE5	phosphodiesterase type 5 inhibitor
PJIA	polyarticular juvenile idiopathic arthritis
PM	post-meridiem, evening
PMDD	premenstrual Dysmorphic Disorder
PMHx	past medical history
PPI	proton pump inhibitor
PO	per oral, by mouth
PO_4^{3-}	phosphate
POC	point of care
Post-op	post-operative
PR	per rectum
PRN	as needed
PTSD	post traumatic stress disorder
PUD	peptic ulcer disease
PVD	peripheral vascular disease
pwdr	powder
pwdr w. diluent	powder with diluent
q	per
qd	once daily
qHS	per hour of sleep, bedtime
qid	quater in die, four times-a-day
RA	rheumatoid arthritis
RAI	reversible anticholinesterase inhibitor
RBC	red blood cell

SC	subcutaneous
sgc	soft-gel capsule
SGOT	serum glutamic-oxaloacetic transaminase
SGPT	serum glutamic-pyruvic transaminase
SL	sublingual, under the tongue
syr	syrup
soln	solution
supp	suppository
susp	suspension
sust-rel	sustained release
SNRI	selective serotonin and norepinephrine reuptake inhibitor
SR	sustained-release
SSRI	selective serotonin reuptake inhibitor
STD	sexually transmitted disease
T1DM	type 1 diabetes mellitus
T2DM	type 2 diabetes mellitus
T3	liothyronine
T4	levothyroxine
tab	tablet
TCA	tricyclic antidepressant
TG	triglyceride
tid	ter in die, three times-a-day
TMP/SMX	trimethoprim-sulfamethoxizole
trans-sys	transdermal system
TRD	treatment-resistant depression
TSH	thyroid stimulating hormone
tsp	teaspoon, 4-5 ml
TSSRI	thienobenzodiazepine-selective serotonin reuptake inhibitor

VVC	vulvovaginal candidiasis
WBC	white blood cell
w.	with
XL	extra long-acting
XOI	xanthine oxidase inhibitor
XR	extended-release

PREFACE

The APRN's Complete Guide to Prescribing Drug Therapy is a prescribing reference intended for use by health care providers in all clinical practice settings who are involved in the primary care management of patients with acute, episodic, and chronic health problems. It is organized in a concise and easy-to-read format. Comments are interspersed throughout, including such clinically useful information as laboratory values to be monitored, patient teaching points, and safety information.

This clinical guide is divided into two sections. **Section I** presents drug treatment regimens for over 500 clinical diagnoses. Each drug is listed alphabetically by generic name, followed by the FDA pregnancy category (A, B, C, D, X, or NR if a pregnancy category has not been assigned), whether the drug is available over-the-counter (OTC), DEA schedule (I, II, III, IV, V), generic availability (G), adult and pediatric dosing regimens, brand names and available dose forms, whether tablets, caplets, or chew tabs are scored (*) or cross-scored (**), flavors of chewable, sublingual, buccal, and liquid forms and information regarding additives (e.g., dye-free, sugar-free, preservative-free or preservative type, and alcohol-free or alcohol content).

Section II presents clinically useful information in convenient table format, including: the JNC-8 recommendations for hypertension management, the U.S. schedule of controlled substances and the FDA pregnancy categories, measurement conversions, childhood and adult immunization recommendations, brand-name drugs (with contents) for the management of common respiratory symptoms, anti-infectives by classification, pediatric dosing by weight for liquid forms, gluco-corticosteroids by potency and route of administration, and contraceptives by route of administration and estrogen and/or progesterone content. An alphabetical cross reference index of drugs by generic and brand name, with FDA pregnancy category and controlled drug schedule, facilitates quick identification of drugs by alternate names, relative safety during pregnancy, and DEA schedule.

Selected diagnoses (e.g., angina, ADD/ADHD, growth failure, glaucoma, Parkinson's disease, CMV retinitis, multiple sclerosis, cystic fibrosis) and selected drugs (e.g., antineoplastics, antipsychotics, anti-arrhythmics, anti-HIV drugs, and anticoagulants) are included as patients are often referred by surgeons and emergency and urgent care providers to the primary care provider for follow-up monitoring and management.

Safe, efficacious, prescribing and monitoring of drug therapy regimens require adequate knowledge about (a) the pharmacodynamics and pharmacokinetics of drugs, (b) concomitant therapies, and (c) individual characteristics of the patient (e.g., current and past medical history, physical examination findings, hepatic and renal function, and co-morbidities). Users of this clinical guide are encouraged to utilize the manufacturer's package insert, recommendations and guidance of specialists, standard of practice protocols, and the current research literature for more comprehensive information about specific drugs (e.g., special precautions, drug-drug and drug-food interactions, risk versus benefit, age-related considerations, adverse reactions) and appropriate use with individual patients.

ACKNOWLEDGMENTS

This publication, which we consider to be a "must have" for students, academicians, and practicing clinicians with prescriptive authority, represents the culmination of Springer Publishing Company's collaborative team effort. Margaret Zuccarini, Publisher, Nursing, and the Editorial Committee, shared my vision for a handy pocket prescribing reference for new and experienced prescribers in primary care. Joanne Jay, Vice President, Production and Manufacturing, designed the contents for ease and efficiency of user navigation. The production team at Exeter Premedia Services, on behalf of Springer Publishing Company, understood the critical nature of exactness in this prescribing resource, and faithfully managed the complex files as content was updated and cross-paginated for the final product. The work of the reviewers from academia and clinical practice was essential to the process and their contributions are greatly appreciated. I am proud of my association with these dedicated professionals and I thank them on behalf of the medical and advanced practice nursing community worldwide, for supporting the end goal of quality health care for all.

SECTION I

DRUG THERAPY BY CLINICAL DIAGNOSIS

ACETAMINOPHEN OVERDOSE

ANTIDOTE/CHELATING AGENT

▷ *acetylcysteine* (B)(G) *Loading Dose:* 150 mg/kg administered over 15 minutes; *Maintenance:* 50 mg/kg administered over 4 hours; then 100 mg/kg administered over 16 hours
Pediatric: same as adult
Acetadote *Vial: soln for IV infusion after dilution:* 200 mg/ml (30 ml; dilute in D₅W (preservative-free)

Comment: *acetaminophen* overdose is a medical emergency due to the risk of irreversible hepatic injury. An IV infusion of *acetylcysteine* should be started as soon as possible and within 24 hours if the exact time of ingestion is unknown. Use a serum *acetaminophen* nomogram to determine need for treatment. Extreme caution is needed if used with concomitant hepatotoxic drugs.

ACNE ROSACEA

Comment: All acne rosacea products should be applied sparingly to clean, dry skin as directed. Avoid use of topical corticosteroids.
▷ *ivermectin* (C) apply bid
Soolantra *Crm:* 1% (30 g)
Comment: **Soolantra** is a macrocyclic lactone. Exactly how it works to treat rosacea is unknown.

TOPICAL ALPHA-2 AGONIST

▷ *brimonidine* (B) apply once daily
Pediatric: <18 years: not recommended
Mirvaso apply to affected area once daily
Gel: 0.33% (30, 45 g tube; 30 g pump)
Comment: For persistant erythema; constricts dilated facial blood vessels to reduce redness.

TOPICAL ANTIMICROBIALS

▷ *azelaic acid* (B) apply bid
Azelex *Crm:* 20% (30, 50 g)
Finacea *Gel:* 15% (30 g); *Foam:* 15% (50 g)
▷ *metronidazole* (B) apply to clean dry skin
MetroCream apply bid
Emol crm: 0.75% (45 g)
MetroGel apply once daily
Gel: 1% (60 g tube; 55 g pump)
MetroLotion apply bid
Lotn: 0.75% (2 oz)
▷ *sodium sulfacetamide* (C)(G) apply 1-3 x daily
Klaron *Lotn:* 10% (2 oz)
▷ *sodium sulfacetamide/sulfur* (C)
Clenia Emollient Cream apply 1-3 x daily
Wash: sod sulfa 10%/sulfur 5% (10 oz)

Clenia Foaming Wash wash affected area once <u>or</u> twice daily
Wash: sod sulfa 10%/*sulfur* 5% (6, 12 oz)
Rosula Gel apply 1-3 x daily
Gel: sod sulfa 10%/*sulfur* 5% (45 ml)
Rosula Lotion apply tid
Lotn: sod sulfa 10%/*sulfur* 5% (45 ml) (alcohol-free)
Rosula Wash wash bid
Clnsr: sod sulfa 10%/*sulfur* 5% (335 ml)

ORAL ANTIMICROBIALS

▷ *doxycycline* (D)(G) 40-100 mg bid
Pediatric: <8 years: not recommended; ≥8 years, <100 lb: 2 mg/lb on first day in 2 divided doses, followed by 1 mg/lb/day in 1-2 divided doses; ≥8 years, ≥100 lb: same as adult; *see page 561 for dose by weight*
Actilate *Tab:* 75, 150** mg
Adoxa *Tab:* 50, 75, 100, 150 mg ent-coat
Doryx *Tab:* 75, 100, 150 mg del-rel
Monodox *Cap:* 50, 75, 100 mg
Oracea *Cap:* 40 mg del-rel
Vibramycin *Cap:* 50, 100 mg; *Syr:* 50 mg/5 ml (raspberry; sulfites); *Oral susp:* 25 mg/5 ml (raspberry-apple)
Vibra-Tab *Tab:* 100 mg film-coat
Comment: *doxycycline* is contraindicated <8 years-of-age, in pregnancy, and lactation (discolors developing tooth enamel). A side effect may be photosensitivity (photophobia). Do not give with antacids, calcium supplements, milk or other dairy, or within two hours of taking another drug.

▷ *minocycline* (D)(G) 200 mg on first day; then 100 mg q 12 hours x 9 more days
Pediatric: <8 years: not recommended; ≥8 years, <100 lb: 2 mg/lb on first day in 2 divided doses, followed by 1 mg/lb q 12 hours x 9 more days; ≥8 years, ≥100 lb: same as adult
Dynacin *Cap:* 50, 100 mg
Minocin *Cap:* 50, 75, 100 mg; *Oral susp:* 50 mg/5 ml (60 ml) (custard) (sulfites, alcohol 5%)
Comment: *minocycline* is contraindicated <8 years-of-age, in pregnancy, and lactation (discolors developing tooth enamel). A side effect may be photosensitivity (photophobia). Do not give with antacids, calcium supplements, milk or other dairy, or within two hours of taking another drug.

ACNE VULGARIS

ANTIBACTERIAL SOAPS

Dial (OTC) wash affected area bid
Lever 2000 Antibacterial (OTC) wash affected area bid

TOPICAL ANTIMICROBIALS

Comment: All topical antimicrobials should be applied sparingly to clean, dry skin.

▷ *azelaic acid* (B) apply bid
    Azelex *Crm:* 20% (30, 50 g)
    Finacea *Gel:* 15% (30 g); *Foam:* 15% (50g)
▷ *benzoyl peroxide* (C)(G)
  Comment: *benzoyl peroxide* may discolor clothing and linens.
    Benzac-W initially apply to affected area once daily; increase to bid-tid as tolerated
      Gel: 2.5, 5, 10% (60 g)
    Benzac-W Wash wash affected area bid
      Wash: 5% (4, 8 oz); 10% (8 oz)
    Benzagel apply to affected area one <u>or</u> more times/day
      Gel: 5, 10% (1.5, 3 oz) (alcohol 14%)
    Benzagel Wash wash affected area bid
      Gel: 10% (6 oz)
    Desquam X⁵ wash affected area bid
      Wash: 5% (5 oz)
    Desquam X¹⁰ wash affected area bid
      Wash: 10% (5 oz)
    Triaz apply to affected area daily bid
      Lotn: 3, 6, 9% (bottle); 3% (tube); *Pads:* 3, 6, 9% (jar)
    ZoDerm apply once <u>or</u> twice daily
      Gel: 4.5, 6.5, 8.5% (125 ml); *Crm:* 4.5, 6.5, 8.5% (125 ml); *Clnsr:* 4.5, 6.5, 8.5% (400 ml)
▷ *clindamycin* topical (B) apply bid
  Pediatric: not recommended
    Cleocin T *Pad:* 1% (60/pck; alcohol 50%); *Lotn:* 1% (60 ml); *Gel:* 1% (30, 60 g);
    Soln w. applicator: 1% (30, 60 ml) (alcohol 50%)
    Clindagel *Gel:* 1% (42, 77 g)
    Evoclin Foam: 1% (50, 100 g) (alcohol)
▷ *clindamycin/benzoyl peroxide* topical (C) apply sparingly to clean dry skin once daily
  Pediatric: <12 years: not recommended; ≥12 years: same as adult
    Acanya *Gel: clin* 1.2%/*benz* 2.5% (50 g)
    BenzaClin (G) *Gel: clin* 1%/*benz* 5% (25, 50 g)
    Duac *Gel: clin* 1%/*benz* 5% (45 g)
    Onexton Gel *Gel: clin* 1.2%/*benz* 3.75% (50 g Pump) (alcohol-free, preservative-free)
▷ *dapsone* topical (C) apply bid
  Pediatric: <12 years: not recommended; ≥12 years: same as adult
    Aczone *Gel:* 5, 7.5% (30, 60, 90 g Pump)
▷ *erythromycin/benzoyl peroxide* (C) initially apply once daily; increase to bid as tolerated
    Benzamycin Topical Gel *Gel: eryth* 3%/*benz* 5% (46.6 g/jar)
▷ *sodium sulfacetamide* (C)(G) apply tid
    Klaron *Lotn:* 10% (2 oz)

ORAL ANTIMICROBIALS

▷ *doxycycline* (D)(G) 100 mg bid
  Pediatric: <8 years: not recommended; ≥8 years, <100 lb: 2 mg/lb on first day in 2
  divided doses, followed by 1 mg/lb/day in 1-2 divided doses; ≥8 years, ≥100 lb: same
  as adult; *see page 561 for dose by weight*
    Actilate *Tab:* 75, 150**mg
    Adoxa *Tab:* 50, 75, 100, 150 mg ent-coat
    Doryx *Tab:* 75, 100, 150 mg del-rel

Monodox *Cap:* 50, 75, 100 mg
Oracea *Cap:* 40 mg del-rel
Vibramycin *Cap:* 50, 100 mg; *Syr:* 50 mg/5 ml (raspberry-apple) (sulfites); *Oral susp:* 25 mg/5 ml (raspberry-apple)
Vibra-Tab *Tab:* 100 mg film coat

Comment: *doxycycline* is contraindicated <8 years-of-age, in pregnancy, and lactation (discolors developing tooth enamel). A side effect may be photo-sensitivity (photophobia). Do not give with antacids, calcium supplements, milk or other dairy, or within two hours of taking another drug.

▶ *erythromycin base* (B)(G) 250 mg qid, 333 mg tid <u>or</u> 500 mg bid x 7-10 days; then taper to lowest effective dose
Pediatric: <45 kg: 30-50 mg in 2-4 divided doses x 7-10 days; ≥45 kg: same as adult
Ery-Tab *Tab:* 250, 333, 500 mg ent-coat
PCE *Tab:* 333, 500 mg

Comment: *erythromycin* may increase INR with concomitant *warfarin*, as well as increase serum level of *digoxin*, benzodiazepines and statins.

▶ *erythromycin ethylsuccinate* (B)(G) 400 mg qid x 7-10 days
Pediatric: 30-50 mg/kg/day in 4 divided doses x 7-10 days; may double dose with severe infection; max 100 mg/kg/day; *see page 563 for dose by weight*
EryPed *Oral susp:* 200 mg/5 ml (100, 200 ml) (fruit); 400 mg/5 ml (60, 100, 200 ml) (banana); *Oral drops:* 200, 400 mg/5 ml (50 ml) (fruit); *Chew tab:* 200 mg wafer (fruit)
E.E.S. *Oral susp:* 200, 400 mg/5 ml (100 ml) (fruit)
E.E.S. Granules *Oral susp:* 200 mg/5 ml (100, 200 ml) (cherry)
E.E.S. 400 Tablets *Tab:* 400 mg

Comment: *erythromycin* may increase INR with concomitant *warfarin*, as well as increase serum level of *digoxin*, benzodiazepines and statins.

▶ *minocycline* (D)(G) initially 50-200 mg/day in 2 divided doses; reduce dose after improvement
Pediatric: <8 years: not recommended; ≥8 years: same as adult
Dynacin *Cap:* 50, 100 mg
Minocin *Cap:* 50, 75, 100 mg; *Oral susp:* 50 mg/5 ml (60 ml) (custard) (sulfites, alcohol 5%)

Comment: *minocycline* is contraindicated <8 years-of-age, in pregnancy, and lactation (discolors developing tooth enamel). A side effect may be photo-sensitivity (photophobia). Do not give with antacids, calcium supplements, milk or other dairy, or within two hours of taking another drug.

▶ *tetracycline* (D)(G) initially 1 g/day in 2-4 divided doses; after improvement, 125-500 mg daily
Pediatric: <8 years: not recommended; ≥8 years, <100 lb: 25-50 mg/kg/day in 2-4 divided doses; ≥8 years, ≥100 lb: same as adult; *see page 574 for dose by weight*
Achromycin V *Cap:* 250, 500 mg
Sumycin *Tab:* 250, 500 mg; *Cap:* 250, 500 mg; *Oral susp:* 125 mg/5 ml (100, 200 ml) (fruit) (sulfites)

Comment: *tetracycline* is contraindicated <8 years-of-age, in pregnancy, and lactation (discolors developing tooth enamel). A side effect may be photo-sensitivity (photophobia). Do not give with antacids, calcium supplements, milk or other dairy, or within two hours of taking another drug.

TOPICAL RETINOIDS

Comment: Wash affected area with a soap-free cleanser; pat dry and wait 20 to 30 minutes; then apply sparingly to affected area; use only once daily in the evening. Avoid applying to eyes, ears, nostrils, and mouth.
Pediatric: <8 years: not recommended; ≥8 years: same as adult
➤ *adapalene* (C) apply once daily at HS
  Differin *Crm:* 0.1% (45 g); *Gel:* 0.1. 0.3% (45 g) (alcohol-free); *Pad:* 0.1% (30/pck) (alcohol 30%); *Ltn:* 0.1% (2, 4 oz)
➤ *tazarotene* (X) apply once daily at HS
  Pediatric: not recommended
  Avage Cream *Crm:* 0.1% (30 g)
  Tazorac Cream *Crm:* 0.05, 0.1% (15, 30, 60 g)
  Tazorac Gel *Gel:* 0.05, 0.1% (30, 100 g)
➤ *tretinoin* (C) apply once daily at HS
  Pediatric: <12 years: not recommended; ≥12 years: same as adult
  Atralin Gel *Gel:* 0.05% (45 g)
  Avita *Crm:* 0.025% (20, 45 g); *Gel:* 0.025% (20, 45 g)
  Renova *Crm:* 0.02% (40 g); 0.05% (40, 60 g)
  Retin-A Cream *Crm:* 0.025, 0.05, 0.1% (20, 45 g)
  Retin-A Gel *Gel:* 0.01, 0.025% (15, 45 g) (alcohol 90%)
  Retin-A Liquid *Soln:* 0.05% (alcohol 55%)
  Retin-A Micro Gel *Gel:* 0.04, 0.08, 0.1% (20, 45 g)
  Tretin-X Cream *Crm:* 0.075% (35 g) (parabens-free, alcohol-free, propylene glycol-free)

TOPICAL RETINOID/ANTIMICROBIAL COMBINATIONS

Comment: Wash affected area with a soap-free cleanser; pat dry and wait 20-30 minutes; then apply sparingly to affected area; use only once daily in the evening. Avoid eyes, ears, nostrils, and mouth.
➤ *adapalene/benzoyl peroxide* (C) apply a thin film once daily
  Pediatric: <18 years: not recommended
  Epiduo Gel *Gel: adap* 0.1%/*benz* 2.5% (45 g)
➤ *tretinoin/clindamycin* (C) apply a thin film once daily
  Pediatric: <18 years: not recommended
  Ziana Gel *Gel: tret* 0.025%/*clin* 1.2% (30, 60 g)

ORAL RETINOID

Comment: Oral retinoids are indicated only for severe recalcitrant nodular acne unresponsive to conventional therapy including systemic antibiotics.
➤ *isotretinoin* (X) initially 0.5-1 mg/kg/day in 2 divided doses; maintenance 0.5-2 mg/kg/day in 2 divided doses x 4-5 months; repeat only if necessary 2 months following cessation of first treatment course
  Pediatric: not recommended
  Accutane *Cap:* 10, 20, 40 mg (parabens)
  Amnesteem *Cap:* 10, 20, 40 mg (soy)
Comment: *isotretinoin* is *highly teratogenic* and, therefore, female patients should be counseled prior to initiation of treatment as follows: Two negative pregnancy

tests are required prior to initiation of treatment and monthly thereafter. Not for use in females who are or who may become pregnant or who are breastfeeding. Two effective methods of contraception should be used for 1 month prior to, during, and continuing for 1 month following completion of treatment. Low-dose *progestin* (mini-pill) may be an *inadequate* form of contraception. No refills; a new prescription is required every 30 days and prescriptions must be filled within 7 days. Serum lipids should be monitored until response is established (usually initially and again after 4 weeks). Bone growth, serum glucose, ESR, RBCs, WBCs, and liver enzymes should be monitored. Blood should not be donated during, or for 1 month after, completion of treatment. Avoid the sun and artificial UV light. *Isotretinoin* should be discontinued if any of the following occurs: visual disturbances, tinnitus, hearing impairment, rectal bleeding, pancreatitis, hepatitis, significant decrease in CBC, hyperlipidemia (particularly hypertriglyceridemia).

ORAL CONTRACEPTIVES

see **Combined Oral Contraceptives** *page* 475
see **Progesterone-only Contraceptives (Mini-Pill)** *page* 484

⬤ ACROMEGALY

GROWTH HORMONE RECEPTOR ANTAGONIST

▶ *pegvisomant* (B) *Loading dose:* 40 mg SC; *Maintenance:* 10 mg SC daily; titrate by 5 mg (increments or decrements, based on IGF-1 levels) every 4 to 6 weeks; max 30 mg/day
Pediatric: not recommended
   Somavert *Inj:* 10, 15, 20 mg
Comment: Prior to initiation of *pegvisomant*, patients should have baseline fasting serum glucose, HgbA1c, serum potassium and magnesium, liver function tests (LFTs), EKG, and gall bladder ultrasound.

Cyclohexapeptide Somatostatin

▶ *pasireotide* (C) administer SC in the thigh or abdomen; initial dose is 0.6 mg or 0.9 mg bid. Titrate dose based on response and tolerability; for patients with moderate hepatic impairment (Child-Pugh B), the recommended initial dosage is 0.3 mg twice daily and max dose 0.6 mg twice daily; avoid use in patients with severe hepatic impairment (Child-Pugh C)
Pediatric: not recommended
   Signifor LAR *Amp:* 0.3, 0.6, 0.9 mg/ml, single-dose, long-act rel (LAR) susp for inj

⬤ ACTINIC KERATOSIS

Comment: *pasireotide* is also indicated for destroying superficial basal cell carcinoma (sBCC) lesions.
▶ *diclofenac sodium* 3% (C; D ≥30 wks) apply to lesions bid x 60-90 days
Pediatric: not recommended

Solaraze Gel *Gel:* 3% (50 g) (benzyl alcohol)
Comment: Contraindicated with **aspirin** allergy. As with other NSAIDs, **Solaraze Gel** should be avoided in late pregnancy (≥30 weeks) because it may cause premature closure of the ductus arteriosus.

▷ *fluorouracil* (X) apply to lesion(s) daily-bid until erosion occurs, usually 2-4 weeks
Pediatric: not recommended
Carac *Crm:* 0.5% (30 g)
Efudex (G) *Crm:* 5% (25 g); *Soln:* 2, 5% (10 ml w. dropper)
Fluoroplex (G) *Crm:* 1% (30 g); *Soln:* 1% (30 ml w. dropper)

▷ *imiquimod* (B)
Pediatric: <18 years: not recommended
Aldara (G) rub into lesions before bedtime and remove with soap and water 8 hours later; treat 2 times per week; max 16 weeks
Crm: 5% (single-use pkts/carton)
Zyclara rub into lesions before bedtime and remove with soap and water 8 hours later; treat for 2-week cycles separated by a 2-week no-treatment cycle; max 2 packs per application; max one treatment course per area
Crm: 3.75% (single-use pkts; 28/carton) (parabens)

▷ *ingenol mebutate* (C) limit application to one contiguous skin area of about 25 cm^2 using one unit dose tube; allow treated area to dry for 15 minutes; wash hands immediately after application; may remove with soapy water after 6 hours; *Face and Scalp:* apply 0.015% gel to lesions daily x 3 days; *Trunk and Extremities:* apply 0.05% gel to lesions daily x 2 days
Pediatric: <18 years: not recommended
Picato *Gel:* 0.015% (3 single-use tubes), 0.05% (2 single-use tubes)

ALCOHOL DEPENDENCE/ALCOHOL WITHDRAWAL SYNDROME

ALCOHOL WITHDRAWAL SYNDROME

Comment: Total length of time of a given detoxification regimen and/or length of time of treatment at any dose reduction level may be extended based on patient-specific factors, including potential or actual seizure, hallucinosis, increased sympathetic nervous system activity (severe anxiety, unwanted elevation in vital signs). If any of these symptoms are anticipated or occur, revert to an earlier step in the dosing regimen to stabilize the patient, extend the detoxification timeline and consider appropriate adjunctive drug treatments (e.g., anti-convulsants, antipsychotic agents, antihypertensive agents, sedative hypnotics agents).

▷ *clorazepate* (D)(IV)(G) in the following dosage schedule: *Day 1:* 30 mg initially, followed by 30-60 mg in divided doses; *Day 2:* 45-90 mg in divided doses; *Day 3:* 22.5-45 mg in divided doses; *Day 4:* 15-30 mg in divided doses; *Thereafter,* gradually reduce the daily dose to 7.5-15 mg; then discontinue when patient's condition is stable; max dose 90 mg/day
Tranxene *Tab:* 3.75, 7.5, 15 mg
Tranxene T-Tab *Tab:* 3.75*, 7.5*, 15*mg

▷ *chlordiazepoxide* (D)(IV)(G)
Librium 50-100 mg q 6 hours x 24-72 hours; then q 8 hours x 24-72 hours; then q 12 hours x 24-72 hours; then daily x 24-72 hours

Cap: 5, 10, 25 mg
Librium Injectable 50-100 mg IM <u>or</u> IV; then 25-50 mg IM tid-qid prn; max 300 mg/day
Inj: 100 mg

▷ *diazepam* (D)(IV)(G) 2-10 mg q 6 hours x 24-72 hours; then q 8 hours x 24-72 hours; then q 12 hours x 24-72 hours; then daily x 24-72 hours
Diastat *Rectal gel delivery system:* 2.5 mg
Diastat Acu Dial *Rectal gel delivery system:* 10, 20 mg
Valium *Tab:* 2*, 5*, 10*mg
Valium Injectable *Vial:* 5 mg/ml (10 ml); *Amp:* 5 mg/ml (2 ml); *Prefilled syringe:* 5 mg/ml (5 ml)
Valium Intensol *Conc oral soln:* 5 mg/ml (30 ml w. dropper) (alcohol 19%)
Valium Oral Solution *Oral soln:* 5 mg/5 ml (500 ml) (wintergreen-spice)

▷ *oxazepam* (C) 10-15 mg tid-qid x 24-72 hours; decrease dose <u>and/or</u> frequency every 24-72 hours; total length of therapy 5-14 days; max 120 mg/day
Cap: 10, 15, 30 mg

ABSTINENCE THERAPY

GABA Taurine Analogue

▷ *acamprosate* (C)(G) 666 mg tid; begin therapy during abstinence; continue during relapse; *CrCl 30-50-mL/min:* max 333 mg tid; *CrCl <30 mL/min:* contraindicated
Campral *Tab:* 333 mg ext-rel
Comment: **Campral** does not eliminate or diminish alcohol withdrawal symptoms.

AVERSION THERAPY

▷ *disulfiram* (X)(G)
Antabuse 500 mg once daily x 1-2 weeks; then 250 mg once daily
Tab: 250, 500 mg; *Chew tab:* 200, 500 mg
Comment: *disulfiram* use requires informed consent. Contraindications: severe cardiac disease, psychosis, concomitant use of *isoniazid, phenytoin, paraldehyde,* and topical and systemic alcohol-containing products. Approximately 20% remains in the system for 1 week after discontinuation.

Nutritional Support

▷ *thiamine* (A)(G) injectable 50-100 mg IM/IV daily (<u>or</u> tid if severely deficient)
Vial: 100 mg/1 ml (1 ml)

⬤ ALLERGIC REACTION: GENERAL

PARENTERAL ANTIHISTAMINE

▷ *diphenhydramine* (C)(G) 25-50 mg IM immediately; then q 6 hours prn
Pediatric: 1.25 mg/kg up to 25 mg IM x 1 dose; then q 6 hours prn
Benadryl Injectable *Vial:* 50 mg/ml (1 ml single-use); 50 mg/ml (10 ml multi-dose); *Amp:* 10 mg/ml (1 ml); *Prefilled syringe:* 50 mg/ml (1 ml)
Oral Drugs for Allergy, Cough, and Cold *see page 524*

Topical Corticosteroids *see page* 494
Parenteral Corticosteroids *see page* 499
Oral Corticosteroids *see page* 497

 ALZHEIMER'S DISEASE

NUTRITIONAL SUPPLEMENT

▷ *L-methylfolate calcium (as metafolin)/methylcobalamin/N-acetyl cysteine* (NR) take 1 cap once daily

Cerefolin *Cap:* metafo 5.6 mg/*methyl* 2 mg/*N-ace* 600 mg (gluten-free, yeast-free, lactose-free)

Comment: **Cerefolin** is indicated in the dietary management of patients treated for early memory loss, with emphasis on those at risk for neurovascular oxidative stress, hyperhomocysteinemia, mild to moderate cognitive impairment with <u>or</u> without vitamin B-12 deficiency, vascular dementia, <u>or</u> Alzheimer's disease.

REVERSIBLE ANTICHOLINESTERASE INHIBITORS (RAIs)

Comment: The RAI drugs do not halt disease progression. They are indicated for early-stage disease; not effective for severe dementia. If treatment is stopped for more than several days, re-titrate from lowest dose. Side effects include nausea, anorexia, dyspepsia, diarrhea, headache, and dizziness. Side effects tend to resolve with continued treatment. Peak cognitive improvements are seen 12 weeks into therapy (increased spontaneity, reduced apathy, lessened confusion, and improved attention, conversational language, and performance of daily routines).

▷ *donepezil* (C) initially 5 mg q HS, increase to 10 mg after 4-6 weeks as needed; max 23 mg/day

Aricept (G) *Tab:* 5, 10, 23 mg
Aricept ODT *ODT tab:* 5, 10 mg orally-disint

▷ *galantamine* (B) initially 4 mg bid x at least 4 weeks; usual maintenance 8 mg bid; max 16 mg bid

Razadyne *Tab:* 4, 8, 12 mg
Razadyne ER *Tab:* 8, 16, 24 mg ext-rel
Razadyne Oral Solution *Oral soln:* 4 mg/ml (100 ml w. calib pipette)

▷ *rivastigmine* (B)(G)

Exelon initially 1.5 mg bid, increase every 2 weeks as needed; max 12 mg/day; take with food
Cap: 1.5, 3, 4.5, 6 mg

Excelon Oral Solution initially 1.5 mg bid; may increase by 1.5 mg bid at intervals of at least 2 weeks; usual range 6-12 mg/day; max 12 mg/day; if stopped, restart at lowest dose and re-titrate; may take directly from syringe <u>or</u> mix with water, fruit juice, <u>or</u> cola
Oral soln: 2 mg/ml (120 ml w. dose syringe)

Excelon Patch initially apply 4.6 mg/24 hours patch; if tolerated, may increase to 9.5mg/24 hours patch after 4 weeks; max 13.3 mg /24 hours; change patch daily; apply to clean, dry, hairless, intact skin; rotate application site; allow 14 days before applying new patch to same site
Patch: 4.6, 9.5, 13.3 mg/24 hours trans-sys (30/carton)

▷ *tacrine* (C) initially 10 mg qid, increase 40 mg/day q 4 weeks as needed; max 160 mg/day

Cognex *Cap:* 10, 20, 30, 40 mg

Comment: Transaminase levels should be checked every 3 months.

N-METHYL-D-ASPARTATE (NMDA) RECEPTOR ANTAGONIST

▷ *memantine* (B)

Namenda initially 5 mg once daily; titrate weekly in 5 mg/day increments; *Week 2:* 5 mg bid; *Week 3:* 5 mg AM and 10 mg PM; *Week 4:* 10 mg bid; *CrCl 5-29 mL/min:* max 5 mg bid

Tab: 5, 10 mg

Namenda Oral Solution initially 5 mg once daily; titrate weekly in 5 mg increments administered bid

Oral soln: 2 mg/ml (360 ml) (peppermint) (sugar-free, alcohol-free)

Namenda Titration Pak

Cap: 7 x 7 mg, 7 x 14 mg, 7 x 21 mg, 7 x 28 mg/pck

Namenda XR initially 7 mg once daily; titrate in 7 mg increments weekly; max 28 mg once daily; do not divide doses

Cap: 7, 14, 21, 28 mg ext-rel

Comment: *memantine* does not halt disease progression. It is indicated for moderate to severe dementia.

N-METHYL-D-ASPARTATE (NMDA) RECEPTOR ANTAGONIST/ACETYLCHOLIN-ESTERASE INHIBITOR COMBINATION

▷ *memantine/donepezil* (C) initiate one 28/10 dose daily in the evening after stabilized on *memantine* and *donepezil* separately; start the day after the last dose of *memantine* and *donepezil* taken separately; swallow whole or open cap and sprinkle on applesauce; *CrCl 5-29 mL/min:* take one 14/10 dose once daily in the evening

Namzaric

Cap: **Namzaric 14/10:** *mem* 14mg/*done* 10mg
Namzaric 28/10: *mem* 28 mg/*done* 10 mg

ERGOT ALKALOID (DOPAMINE AGONIST)

▷ *ergoloid mesylate* (C) 1 mg tid

Hydergine *Tab:* 1 mg
Hydergine LC *Cap:* 1 mg
Hydergine Liquid *Liq:* 1 mg/ml (100 ml w. calib dropper) (alcohol 28.5%)

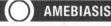 **AMEBIASIS**

AMEBIASIS (INTESTINAL)

▷ *diiodohydroxyquin (iodoquinol)* (C)(G) 650 mg tid pc x 20 days
Pediatric: <6 years: 40 mg/kg/day in 3 divided doses pc x 20 days; max 1.95 g; 6-12 years: 420 mg tid pc x 20 days
Tab: 210, 650 mg

▷ *metronidazole* (not for use in 1st; B in 2nd, 3rd)(G) 750 mg tid x 5-10 days
Pediatric: 35-50 mg/kg/day in 3 divided doses x 10 days

> **Flagyl** *Tab:* 250*, 500*mg
> **Flagyl 375** *Cap:* 375 mg
> **Flagyl ER** *Tab:* 750 mg ext-rel

Comment: Alcohol is contraindicated during treatment with oral ***metronidazole*** and for 72 hours after therapy due to a possible ***disulfiram***-like reaction (nausea, vomiting, flushing, headache).

▶ ***tinidazole* (not for use in 1st; B in 2nd, 3rd)** 2 g daily x 3 days; take with food
Pediatric: <3 years: not recommended; ≥3 years: 50 mg/kg daily x 3 days; take with food; max 2 g/day
> **Tindamax** *Tab:* 250*, 500*mg

Comment: Alcohol is contraindicated during treatment with oral ***tinidazole*** and for 72 hours after therapy due to a possible ***disulfiram***-like reaction (nausea, vomiting, flushing, headache).

▶ ***paromomycin*** 25-35 mg/kg/day in 3 divided doses x 5-10 days
Pediatric: same as adult
> **Humatin** *Cap:* 250 mg

AMEBIASIS (EXTRAINTESTINAL)

▶ ***chloroquine phosphate*** (C)(G) 1 g PO daily x 2 days; then 500 mg daily x 2 to 3 weeks or 200-250 mg IM daily x 10-12 days (when oral therapy is impossible); use with intestinal amebicide
Pediatric: see mfr literature
> **Aralen** *Tab:* 500 mg; *Amp:* 50 mg/ml (5 ml)

○ AMEBIC LIVER ABSCESS

ANTI-INFECTIVES

▶ ***metronidazole* (not for use in 1st; B in 2nd, 3rd)(G)** 250 mg tid or 500 mg bid or 750 mg daily x 7 days
Pediatric: not recommended
> **Flagyl** *Tab:* 250*, 500*mg
> **Flagyl 375** *Cap:* 375 mg
> **Flagyl ER** *Tab:* 750 mg ext-rel

Comment: Alcohol is contraindicated during treatment with oral ***metronidazole*** and for 72 hours after therapy due to a possible ***disulfiram***-like reaction (nausea, vomiting, flushing, headache).

▶ ***tinidazole* (not for use in 1st; B in 2nd, 3rd)** 2 g once daily x 3-5 days; take with food
Pediatric: <3 years: not recommended; ≥3 years: 50 mg/kg once daily x 3-5 days; take with food; max 2 g/day
> **Tindamax** *Tab:* 250*, 500*mg

Comment: Alcohol is contraindicated during treatment with oral ***tinidazole*** and for 72 hours after therapy due to a possible ***disulfiram***-like reaction (nausea, vomiting, flushing, headache).

◯ AMENORRHEA: SECONDARY

▷ *estrogen/progesterone* (X)
   Premarin (*estrogen*) 0.625 mg daily x 25 days; then 5 days off; repeat monthly
   Provera (*progesterone*) 5-10 mg last 10 days of cycle; repeat monthly
▷ *estrogen replacement* (X)
   see **Menopause** page 254
▷ *human chorionic gonadotropin* 5,000-10,000 units IM x 1 dose following last dose
   of menotropins
   Pregnyl *Vial:* 10,000 units (10 ml) w. diluent (10 ml)
▷ *medroxyprogesterone* (X) *Monthly:* 5-10 mg last 5-10 days of cycle; begin on the
   16th or 21st day of cycle; repeat monthly; *One-time only:* 10 mg once daily x 10 days
   Amen *Tab:* 10 mg
   Provera *Tab:* 2.5, 5, 10 mg
▷ *norethindrone* (X) 2.5-10 mg daily x 5-10 days
   Aygestin *Tab:* 5 mg
▷ *progesterone, micronized* (X)(G) 400 mg q HS x 10 days
   Prometrium *Cap:* 100, 200 mg

   Comment: Administration of *progesterone* induces optimum secretory
   transformation of the *estrogen*-primed endometrium. Administration of
   progesterone is contraindicated with breast cancer, undiagnosed vaginal
   bleeding, genital cancer, severe liver dysfunction or disease, missed abortion,
   thrombophlebitis, thromboembolic disorders, cerebral apoplexy, and pregnancy.

◯ ANAPHYLAXIS

▷ *epinephrine* (C)(G) 0.3-0.5 mg (0.3-0.5 ml of a 1:1000 soln) SC q 20-30 minutes as
   needed up to 3 doses
   Pediatric: <2 years: 0.05-0.1 ml; 2-6 years: 0.1 ml; ≥6-12 years: 0.2 ml; All: q 20-30
   minutes as needed up to 3 doses; >12 years: same as adult
Parenteral Corticosteroids *see page* 499
Oral Corticosteroids *see page* 497

ANAPHYLAXIS EMERGENCY TREATMENT KITS

▷ *epinephrine* (C) 0.3 ml IM or SC in thigh; may repeat if needed
   Pediatric: 0.01 mg/kg SC or IM in thigh; may repeat if needed; <15 kg: not estab-
   lished; 15-30 kg: 0.15 mg; >30 kg: same as adult
   Adrenaclick *Auto-injector:* 0.15, 0.3 mg (1 mg/ml; 1, 2/carton) (sulfites)
   Auvi-Q *Auto-injector:* 0.15, 0.3 mg (1 mg/ml; 1/pck w. 1 non-active training
   device) (sulfites)
   EpiPen *Auto-injector 0.3 mg* (*epi* 1:1000, 0.3 ml (1, 2/carton) (sulfites)
   EpiPen Jr *Auto-injector 0.15 mg* (*epi* 1:2000, 0.3 ml) (1, 2/carton) (sulfites)
   Twinject *Auto-injector:* 0.15, 0.3 mg (epi 1:1000) (1, 2/carton) (sulfites)
▷ *epinephrine/chlorpheniramine* (C) epinephrine 0.3 ml SC or IM plus 4 tabs *chlor-
   pheniramine* by mouth
   Pediatric: infants to 2 years: 0.05-0.1 ml SC or IM; ≥2-6 years: 0.15 ml SC or IM plus
   1 tab *chlor*; ≥6-12 years: 0.2 ml SC or IM plus 2 tabs *chlor*
   Ana-Kit: two 0.3 ml syringes of *epi* 1:1000 for self-injection plus *chlor* 2 mg
   chewable tabs x 4

ANEMIA OF CHRONIC KIDNEY DISEASE (CKD) AND CHRONIC RENAL FAILURE (CRF)

ERYTHROPOIESIS STIMULATING AGENTS (ESAs)

▷ *darbepoetin alpha* (erythropoiesis stimulating protein) **(C)** administer IV or SC q 1-2 weeks; do not increase more frequently than once per month; *Not currently receiving epoetin alpha:* initially 0.75 mcg/kg once weekly; adjust based on Hgb levels (target not to exceed 12 g/dL); reduce dose if Hgb increases more than 1 g/dL in any 2-week period; suspend therapy if polycythemia occurs; *Converting from epoetin alpha and for dose titration:* see mfr literature
Pediatric: not recommended

    Aranesp *Vial:* 25, 40, 60, 100, 150, 200, 300, 500 mcg/ml (single-dose) for IV or SC administration (preservative-free, albumin [human] or polysorbate 80)

    Aranesp Singleject, Aranesp Sureclick Singleject *Prefilled syringe:* 25, 40, 60, 100, 150, 200, 300, 500 mcg (single-dose) for IV or SC administration (preservative-free, albumin [human] or polysorbate 80)

▷ *peginesatide* **(C)** use lowest effective dose; initiate when Hgb <10 g/dL; do not increase dose more often than every 4 weeks; if Hgb rises rapidly (i.e., >1 g/dL in 2 weeks or >2 g/dL in 4 weeks), reduce dose by 25% or more; if Hgb approaches or exceeds 11 g/dL, reduce or interrupt dose and then when Hgb decreases, resume dose at approximately 25% below previous dose; if Hgb does not increase by >1 g/dL after 4 weeks, increase dose by 25%; if response inadequate after a 12-week escalation period, use lowest dose that will maintain Hgb sufficient to reduce need for RBC transfusion; discontinue if response does not improve; *Not currently on ESA:* initially 0.04 mg/kg as a single IV or SC dose once monthly; *Converting from epoetin alfa:* administer first dose 1 week after last epoetin alfa; *Converting from darbepoetin alfa:* administer first dose at next scheduled dose of darbepoetin alfa
Pediatric: not established

    Omontys *Vial, single-use:* 2, 3, 4, 5, 6 mg (0.5 ml) (preservative-free); *Vial, multi-use:* 10, 20 mg (2 ml) (preservatives); *Prefilled syringe:* 2, 3, 4, 5, 6 mg (0.5 ml) (preservative-free)

ERYTHROPOIETIN HUMAN, RECOMBINANT

▷ *epoetin alpha* **(C)** individualize; initially 50-100 units/kg 3 x/week; IV (dialysis or nondialysis) or SC (nondialysis); usual max 200 units/kg 3 x/week (dialysis) or 150 units/kg 3 x/week (non-dialysis); target Hct 30-36%
Pediatric: <1 month: not recommended; ≥1 month: individualize; *Dialysis:* initially 50 units/kg 3 x/week IV or SC; target Hct 30-36%

    Epogen *Vial:* 2,000, 3,000, 4,000, 10,000, 40,000 units/ml (1 ml) single-use for IV or SC administration (albumin [human]; preservative-free)

    Epogen Multidose *Vial:* 10,000 units/ml (2 ml); 20,000 units/ml, (1 ml) for IV or SC administration (albumin [human]; benzoyl alcohol)

    Procrit *Vial:* 2,000, 3,000, 4,000, 10,000, 40,000 units/ml (1 ml) single-use for IV or SC administration (albumin [human]) (preservative-free)

    Procrit Multidose *Vial:* 10,000 units/ml (2 ml); 20,000 units/ml, (1 ml) for IV or SC administration (albumin [human]; benzoyl alcohol)

ANEMIA: FOLIC ACID DEFICIENCY

> *folic acid* (A)(OTC) 0.4-1 mg once daily

Comment: *folic acid (vitamin B-9)* 400 mcg daily is recommended during pregnancy to prevent neural tube defects. Women who have had a baby with a neural tube defect should take 400 mcg every day, even when not planning to become pregnant, and if planning to become pregnant should take 4 mg daily during the month before becoming pregnant until at least the 12th week of pregnancy.

ANEMIA: IRON DEFICIENCY

Comment: Hemochromatosis and hemosiderosis are contraindications to iron therapy. *Iron* supplements are best absorbed when taken between meals and with *vitamin C*-rich foods. Excessive *iron* may be extremely hazardous to infants and young children. All vitamin and mineral supplements should be kept out of the reach of children.

IRON PREPARATIONS

> *ferrous gluconate* (A)(G) 1 tab once daily
>> Fergon (OTC)
>>> *Pediatric:* not recommended
>>> *Tab:* iron 27 mg (240 mg as gluconate)
> *ferrous sulfate* (A)(G)
>> Feosol Tablets (OTC) 1 tab tid-qid pc and HS
>>> *Pediatric:* <6 years: use elixir; ≥6-12 years: 1 tab tid pc
>>> *Tab:* iron 65 mg (200 mg as sulfate)
>> Feosol Capsules (OTC) 1-2 caps daily
>>> *Pediatric:* not recommended
>>> *Cap:* iron 50 mg (169 mg as sulfate) sust-rel
>> Feosol Elixir (OTC) 5-10 ml tid
>>> *Pediatric:* >1 year: 2.5-5 ml tid between meals
>>> *Elix:* iron 44 mg (220 mg as sulfate) per 5 ml
>> Fer-In-Sol (OTC) 5 ml daily
>>> *Pediatric:* <4 years, use drops; ≥4 years: 5 ml once daily
>>> *Syr:* iron 18 mg (90 mg as sulfate) per 5 ml (480 ml)
>> Fer-In-Sol Drops (OTC)
>>> *Pediatric:* <4 years: 0.6 ml daily; ≥4 years: use syrup
>>> *Oral drops:* iron 15 mg (75 mg as sulfate) per 5 ml (50 ml)

ANEMIA: MEGALOBLASTIC/ANEMIA: PERNICIOUS

Comment: Signs of *vitamin B-12* deficiency include megaloblastic anemia, glossitis, paresthesias, ataxia, spastic motor weakness, and reduced mentation.

> *vitamin B-12 (cyanocobalamin)* (A)(G) 500 mcg intranasally once a week; may increase dose if serum B-12 levels decline; adjust dose in 500 mcg increments
>> Nascobal Nasal Spray

Intranasal gel: 500 mcg/0.1 ml (1.3 ml, 4 doses) (citric acid, benzalkonium chloride)
Comment: **Nascobal Nasal Spray** is indicated for maintenance of hematologic remission following IM B-12 therapy without nervous system involvement. Must be primed before each use.

⬭ ANGINA PECTORIS: STABLE

▷ *aspirin* (D) 325 mg (range 75-325 mg) once daily
Comment: Daily ASA dose is contingent upon whether the patient is also taking an anticoagulant or antiplatelet agent.

CALCIUM ANTAGONISTS

Comment: Calcium antagonists are contraindicated with history of ventricular arrhythmias, sick sinus syndrome, 2nd or 3rd degree heart block, cardiogenic shock, acute myocardial infarction, and pulmonary congestion.

▷ *amlodipine* (C)(G) 5-10 mg daily
Pediatric: not recommended
    Norvasc *Tab:* 2.5, 5, 10 mg

▷ *diltiazem* (C)(G)
    Cardizem initially 30 mg qid; may increase gradually every 1-2 days; max 360 mg/day in divided doses
      Pediatric: not recommended
      Tab: 30, 60, 90, 120 mg
    Cardizem CD initially 120-180 mg daily; adjust at 1- to 2-week intervals; max 480 mg/day
      Pediatric: not recommended
      Cap: 120, 180, 240, 300, 360 mg ext-rel
    Cardizem LA initially 180-240 mg daily; titrate at 2 week intervals; max 540 mg/day
      Pediatric: not recommended
      Tab: 120, 180, 240, 300, 360, 420 mg ext-rel
    Cartia XT initially 180 mg or 240 mg once daily; max 540 mg once daily
      Cap: 120, 180, 240, 300 mg ext-rel
    Dilacor XR initially 180 mg or 240 mg once daily; max 540 mg once daily
      Cap: 180, 240 mg ext-rel
    Tiazac initially 120-180 mg daily; max 540 mg/day
      Cap: 120, 180, 240, 300, 360, 420 mg ext-rel

▷ *nicardipine* (C)(G) initially 20 mg tid; adjust q 3 days; max 120 mg/day
Pediatric: not recommended
    Cardene *Cap:* 20, 30 mg

▷ *nifedipine* (C)(G)
Pediatric: not recommended
    Adalat CC initially 30 mg once daily; usual range 30-60 mg tid; max 90 mg/day
      Tab: 30, 60, 90 mg ext-rel
    Procardia initially 10 mg tid; titrate over 7-14 days: max 30 mg/dose and 180 mg/day in divided doses
      Cap: 10, 20 mg
    Procardia XL initially 30-60 mg daily; titrate over 7-14 days; max dose 90 mg/day
      Tab: 30, 60, 90 mg ext-rel

▷ *verapamil* (C)(G)
  Pediatric: not recommended
    Calan 80-120 mg tid; increase daily <u>or</u> weekly if needed
      Tab: 40, 80*, 120*mg
    Calan SR initially 120 mg once daily; increase weekly if needed
      Tab: 120, 180, 240 mg
    Covera HS initially 180 mg q HS; titrate in steps to 240 mg; then to 360 mg; then to 480 mg if needed
      Tab: 180, 240 mg ext-rel
    Isoptin SR initially 120-180 mg in the AM; may increase to 240 mg in the AM; then 180 mg q 12 hours <u>or</u> 240 mg in the AM and 120 mg in the PM; then 240 mg q 12 hours
      Tab: 120, 180*, 240*mg sust-rel

BETA-BLOCKERS

Comment: Beta-blockers are contraindicated with history of sick sinus syndrome (SSS), 2nd <u>or</u> 3rd degree heart block, cardiogenic shock, pulmonary congestion, asthma, moderate to severe COPD with FEV1 <50% predicted, patients with chronic bronchodilator treatment.

▷ *atenolol* (D)(G) initially 25-50 mg daily; increase weekly if needed; max 200 mg daily
  Pediatric: not recommended
    Tenormin *Tab:* 25, 50, 100 mg
▷ *metoprolol succinate* (C)
  Pediatric: not recommended
    Toprol-XL initially 100 mg in a single dose once daily; increase weekly if needed; max 400 mg/day
      Tab: 25*, 50*, 100*, 200*mg ext-rel
▷ *metoprolol tartrate* (C)
  Pediatric: not recommended
    Lopressor (G) initially 25-50 mg bid; increase weekly if needed; max 400 mg/day
      Tab: 25, 37.5, 50, 75, 100 mg
▷ *nadolol* (C)(G) initially 40 mg daily; increase q 3-7 days; max 240 mg/day
  Pediatric: not recommended
    Corgard *Tab:* 20*, 40*, 80*, 120*, 160*mg
▷ *propranolol* (C)(G)
  Pediatric: not recommended
    Inderal LA initially 80 mg daily in a single dose; increase q 3-7 days; usual range 120-160 mg/day; max 320 mg/day in a single dose
      Cap: 60, 80, 120, 160 mg sust-rel
    InnoPran XL initially 80 mg q HS; max 120 mg/day
      Cap: 80, 120 mg ext-rel

NITRATES

Comment: Use a daily nitrate dosing schedule that provides a dose-free period of 14 hours <u>or</u> more to prevent tolerance. *aspirin* and *acetaminophen* may relieve nitrate-induced headache. *Isosorbide* is not recommended for use in MI <u>and/or</u> CHF. Nitrate use is a contraindication for using phosphodiesterase type 5 inhibitors: *sildenafil* (Viagra), *tadalafil* (Cialis), *vardenafil* (Levitra).

▷ *isosorbide dinitrate* (C)
  Pediatric: not recommended
      Dilatrate-SR 40 mg once daily; max 160 mg/day
          Cap: 40 mg sust-rel
      Isordil Titradose initially 5-20 mg q 6 hours; maintenance 10-40 mg q 6 hours
          Tab: 5, 10, 20, 30, 40 mg
▷ *isosorbide mononitrate* (C)
  Pediatric: not recommended
      Imdur initially 30-60 mg q AM; may increase to 120 mg daily; max 240 mg/day
          Tab: 30*, 60*, 120 mg ext-rel
      Ismo 20 mg upon awakening; then 20 mg 7 hours later
          Tab: 20*mg
▷ *nitroglycerin* (C)(G)
  Pediatric: not recommended
      Nitro-Bid Ointment initially 1/2 inch q 8 hours; titrate in 1/2 inch increments
          Oint: 2% (20, 60 g)
      Nitrodisc initially one 0.2-0.4 mg/hour patch for 12-14 hours/day
          Transdermal disc: 0.2, 0.3, 0.4 mg/hour (30, 100/carton)
      Nitro-Dur initially 0.2-0.4 mg/hour patch for 12-14 hours/day
          Transdermal patch: 0.1, 0.2, 0.3, 0.4, 0.6, 0.8 mg/hour
      Nitrolingual 1-2 sprays on <u>or</u> under tongue; max 3 sprays/15 minutes
          Spray: 0.4 mg/dose (14.5 g, 200 doses)
      Nitromist 1-2 sprays at onset of attack, on <u>or</u> under the tongue while sitting;
      may repeat q 5 minutes as needed; max 3 sprays/15 minutes; may use pro-
      phylactically 5-10 minutes prior to exertion; do not inhale spray; do not rinse
      mouth for 5-10 minutes after use
          Lingual aerosol spray: 0.4 mg/actuation (230 metered sprays)
      Nitrostat 1 tab SL; may repeat q 5 minutes x 3
          SL tab: 0.3 (1/100 gr), 0.4 (1/150 gr), 0.6 (1/4 gr) mg
      Transderm-Nitro initially one 0.2 mg/hour <u>or</u> 0.4 mg/hour patch for 12-14
      hours/day
          Transdermal patch: 0.1, 0.2, 0.4, 0.6, 0.8 mg/hour

NON-NITRATE PERIPHERAL VASODILATOR

▷ *hydralazine* (C)(G) initially 10 mg qid x 2-4 days; then increase to 25 mg qid for
  remainder of first week; then increase to 50 mg qid; max 300 mg/day
  Tab: 10, 25, 50, 100 mg

NITRATE/PERIPHERAL VASODILATOR COMBINATION

▷ *isosorbide/hydralazine HCl* (C) initially 1 tab tid; max 2 tabs tid
  Bidil *Tab:* isosorb 20 mg/hydral 37.5 mg

NON-NITRATE ANTI-ANGINAL

▷ *ranolazine* (C) initially 500 mg bid; may increase to max 1 g bid
      Ranexa *Tab:* 500, 1000 mg ext-rel
      Comment: **Ranexa** is indicated for the treatment chronic angina that is inade-
      quately controlled with other antianginals. Use with amlodipine, beta-blocker,
      <u>or</u> nitrate.

ANOREXIA/CACHEXIA

APPETITE STIMULANTS

➤ *cyproheptadine* (B)(G) initially 4 mg tid prn; then adjust as needed; usual range 12-16 mg/day; max 32 mg/day
   Pediatric: <2 years: not recommended; ≥2-6 years: 2 mg bid-tid prn; max 12 mg/day; 7-14 years: 4 mg bid-tid prn; max 16 mg/day; >14 years: same as adult
      Periactin *Tab:* cypro 4*mg; *Syr:* cypro 2 mg/5 ml
➤ *dronabinol* (cannabinoid) (B)(III) initially 2.5 mg bid before lunch and dinner; may reduce to 2.5 mg q HS or increase to 2.5 mg before lunch and 5 mg before dinner; max 20 mg/day in divided doses
   Pediatric: not recommended
      Marinol *Cap:* 2.5, 5, 10 mg (sesame oil)
➤ *megestrol* (progestin) (X) 40 mg qid
   Pediatric: not recommended
      Megace *Tab:* 20*, 40*mg
      Megace ES *Oral susp (concentrate):* 125 mg/ml; 625 mg/5 ml (5 oz) (lemon-lime)
      Megace Oral Suspension *Oral susp:* 40 mg/ml (8 oz); 820 mg/20 ml) (lemon-lime)
      Megestrol Acetate Oral Suspension (G) 125 mg/ml

Comment: *megestrol* is indicated for the treatment of anorexia, cachexia, or an unexplained, significant weight loss in patients with a diagnosis of AIDS.

 ANTHRAX (*BACILLUS ANTHRACIS*)

POSTEXPOSURE PROPHYLAXIS OF INHALATIONAL ANTHRAX AND TREATMENT OF INHALED AND CUTANEOUS ANTHRAX INFECTION

IMMUNE GLOBULIN

➤ *bacillus athracis immune globulin intravenous (human)* (NR) administer via IV infusion at a maximum rate of 2 ml/min; dose is weight-based as follows, but may doubled in severe cases if weight >5 kg:
   Pediatric: <16 years: not established; 5-<10 kg: 1 vial; 10-<18 kg: 2 vials; 18-<25 kg: 3 vials; 25-<35 kg: 4 vials; 35-<50 kg: 5 vials; 50-<60 kg: 6 vials; ≥60 kg: 7 vials
      Anthrasil *Vial:* (60 units) sterile solution of purified human immune globulin G (IgG) containing polyclonal antibodies that target the anthrax toxins of *Bacillus anthracis* for IV infusion

      Comment: **Anthrasil** is indicated for the emergent treatment of inhaled anthrax in combination with appropriate antibacterial agents
➤ *ciprofloxacin* (C) 500 mg (or 10-15 mg/kg/day) q 12 hours for 60 days (start as soon as possible after exposure)
   Pediatric: <18 years: usually not recommended
      Cipro (G) *Tab:* 250, 500, 750 mg; *Oral susp:* 250, 500 mg/5 ml (100 ml) (strawberry)
      Cipro XR *Tab:* 500, 1000 mg ext-rel
      ProQuin XR *Tab:* 500 mg ext-rel

Comment: *ciprofloxacin* is contraindicated <18 years-of-age, and during pregnancy and lactation. Risk of tendonitis or tendon rupture, especially 60 years-of-age and older.

▷ *doxycycline* (D)(G) 100 mg daily bid
Pediatric: <8 years: not recommended ≥8 years, <100 lb: 2 mg/lb on first day in 2 divided doses, followed by 1 mg/lb/day in a single or divided doses; ≥8 years, ≥100 lb: same as adult; *see page 561 for dose by weight*

    Actilate *Tab:* 75, 150**mg
    Adoxa *Tab:* 50, 75, 100, 150 mg ent-coat
    Doryx *Tab:* 75, 100, 150 mg del-rel
    Monodox *Cap:* 50, 75, 100 mg
    Oracea *Cap:* 40 mg del-rel
    Vibramycin *Cap:* 50, 100 mg; *Syr:* 50 mg/5 ml (raspberry; sulfites); *Oral susp:* 25 mg/5 ml (raspberry-apple)
    Vibra-Tab *Tab:* 100 mg film-coat

Comment: *doxycycline* is contraindicated <8 years-of-age, in pregnancy, and lactation (discolors developing tooth enamel). A side effect may be photosensitivity (photophobia). Do not give with antacids, calcium supplements, milk or other dairy, or within two hours of taking another drug.

▷ *minocycline* (D)(G) 100 mg q 12 hours
Pediatric: <8 years: not recommended; ≥8 years, <100 lb: 2 mg/lb on first day in 2 divided doses, followed by 1 mg/lb q 12 hours x 9 more days; ≥8 years, ≥100 lb: same as adult

    Dynacin *Cap:* 50, 100 mg
    Minocin *Cap:* 50, 75, 100 mg; *Oral susp:* 50 mg/5 ml (60 ml) (custard) (sulfites, alcohol 5%)

Comment: *minocycline* is contraindicated <8 years-of-age, in pregnancy, and lactation (discolors developing tooth enamel). A side effect may be photosensitivity (photophobia). Do not give with antacids, calcium supplements, milk or other dairy, or within two hours of taking another drug.

TREATMENT OF INHALATIONAL, GI, AND OROPHARYNGEAL ANTHRAX

▷ *ciprofloxacin* (C) 400 mg IV q 12 hours (start as soon as possible); then, switch to 500 mg PO q 12 hours for total 60 days
Pediatric: <18 years: usually not recommended; 10-15 mg/kg IV q 12 hours (start as soon as possible); then switch to 10-15 mg/kg PO q 12 hours for 60 days

    Cipro (G) *Tab:* 250, 500, 750 mg; *Oral susp:* 250, 500 mg/5 ml (100 ml) (strawberry); *IV conc:* 10 mg/ml after dilution (20, 40 ml); *IV premix:* 2 mg/ml (100, 200 ml)
    Cipro XR *Tab:* 500, 1000 mg ext-rel
    ProQuin XR *Tab:* 500 mg ext-rel

Comment: *ciprofloxacin* is contraindicated <18 years-of-age, and during pregnancy and lactation. Risk of tendonitis or tendon rupture, especially 60 years-of-age and older. Infuse IV *ciprofloxacin* over 60 minutes.

▷ *doxycycline* (D)(G) 100 mg daily bid
Pediatric: <8 years: not recommended ≥8 years, <100 lb: 2 mg/lb on first day in 2 divided doses, followed by 1 mg/lb/day in a single or divided doses; ≥8 years, ≥100 lb: same as adult; *see page 561 for dose by weight*

    Actilate *Tab:* 75, 150**mg
    Adoxa *Tab:* 50, 75, 100, 150 mg ent-coat
    Doryx *Tab:* 75, 100, 150 mg del-rel
    Monodox *Cap:* 50, 75, 100 mg

Oracea *Cap:* 40 mg del-rel
Vibramycin *Cap:* 50, 100 mg; *Syr:* 50 mg/5 ml (raspberry; sulfites); *Oral susp:* 25 mg/5 ml (raspberry-apple)
Vibra-Tab *Tab:* 100 mg film-coat

Comment: *doxycycline* is contraindicated <8 years-of-age, in pregnancy, and lactation (discolors developing tooth enamel). A side effect may be photo-sensitivity (photophobia). Do not give with antacids, calcium supplements, milk <u>or</u> other dairy, <u>or</u> within two hours of taking another drug.

▶ *minocycline* **(D)(G)** 100 mg q 12 hours
Pediatric: <8 years: not recommended; ≥8 years, <100 lb: 2 mg/lb on first day in 2 divided divided doses, followed by 1 mg/lb q 12 hours x 9 more days; ≥8 years, ≥100 lb: same as adult

Dynacin *Cap:* 50, 100 mg
Minocin *Cap:* 50, 75, 100 mg; *Oral susp:* 50 mg/5 ml (60 ml) (custard) (sulfites, alcohol 5%)

Comment: *minocycline* is contraindicated <8-years-of-age, in pregnancy, and lactation (discolors developing tooth enamel). A side effect may be photo-sensitivity (photophobia). Do not give with antacids, calcium supplements, milk <u>or</u> other dairy, <u>or</u> within two hours of taking another drug.

ANXIETY DISORDER: GENERALIZED (GAD)/ ANXIETY DISORDER: SOCIAL (SAD)

1ST GENERATION ANTIHISTAMINE

▶ *hydroxyzine* **(C)(G)** 50-100 mg qid; max 600 mg/day
Pediatric: <6 years: 50 mg/day divided qid; ≥6 years: 50-100 mg/day divided qid
Atarax *Tab:* 10, 25, 50, 100 mg; *Syr:* 10 mg/5 ml (alcohol 0.5%)
Vistaril *Cap:* 25, 50, 100 mg; *Oral susp:* 25 mg/5 ml (4 oz) (lemon)

AZASPIRONES

▶ *buspirone* **(B)** initially 7.5 mg bid; may increase by 5 mg/day q 2-3 days; max 60 mg/day
Pediatric: <6 years: not recommended; 6-17 years: same as adult
BuSpar *Tab:* 5, 10, 15*, 30* mg

BENZODIAZEPINES

Comment: If possible when considering a benzodiazepine to treat anxiety, a short-acting benzodiazepines should be used only prn to avert intense anxiety and panic for the least time necessary while a different non-addictive antianxiety regimen (e.g., SSRI, SNRI, TCA, *buspirone*, beta-blocker) is established and effective treatment goals achieved. Benzodiazepines have a high addiction potential when they are chronically used and are common drugs of abuse. *Benzodiazepine withdrawal syndrome* may include restlessness, agitation, anxiety, insomnia, tachycardia, tachypnea, diaphoresis, and may be potentially life threatening depending on the benzodiazepine and the length of use. Symptoms of withdrawal from short-acting benzodiazepines, such as *alprazolam* (Xanax), *oxazepam*, *lorazepam* (Ativan), *triazolam* (Halcion), usually appear within 6-8 hours after the last dose and may continue 10-14 days. Symptoms of withdrawal from long-acting benzodiazepines, such as *diazepam* (**Valium**), *clonazepam* (**Klonopin**), *chlordiazepam* (**Librium**), usually appear within 24-96 hours after the last dose and may continue from 3-4 weeks to 3 months. People who are heavily dependent on benzodiazepines may experience *protracted withdrawal syndrome* (PAWS), random periods of sharp withdrawal symptoms months after quitting. A closely monitored medical detoxification regimen may be required for a safe withdrawal and to prevent PAWS. Detoxification includes gradual tapering of the benzodiazepine along with other medications to manage the withdrawal symptoms.

Short Acting

▷ *alprazolam* (D)(IV)(G)
  Pediatric: <18 years: not recommended
    Niravam initially 0.25-0.5 mg tid; may titrate every 3-4 days; max 4 mg/day
      Tab: 0.25*, 0.5*, 1*, 2*mg orally-disint
    Xanax initially 0.25-0.5 mg tid; may titrate every 3-4 days; max 4 mg/day
      Tab: 0.25*, 0.5*, 1*, 2*mg
    Xanax XR initially 0.5-1 mg once daily, preferably in the AM; increase at intervals of at least 3-4 days by up to 1 mg/day. Taper no faster than 0.5 mg every 3 days; max 10 mg/day. When switching from immediate-release *alprazolam*, give total daily dose of immediate-release once daily.
      Tab: 0.5, 1, 2, 3 mg ext-rel
▷ *oxazepam* (C)(IV)(G) 10-15 mg tid-qid for moderate symptoms; 15-30 mg tid-qid for severe symptoms
  Pediatric: not recommended
  Cap: 10, 15, 30 mg

Intermediate Acting

▷ *lorazepam* (D)(IV)(G) 1-10 mg/day in 2-3 divided doses
  Pediatric: not recommended
    Ativan *Tab:* 0.5, 1*, 2*mg
    Lorazepam Intensol *Oral conc:* 2 mg/ml (30 ml w. graduated dropper)

Long Acting

▷ *chlordiazepoxide* (D)(IV)(G)
  Pediatric: <6 years: not recommended; ≥6 years: 5 mg bid-qid; increase to 10 mg bid-tid
    Librium 5-10 mg tid-qid for moderate symptoms; 20-25 mg tid-qid for severe symptoms
      Cap: 5, 10, 25 mg
    Librium Injectable 50-100 mg IM <u>or</u> IV; then 25-50 mg IM tid-qid prn; max 300 mg/day
      Inj: 100 mg
▷ *chlordiazepoxide/clidinium* (D)(IV) 1-2 caps tid-qid: max 8 caps/day
  Pediatric: not recommended
    Librax *Cap: chlor* 5 mg/*clid* 2.5 mg
▷ *clonazepam* (D)(IV)(G) initially 0.25 mg bid; increase to 1 mg/day after 3 days
  Pediatric: <18 years: not recommended
    Klonopin *Tab:* 0.5*, 1, 2 mg

      Klonopin Wafers dissolve in mouth with <u>or</u> without water
        Wafer: 0.125, 0.25, 0.5, 1, 2 mg orally-disint
▷ *clorazepate* (D)(IV)(G) 30 mg/day in divided doses; max 60 mg/day
   Pediatric: <9 years: not recommended; ≥9 years: same as adult
      Tranxene *Tab:* 3.75, 7.5, 15 mg
      Tranxene SD do not use for initial therapy
        Tab: 22.5 mg ext-rel
      Tranxene SD Half Strength do not use for initial therapy
        Tab: 11.25 mg ext-rel
      Tranxene T-Tab *Tab:* 3.75*, 7.5*, 15*mg
▷ *diazepam* (D)(IV)(G) 2-10 mg bid to qid
   Pediatric: not recommended
      Diastat *Rectal gel delivery system:* 2.5 mg
      Diastat AcuDial *Rectal gel delivery system:* 10, 20 mg
      Valium *Tab:* 2*, 5*, 10*mg
      Valium Injectable *Vial:* 5 mg/ml (10 ml); *Amp:* 5 mg/ml (2 ml); *Prefilled syringe:* 5 mg/ml (5 ml)
      Valium Intensol *Conc oral soln:* 5 mg/ml (30 ml w. dropper) (alcohol 19%)
      Valium Oral Solution *Oral soln:* 5 mg/5 ml (500 ml) (wintergreen spice)

TRICYCLIC ANTIDEPRESSANTS (TCAs)

Comment: Co-administration of TCAs with SSRIs requires extreme caution.
▷ *doxepin* (C)(G) usual optimum dose 75-150 mg/day; elderly lower initial dose and therapeutic dose; max single dose 150 mg; max 300 mg/day in divided doses
      Sinequan
      Pediatric: not recommended
      Cap: 10, 25, 50, 75, 100, 150 mg; *Oral conc:* 10 mg/ml (4 oz w. dropper)
   Comment: Glaucoma, urinary retention, and bipolar disorder are contraindications to *doxepin*. Separate from MAOIs by at least 14 days. Separate from *fluoxetine* by at least 5 weeks. Avoid abrupt cessation. doxepin is potentiated by CYP2D6 inhibitors (e.g., *cimetidine*, SSRIs, phenothiazines, type 1C antiarrhythmics).

PHENOTHIAZINES

▷ *prochlorperazine* (C)(G)
      Compazine 5 mg tid-qid
      Pediatric: not recommended
      Tab: 5 mg; *Syr:* 5 mg/5 ml (4 oz) (fruit); *Rectal supp:* 2.5, 5, 25 mg
      Compazine Spansule 15 mg q AM <u>or</u> 10 mg q 12 hours
      Pediatric: not recommended
      Spansule: 10, 15 mg sust-rel
▷ *trifluoperazine* (C)(G) 1-2 mg bid; max 6 mg/day; max 12 weeks
   Pediatric: not recommended
      Stelazine *Tab:* 1, 2, 5, 10 mg

SELECTIVE SEROTONIN REUPTAKE INHIBITORS (SSRIs)

Comment: Co-administration of SSRIs with TCAs requires extreme caution.
Concomitant use of MAOIs and SSRIs is absolutely contraindicated. Avoid St. John's

wort and other serotonergic agents. A potentially fatal adverse event is *serotonin syndrome*, caused by serotonin excess. Milder symptoms require HCP intervention to avert severe symptoms that can be rapidly fatal without urgent/emergent medical care. Symptoms include restlessness, agitation, confusion, tachycardia, hypertension, dilated pupils, muscle twitching, muscle rigidity, loss of muscle coordination, diaphoresis, diarrhea, headache, shivering, piloerection, hyperpyrexia, cardiac arrhythmias, seizures, loss of consciousness, coma, death. Common symptoms of the *serotonin discontinuation syndrome* include flu-like symptoms (nausea, vomiting, diarrhea, headaches, diaphoresis); sleep disturbances (insomnia, nightmares, constant sleepiness); mood disturbances (dysphoria, anxiety, agitation); cognitive disturbances (mental confusion, hyperarousal); and sensory and movement disturbances (imbalance, tremors, vertigo, dizziness, electric-shock-like sensations in the brain often described by sufferers as "brain zaps").

▷ *escitalopram* (C)(G) initially 10 mg daily; may increase to 20 mg daily after 1 week; elderly or hepatic impairment, 10 mg once daily
  Pediatric: <12 years: not recommended; 12-17 years: initially 10 mg once daily; may increase to 20 mg once daily after 3 weeks
  Lexapro *Tab:* 5, 10*, 20*mg
  Lexapro Oral Solution *Oral soln:* 1 mg/ml (240 ml) (peppermint) (parabens)

▷ *fluoxetine* (C)(G)
  Prozac initially 20 mg daily; may increase after 1 week; doses >20 mg/day may be divided into AM and noon doses; max 80 mg/day
    Pediatric: <8 years: not recommended; 8-17 years: initially 10-20 mg once daily; start lower weight children at 10 mg once daily; if starting at 10 mg once daily, may increase after 1 week to 20 mg once daily
    Cap: 10, 20, 40 mg; *Tab:* 30*, 60*mg; *Oral soln:* 20 mg/5 ml (4 oz) (mint)
  Prozac Weekly following daily *fluoxetine* therapy at 20 mg/day x 13 weeks, may initiate **Prozac Weekly** 7 days after the last 20 mg *fluoxetine* dose
    Pediatric: not recommended
    Cap: 90 mg ent-coat del-rel pellets

▷ *paroxetine maleate* (D)(G)
  Pediatric: not recommended
    Paxil initially 10-20 mg daily in AM; may increase by 10 mg/day at weekly intervals as needed; max 60 mg/day
    Tab: 10*, 20*, 30, 40 mg
    Paxil CR initially 12.5-25 mg daily in AM; may increase by 12.5 mg at weekly intervals as needed; max 62.5 mg/day
    Tab: 12.5, 25, 37.5 mg ent-coat cont-rel
    Paxil Suspension initially 10-20 mg daily in AM; may increase by 10 mg/day at weekly intervals as needed; max 60 mg/day
    Oral susp: 10 mg/5 ml (250 ml) (orange)

▷ *sertraline* (C) initially 50 mg daily; increase at 1 week intervals if needed; max 200 mg daily
  Pediatric: <6 years: not recommended; 6-12 years: initially 25 mg daily; max 200 mg/day; 13-17 years: initially 50 mg daily; max 200 mg/day
    Zoloft *Tab:* 15*, 50*, 100*mg; *Oral conc:* 20 mg per ml (60 ml [dilute just before administering in 4 oz water, ginger ale, lemon-lime soda, lemonade, or orange juice]) (alcohol 12%)

SEROTONIN AND NOREPINEPHRINE REUPTAKE INHIBITORS (SNRIs)

➤ *venlafaxine* (C)(G)
    Effexor initially 75 mg/day in 2-3 divided doses; may increase at 4 day intervals in 75 mg increments to 150 mg/day; max 225 mg/day
    Pediatric: <18 years: not recommended
    Tab: 37.5, 75, 150, 225 mg
    Effexor XR initially 75 mg q AM; may start at 37.5 mg daily x 4-7 days; then increase by increments of up to 75 mg/day at intervals of at least 4 days; usual max 375 mg/day
    Pediatric: not recommended
    Tab: Cap: 37.5, 75, 150 mg ext-rel

COMBINATION AGENTS

➤ *chlordiazepoxide/amitriptyline* (D)(G)
    Pediatric: not recommended
    Limbitrol 3-4 tabs/day in divided doses
    Tab: chlor 5 mg/*amit* 12.5 mg
    Limbitrol DS 3-4 tabs/day in divided doses; max 6 tabs/day
    Tab: chlor 10 mg/*amit* 25 mg
➤ *perphenazine/amitriptyline* (C)(G) 1 tab bid-qid
    Pediatric: not recommended
    Tab: **Etrafon 2-10:** *perph* 2 mg/*amit* 10 mg
        Etrafon 2-25: *perph* 2 mg/*amit* 25 mg
        Etrafon 4-25: *perph* 4 mg/*amit* 25 mg

APHTHOUS STOMATITIS (MOUTH ULCER, CANKER SORE)

ANTI-INFLAMMATORY AGENTS

➤ *dexamethasone* elixir (B) 5 ml swish and spit q 12 hours
    Pediatric: not recommended
    Elix: 0.5 mg/ml
➤ *triamcinolone acetonide* 0.1% dental paste (NR)(G) press (do not rub) thin film onto lesion at bedtime and, if needed, 2-3 x daily after meals; re-evaluate if no improvement in 7 days
    Oralone *Dental paste:* 0.1% (5 g)
➤ *triamcinolone* 1% in **Orabase** (B) apply 1/4 inch to each ulcer bid-qid until ulcer heals
    Pediatric: not recommended
    Kenalog in Orabase *Crm:* 1% (15, 60, 80 g)

TOPICAL ANESTHETICS

➤ *benzocaine* topical gel (C)(G) apply tid-qid
➤ *benzocaine* topical spray (C)(G) 1 spray to painful area every 2 hours as needed; retain for 15 seconds, then spit
    Cepocal Spray (OTC), **Chloraseptic Spray** (OTC)

➤ *lidocaine* viscous soln **(B)(G)** 15 ml gargle <u>or</u> swish, then spit; repeat after 3 hours; max 8 doses/day
Pediatric: <3 years: 1.25 ml; apply with cotton-tipped applicator; may repeat after 3 hours; max 8 doses/day
   Xylocaine Viscous Solution *Viscous soln:* 2% (20, 100, 450 ml)
➤ *triamcinolone* **(Kenalog)** in **Orabase (C)** apply with swab

DEBRIDING AGENT/CLEANSER

➤ *carbamide peroxide 10%* **(NR)(OTC)** apply 10 drops to affected area; swish x 2-3 minutes, then spit; do not rinse; repeat treatment qid
   Gly-Oxide *Liq:* 10% (50, 60 ml squeeze bottle w. applicator)

ANTI-INFECTIVES

➤ *minocycline* **(D)(G)** swish and spit 10 ml susp (50 mg/5 ml) <u>or</u> 1 x 100 mg cap <u>or</u> 2 x 50 mg caps dissolved in 180 ml water, bid x 4-5 days
Pediatric: <8 years: not recommended; ≥8 years: same as adult
   Dynacin *Cap:* 50, 100 mg
   Minocin *Cap:* 50, 75, 100 mg; *Oral susp:* 50 mg/5 ml (60 ml) (custard) (sulfites, alcohol 5%)
Comment: *minocycline* is contraindicated <8 years-of-age, in pregnancy, and lactation (discolors developing tooth enamel). A side effect may be photo-sensitivity (photophobia). Do not give with antacids, calcium supplements, milk or other dairy, or within two hours of taking another drug.
➤ *tetracycline* **(D)** swish and spit 10 ml susp (125 mg/5 ml) <u>or</u> one 250 mg tab/cap dissolved in 180 ml water qid x 4-5 days
Pediatric: <8 years: not recommended; ≥8 years: same as adult; *see page 574 for dose by weight*
   Achromycin V *Cap:* 250, 500 mg
   Sumycin *Tab:* 250, 500 mg; *Cap:* 250, 500 mg; *Oral susp:* 125 mg/5 ml (100, 200 ml) (fruit) (sulfites)
Comment: *tetracycline* is contraindicated <8 years-of-age, in pregnancy, and lactation (discolors developing tooth enamel). A side effect may be photo-sensitivity (photophobia). Do not give with antacids, calcium supplements, milk or other dairy, or within two hours of taking another drug.

ASPERGILLOSIS (*SCEDOSPORIUM APIOSPERMUM, FUSARIUM* SPP.)

INVASIVE INFECTION

➤ *isavuconazonium* **(C)** swallow cap whole; *Loading dose:* 372 mg q 8 hours x 6 doses (48 hours); *Maintenance:* 372 mg once daily starting 12-24 hours after last loading dose
Pediatric: <18 years: not established
   Cresemba *Cap:* 186 mg; *Vial:* 372 mg pwdr for reconstitution (7/blister pck) (preservative-free)

Comment: **Cresemba** is indicated for the treatment of invasive aspergillus and mucormycosis in patients >18-years-old who are at high risk due to being severely compromised.

▷ *posaconazole* (D) take with food; swallow tab whole; *Day 1*: 300 mg bid; then 300 mg once daily for duration of treatment (e.g., resolution of neutropenia or immunosuppression)
Pediatric: <13 years: not recommended; ≥13 years: same as adult
    Noxafil *Tab*: 100 mg del-rel; *Oral susp*: 40 mg/ml (105 oz w. dosing spoon) (cherry)
    Comment: **Noxafil** is indicated as prophylaxis for invasive aspergillus and candida infections in patients >13-years-old who are at high risk due to being severely compromised.

▷ *voriconazole* (D) *IV*: 6 mg/kg q 12 hours x 2 doses; then 4 mg/kg q 12 hour; max rate 3 mg/kg/hour over 1-2 hours; *PO*: <40 kg: 100 mg q 12 hours; may increase to 150 mg q 12 hours if inadequate response; >40 kg: 200 mg q 12 hours; may increase to 300 mg q 12 hours if inadequate response
Pediatric: not recommended
    Vfend *Tab*: 50, 200 mg
    Vfend I.V. for Injection *Vial*: 200 mg pwdr for reconstitution (preservative-free)

⃝ ASTHMA

Parenteral Corticosteroids *see page* 499
Oral Corticosteroids *see page* 497

LEUKOTRIENE RECEPTOR ANTAGONISTS (LRAs)

Comment: The LRAs are indicated for prophylaxis and chronic treatment, only. Not for primary (rescue) treatment of acute asthma attack.

▷ *montelukast* (B)(G) 10 mg once daily in the PM; for EIB, take at least 2 hours before exercise; max 1 dose/day
Pediatric: <12 months: not recommended; 12-23 months: one 4 mg granule pkt daily; 2-5 years: one 4 mg chew tab or granule pkt daily; 6-14 years: one 5 mg chew tab daily; ≥15 years: same as adult
    Singulair *Tab*: 10 mg
    Singulair Chewable *Chew tab*: 4, 5 mg (cherry) (phenylalanine)
    Singulair Oral Granules *Granules*: 4 mg/pkt; take within 15 minutes of opening pkt; may mix with applesauce, carrots, rice, or ice cream

▷ *zafirlukast* (B) 20 mg bid, 1 hour ac or 2 hours pc
Pediatric: <7 years: not recommended; 7-11 years: 10 mg bid 1 hour ac or 2 hours pc; ≥12 years: same as adult
    Accolate *Tab*: 10, 20 mg

▷ *zileuton* (C)
Pediatric: <12 years: not recommended; ≥12 years: same as adult
    Zyflo 1 tab qid
        Tab: 600 mg
    Zyflo CR 2 tabs bid
        Tab: 600 mg ext-rel

IGE BLOCKER (IGG1K MONOCLONAL ANTIBODY)

▷ *omalizumab* (B) 150-375 mg SC every 2-4 weeks based on body weight and pre-treatment serum total IgE level; max 150 mg/injection site
Pediatric: <12 years: not recommended; 30-90 kg + IgE >30-100 IU/ml 150 mg q 4 weeks; 90-150 kg + IgE >30-100 IU/ml or 30-90 kg + IgE >100-200 IU/ml or 30-60 kg + IgE >200-300 IU/ml 300 mg q 4 hours; >90-150 kg + IgE >100-200 IU/ml or >60-90 kg + IgE >200-300 IU/ml or 30-70 kg + IgE >300-400 IU/ml 225 mg q 2 weeks; >90-150 kg + IgE >200-300 IU/ml or >70-90 kg + IgE >300-400 IU/ml or 30-70 kg + IgE >400-500 IU/ml or 30-60 kg + IgE >500-600 IU/ml or 30-60 kg + IgE >600-700 IU/ml 375 mg q 2 weeks
  Xolair *Vial:* 150 mg pwdr for SC injection after reconstitution (preservative-free)

INHALED ANTICHOLINERGICS

▷ *ipratropium bromide* (C)(G)
  Atrovent 2 inhalations qid; additional inhalations as required; max 12 inhalations/day
    Pediatric: not recommended
    Inhaler: 18 mcg/actuation (14 g, 200 inh)
  Atrovent Inhalation Solution 500 mcg tid-qid prn by nebulizer
    Pediatric: not recommended
    Inhal soln: 0.02% (500 mcg in 2.5 ml; 25/carton)

INHALED CORTICOSTEROIDS

Comment: Instruct patient to rinse mouth after using an inhaled steroid to reduce risk of oral candidiasis. Not for primary (rescue) treatment of acute asthma attack.
▷ *beclomethasone dipropionate* (C)(G) *Previously using only bronchodilators:* initiate 40-80 mcg bid; max 320 mcg bid; *Previously using inhaled corticosteroid:* initiate 40-160 mcg bid; max 320 mcg/day; *Previously taking a systemic corticosteroid:* attempt to to wean off the systemic drug after approximately 1 week after initiating; rinse mouth after use
Pediatric: not recommended
  Qvar
    Inhal aerosol: 40, 80 mcg/metered dose actuation (8.7 g, 120 inh) metered dose inhaler (chlorofluorocarbon [CFC]-free)
▷ *budesonide* (B)
  Pulmicort Flexhaler initially 180-360 mcg bid; max 360 mcg bid; rinse mouth after use
    Pediatric: <6 years: not recommended; ≥6 years: 1-2 inhalations bid
    Flexhaler: 90 mcg/actuation (60 inh); 180 mcg/actuation (120 inh)
  Pulmicort Respules (G) adult use flexhaler
    Pediatric: <12 months: not recommended; 12 months-8 years: *Previously using only bronchodilators:* initiate 0.5 mg/day once daily or in 2 divided doses; may start at 0.25 mg daily; *Previously using inhaled corticosteroids:* initiate 0.5 mg once daily or in 2 divided doses; max 1 mg/day; *Previously taking oral corticosteroids:* initiate 1 mg/day daily or in 2 divided doses; >8 years: use flexhaler; rinse mouth after use
    Inhal susp: 0.25, 0.5, 1 mg/2 ml (30/carton)

▷ *ciclesonide* (C) initially 80 mcg bid; max 320 mcg/day; rinse mouth after use; *Previously on inhaled corticosteroid:* initially 80 mcg bid; *Previously on oral steroid:* 320 mg bid
Pediatric: <12 years: not recommended; ≥12 years: same as adult
    Alvesco
        Inhal aerosol: 80, 160 mcg/actuation (6.1 g, 60 inh)
▷ *flunisolide* (C) rinse mouth after use
    AeroBid, AeroBid-M initially 2 inhalations bid; max 8 inhalations/day; rinse mouth after use
        Pediatric: <6 years: not recommended; 6-15 years: 2 inhalations bid; ≥15 years: same as adult
        Inhaler: 250 mcg/actuation (7 g, 100 inh)
    Aerospan HFA initially 160 mcg bid; max 320 mcg bid
        Pediatric: <6 years: not recommended; 6-11 years: 80 mcg bid; max 160 mcg bid; ≥12 years: same as adult
        Inhaler: 80 mcg (5.1 g, 60 doses; 80 mcg, 120 doses)
▷ *fluticasone furoate* (C) *currently not on inhaled corticosteroid:* usually initiate at 100 mcg once daily at the same time each day; may increase to 200 mcg once daily if inadequate response after 2 weeks; max 200 mcg/day; rinse mouth after use
Pediatric: not established
    Arnuity Ellipta *Inhal:* 100, 200 mcg/dry pwdr per inhalation (30 doses)
    Comment: **Arnuity Ellipta** is not for primary treatment of status asthmaticus or acute asthma episodes. **Arnuity Ellipta** is contraindicated with severe hypersensitivity to milk proteins.
▷ *fluticasone propionate* (C)
    Flovent, Flovent HFA initially 88 mcg bid; *Previously using an inhaled corticosteroid:* initially 88-220 mcg bid; *Previously taking an oral corticosteroid:* 880 mcg bid; rinse mouth after use
        Pediatric: use **Flovent Diskus**
        Inhaler: 44 mcg/actuation (7.9 g, 60 inh; 13 g, 120 inh); 110 mcg/actuation (13 g, 120 inh); 220 mcg/actuation (13 g, 120 inh)
    Flovent Diskus initially 100 mcg bid; max 500 mcg bid; *Previously using an inhaled corticosteroid:* initially 100-250 mcg bid; max 500 mcg bid; *Previously taking an oral corticosteroid:* 1000 mcg bid
        Pediatric: <4 years: not recommended; 4-11 years: initially 50 mcg bid; max 100 mcg bid; rinse mouth after use; ≥12 years: same as adult
        Diskus: 50, 100, 250 mcg/inh dry pwdr (60 blisters w. diskus)
▷ *mometasone furoate* (C) 220-440 mcg once daily or bid; max 880 mcg/day; rinse mouth after use
    Asmanex HFA *Inhaler:* 100, 200 mcg/actuation (13 g, 120 inh)
        Pediatric: not established
    Asmanex Twisthaler *Inhaler:* 110 mcg/actuation (30 inh), 220 mcg/actuation (30, 60, 120 inh)
        Pediatric: <4 years: not recommended; 4-11 years: 110 mcg once daily in the PM; rinse mouth after use
▷ *triamcinolone* (C)
    Azmacort 2 inhalations tid-qid or 4 inhalations bid; rinse mouth after use
        Pediatric: <6 years: not recommended; 6-12 years: 1-2 inhalations tid or 2-4 inhalations bid; >12 years: same as adult
        Inhaler: 100 mcg/actuation (20 g, 240 inh)

INHALED MAST CELL STABILIZERS (PROPHYLAXIS)

Comment: IMCSs are for prophylaxis and chronic treatment, only. Not for primary (rescue) treatment of acute asthma attack.

▷ *cromolyn sodium* (B)(G)
    Intal 2 inhalations qid; 2 inhalations up to 10-60 minutes before precipitant as prophylaxis; rinse mouth after use
        Pediatric: <2 years: not recommended; 2-5 years: use inhal soln via nebulizer; >5 years: 2 inhalations qid via inhaler
        Inhaler: 0.8 mg/actuation (8.1, 14.2 g; 112, 200 inh)
    Intal Inhalation Solution 20 mg by nebulizer qid; 20 mg up to 10-60 minutes before precipitant as prophylaxis
        Pediatric: <2 years: not recommended; ≥2 years: same as adult
        Inhal soln: 20 mg/2 ml (60, 120/carton)
▷ *nedocromil sodium* (B)
    Tilade 2 sprays qid; rinse mouth after use
        Pediatric: <6 years: not recommended; ≥6 years: 2 sprays qid
        Inhaler: 1.75 mg/spray (16.2 g; 104 sprays)
    Tilade Nebulizer Solution 0.5% 1 amp qid by nebulizer
        Pediatric: <2 years: not recommended; ≥2 years: initially 1 amp qid by nebulizer; 2-5 years: initially 1 amp tid by nebulizer; ≥5 years: same as adult
        Inhal soln: 11 mg/2.2 ml (2 ml; 60, 120/carton)

INHALED BETA AGONISTS (BRONCHODILATORS)

▷ *albuterol sulfate* (C)(G)
    AccuNeb Inhalation Solution 1 unit-dose vial tid-qid prn by nebulizer; ages 2-12 years only; not for adult
        Pediatric: <2 years: not recommended; 2-12 years: initially 0.63 mg or 1.25 mg tid-qid; 6-12 years: with severe asthma, or >40 kg, or 11-12 years: initially 1.25 mg tid-qid
        Inhal soln: 0.63, 1.25 mg/3ml (3 ml, 25/carton) (preservative-free)
    Albuterol Inhalation Solution (G) not recommended
        Pediatric: <2 years: not recommended; ≥2 years: 1 vial via nebulizer over 5-15 minutes
        Inhal soln: 0.63 mg/3 ml (0.021%); 1.25 mg/3 ml (0.042%) (25/carton)
    Albuterol Inhalation Solution 0.5% (G) not recommended
        Pediatric: <4 years: not recommended; ≥4 years: same as adult
        Inhal soln: 0.083% (25/carton)
    Albuterol Nebules (G) 2.5 mg (0.5 ml of 5% diluted to 3 ml with sterile NS or 3 ml of 0.083%) tid-qid
        Pediatric: use other forms
        Inhal soln: 0.083% (25/carton)
    Proair HFA Inhaler 1-2 inhalations q 4-6 hours prn; 2 inhalations 15 minutes before exercise as prophylaxis for exercise-induced asthma (EIA)
        Pediatric: <4 years: not established; ≥4 years: same as adult
        Inhaler: 90 mcg/actuation (0.65 g, 200 inh) (CFC-free)
    Proair RespiClick 1-2 inhalations q 4-6 hours prn; 2 inhalations 15-30 minutes before exercise as prophylaxis for exercise-induced asthma (EIA)
        Pediatric: not established

Inhaler: 90 mcg/actuation (8.5 g, 200 inh)

Proventil HFA Inhaler 1-2 inhalations q 4-6 hours prn; 2 inhalations 15 minutes before exercise as prophylaxis for exercise-induced asthma (EIA)

Pediatric: <4 years: use syrup; ≥4 years: same as adult

Inhaler: 90 mcg/actuation with a dose counter (6.7 g, 200 inh)

Proventil Inhalation Solution 2.5 mg diluted to 3 ml with normal saline tid-qid prn by nebulizer

Pediatric: use syrup

Inhal soln: 0.5% (20 ml w. dropper); 0.083% (3 ml; 25/carton)

Ventolin Inhaler 2 inhalations q 4-6 hours prn; 2 inhalations 15 minutes before exercise as prophylaxis for exercise-induced asthma

Pediatric: <2 years: not recommended; 2-4 years: use syrup; >4 years: same as adult

Inhaler: 90 mcg/actuation (17 g, 220 inh)

Ventolin Rotacaps 1-2 cap inhalations q 4-6 hours prn; 2 inhalations 15 minutes before exercise as prophylaxis for exercise-induced asthma (EIA)

Pediatric: <4 years: not recommended; ≥4 years 1-2 caps q 4-6 hours prn

Rotacaps: 200 mcg/Rotacaps (100 doses/Rotacaps)

Ventolin 0.5% Inhalation Solution

Pediatric: <2 years: not recommended; ≥2 years: initially 0.1-0.15 mg/kg/dose tid-qid prn; 10-15 kg: 0.25 ml diluted to 3 ml with normal saline by nebulizer tid-qid prn; >15 kg: 0.5 ml diluted to 3 ml with normal saline by nebulizer tid-qid prn

Inhal soln: 20 ml w. dropper

Ventolin Nebules

Pediatric: <2 years: not recommended; ≥2 years: initially 0.1-0.15 mg/kg/dose tid-qid prn; 10-15 kg: 1.25 mg or 1/2 nebule tid-qid prn; >15 kg: 2.5 mg or 1 nebule tid-qid prn

Inhal soln: 0.083% (3 ml; 25/carton)

▷ *isoproterenol* (B) *Rescue:* 1 inhalation prn; repeat if no relief in 2-5 minutes; *Maintenance:* 1-2 inhalations q 4-6 hours

Pediatric: <12 years: not recommended; ≥12 years: same as adult

Medihaler-ISO *Inhaler:* 80 mcg/actuation (15 ml, 30 inh)

▷ *levalbuterol* (C)(G) initially 0.63 mg tid q 6-8 hours prn by nebulizer; may increase to 1.25 mg tid at 6-8 hour intervals as needed

Pediatric: not recommended

Xopenex *Inhal soln:* 0.31, 0.63, 1.25 mg/3 ml (24/carton) (preservative-free)

Xopenex HFA *Inh:* 45 mg (15 g, 200 inh) (preservative-free)

Xopenex Concentrate *Vial:* 1.25 mg/0.5 ml (30/carton) (preservative-free)

▷ *metaproterenol* (C)(G)

Alupent 2-3 inhalations tid-qid prn; max 12 inhalations/day

Pediatric: <6 years: use syrup; ≥6 years: via nebulizer 0.1-0.2 ml diluted with normal saline to 3 ml, up to q 4 hours prn

Inhaler: 0.65 mg/actuation (14 g, 200 doses)

Alupent Inhalation Solution 5-15 inhalations tid-qid prn; q 4 hours prn for acute attack

Pediatric: <6 years: use syrup ≥6 years: via nebulizer 0.1-0.2 ml diluted with normal saline to 3 ml, up to q 4 hours prn

Inhal soln: 5% (10, 30 ml w. dropper)

▷ *pirbuterol* (C) 1-2 inhalations q 4-6 hours prn; max 12 inhalations/day
    Maxair
        Pediatric: <12 years: not recommended
        Autohaler: 200 mcg/actuation (14 g, 400 inh); *Inhaler:* 200 mcg/actuation
        (25.6 g, 300 inh)
▷ *terbutaline* (B) 2 inhalations q 4-6 hours prn
    Pediatric: not recommended
    Inhaler: 0.2 mg/actuation (10.5 g, 300 inh)

INHALED RACEPINEPHRINE (BRONCHODILATOR)

▷ *racepinephrine* (C)(OTC)(G) 1-3 inhalations not more than every 3 hours; max 12
inhalations/24 hours
    Pediatric: <4 years: not recommended; ≥4 years: same as adult
        Asthmanephrin Inhaler *Starter kit:* 10 x 0.5 ml vials 2.25% solution for atom-
        ized inhalation w. EZ Breathe Atomizer; *Refills:* 30 x 0.5 ml vials 2.25% solution
        for atomized inhalation
Comment: Inhalational epinephrine is only recommended for use during pregnancy
when there are no alternatives and benefit outweighs risk.

INHALED LONG-ACTING ANTICHOLINERGIC

▷ *tiotropium (as bromide monohydrate)* (C) 2 inhalations once daily using inhalation
device; do not swallow caps
    Pediatric: <12 years: not recommended; ≥12 years: same as adult
        Spiriva HandiHaler *Inhal device:* 18 mcg/cap pwdr for inhalation (5, 30, 90 caps
        w. inhalation device)
        Spiriva Respimat *Inhal device:* 1.25, 2.5 mcg/actuation cartridge w. inhalation
        device (4 g, 60 metered actuations) (benzylkonian chloride)
Comment: *tiotropium is f*or prophylaxis and chronic treatment, only. Not for
primary (rescue) treatment of acute attack. Avoid getting powder in eyes. Caution
with narrow-angle glaucoma, BPH, bladder neck obstruction, and pregnancy.
Contraindicated with allergy to *atropine* or its derivatives (e.g., *ipratropium*).

INHALED ANTICHOLINERGIC/BETA AGONIST

▷ *ipratropium bromide/albuterol sulfate* (C) 2 inhalations qid
        Combivent 2 inhalations qid; additional inhalations as required; max 12
        inhalations/day
            Pediatric: not recommended
            Inhaler: ipra 18 mcg/*albu* 90 mcg/actuation (14.7 g, 200 inh)
        Duoneb 1 vial via nebulizer 4-6 times daily prn
            Pediatric: <18 years: not recommended
            Inhal soln: ipra 0.5 mg (0.017%)/*albu* 2.5 mg (0.083%) per 3 ml (23/carton)

INHALED BETA AGONIST (LONG-ACTING) (LABA)

▷ *arformoterol* (C) 15 mcg bid via nebulizer
    Pediatric: not recommended
        Brovana *Inhal soln:* 15 mcg/2 ml (2 ml; 30/carton)

Comment: *arformoterol* is indicated for the treatment of COPD but is used off-label for the treatment of asthma. It is used for prophylaxis and chronic treatment, only. Not for primary (rescue) treatment of acute attack.

▷ *formoterol fumarate* (C)

> **Foradil Aerolizer** 12 mcg q 12 hours
>> *Pediatric:* <5 years: not recommended; ≥5 years: same as adult
>> *Inhaler:* 12 mcg/cap (12, 60 caps w. device)
>
> **Perforomist** 20 mcg q 12 hours
>> *Pediatric:* not recommended
>> *Inhal soln:* 20 mcg/2 ml (60/carton)

Comment: *formoterol* is for prophylaxis and chronic treatment, only. Not for primary (rescue) treatment of acute attack. Do not mix *formoterol* with other drugs. *formoterol* off-label for asthma.

▷ *olodaterol* (C)

Pediatric: not established

> **Striverdi Respimat** 12 mcg q 12 hours
>> *Inhal soln:* 2.5 mcg/cartridge (metered actuation) (40 g, 60 metered actuations) (benzalkonium chloride)

Comment: **Striverdi Respimat** is contraindicated in persons with asthma without use of long-term control medication.

▷ *salmeterol* (C)(G) 2 inhalations q 12 hours prn; 2 inhalations at least 30-60 minutes before exercise as prophylaxis for exercise-induced asthma; do not use extra doses for exercise-induced bronchospasm if already using regular dose

> **Serevent Diskus**
>> *Pediatric:* <4 years: not recommended; ≥4 years: 1 inhalation q 12 hours prn; 1 inhalation at least 30-60 minutes before exercise as prophylaxis for exercise-induced asthma; do not use extra doses for exercise-induced bronchospasm if already using regular dose
>> *Diskus (pwdr):* 50 mcg/actuation (60 doses/disk)

CORTICOSTEROID/INHALED LONG-ACTING BETA AGONIST (LABA)

▷ *budesonide/formoterol* (C) 1 inhalation bid; rinse mouth after use

Pediatric: <12 years: not recommended; ≥12 years: same as adult

> **Symbicort 80/4.5**
>> *Inhaler: bud* 80 mcg/*for* 4.5 mcg
>
> **Symbicort 160/4.5**
>> *Inhaler: bud* 160 mcg/*for* 4.5 mcg

▷ *fluticasone propionate/salmeterol* (C)

> **Advair HFA** *Not previously using inhaled steroid:* start with 2 inh 45/21 or 115/21 bid; if insufficient response after 2 weeks, use next higher strength; max 2 inh 230/50 bid; *Already using inhaled steroid;* see mfr literature; rinse mouth after use
>
> **Advair HFA 45/21**
>> *Pediatric:* not recommended
>> *Inhaler: flu pro* 45 mcg/*sal* 21 mcg/actuation (CFC-free)
>
> **Advair HFA 115/21**
>> *Pediatric:* not recommended
>> *Inhaler: flu pro* 115 mcg/*sal* 21 mcg/actuation (CFC-free)
>
> **Advair HFA 230/21**

    Pediatric: not recommended
    Inhaler: flu pro 230 mcg/*sal* 21 mcg/actuation (CFC-free)
Advair Diskus *Not previously using inhaled steroid:* start with 1 inh 100/50 bid; *Already using inhaled steroid:* see mfr literature; rinse mouth after use
Advair Diskus 100/50
    Pediatric: <4 years: not recommended; 4-11 years: 1 inhalation bid; >11 years: 1 inhalation bid
    Diskus: flu pro 100 mcg/*sal* 50 mcg/actuation (60 blisters)
Advair Diskus 250/50 1 inhalation bid; rinse mouth after use
    Pediatric: 4-12 years: use 100/50 strength; >12 years: same as adult
    Diskus: flu pro 250 mcg/*sal* 50 mcg/actuation (60 blisters)
Advair Diskus 500/50
    Pediatric: 4-12 years: use 100/50 strength; >12 years: same as adult
    Diskus: fluticasone propionate 500 mcg/salmeterol 50 mcg/actuation (60 blisters)
Comment: **Advair Diskus** is not a rescue inhaler. Allow 12 hours between doses.

▷ *fluticasone furoate/vilanterol* (C) 1 inhalation 100/25 once daily at the same time each day
Pediatric: <17 years: not established
    Breo Ellipta 100/25 *Inhal pwdr: flu* 100 mcg/*vil* 25 mcg dry pwdr per inhal (30 doses)
    Breo Ellipta 200/25 *Inhal pwdr: flu* 200 mcg/*vil* 25 mcg dry pwdr per inhal (30 doses)
    Comment: **Breo Ellipta** is contraindicated with severe hypersensitivity to milk proteins.

▷ *mometasone furoate/formoterol fumarate* (C) 2 inhalations bid; rinse mouth after use
Pediatric: not established
    Dulera 100/5 *Inhaler: mom* 100 mcg/*for* 5 mcg (HFA)
    Dulera 200/5 *Inhaler: mom* 200 mcg/*for* 5 mcg (HFA)
    Comment: **Dulera** is not a rescue inhaler.

ORAL BETA2-AGONISTS (BRONCHODILATORS)

▷ *albuterol* (C)
    Albuterol Syrup (G) *Adults:* 2-4 mg tid-qid; may increase gradually; max 8 mg qid; *Elderly:* initially 2-3 mg tid-qid; may increase gradually; max 8 mg qid
        Pediatric: <2 years: not recommended; ≥2-6 years: 0.1 mg/kg tid; initially max 2 mg tid; may increase gradually to 0.2 mg/kg tid; max 4 mg tid; >6-12 years: 2 mg tid-qid; may increase gradually; max 6 mg qid; ≥12 years: same as adult
        Syr: 2 mg/5 ml
    Proventil 2-4 mg tid-qid prn
        Pediatric: <6 years: not recommended; ≥6 years: same as adult
        Tab: 2, 4 mg
    Proventil Repetabs 4-8 mg q 12 hours prn
        Pediatric: use syrup
        Repetab: 4 mg sust-rel
    Proventil Syrup 5-10 ml tid-qid prn; may increase gradually; max 20 ml qid prn
        Pediatric: <2 years: not recommended; ≥2-6 years: 0.1 mg/kg tid; max initially 5 ml tid prn; may increase gradually to 0.2 mg/kg tid prn; max 10 ml tid; >6-14 years: 5 ml tid-qid prn; may increase gradually; max 60 ml/day in divided doses; >14 years: same as adult
        Syr: 2 mg/5 ml

Ventolin 2-4 mg tid-qid prn; may increase gradually; max 8 mg qid
Pediatric: <2 years: not recommended; ≥2-6 years: 0.1 mg/kg tid prn; max initially 2 mg tid prn; may increase gradually to 0.2 mg/kg tid; max 4 mg tid; >6-14 years: 2 mg tid-qid prn; may increase gradually; max 6 mg tid
Tab: 2, 4 mg; *Syr:* 2 mg/5 ml (strawberry)
VoSpire ER 4-8 mg q 12 hours prn; max 32 mg/day divided q 12 hours; swallow whole
Pediatric: <6 years: not recommended; ≥6-12 years: 4 mg q 12 hours; max 24 mg/day q 12 hours; >12 years: same as adult
Tab: 4, 8 mg ext-rel
▷ *metaproterenol* (C)
Alupent 20 mg tid-qid prn
Pediatric: <6 years: not recommended (doses of 1.3-2.6 mg/kg/day have been used); ≥6-9 years (<60 lb): 10 mg tid-qid prn; >9-12 years (>60 lb): 20 mg tid-qid prn; >12 years: same as adult
Tab: 10, 20 mg; *Syr:* 10 mg/5 ml

METHYLXANTHINES

Comment: Check serum theophylline level just before 5th dose is administered. Therapeutic theophylline level: 10-20 mcg/ml.
▷ *theophylline* (C)(G)
Theo-24 initially 300-400 mg once daily at HS; after 3 days, increase to 400-600 mg once daily at HS; max 600 mg/day
Pediatric: <45 kg: initially 12-14 mg/kg/day; max 300 mg/day; increase after 3 days to 16 mg/kg/day to max 400 mg; after 3 more days increase to 30 mg/kg/day to max 600 mg/day; ≥45 kg: same as adult
Cap: 100, 200, 300, 400 mg ext-rel
Theo-Dur initially 150 mg bid; increase to 200 mg bid after 3 days; then to 300 mg bid after 3 more days
Pediatric: <6 years: not recommended; 6-15 years: initially 12-14 mg/kg/day in 2 divided doses; max 300 mg/day; then increase to 16 mg/kg in 2 divided doses; max 400 mg/day; then to 20 mg/kg/day in 2 divided doses; max 600 mg/day; ≥15 years: same as adult
Tab: 100, 200, 300 mg ext-rel
Theolair-SR
Pediatric: not recommended
Tab: 200, 250, 300, 500 mg sust-rel
Uniphyl 400-600 mg daily with meals
Pediatric: not recommended
Tab: 400*, 600*mg cont-rel

METHYLXANTHINE/EXPECTORANT

▷ *dyphylline/guaifenesin* (C) 1 tab qid
Lufyllin GG *Tab:* dyphy 200 mg/*guaif* 200 mg; *Elix:* dyphy 100 mg/*guaif* 100 mg per 15 ml

HUMANIZED INTERLEUKIN-5 ANTAGONIST MONICLONAL ANTIBODY

▷ *mepolizumab* (NR) 100 mg SC once every 4 weeks in upper arm, abdomen, or thigh
Pediatric: <12 years: not recommended; ≥12 years: same as adult

Nucala *Vial:* 100 mg pwdr for reconstitution, single-use (preservative-free)
Comment: **Nucala** is an add-on maintenance treatment for severe asthma.
There is a pregnancy exposure registry that monitors pregnancy outcomes in
women exposed to **Nucala** during pregnancy. Healthcare providers can enroll
patients <u>or</u> encourage patients to enroll themselves by calling 1-877-311-8972
<u>or</u> visiting www.mothertobaby.org/asthma.

 ATROPHIC VAGINITIS

Oral Estrogens *see Menopause* page 254

VAGINAL ESTROGEN PREPARATIONS

▷ *estradiol* (X)
   Vagifem Vaginal Tablet 1 tab intravaginally daily x 2 weeks; then 1 tab intravaginally twice weekly
      Vag tab: 10 mcg (15 tabs w. applicators)
▷ *estradiol* (X)
   Estrace Vaginal Cream 2-4 g daily x 1-2 weeks; then gradually reduce to 1/2
   initial dose x 1-2 weeks; then maintenance dose of 1 g 1-3 times/week
      Vag crm: 0.01% (1 oz tube w. calib applicator)
▷ *estrogens, conjugated* (X)
   Premarin Cream 2 g/day intravaginally
      Vag crm: 1.5 oz w. applicator marked in 1/2 g increments to max 2 g
▷ *estropipate* (X)
   Ogen Cream 2-4 g intravaginally daily x 3 weeks; discontinue 4th week;
   continue in this cyclical pattern
      Vag crm: 1.5 mg/g (42.5 g w. calib applicator)

 **ATTENTION DEFICIT DISORDER (ADD)/
ATTENTION DEFICIT HYPERACTIVITY
DISORDER (ADHD)**

SELECTIVE NOREPINEPHRINE REUPTAKE INHIBITOR (SNRI)

▷ *atomoxetine* (C) take one dose daily in the morning <u>or</u> in two divided doses in the
   morning and late afternoon <u>or</u> early evening; initially 40 mg/kg; increase after at
   least 3 days to 80 mg/kg; then after 2-4 weeks may increase to max 100 mg/day
   Pediatric: <6 years: not recommended; ≥6 years, <70 kg: initially 0.5 mg/kg/day:
   increase after at least 3 days to 1.2 mg/kg/day; max 1.4 mg/ kg/day <u>or</u> 100 mg/day
   (whichever is less); ≥6 years, >70 kg: same as adult
      Strattera *Cap:* 10, 18, 25, 40, 60, 80, 100 mg
Comment: Not associated with stimulant <u>or</u> euphoric effects. May discontinue without
tapering.

STIMULANTS

▷ *amphetamine sulfate* (C)(II)

    Adzenys XT-ODT take with <u>or</u> without food; individualize the dosage according to the therapeutic needs and response; initially 6.3 mg once daily in the morning; increase in increments of 3.1 mg <u>or</u> 6.3 mg at weekly intervals; max recommended dose 18.8 mg once daily (6-12 years-of-age) and 12.5 mg once daily (13-17 years-of-age);

    Pediatric: <6 years: not recommended; ≥6 years: same as adult

    Comment: Patients taking **Adderall XR** may be switched to **Adzenys XR-ODT** at the equivalent dose taken once daily; switching from any other amphetamine products (e.g., **Adderall** immediate-release), discontinue that treatment, and titrate with **Adzenys XR-ODT** using the titration schedule (see mfr literature)

    ODT: 3.1, 6.3, 9.4, 12.5, 15.7, 18.8 mg orally-disint (orange) (fructose)

    Dyanavel XR Oral Suspension initially 2.5 mg <u>or</u> 5 mg once daily in the morning; may increase in increments of 2.5 mg to 5 mg per day every 4-7 days; max 20 mg per day; shake bottle prior to administration

    Pediatric: <6 years: not recommended; ≥6 years: same as adult

    Oral susp: 2.5 mg/ml (464 ml)

    Evekeo initially 5 mg once <u>or</u> twice daily at the same time(s) each day; may increase by 5 mg/day at weekly intervals; max 40 mg/day

    Pediatric: <3 years: not recommended; ≥3-5 years: initially 2.5 mg once <u>or</u> twice daily at the same time(s) each day; may increase by 2.5 mg/day at weekly intervals; max 40 mg/day; ≥6 years: same as adult

    Tab: 5, 10 mg

▷ *dextroamphetamine sulfate* (C)(II)(G) initially start with 10 mg daily; increase by 10 mg at weekly intervals if needed; may switch to daily dose with sust-rel spansules when titrated

Pediatric: <3 years: not recommended; ≥3-5 years: 2.5 mg daily; may increase by 2.5 mg daily at weekly intervals if needed; 6-12 years: initially 5 mg daily <u>or</u> bid; may increase by 5 mg/day at weekly intervals; usual max 40 mg/day; >12 years: initially 10 mg daily; may increase by 10 mg/day at weekly intervals; max 40 mg/day

    Dexedrine *Tab:* 5*mg (tartrazine)

    Dexedrine Spansule *Cap:* 5, 10, 15 mg sust-rel

    Dextrostat *Tab:* 5, 10 mg (tartrazine)

▷ *dextroamphetamine saccharate/dextroamphetamine sulfate/amphetamine aspartate/ amphetamine sulfate* (C)(II)(G) not indicated for adults

    Adderall initially 10 mg daily; may increase weekly by 10 mg/day; usual max 60 mg/day in 2-3 divided doses; first dose on awakening; then q 4-6 hours prn

    Pediatric: <6 years: not indicated; ≥6-12 years: initially 5 mg daily; may increase by 5 mg/day at weekly intervals; >12 years: same as adult

    Tab: 5**, 7.5**, 10**, 12.5**, 15**mg, 3.75 mg, 20**, 30**mg

    Adderall XR 20 mg by mouth once daily in AM; may increase by 10 mg/day at weekly intervals; max: 60 mg/day

    Pediatric: <6 years: not recommended; ≥6 years: initially 10 mg daily in the AM; may increase by 10 mg/day at weekly intervals; max 30 mg/day; 13-17 years: 10-20 mg by mouth daily in the AM; may increase by 10 mg/day at weekly intervals; max 40 mg/day; Do not chew; may sprinkle on apple sauce

    Cap: 5, 10, 15, 20, 25, 30 mg ext-rel

▷ *dexmethylphenidate* (C)(II)(G) not indicated for adults
  Pediatric: <6 years: not recommended; ≥6 years: initially 2.5 mg bid; allow at least 4 hours between doses; may increase at 1 week intervals; max 20 mg/day
  Focalin *Tab:* 2.5, 5, 10*mg (dye-free)
  Focalin ER *Cap:* 15, 30 mg ext-rel
  Focalin XR *Cap:* 5, 10, 15, 20, 25, 30, 35, 40 mg ext-rel
▷ *lisdexamphetamine dimesylate* (C)(II) 30 mg once daily in the AM; may increase by 10-20 mg/day at weekly intervals; max 70 mg/day
  Pediatric: <6 years: not recommended; ≥6 years: same as adult
  Vyvanse *Cap:* 20, 30, 40, 50, 60, 70 mg
  Comment: May dissolve **Vyvanse** capsule contents in water; take immediately.
▷ *methamphetamine* (C)(II)(G) initially 5 mg once daily to bid; may increase by 5 mg/day at weekly intervals; usual effective dose 20-25 mg/day
  Desoxyn Granumets
    Pediatric: <6 years: not recommended; ≥6 years: same as adult
    Tab: 5, 10, 15 mg sust-rel
▷ *methylphenidate (regular-acting)* (C)(II)(G)
  Methylin, Methylin Chewable, Methylin Oral Solution usual dose 20-30 mg/day in 2-3 divided doses 30-45 minutes before a meal; max 60 mg/day
    Pediatric: <6 years: not recommended; ≥6 years: initially 5 mg bid ac (breakfast and lunch); may increase 5-10 mg/day at weekly intervals; max 60 mg/day
    Tab: 5, 10*, 20*mg; *Chew tab:* 2.5, 5, 10 mg; (grape; phenylalanine); *Oral soln:* 5, 10 mg/5 ml (grape)
  Ritalin 10-60 mg/day in 2-3 divided doses 30-45 minutes ac; max 60 mg/day
    Pediatric: <6 years: not recommended; ≥6 years: initially 5 mg bid ac (breakfast and lunch); may increase by 5-10 mg at weekly intervals as needed; max 60 mg/day
    Tab: 5, 10*, 20*mg
▷ *methylphenidate (long-acting)* (C)(II)
  Concerta initially 18 mg q AM; may increase in 18 mg increments as needed; max 54 mg/ day; do not crush or chew
    Pediatric: <6 years: not recommended; ≥6-12 years: initially 18 mg daily; max 54 mg/day; ≥13-17 years: initially 18 mg daily; max 72 mg/day or 2 mg/kg, whichever is less
    Tab: 18, 27, 36, 54 mg sust-rel
  Metadate CD (G) 1 cap daily in the AM; may sprinkle on food; do not crush or chew
    Pediatric: <6 years: not recommended; ≥6 years: initially 20 mg daily; may gradually increase by 20 mg/day at weekly intervals as needed; max 60 mg/day
    Cap: 10, 20, 30, 40, 50, 60 mg immed- and ext-rel beads
  Metadate ER 1 tab daily in the AM; do not crush or chew
    Pediatric: <6 years: not recommended; >6 years: use in place of regular-acting *methylpheni- date* when the 8-hour dose of **Metadate-ER** corresponds to the titrated 8-hour dose of regular-acting *methylphenidate*
    Tab: 10, 20 mg ext-rel (dye-free)
  QuilliChew ER initially 1 x 10 mg chew tab once daily in the AM
    Pediatric: <6 years: not recommended; initially 10 mg daily; may gradually increase by 20 mg/day at weekly intervals as needed; max 60 mg/day
    Chew tab: 20*, 30*, 40 mg ext-rel

Quillivant XR initially 20 mg once daily in the AM, with <u>or</u> without food; may be titrated in increments of 10-20 mg/day at weekly intervals; daily doses above 60 mg have not been studied and are not recommended; shake the bottle vigorously for at least 10 seconds to ensure that the correct dose is administered
> *Pediatric:* <6 years: not recommended; ≥6 years: same as adult
> *Bottle:* 5 mg/ml, 25 mg/5 ml pwdr for reconstitution; 300 mg (60 ml), 600 mg (120 ml), 750 mg (150 ml), 900 mg (180 ml)

Comment: **Quillivant XR** must be reconstituted by a pharmacist, not by the patient <u>or</u> caregiver.

Ritalin LA (G) 1 cap daily in the AM
> *Pediatric:* <6 years: not recommended; ≥6 years: use in place of regular-acting *methylphenidate* when the 8-hour dose of **Ritalin LA** corresponds to the titrated 8-hour dose of regular-acting *methylphenidate*; max 60 mg/day
> *Cap:* 10, 20, 30, 40 mg ext-rel (immed- and ext-rel beads)

Ritalin SR 1 cap daily in the AM
> *Pediatric:* <6 years: not recommended; ≥6 years: use in place of regular-acting *methylphenidate* when the 8-hour dose of **Ritalin SR** corresponds to the titrated 8-hour dose of regular-acting *methylphenidate*; max 60 mg/day
> *Tab:* 20 mg sust-rel (dye-free)

➤ *methylphenidate* (transdermal patch) **(C)(II)(G)** not applicable >17 years
> *Pediatric:* <6 years: not recommended; ≥6-17 years: initially 10 mg patch applied to hip 2 hours before desired effect daily in the AM; may increase by 5-10 mg at weekly intervals; max 60 mg/day
> **Daytrana** *Transdermal patch:* 10, 15, 20, 30 mg

➤ *pemoline* **(B)(IV)** 18.75-112.5 mg/day; usually start with 37.5 mg in AM; may increase 18.75 mg/day at weekly intervals; max 112.5 g/day
> *Pediatric:* <6 years: not recommended; ≥6 years: same as adult
> **Cylert** *Tab:* 18.75*, 37.5*, 75*mg
> **Cylert Chewable** *Chew tab:* 37.5*mg

Comment: Check baseline serum ALT and monitor every 2 weeks thereafter.

CENTRAL ALPHA2A-AGONIST

➤ *guanfacine* **(B)(G)** not applicable >17 years
> *Pediatric:* <6 years: not recommended; ≥6-17 years: initially 1 mg once daily; may increase by 1 mg/day at weekly intervals; usual max 4 mg/day
> **Intuniv** *Tab:* 1, 2, 3, 4 mg ext-rel
> Comment: Take **Intuniv** with water, milk, <u>or</u> other liquid. Do not take with a high-fat meal. Withdraw gradually by 1 mg every 3-7 days.

TRICYCLIC ANTIDEPRESSANTS (TCAs)

see Depression page 105

OTHER AGENTS

➤ *clonidine* **(C)(G)**
> **Catapres** 4-5 mcg/kg/day
> > *Pediatric:* <12 years: not recommended; ≥12 years: same as adult
> > *Tab:* 0.1*, 0.2*, 0.3*mg

Kapvay not indicated for adults
> *Pediatric:* <6 years: not recommended; ≥6-12 years: initially 0.1 mg at bed-
> time x 1 week; then 0.1 mg bid x 1 week; then 0.1 mg AM and 0.2 mg PM x 1
> week; then 0.2 mg bid; withdraw gradually by 0.1 mg/day at 3-7 day intervals
> *Tab:* 0.1, 0.2 mg ext-rel

AMINOKETONES (FOR THE TREATMENT OF ADHD)

▷ *bupropion HCl* (B)(G)
Pediatric: <18 years: not recommended
> **Wellbutrin** initially 100 mg bid for at least 3 days; may increase to 375 or 400
> mg/day after several weeks; then after at least 3 more days, 450 mg in 4 divided
> doses; max 450 mg/day, 150 mg/single dose
> *Tab:* 75, 100 mg
> **Wellbutrin SR** initially 150 mg in AM for at least 3 days; may increase to 150
> mg bid if well tolerated; usual dose 300 mg/day; max 400 mg/day
> *Tab:* 100, 150 mg sust-rel
> **Wellbutrin XL** initially 150 mg in AM for at least 3 days; increase to 150 mg bid
> if well tolerated; usual dose 300 mg/day; max 400 mg/day
> *Tab:* 150, 300 mg sust-rel

◯ BACTERIAL ENDOCARDITIS: PROPHYLAXIS

Comment: Bacterial endocarditis prophylaxis is appropriate for persons with a history
of previous infective endocarditis, persons with a prosthetic cardiac valve or prosthetic
material used for valve repair, cardiac transplant patients who develop cardiac
valvulopathy, congenital heart disease (CHD), unrepaired cyanotic CHD including
palliative shunts and conduits, completely repaired congenital heart defect(s) with
prosthetic material or device, whether placed by surgery or by catheter intervention,
during the first 6 months after the procedure, repaired CHD with residual defects at the
site or adjacent to the site of a prosthetic patch or prosthetic device (which may inhibit
endothelialization), or any other condition deemed to place a patient at high risk.

DENTAL, ORAL, RESPIRATORY TRACT, OR ESOPHAGEAL PROCEDURES

▷ *amoxicillin* (B)(G) 2 g PO 30-60 minutes before procedure as a single dose or 3 g
1 hour before procedure and 1.5 g 6 hours later
Pediatric: 50 mg/kg as a single dose or 50 mg/kg (max 3 g) 1 hour before procedure
and (max 1.5 g) 25 mg/kg 6 hours later; ≥40 kg: same as adult; *see pages 543-546 for
dose by weight*
> **Amoxil** *Cap:* 250, 500 mg; *Tab:* 875*mg; *Chew tab:* 125, 200, 250, 400 mg (cher-
> ry-banana-peppermint) (phenylalanine); *Oral susp:* 125, 250 mg/5 ml (80, 100,
> 150 ml) (strawberry); 200, 400 mg/5 ml (50, 75, 100 ml) (bubble gum); *Oral
> drops:* 50 mg/ml (30 ml) (bubble gum)
> **Trimox** *Tab:* 125, 250 mg; *Cap:* 250, 500 mg; *Oral susp:* 125, 250 mg/5 ml (80,
> 100, 150 ml) (raspberry-strawberry)
▷ *ampicillin* (B)(G) 2 g PO/IM/IV 30-60 minutes before procedure
Pediatric: 50 mg/kg PO/IM/IV 30-60 minutes before procedure

Omnipen, Principen *Cap:* 250, 500 mg; *Oral susp:* 125, 250 mg/5 ml (100, 150, 200 ml) (fruit)
Unisyn Vial: 1.5, 3 g

▷ *azithromycin* **(B)** 500 mg 30-60 minutes before procedure
Pediatric: 15 mg/kg 30-60 minutes before procedure; max 500 mg; *see page 548 for dose by weight*
Zithromax *Tab:* 250, 500, 600 mg; *Oral susp:* 100 mg/5 ml (15 ml); 200 mg/5 ml (15, 22.5, 30 ml) (cherry)

▷ *cefazolin* **(B)** 1 g IM/IV 30-60 minutes before procedure
Pediatric: 25 mg/kg IM/IV 30-60 minutes before procedure
Ancef *Vial:* 250, 500 mg; 1, 5 g
Kefzol *Vial:* 500 mg; 1 g

▷ *ceftriaxone* **(B)(G)** 1 g IM/IV as a single dose
Pediatric: 50 mg/kg IM/IV as a single dose
Rocephin Vial: 250, 500 mg; 1, 2 g

▷ *cephalexin* **(B)(G)** 2 g as a single dose 30-60 minutes before procedure
Pediatric: 50 mg/kg as a single dose 30-60 minutes before procedure; *see page 557 for dose by weight*
Keflex *Cap:* 250, 333, 500, 750 mg; *Oral susp:* 125, 250 mg/5 ml (100, 200 ml) (strawberry)

▷ *clarithromycin* **(C)(G)** 500 mg or 500 mg ext-rel as a single dose 30-60 minutes before procedure
Pediatric: 15 mg/kg as a single dose 30-60 minutes before procedure; *see page 558 for dose by weight*
Biaxin *Tab:* 250, 500 mg
Biaxin Oral Suspension *Oral susp:* 125, 250 mg/5 ml (50, 100 ml) (fruit-punch)
Biaxin XL *Tab:* 500 mg ext-rel

▷ *clindamycin* **(B)(G)** 600 mg PO as a one time single dose or 300 mg 30-60 minutes before procedure and 150 mg 6 hours later; take with a full glass of water
Pediatric: 20 mg/kg (max 300 mg) 1 hour before procedure and 10 mg/kg (max 150 mg) 6 hours later; take with a full glass of water; *see page 559 for dose by weight*
Cleocin **(G)** *Cap:* 75 (tartrazine), 150 (tartrazine), 300 mg; *Vial:* 150 mg/ml (2, 4 ml) (benzyl alcohol)
Cleocin Pediatric Granules **(G)** *Oral susp:* 75 mg/ml (100 ml)(cherry)

▷ *erythromycin estolate* **(B)(G)** 1 g 1 hour before procedure; then 500 mg 6 hours later
Pediatric: 20 mg/kg 1 hour before procedure; then 10 mg/kg 6 hours later; *see page 562 for dose by weight*
Ilosone *Pulvule:* 250 mg; *Tab:* 500 mg; *Liq:* 125, 250 mg/5 ml (100 ml)
Comment: *erythromycin* may increase INR with concomitant *warfarin*, as well as increase serum level of *digoxin*, benzodiazepines and statins.

▷ *penicillin V potassium* **(B)(G)** 2 g 1 hour before procedure; then 1 g 6 hours later or 2 g 1 hour before procedure; then 1 g q 6 hours x 8 doses
Pediatric: <60 lb: 1 g 1 hour before procedure; then 500 mg 6 hours later or 1 g 1 hour before procedure; then 500 mg q 6 hours x 8 doses; >12 years: same as adult; *see page 572 for dose by weight*
Pen-Vee K *Tab:* 250, 500 mg; *Oral soln:* 125 mg/5 ml (100, 200 ml); 250 mg/5 ml (100, 150, 200 ml)

BACTERIAL VAGINOSIS (BV; GARDNERELLA VAGINALIS)

PROPHYLAXIS AND RESTORATION OF VAGINAL ACIDITY

▷ *acetic acid/oxyquinolone* (C) one full applicator intravaginally bid for up to 30 days
  Pediatric: not recommended
    Relagard *Gel:* acet acid 0.9%/oxyq 0.025% (50 g tube w. applicator)

Comment: The following treatment regimens for *bacterial vaginosis* are published in the **2015 CDC Sexually Transmitted Diseases Treatment Guidelines**. Treatment regimens are presented by generic drug name first, followed by information about brands and dose forms. BV is associated with adverse pregnancy outcomes, including premature rupture of the membranes, preterm labor, preterm birth, intraamniotic infection, and postpartum endometritis. Therefore, treatment is recommended for all pregnant women with symptoms _or_ positive screen.

RECOMMENDED REGIMENS

Regimen 1
▷ *metronidazole* 500 mg bid x 7 days

Regimen 2
▷ *metronidazole* gel 0.75% one full applicatorful (5 g) once daily x 5 days

Regimen 3
▷ *clindamycin* cream 2% one full applicatorful (5 g) intravaginally once daily at bedtime x 5 days

CDC Alternate Regimens

Regimen 1
▷ *tinidazole* 2 g once daily x 2 days

Regimen 2
▷ *tinidazole* 1 g once daily x 5 days

Regimen 3
▷ *clindamycin* 300 mg bid x 7 days

Regimen 4
▷ *clindamycin* ovules 100 mg intravaginally once daily at bedtime x 3 days

Drug Brands and Dose Forms

▷ *clindamycin* (B)
    Cleocin (G) *Cap:* 75 (tartrazine), 150 (tartrazine), 300 mg
    Cleocin Pediatric Granules (G) *Oral susp:* 75 mg/5 ml (100 ml) (cherry)
    Cleocin Vaginal Cream *Vag crm:* 2% (21, 40 g tubes w. applicator)
    Cleocin Vaginal Ovules *Vag supp:* 100 mg
▷ *metronidazole* (not for use in 1st; B in 2nd, 3rd)
    Flagyl *Tab:* 250*, 500* mg
    Flagyl 375 *Cap:* 375 mg
    Flagyl ER *Tab:* 750 mg ext-rel
    MetroGel-Vaginal, Vandazole *Vag gel:* 0.75% (70 g w. applicator) (parabens)

Comment: Alcohol is contraindicated during treatment with oral *metronidazole* and for 72 hours after therapy due to a possible *disulfiram*-like reaction (nausea, vomiting, flushing, headache).

▶ *tinidazole* (not for use in 1st; B in 2nd, 3rd)
> Tindamax *Tab:* 250*, 500*mg

Comment: Alcohol is contraindicated during treatment with oral *tinidazole* and for 72 hours after therapy due to a possible *disulfiram*-like reaction (nausea, vomiting, flushing, headache).

 BALDNESS: MALE PATTERN

TYPE II 5-ALPHA-REDUCTASE SPECIFIC INHIBITOR

▶ *finasteride* (X)(G) 1 mg daily
> Propecia *Tab:* 1 mg

Comment: Pregnant women should not touch broken *finasteride* tabs. Use of **Propecia**, a 5-alpha reductase inhibitor, is associated with low but increased risk of high-grade prostate cancer.

PERIPHERAL VASODILATOR

▶ *minoxidil* topical soln (C) 1 ml from dropper <u>or</u> 6 sprays bid
> *Pediatric:* <18 years: not recommended
> **Rogaine for Men** (OTC) *Regular soln:* 2% (60 ml w. applicator) (alcohol 60%);
> *Extra strength soln:* 5% (60 ml w. applicator) (alcohol 30%)
> **Rogaine for Women** (OTC) Regular soln: 2% (60 ml w. applicator) (alcohol 60%)

Comment: Do not use *minoxidil* on abraded <u>or</u> inflamed scalp.

 BELL'S PALSY

▶ *prednisone* (C)(G) 80 mg once daily x 3 days; then 60 mg daily x 3 days; then 40 mg daily x 3 days; then 20 mg x 1 dose; then discontinue
> **Deltasone** *Tab:* 2.5*, 5*, 10*, 20*, 50*mg

BENIGN ESSENTIAL TREMOR

ANTI-PARKINSON'S AGENT

▶ *amantadine* (C)(G) 200 mg daily <u>or</u> 100 mg bid; 4 tsp of syrup once daily <u>or</u> 2 tsp bid
> **Symmetrel** *Tab:* 100 mg; *Syr:* 50 mg/5 ml (raspberry)

BETA-BLOCKER

▶ *propranolol* (C)(G)
> **Inderal** initially 40 mg bid; usual range 160-240 mg/day
> *Tab:* 10*, 20*, 40*, 60*, 80*mg
> **Inderal LA** initially 80 mg once daily in a single dose; increase q 3-7 days; usual range 120-160 mg/day; max 320 mg/day in a single dose

Cap: 60, 80, 120, 160 mg sust-rel
InnoPran XL initially 80 mg q HS; max 120 mg/day
Cap: 80, 120 mg ext-rel

⭕ BENIGN PROSTATIC HYPERPLASIA (BPH)

ALPHA-1 BLOCKERS

Comment: Educate patient regarding potential side effect of hypotension especially with first dose. Usually start at lowest dose and titrate upward.
▷ *doxazosin* (C)
    Cardura initially 1 mg daily; may double dose every 1-2 weeks; max 8 mg/day
      Tab: 1*, 2*, 4*, 8*mg
    Cardura XL initially 4 mg once daily with breakfast; may titrate after 3-4 weeks; max 8 mg/day
      Tab: 4, 8 mg ext-rel
▷ *silodosin* (B) 8 mg once daily; *CrCl 30-50 mL/min:* 4 mg once daily
    Rapaflo *Cap:* 4, 8 mg
▷ *terazosin* (C)(G) initially 1 mg q HS; titrate up to 10 mg once daily; max 20 mg/day
    Hytrin *Cap:* 1, 2, 5, 10 mg

ALPHA-1A BLOCKERS

▷ *alfuzosin* (B)(G) 10 mg once daily taken immediately after the same meal each day
    UroXatral *Tab:* 10 mg ext-rel
▷ *tamsulosin* (B)(G) initially 0.4 mg once daily; may increase to 0.8 mg daily after 2-4 weeks if needed
    Flomax *Cap:* 0.4 mg
    Comment: May take **Flomax** 0.4 mg with **Avodart** 0.5 mg once daily as combination therapy.

TYPE II 5-ALPHA-REDUCTASE INHIBITOR

Comment: Pregnant women and women of childbearing age should not handle *finasteride*. Monitor for potential side effects of decreased libido and/or impotence. Low, but increased risk of being diagnosed with high-grade prostate cancer.
▷ *finasteride* (X) 5 mg once daily
    Proscar *Tab:* 5 mg

TYPES I AND II 5-ALPHA-REDUCTASE INHIBITOR

Comment: Pregnant women and women of childbearing age should not handle *dutasteride*. Monitor for potential side effects of decreased libido and/or impotence. Low, but increased risk of being diagnosed with high-grade prostate cancer.
▷ *dutasteride* (X) 0.5 mg once daily
    Avodart *Cap:* 0.5 mg
    Comment: May take **Avodart** 0.5 mg with **Flomax** 0.4 mg once daily as combination therapy.

TYPE I AND II 5-ALPHA-REDUCTASE INHIBITOR/ALPHA-1A BLOCKER

▷ *dutasteride/tamsulosin* (X) take 1 cap once daily after the same meal each day
    Jalyn *Cap:* duta 0.5 mg/*tam* 0.4 mg

PHOSPHODIESTERASE TYPE 5 (PDE5) INHIBITORS, CGMP-SPECIFIC

Comment: Oral PDE5 inhibitors are contraindicated in patients taking nitrates.
Caution with history of recent MI, stroke, life-threatening arrhythmia, hypotension,
hypertension, cardiac failure, unstable angina, retinitis pigmentosa, CYP3A4 inhibitors
(e.g., *cimetidine*, the azoles, *erythromycin*, grapefruit juice), protease inhibitors (e.g.,
ritonavir), CYP3A4 inducers (e.g., *rifampin*, *carbamaepine*, *phenytoin*, *phenobarbital*),
alcohol, antihypertensive agents. Side effects include headache, flushing, nasal
congestion, rhinitis, dyspepsia, and diarrhea.

▷ *tadalafil* (B) 5 mg once daily at the same time each day; *CrCl 30-50 mL/min:* initially
2.5 mg; *CrCl <30 mL/min:* not recommended; *Concomitant alpha blockers:* not recommended
    Cialis *Tab:* 2.5, 5, 10, 20 mg

◯ BILE ACID DEFICIENCY

BILE ACID

▷ *ursodiol* (B)
    Dissolution of radiolucent non-calcified gallstones <20 mm diameter: 8-10 mg/kg/
    day in 2-3 divided doses; *Prevention:* 13-15 mg/kg/day in 4 divided doses
    Pediatric: not recommended
    Actigall *Cap:* 300 mg

Comment: *ursodiol* decreases the amount of cholesterol produced by the liver
and absorbed by the intestines. It helps break down cholesterol that has formed
into stones in the gallbladder. *ursodiol* increases bile flow in patients with
primary biliary cirrhosis. It is used to treat small gallstones in people who cannot
have cholecystectomy surgery and to prevent gallstones in overweight patients
undergoing rapid weight loss. *ursodiol* is not for treating gallstones that are
calcified.

◯ BINGE EATING DISORDER

CENTRAL NERVOUS SYSTEM (CNS) STIMULANT

▷ *lisdexamfetamine dimesylate* (C)(II) swallow whole or may open and mix/dissolve
contents of cap in yogurt, water, orange juice and take immediately; 30 mg once daily
in the AM; may adjust in increments of 20 mg at weekly intervals; target dose 50-70
mg/day; max 70 mg/day; *GFR 15-<30 mL/min:* max 50 mg/day; *GFR <15 mL/min,
ESRD:* max 30 mg/day
    Vyvanse *Cap:* 10, 20, 30, 40, 50, 60 70 mg
    Comment: **Vyvanse** is not approved or recommended for weight loss treatment
    of obesity.

BIPOLAR I DISORDER: DEPRESSION

Comment: The cornerstone of treatment for Bipolar I Disorder: Depression is mood-stabilizers (*lithium* and *valproate*). Common adjunctive agents include antiepileptics, antipsychotics, and combination agents. Mounting evidence suggests that antidepressants aren't effective in the treatment of bipolar depression. A major study funded by the National Institute of Mental Health (NIMH) showed that adding an antidepressant to a mood stabilizer was no more effective in treating bipolar I depression than using a mood stabilizer alone. Another NIMH study found that antidepressants work no better than placebo. If antidepressants are used at all, they should be combined with a mood stabilizer such as *lithium* <u>or</u> *valproic acid*. Taking an antidepressant without a mood stabilizer is likely to trigger a manic episode. Antidepressants can increase mood cycling. Many experts believe that over time, antidepressant use in people with bipolar disorder has a mood destabilizing effect, increasing the frequency of manic and depressive episodes. Drugs and conditions that can mimic bipolar I disorder include thyroid disorders, corticosteroids, antidepressants, adrenal disorders (e.g. Addison's disease, Cushing's syndrome), antianxiety drugs, drugs for Parkinson's disease, vitamin B12 deficiency, neurological disorders (e.g. epilepsy, multiple sclerosis).

MOOD STABILIZERS

Lithium Salts Mood Stabilizer

▷ *lithium carbonate* (D)(G) swallow whole; *Usual maintenance:* 900-1200 mg/day in 2-3 divided doses
Pediatric: not recommended
   Lithobid *Tab:* 300 mg slow-rel
   Comment: Signs and symptoms of *lithium* toxicity can occur below 2 mEq/L and include blurred vision, tinnitus, weakness, dizziness, nausea, abdominal pains, vomiting, diarrhea to (severe) hand tremors, ataxia, muscle twitches, nystagmus, seizures, slurred speech, decreased level of consciousness, coma, death.

Valproate Mood Stabilizer

▷ *divalproex sodium* (D)(G) take once daily; swallow ext-rel form whole; initially 25 mg/kg/day in divided doses; max 60 mg/kg/day; *Elderly:* reduce initial dose and titrate slowly
Pediatric: not recommended
   Depakene *Cap:* 250 mg; *Syr:* 250 mg/5 ml (16 oz)
   Depakote *Tab:* 125, 250 mg
   Depakote ER *Tab:* 250, 500 mg ext-rel
   Depakote Sprinkle *Cap:* 125 mg

ANTIEPILEPTICS

▷ *carbamazepine* (D)(G) swallow ext-rel form whole; may open caps and sprinkle on applesauce (do not crush <u>or</u> chew beads); initially 400 mg/day in 2 divided doses; adjust in increments of 200 mg/day; max 1.6 g/day. *Elderly:* reduce initial dose and titrate slowly
Pediatric: not recommended

Carbatrol *Cap:* 200, 300 mg ext-rel
Equetro (G) *Cap:* 100, 200, 300 mg ext-rel
Tegretol *Tab:* 200*mg; *Chew tab:* 100*mg; *Oral susp:* 100 mg/5 ml (450 ml; citrus-vanilla)
Tegretol XR *Tab:* 100, 200, 400 mg ext-rel
Comment: *carbamazepine* is indicated in mixed episodes in bipolar I disorder.

➢ *lamotrigine* (C)(G) *Not taking an enzyme-inducing antiepileptic drug (EIAED) (e.g., phenytoin, carbamazepine, phenobarbital, primidone, valproic acid):* 25 mg once daily x 2 weeks; then 50 mg once daily x 2 weeks; then 100 mg once daily x 2 weeks; then target dose 200 mg once daily; *Concomitant* **valprooic acid:** 25 mg every other day x 2 weeks; then 25 mg once daily x 2 weeks; then 50 mg once daily x 1 week; then target dose 100 mg once daily; *Concomitant EIAED, not valproic acid:* 50 mg once daily x 2 weeks; then 100 mg daily in divided doses; then increase weekly by 100 mg in divided doses to target dose 400 mg/day in divided doses daily
Pediatric: not recommended
Lamictal *Tab:* 25*, 100*, 150*, 200*mg
Lamictal Chewable Dispersible Tab *Chew tab:* 2, 5, 25, 50 mg (black current)
Lamictal ODT *ODT:* 25, 50, 100, 200 mg
Lamictal XR *Tab:* 25, 50, 100, 200 mg ext-rel
Comment: *lamotrigine* is indicated for maintenance treatment of bipolar I disorder. See mfr literature for drug interactions, interactions with contraceptives and hormone replacement therapy, and discontinuation protocol

ANTIPSYCHOTICS

Comment: Side effects of antipsychotics include drowsiness, weight gain, sexual dysfunction, dry mouth, constipation, blurred vision.

➢ *aripiprazole* (C) initially 15 mg once daily; may increase to max 30 mg/day
Pediatric: <10 years: not recommended; ≥10-17 years: initially 2 mg/day in a single dose for 2 days; then increase to 5 mg/day in a single dose for 2 days; then increase to target dose of 10 mg/day in a single dose; may increase by 5 mg/day at weekly intervals as needed to max 30 mg/day
Abilify *Tab:* 2, 5, 10, 15, 20, 30 mg
Abilify Discmelt *Tab:* 15 mg orally-disint (vanilla) (phenylalanine)
Abilify Maintena *Vial:* 300, 400 mg ext-rel pwdr for IM injection after reconstitution; 300, 400 mg single-dose prefilled dual-chamber syringes w. supplies
Comment: **Abilify** is indicated for acute and maintenance treatment of mixed episodes in bipolar I disorder, as monotherapy or as adjunct to *lithium* or *valproic acid.*

➢ *asenapine* (C) allow SL tab to dissolve on tongue; do not split, crush, chew, or swallow; do not eat or drink for 10 minutes after administration; *Monotherapy:* 10 mg bid; *Adjunctive therapy:* 5 mg bid; may increase to max 10 mg bid
Pediatric: <10 years: not established; 10-17 years: *Monotherapy:* initially 2.5 mg bid; may increase to 5 mg bid after 3 days; then to 10 mg bid after 3 more days; max 10 mg bid
Saphris *SL tab:* 2, 5, 5, 10 mg (black cherry)
Comment: **Saphris** is indicated for acute treatment of manic or mixed episodes in bipolar I disorder, as monotherapy or as adjunct to *lithium* or *valproic acid.*

➢ *cariprazine* (NR)
Pediatric: NR

Vraylar *Cap:* 1.5, 3, 4.5, 6 mg; 7-count (1 x 1.5 mg, 6 x 3 mg) mixed blister pck
Comment: **Vraylar** is an atypical antipsychotic with partial agonist activity at
D2 and 5-HT1A receptors and antagonist activity at 5-HT2A receptors. It is
indicated for acute treatment of mixed episodes in bipolar I disorder. There is
a **Vraylar** pregnancy exposure registry that monitors pregnancy outcomes in
women exposed to **Vraylar** during pregnancy. For more information, contact
the National Pregnancy Registry for Atypical Antipsychotics at 1-866-961-2388
or visit https://womensmentalhealth.org/clinical-and-research-programs/
pregnancyregistry. Safety and effectiveness in pediatric patients have not been
established.

➤ *lurasidone* (B) initially 20 mg once daily; usual range 20 to max 120 mg/day; take
with food; *CrCl <50 mL/min, moderate hepatic impairment (Child Pugh 7-9):* max 80
mg/day; *Child Pugh 10-15):* max 40 mg/day
Pediatric: not established
    Latuda *Tab:* 20, 40, 60, 80, 120 mg
    Comment: **Latuda** is indicated for major depressive episodes associated with
bipolar I disorder as monotherapy and as adjunctive therapy with *lithium* or
valproic acid. Contraindicated with concomitant strong CYP3A4 inhibitors
(e.g., *ketoconazole, voriconazole, clarithromycin, ritonavir*) and inducers
(e.g., *phenytoin, carbamazepine, rifampin, St. John's wort*); see mfr literature
if patient taking moderate CYP3A4 inhibitors (e.g., *diltiazem, atazanavir,
erythromycin, fluconazole, verapamil*)

➤ *quetiapine fumarate* (C)
    SeroQUEL initially 25 mg bid, titrate q 2nd or 3rd day in increments of 25-50
mg bid-tid; usual maintenance 400-600 mg/day in 2-3 divided doses
    Pediatric: <10 years: not recommended; ≥10-17 years: initially 25 mg bid, titrate
q 2nd or 3rd day in increments of 25-50 mg bid-tid; max 600 mg/day in 2-3
divided doses
        Tab: 25, 50, 100, 200, 300, 400 mg
    SeroQUEL XR swallow whole; administer once daily in the PM; *Day 1:* 50 mg;
Day 2: 100 mg; *Day 3:* 200 mg; *Day 4:* 300 mg; usual range 400-600 mg/day
    Pediatric: <18 years: not recommended
        Tab: 50, 150, 200, 300, 400 mg ext-rel

➤ *risperidone* (C) *Tab:* initially 2-3 mg once daily; may adjust at 24 hour intervals by
1 mg/ day; usual range 1-6 mg/day; max 6 mg/day; *Oral soln:* do not take with cola
or tea; *M-tab:* dissolve on tongue with or without fluid; *Consta:* administer deep IM
in the deltoid or gluteal; give with oral *respirodone* or other antipsychotic x 3 weeks;
then stop oral form; 25 mg IM every 2 weeks; max 50 mg every 2 weeks
    Risperdal
    Pediatric: <5 years: not established; 5-10 years: initially 0.5 mg once daily at the
same time each day adjust at 24 hour intervals by 0.5-1 mg to target dose 1-2.5
mg/day; usual range 1-6 mg/day; max 6 mg/day; >10 years: same as adult
        Tab: 0.25, 0.5, 1, 2, 3, 4 mg; *Oral soln:* 1 mg/ml (100 ml)
    Risperdal Consta
    Pediatric: <18 years: not established
        Vial: 12.5, 25, 37.5, 50 mg pwdr for long-acting IM inj after reconstitution,
single-use, w. diluent and supplies
    Risperdal M-Tab
    Pediatric: <10 years: not established; ≥10 years: same as adult
        Tab: 0.5, 1, 2, 3, 4 mg orally-disint (phenylalanine)

Comment: **Risperdol** tabs, oral solution, and M-tabs are indicated for the short-term monotherapy of acute mania or mixed episodes associated with bipolar I disorder, or in combination with *lithium* or *valproic acid* in adults
Risperdol Consta is indicated as monotherapy or adjunctive therapy to *lithium* or *valproic*
Acid for the maintenance treatment mania and mixed episodes in bipolar I disorder.

▷ *ziprasidone* (C)(G) *Adult*: take with food; initially 40 mg bid; on day 2, may increase to 60-80 mg bid; *Elderly*: lower initial dose and titrate slowly
Pediatric: not recommended
    Geodon *Cap*: 20, 40, 60, 80 mg
    Comment: **Geodon** is indicated for acute and maintenance treatment of mixed episodes in bipolar I disorder, as monotherapy or as adjunct to *lithium* or *valproic acid*.

COMBINATION AGENTS

Thienobenzodiazepine/Selective Serotonin Reuptake Inhibitor Combinations

▷ *fluoxetine* (C)(G)
    Prozac initially *olanzapine* 5 mg plus fluoxetine 20 mg daily in the PM; range *olanzapine* 5-12.5 mg plus *fluoxetine* 20-50 mg; risk of hypotension, or hepatic impairment, slow metabolizers, or sensitive to *olanzapine*, initially *olanzapine* 2.5-5 mg plus *fluoxetine* 20 mg daily in the PM; *fluoxetine* doses >20 mg/day may be divided into AM and noon doses
    Pediatric: not recommended
        Cap: 10, 20, 40 mg; *Tab*: 30*, 60*mg; *Oral soln*: 20 mg/5 ml (4 oz) (mint)
    Prozac Weekly following daily *fluoxetine* therapy at 20 mg/day for 13 weeks, may initiate
    Prozac Weekly 7 days after the last 20 mg *fluoxetine* dose
    Pediatric: not recommended

▷ *olanzapine/fluoxetine* (C) initially 1 x 6/25 cap once daily in the PM; titrate; max 1 x 12/50 cap once daily in the PM
Pediatric: <10 years: not recommended; 10-17 years: initially 1 x 3/25 cap once daily in the PM; max 1 x 12/50 cap once daily in the PM
    Symbyax
        Cap: **Symbyax 3/25**: *olan* 3 mg/*fluo* 25 mg
            Symbyax 6/25: *olan* 6 mg/*fluo* 25 mg
            Symbyax 6/50: *olan* 6 mg/*fluo* 50 mg
            Symbyax 12/25: *olan* 12 mg/*fluo* 25 mg
            Symbyax 12/50: *olan* 12 mg/*fluo* 50 mg
    Comment: **Symbyax** is indicated for the treatment of depressive episodes associated with bipolar I disorder and treatment-resistant depression (TRD).

◯ BIPOLAR I DISORDER: MANIA

Comment: The cornerstone of treatment for Bipolar I Disorder: Mania is mood-stabilizers (*lithium* and *valproic acid*). Common adjunctive agents include antiepileptics and antipsychotics. Drugs and conditions that can mimic bipolar I disorder include thyroid disorders, corticosteroids, antidepressants, adrenal disorders (e.g. Addison's disease, Cushing's syndrome), antianxiety drugs, drugs for Parkinson's disease, vitamin B12 deficiency, neurological disorders (e.g. epilepsy, multiple sclerosis).

MOOD STABILIZERS

Lithium Salts Mood Stabilizer

▷ *lithium carbonate* (D)(G) swallow whole; *Usual maintenance:* 900-1200 mg/day in 2-3 divided doses
  Pediatric: not recommended
    Lithobid *Tab:* 300 mg slow-rel
  Comment: Signs and symptoms of *lithium* toxicity can occur below 2 mEq/L and include blurred vision, tinnitus, weakness, dizziness, nausea, abdominal pains, vomiting, diarrhea to (severe) hand tremors, ataxia, muscle twitches, nystagmus, seizures, slurred speech, decreased level of consciousness, coma, death.

Valproate Mood Stabilizer

▷ *divalproex sodium* (D)(G) take once daily; swallow ext-rel form whole; initially 25 mg/kg/day in divided doses; max 60 mg/kg/day; *Elderly:* reduce initial dose and titrate slowly
  Pediatric: not recommended
    Depakene *Cap:* 250 mg; *Syr:* 250 mg/5 ml (16 oz)
    Depakote *Tab:* 125, 250 mg
    Depakote ER *Tab:* 250, 500 mg ext-rel
    Depakote Sprinkle *Cap:* 125 mg

ANTIEPILEPTICS

▷ *carbamazepine* (D)(G) swallow ext-rel form whole; may open caps and sprinkle on applesauce (do not crush or chew beads); initially 400 mg/day in 2 divided doses; adjust in increments of 200 mg/day; max 1.6 g/day. *Elderly:* reduce initial dose and titrate slowly
  Pediatric: not recommended
    Carbatrol *Cap:* 200, 300 mg ext-rel
    Equetro (G) *Cap:* 100, 200, 300 mg ext-rel
    Tegretol *Tab:* 200*mg; *Chew tab:* 100*mg; *Oral susp:* 100 mg/5 ml (450 ml; citrus-vanilla)
    Tegretol XR *Tab:* 100, 200, 400 mg ext-rel
  Comment: *carbamazepine* is indicated in mixed episodes in bipolar I disorder.
▷ *lamotrigine* (C)(G) *Not taking an enzyme-inducing antiepileptic drug (EIAED)* (*e.g., phenytoin, carbamazepine, phenobarbital, primidone, valproic acid*): 25 mg once daily x 2 weeks; then 50 mg once daily x 2 weeks; then 100 mg once daily x 2 weeks; then target dose 200 mg once daily; *Concomitant valproic acid:* 25 mg every other day x 2 weeks; then 25 mg once daily x 2 weeks; then 50 mg once daily x 1 week; then target dose 100 mg once daily; *Concomitant EIAED, not valproic acid:* 50 mg once daily x 2 weeks; then 100 mg daily in divided doses; then increase weekly by 100 mg in divided doses to target dose 400 mg/day in divided doses daily
  Pediatric: not recommended
    Lamictal *Tab:* 25*, 100*, 150*, 200*mg
    Lamictal Chewable Dispersible Tab *Chew tab:* 2, 5, 25, 50 mg (black current)

>> **Lamictal ODT** *ODT:* 25, 50, 100, 200 mg
>> **Lamictal XR** *Tab:* 25, 50, 100, 200 mg ext-rel

Comment: *lamotrigine* is indicated for maintenance treatment of bipolar I disorder. See mfr literature for drug interactions, interactions with contraceptives and hormone replacement therapy, and discontinuation protocol

▷ *topiramate* (D)(G) initially 25 mg daily in the PM; then 25 mg bid; then, 25 mg in the AM and 50 mg in the PM; then, 50 mg bid
   Pediatric: <12 years: not recommended
>> **Topamax** *Tab:* 25, 50, 100, 200 mg
>> **Topamax Sprinkle Caps** *Cap:* 15, 25 mg

ANTIPSYCHOTICS

Comment: Side effects of antipsychotics include drowsiness, weight gain, sexual dysfunction, dry mouth, constipation, blurred vision.

▷ *aripiprazole* (C) initially 15 mg once daily; may increase to max 30 mg/day
   Pediatric: <10 years: not recommended; ≥10-17 years: initially 2 mg/day in a single dose for 2 days; then increase to 5 mg/day in a single dose for 2 days; then increase to target dose of 10 mg/day in a single dose; may increase by 5 mg/day at weekly intervals as needed to max 30 mg/day
>> **Abilify** *Tab:* 2, 5, 10, 15, 20, 30 mg
>> **Abilify Discmelt** *Tab:* 15 mg orally-disint (vanilla) (phenylalanine)
>> **Abilify Maintena** *Vial:* 300, 400 mg ext-rel pwdr for IM injection after reconstitution; 300, 400 mg single-dose prefilled dual-chamber syringes w. supplies
>> Comment: **Abilify** is indicated for acute and maintenance treatment of mixed episodes in bipolar I disorder, as monotherapy or as adjunct to **lithium** or **valproic acid.**

▷ *asenapine* (C) allow SL tab to dissolve on tongue; do not split, crush, chew, or swallow; do not eat or drink for 10 minutes after administration; *Monotherapy:* 10 mg bid; *Adjunctive therapy:* 5 mg bid; may increase to max 10 mg bid
   Pediatric: <10 years: not established; 10-17 years: *Monotherapy:* initially 2.5 mg bid; may increase to 5 mg bid after 3 days; then to 10 mg bid after 3 more days; max 10 mg bid
>> **Saphris** *SL tab:* 2, 5, 5, 10 mg (black cherry)
>> Comment: **Saphris** is indicated for acute treatment of manic or mixed episodes in bipolar I disorder, as monotherapy or as adjunct to **lithium** or **valproic acid.**

▷ *cariprazine* (NR)
   Pediatric: NR
>> **Vraylar** *Cap:* 1.5, 3, 4.5, 6 mg; 7-count (1 x 1.5 mg, 6 x 3 mg) mixed blister pck
>> Comment: **Vraylar** is an atypical antipsychotic with partial agonist activity at D2 and 5-HT1A receptors and antagonist activity at 5-HT2A receptors. It is indicated for acute treatment of mixed episodes in bipolar I disorder. There is a **Vraylar** pregnancy exposure registry that monitors pregnancy outcomes in women exposed to **Vraylar** during pregnancy. For more information, contact the National Pregnancy Registry for Atypical Antipsychotics at 1-866-961-2388 or visit https:// womensmentalhealth.org/clinical-and-research-programs/pregnancyregistry. Safety and effectiveness in pediatric patients have not been established.

▷ *chlorpromazine* (C)(G) initially 10 mg tid-qid; may increase semi-weekly by 25-50 mg/day
   Pediatric: ≥6 months: initially 0.25 mg/lb every 4-6 hours prn or 0.5 mg/lb rectally q 6-8 hours prn

Thorazine *Tab:* 10, 25, 50, 100, 200 mg; *Spansule:* 30, 75, 150 mg sust-rel; *Syr:* 10 mg/5 ml (4 oz) (orange custard); *Oral conc:* 30 mg/ml (4 oz); 100 mg/ml (2, 8 oz); *Supp:* 25, 100 mg

Comment: *chlorpromazine* is indicated for rapid control of severe psychotic symptoms.

▷ *lurasidone* **(B)** initially 20 mg once daily; usual range 20 to max 120 mg/day; take with food; *CrCl <50 mL/min, moderate hepatic impairment (Child Pugh 7-9):* max 80 mg/day; *Child Pugh 10-15):* max 40 mg/day
Pediatric: not established

Latuda *Tab:* 20, 40, 60, 80, 120 mg

Comment: **Latuda** is indicated for major depressive episodes associated with bipolar I disorder as monotherapy and as adjunctive therapy with *lithium* or *valproic acid*. Contraindicated with concomitant strong CYP3A4 inhibitors (e.g., *ketoconazole, voriconazole, clarithromycin, ritonavir*) and inducers (e.g., *phenytoin, carbamazepine, rifampin, St. John's wort*); see mfr literature if patient taking moderate CYP3A4 inhibitors (e.g., *diltiazem, atazanavir, erythromycin, fluconazole, verapamil*)

▷ *quetiapine fumarate* **(C)**
SeroQUEL initially 25 mg bid, titrate q 2nd or 3rd day in increments of 25-50 mg bid-tid; usual maintenance 400-600 mg/day in 2-3 divided doses
Pediatric: <10 years: not recommended; ≥10-17 years: initially 25 mg bid, titrate q 2nd or 3rd day in increments of 25-50 mg bid-tid; max 600 mg/day in 2-3 divided doses
Tab: 25, 50, 100, 200, 300, 400 mg
SeroQUEL XR swallow whole; administer once daily in the PM; *Day 1:* 50 mg; *Day 2:* 100 mg; *Day 3:* 200 mg; *Day 4:* 300 mg; usual range 400-600 mg/day
Pediatric: <18 years: not recommended
Tab: 50, 150, 200, 300, 400 mg ext-rel

▷ *risperidone* **(C)** *Tab:* initially 2-3 mg once daily; may adjust at 24 hour intervals by 1 mg/ day; usual range 1-6 mg/day; max 6 mg/day; *Oral soln:* do not take with cola or tea; *M-tab:* dissolve on tongue with or without fluid; *Consta:* administer deep IM in the deltoid or gluteal; give with oral *rispirodone* or other antipsychotic x 3 weeks; then stop oral form; 25 mg IM every 2 weeks; max 50 mg every 2 weeks

Risperdal
Pediatric: <5 years: not established; 5-10 years: initially 0.5 mg once daily at the same time each day adjust at 24 hour intervals by 0.5-1 mg to target dose 1-2.5 mg/day; usual range 1-6 mg/day; max 6 mg/day; >10 years: same as adult
Tab: 0.25, 0.5, 1, 2, 3, 4 mg; *Oral soln:* 1 mg/ml (100 ml)

Risperdal Consta
Pediatric: <18 years: not established
Vial: 12.5, 25, 37.5, 50 mg pwdr for long-acting IM inj after reconstitution, single-use, w. diluent and supplies

Risperdal M-Tab
Pediatric: <10 years: not established; ≥10 years: same as adult
Tab: 0.5, 1, 2, 3, 4 mg orally-disint (phenylalanine)

Comment: **Risperdol** tabs, oral solution, and M-tabs are indicated for the short-term monotherapy of acute mania or mixed episodes associated with bipolar I disorder, or in combination with *lithium* or *valproic acid* in adults **Risperdol Consta** is indicated as monotherapy or adjunctive therapy to *lithium* or *valproic*

Acid for the maintenance treatment mania and mixed episodes in bipolar I disorder.

▷ **ziprasidone** (C)(G) *Adult*: take with food; initially 40 mg bid; on day 2, may increase to 60-80 mg bid; *Elderly:* lower initial dose and titrate slowly
  Pediatric: not recommended
  Geodon *Cap:* 20, 40, 60, 80 mg
  Comment: **Geodon** is indicated for acute and maintenance treatment of mania and mixed episodes in bipolar I disorder, as monotherapy or as adjunct to **lithium** or **valproic acid**.

 BITE: CAT

TETANUS PROPHYLAXIS

▷ **tetanus toxoid** vaccine (C) 0.5 ml IM x 1 dose if previously immunized
  Vial: 5 Lf units/0.5 ml (0.5, 5 ml); *Prefilled syringe:* 5 Lf units/0.5 ml (0.5 ml)
  see *Tetanus page 398* for patients not previously immunized

ANTI-INFECTIVES

▷ **amoxicillin/clavulanate** (B)(G) 500 mg tid or 875 mg bid x 10 days
  Augmentin *Tab:* 250, 500, 875 mg; *Chew tab:* 125, 250 mg (lemon-lime); 200, 400 mg (cherry-banana) (phenylalanine); *Oral susp:* 125 mg/5 ml (banana), 250 mg/5 ml (75, 100, 150 ml) (orange); 200, 400 mg/5 ml (50, 75, 100 ml) (orange) (phenylalanine)
    Pediatric: 40-45 mg/kg/day divided tid x 10 days or 90 mg/kg/day divided bid x 10 days *see page 545 for dose by weight*
  Augmentin ES-600 *Oral susp:* 600 mg/5 ml (50, 75, 100, 125, 150, 200 ml) (strawberry cream) (phenylalanine) every 12 hours
    Pediatric: <3 months: not recommended; ≥3 months, <40 kg: 90 mg/kg/day in 2 divided doses; ≥40 kg: not recommended
  Augmentin XR 2 tabs q 12 hours x 7-10 days
    Pediatric: <16 years: use other forms; ≥16 years: same as adult
    Tab: 1000*mg ext-rel
▷ **cefuroxime axetil** (B)(G) 500 mg bid x 10 days
  Pediatric: 15 mg/kg bid x 10 days; *see page 556 for dose by weight*
  Ceftin *Tab:* 250, 500 mg; *Oral susp:* 125, 250 mg/5 ml (50, 100 ml) (tutti-frutti)
▷ **doxycycline** (D)(G) 100 mg bid day 1; then 100 mg daily x 10 days
  Pediatric: <8 years: not recommended ≥8 years, <100 lb: 2 mg/lb on first day in 2 divided doses, followed by 1 mg/lb/day in 1-2 divided doses; ≥8 years, ≥100 lb: same as adult; *see page 561 for dose by weight*
    Actilate *Tab:* 75, 150**mg
    Adoxa *Tab:* 50, 75, 100, 150 mg ent-coat
    Doryx *Tab:* 75, 100, 150 mg del-rel
    Monodox *Cap:* 50, 75, 100 mg
    Oracea *Cap:* 40 mg del-rel
    Vibramycin *Cap:* 50, 100 mg; *Syr:* 50 mg/5 ml (raspberry; sulfites); *Oral susp:* 25 mg/5 ml (raspberry-apple)
    Vibra-Tab *Tab:* 100 mg film-coat
  Comment: **doxycycline** is contraindicated <8-years-of-age, in pregnancy, and lactation (discolors developing tooth enamel). A side effect may be photo-sensitivity

(photophobia). Do not give with antacids, calcium supplements, milk or other dairy, or within two hours of taking another drug.

▷ *penicillin V potassium* (B)(G) 500 mg PO qid x 3 days
Pediatric: 15-50 mg/kg/day in 3-6 divided doses x 3 days; ≥12 years: same as adult; *see page 572 for dose by weight*
  Pen-Vee K *Tab:* 250, 500 mg; *Oral soln:* 125 mg/5 ml (100, 200 ml); 250 mg/5 ml (100, 150, 200 ml)

 BITE: DOG

TETANUS PROPHYLAXIS

▷ *tetanus toxoid* vaccine (C) 0.5 ml IM x 1 dose if previously immunized
Vial: 5 Lf units/0.5 ml (0.5, 5 ml)
Prefilled syringe: 5 Lf units/0.5 ml (0.5 ml)
see Tetanus page 398 for patients not previously immunized

ANTI-INFECTIVES

▷ *amoxicillin/clavulanate* (B)(G) 500 mg tid <u>or</u> 875 mg bid x 10 days
  Augmentin *Tab:* 250, 500, 875 mg; *Chew tab:* 125, 250 mg (lemon-lime); 200, 400 mg (cherry-banana) (phenylalanine); *Oral susp:* 125 mg/5 ml (banana); 250 mg/5 ml (75, 100, 150 ml) (orange); 200, 400 mg/5 ml (50, 75, 100 ml) (orange) (phenylalanine)
    Pediatric: 40-45 mg/kg/day divided tid x 10 days <u>or</u> 90 mg/kg/day divided bid x 10 days *see page 545 for dose by weight*
  Augmentin ES-600 *Oral susp:* 600 mg/5 ml (50, 75, 100, 125, 150, 200 ml) (strawberry cream) (phenylalanine) every 12 hours
    Pediatric: <3 months: not recommended; ≥3 months, <40 kg: 90 mg/kg/day in 2 divided doses; ≥40 kg: not recommended
  Augmentin XR 2 tabs q 12 hours x 7-10 days
    Pediatric: <16 years: use other forms; ≥16 years: same as adult
    Tab: 1000*mg ext-rel

▷ *clindamycin* (B) (administer with fluoroquinolone in adult and TMP-SMX in children) 300 mg qid x 10 days
Pediatric: 8-16 mg/kg/day in 3-4 divided doses x 10 days; *see page 559 for dose by weight*
  Cleocin (G) *Cap:* 75 (tartrazine), 150 (tartrazine), 300 mg
  Cleocin Pediatric Granules (G) *Oral susp:* 75 mg/5 ml (100 ml)(cherry)

▷ *doxycycline* (D)(G) 100 mg bid
Pediatric: <8 years: not recommended ≥8 years, <100 lb: 2 mg/lb on first day in 2 divided doses, followed by 1 mg/lb/day in 1-2 divided doses; ≥8 years, ≥100 lb: same as adult; *see page 561 for dose by weight*
  Actilate *Tab:* 75, 150**mg
  Adoxa *Tab:* 50, 75, 100, 150 mg ent-coat
  Doryx *Tab:* 75, 100, 150 mg del-rel
  Monodox *Cap:* 50, 75, 100 mg
  Oracea *Cap:* 40 mg del-rel
  Vibramycin *Cap:* 50, 100 mg; *Syr:* 50 mg/5 ml (raspberry; sulfites); *Oral susp:* 25 mg/5 ml (raspberry-apple)
  Vibra-Tab *Tab:* 100 mg film-coat

Comment: *doxycycline* is contraindicated <8 years-of-age, in pregnancy, and lactation (discolors developing tooth enamel). A side effect may be photo-sensitivity (photophobia). Do not give with antacids, calcium supplements, milk or other dairy, or within two hours of taking another drug.

▷ *penicillin V potassium* (B)(G) 500 mg PO qid x 3 days
  Pediatric: 50 mg/kg/day in 4 divided doses x 3 days; ≥12 years: same as adult; *see page* 572 *for dose by weight*
  Pen-Vee K *Tab:* 250, 500 mg; *Oral soln:* 125 mg/5 ml (100, 200 ml); 250 mg/5 ml (100, 150, 200 ml)

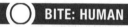

BITE: HUMAN

TETANUS PROPHYLAXIS

▷ *tetanus toxoid* vaccine (C) 0.5 ml IM x 1 dose if previously immunized
  Vial: 5 Lf units/0.5 ml (0.5, 5 ml)
  Prefilled syringe: 5 Lf units/0.5 ml (0.5 ml)
  see **Tetanus** *page* 398 for patients not previously immunized

ANTI-INFECTIVES

▷ *amoxicillin/clavulanate* (B)(G) 500 mg tid or 875 mg bid x 10 days
  Augmentin *Tab:* 250, 500, 875 mg; *Chew tab:* 125, 250 mg (lemon-lime); 200, 400 mg (cherry-banana) (phenylalanine); *Oral susp:* 125 mg/5 ml (banana), 250 mg/5 ml (75, 100, 150 ml) (orange); 200, 400 mg/5 ml (50, 75, 100 ml) (orange) (phenylalanine)
    Pediatric: 40-45 mg/kg/day divided tid x 10 days or 90 mg/kg/day divided bid x 10 days *see page* 545 *for dose by weight*
  Augmentin ES-600 *Oral susp:* 600 mg/5 ml (50, 75, 100, 125, 150, 200 ml) (strawberry cream) (phenylalanine) every 12 hours
    Pediatric: <3 months: not recommended; ≥3 months, <40 kg: 90 mg/kg/day in 2 divided doses; ≥40 kg: not recommended
  Augmentin XR 2 tabs q 12 hours x 7-10 days
    Pediatric: <16 years: use other forms; ≥16 years: same as adult
    Tab: 1000*mg ext-rel
▷ *cefoxitin* (B) 80-160 mg/kg/day IM in 3-4 divided doses x 10 days; max 12 g/day
  Pediatric: <3 months: not recommended; ≥3 months: same as adult
  Mefoxin Injectable *Vial:* 1, 2 g
▷ *ciprofloxacin* (C) 500 mg bid x 10 days
  Pediatric: <18 years: not recommended
  Cipro (G) *Tab:* 250, 500, 750 mg; *Oral susp:* 250, 500 mg/5 ml (100 ml) (strawberry)
  Cipro XR *Tab:* 500, 1000 mg ext-rel
  ProQuin XR *Tab:* 500 mg ext-rel
  Comment: *ciprofloxacin* is contraindicated <18 years-of-age, and during pregnancy and lactation. Risk of tendonitis or tendon rupture, especially 60 years-of-age and older.
▷ *erythromycin base* (B)(G) 250 mg qid x 10 days
  Pediatric: <45 kg: 30-40 mg/kg/day in 4 divided doses x 10 days; ≥45 kg: same as adult

Ery-Tab *Tab:* 250, 333, 500 mg ent-coat
PCE *Tab:* 333, 500 mg

Comment: *erythromycin* may increase INR with concomitant **warfarin**, as well as increase serum level of **digoxin**, benzodiazepines and statins.

▷ *erythromycin ethylsuccinate* (B)(G) 400 mg qid x 10 days
Pediatric: 30-50 mg/kg/day in 4 divided doses x 10 days; may double dose with severe infection; max 100 mg/kg/day; *see page 563 for dose by weight*

EryPed *Oral susp:* 200 mg/5 ml (100, 200 ml) (fruit); 400 mg/5 ml (60, 100, 200 ml) (banana); *Oral drops:* 200, 400 mg/5 ml (50 ml) (fruit); *Chew tab:* 200 mg wafer (fruit)
E.E.S. *Oral susp:* 200 mg/5 ml (100 ml) (fruit)
E.E.S. Granules *Oral susp:* 200 mg/5 ml (100, 200 ml) (cherry)
E.E.S. 400 Tablets *Tab:* 400 mg

Comment: *erythromycin* may increase INR with concomitant **warfarin**, as well as increase serum level of **digoxin**, benzodiazepines and statins.

▷ *trimethoprim/sulfamethoxazole* (D)(G) bid x 10 days
Pediatric: <2 months: not recommended; ≥2 months: 40 mg/kg/day of **sulfamethoxazole** in 2 divided doses bid x 10 days; *see page 576 for dose by weight*

Bactrim, Septra 2 tabs bid x 10 days
Tab: trim 80 mg/*sulfa* 400 mg*
Bactrim DS, Septra DS 1 tab bid x 10 days
Tab: trim 160 mg/*sulfa* 800 mg*
Bactrim Pediatric Suspension, Septra Pediatric Suspension
Oral susp: trim 40 mg/*sulfa* 200 mg per 5 ml (100 ml) (cherry) (alcohol 0.3%)

Comment: *trimethoprim/sulfamethoxazole* is not recommended in pregnancy or lactation. *CrCl 15-30 mL/min:* reduce dose by 1/2; *CrCl <15 mL/min:* not recommended

◯ BLEPHARITIS

OPHTHALMIC AGENTS

▷ *erythromycin* ophthalmic ointment (B) apply 1/2 inch bid-qid x 14 days; then q HS x 10 days
Pediatric: same as adult
Ilotycin *Oint:* 5 mg/g (1/2 oz)

▷ *polymyxin/bacitracin* ophthalmic ointment (C) apply 1/2 inch bid-qid x 14 days; then q HS
Pediatric: same as adult
Polysporin *Oint:* poly B 10,000 U/*baci* 500 U (3.75 g)

▷ *polymyxin B/bacitracin/neomycin* ophthalmic ointment (C) apply 1/2 inch bid-qid x 14 days; then q HS
Pediatric: same as adult
Neosporin *Oint:* poly B 10,000 U/*baci* 400 U/*neo* 3.5 mg/g (3.75 g)

▷ *sodium sulfacetamide* (C)
Bleph-10 Ophthalmic Solution 2 drops q 4 hours x 7-14 days
Pediatric: <2 years: not recommended; ≥2 years: 1-2 drops q 2-3 hours during the day x 7-14 days
Ophth soln: 10% (2.5, 5, 15 ml) (benzalkonium chloride)
Bleph-10 Ophthalmic Ointment apply 1/2 inch qid and HS x 7-14 days
Pediatric: <2 years: not recommended; >2 years: same as adult

Ophth oint: 10% (3.5 g) (phenylmercuric acetate)

SYSTEMIC AGENTS

▷ *tetracycline* (D)(G) 250 mg qid x 7 days
Pediatric: <8 years: not recommended; ≥8 years, <100 lb: 25-50 mg/kg/day in
2-4 divided doses x 7-10 days; ≥100 lb: same as adult; *see page 574 for dose by
weight*

  Achromycin V *Cap:* 250, 500 mg
  Sumycin *Tab:* 250, 500 mg; *Cap:* 250, 500 mg; *Oral susp:* 125 mg/5 ml (100,
  200 ml) (fruit) (sulfites)
Comment: *tetracycline* is contraindicated <8 years-of-age, in pregnancy, and
lactation (discolors developing tooth enamel). A side effect may be photo-
sensitivity (photophobia). Do not give with antacids, calcium supplements, milk or
other dairy, or within two hours of taking another drug.

◯ BREAST CANCER: PROPHYLAXIS

ANTI-ESTROGEN AGENTS

▷ *fulvestrant* (D) 250 mg IM once monthly; administer 2.5 ml IM in each buttock concurrently
  Faslodex *Prefilled syringe:* 50 mg/ml (2 x 2.5 ml, 1 x 5 ml)
▷ *letrozole* (D)(G) 2.5 mg daily
  Femara *Tab:* 2.5 mg film-coat
Comment: *letrozole* is indicated for the extended adjuvant treatment of early breast
cancer in postmenopausal women, who have received 5 years of adjuvant *tamoxifen*
therapy.
▷ *tamoxifen citrate* (D)(G) 20 mg once daily x 5 years
  Tab: 10, 20 mg
Comment: Cautious use of *tamoxifen* with concomitant *coumarin*-type
anticoagulation therapy, history of DVT, <u>or</u> history of pulmonary embolus.

◯ BRONCHIOLITIS

Inhaled Beta₂-Agonists (Bronchodilators) *see Asthma page* 29
Oral Beta₂-Agonists (Bronchodilators) *see Asthma page* 35
Inhaled Corticosteroids *see Asthma page* 29
Parenteral Corticosteroids *see page* 499
Oral Corticosteroids *see page* 497

◯ BRONCHITIS: ACUTE
ACUTE EXACERBATION OF CHRONIC
BRONCHITIS (AECB)

Comment: Antibiotics are seldom needed for treatment of acute bronchitis because the
etiology is usually viral.

Inhaled Beta₂-Agonists (Bronchodilators) *see Asthma page 29*
Oral Beta₂-Agonists (Bronchodilators) *see Asthma page 35*
Decongestants *see page 524*
Expectorants *see page 524*
Antitussives *see page 524*

ANTI-INFECTIVES FOR SECONDARY BACTERIAL INFECTION

▷ *amoxicillin* (B)(G) 500-875 mg bid or 250-500 mg tid x 10 days
  Pediatric: <40 kg (88 lb): 20-40 mg/kg/day in 3 divided doses x 10 days or 25-45 mg/kg/day in 2 divided doses x 10 days; ≥40 kg: same as adult; *see page 543 for dose by weight*
      Amoxil *Cap:* 250, 500 mg; *Tab:* 875*mg; *Chew tab:* 125, 200, 250, 400 mg (cherry-banana-peppermint) (phenylalanine); *Oral susp:* 125, 250 mg/5 ml (80, 100, 150 ml) (strawberry); 200, 400 mg/5 ml (50, 75, 100 ml) (bubble gum); *Oral drops:* 50 mg/ml (30 ml) (bubble gum)
      Moxatag *Tab:* 775 mg ext-rel
      Trimox *Tab:* 125, 250 mg; *Cap:* 250, 500 mg; *Oral susp:* 125, 250 mg/5 ml (80, 100, 150 ml) (raspberry-strawberry)
▷ *amoxicillin/clavulanate* (B)(G) 500 mg tid or 875 mg bid x 10 days
      Augmentin *Tab:* 250, 500, 875 mg; *Chew tab:* 125, 250 mg (lemon-lime); 200, 400 mg (cherry-banana) (phenylalanine); *Oral susp:* 125 mg/5 ml (banana), 250 mg/5 ml (75, 100, 150 ml) (orange); 200, 400 mg/5 ml (50, 75, 100 ml) (orange) (phenylalanine)
          Pediatric: 40-45 mg/kg/day divided tid x 10 days or 90 mg/kg/day divided bid x 10 days *see page 545 for dose by weight*
      Augmentin ES-600 *Oral susp:* 600 mg/5 ml (50, 75, 100, 125, 150, 200 ml) (strawberry cream) (phenylalanine) every 12 hours
          Pediatric: <3 months: not recommended; ≥3 months, <40 kg: 90 mg/kg/day in 2 divided doses; ≥40 kg: not recommended
      Augmentin XR 2 tabs q 12 hours x 7-10 days
          Pediatric: <16 years: use other forms; ≥16 years: same as adult
          Tab: 1000*mg ext-rel
▷ *ampicillin* (B) 250-500 mg qid x 10 days
  Pediatric: not recommended for bronchitis in children
      Omnipen, Principen *Cap:* 250, 500 mg; *Oral susp:* 125, 250 mg/5 ml (100, 150, 200 ml) (fruit)
▷ *azithromycin* (B) 500 mg x 1 dose on day 1, then 250 mg daily on days 2-5 or 500 mg once daily x 3 days or 2 g in a single dose
  Pediatric: not recommended for bronchitis in children
      Zithromax *Tab:* 250, 500, 600 mg; *Oral susp:* 100 mg/5 ml (15 ml); 200 mg/5 ml (15, 22.5, 30 ml) (cherry); *Pkt:* 1 g for reconstitution (cherry-banana)
      Zithromax Tri-pak *Tab:* 3 x 500 mg tabs/pck
      Zithromax Z-pak *Tab:* 6 x 250 mg tabs/pck
      Zmax *Oral susp:* 2 g ext-rel for reconstitution (cherry-banana) (148 mg Na⁺)
▷ *cefaclor* (B)(G) 250-500 mg q 8 hours x 10 days; max 2 g/day
      Tab: 500 mg; *Cap:* 250, 500 mg; *Susp:* 125 mg/5 ml (75, 150 ml) (strawberry); 187 mg/5 ml (50, 100 ml) (strawberry); 250 mg/5 ml (75, 150 ml) (strawberry); 375 mg/5 ml (50, 100 ml) (strawberry)
      Pediatric: <16 years: ext-rel not recommended; ≥16 years: same as adult
      Cefaclor Extended Release *Tab:* 375, 500 mg ext-rel

▷ *cefadroxil* (B) 1-2 g in 1-2 divided doses x 10 days
  Pediatric: 30 mg/kg/day in 2 divided doses x 10 days; *see page 550 for dose by weight*
    Duricef *Tab:* 1 g; *Cap:* 500 mg; *Oral susp:* 250 mg/5 ml (100 ml); 500 mg/5 ml (75, 100 ml) (orange-pineapple)

▷ *cefdinir* (B) 300 mg bid x 5-10 days or 600 mg daily x 10 days
  Pediatric: <6 months: not recommended; 6 months-12 years: 14 mg/kg/day in 1-2 divided doses x 10 days; ≥12 years: same as adult; *see page 551 for dose by weight*
    Omnicef *Cap:* 300 mg; *Oral susp:* 125 mg/5 ml (60, 100 ml) (strawberry)

▷ *cefditoren pivoxil* (B) 400 mg bid x 10 days
  Pediatric: not recommended
    Spectracef *Tab:* 200 mg
    Comment: Spectracef is contraindicated with milk protein allergy or carnitine deficiency.

▷ *cefixime* (B)(G)
  Pediatric: <6 months: not recommended; ≥6 months-12 years, <50 kg: 8 mg/kg/day in 1-2 divided doses x 10 days; ≥12 years, >50 kg: same as adult; *see page 552 for dose by weight*
    Suprax *Tab:* 400 mg; *Cap:* 400 mg; *Oral susp:* 100, 200 mg/5 ml (50, 75, 100 ml) (strawberry)

▷ *cefpodoxime proxetil* (B) 200 mg bid x 10 days
  Pediatric: <2 months: not recommended; ≥2 months-12 years: 10 mg/kg/day (max 400 mg/dose) or 5 mg/kg/day bid (max 200 mg/dose) x 10 days; >12 years: same as adult; *see page 553 for dose by weight*
    Vantin *Tab:* 100, 200 mg; *Oral susp:* 50, 100 mg/5 ml (50, 75, 100 mg) (lemon creme)

▷ *cefprozil* (B) 500 mg q 12 hours x 10 days
  Pediatric: <2 years: not recommended; 2-12 years: 15 mg/kg q 12 hours x 10 days; >12 years: same as adult; *see page 554 for dose by weight*
    Cefzil *Tab:* 250, 500 mg; *Oral susp:* 125, 250 mg/5 ml (50, 75, 100 ml) (bubble gum) (phenylalanine)

▷ *ceftibuten* (B) 400 mg daily x 10 days
  Pediatric: 9 mg/kg daily x 10 days; max 400 mg/day; *see page 555 for dose by weight*
    Cedax *Cap:* 400 mg; *Oral susp:* 90 mg/5 ml (30, 60, 90, 120 ml); 180 mg/5 ml (30, 60, 120 ml) (cherry)

▷ *ceftriaxone* (B)(G) 1-2 g IM daily continued 2 days after signs of infection have disappeared; max 4 g/day
  Pediatric: 50 mg/kg IM daily and continued 2 days after clinical stability
    Rocephin *Vial:* 250, 500 mg; 1, 2 g

▷ *cefuroxime axetil* (B)(G) 250-500 mg bid x 10 days
  Pediatric: 15 mg/kg bid x 10 days; ≥12 years: same as adult; *see page 556 for dose by weight*
    Ceftin *Tab:* 250, 500 mg; *Oral susp:* 125, 250 mg/5 ml (50, 100 ml) (tutti-frutti)

▷ *cephalexin* (B)(G) 250-500 mg qid or 500 mg bid x 10 days
  Pediatric: 25-50 mg/kg/day in 4 divided doses x 10 days; ≥12 years: same as adult; *see page 557 for dose by weight*
    Keflex *Cap:* 250, 333, 500, 750 mg; *Oral susp:* 125, 250 mg/5 ml (100, 200 ml) (strawberry)

▶ *clarithromycin* (C)(G) 500 mg or 500 mg ext-rel once daily x 7 days
Pediatric: <6 months: not recommended; ≥6 months: 7.5 mg/kg bid x 7 days; ≥12 years: same as adult; *see page 558 for dose by weight*
    Biaxin *Tab:* 250, 500 mg
    Biaxin Oral Suspension *Oral susp:* 125, 250 mg/5 ml (50, 100 ml) (fruit-punch)
    Biaxin XL *Tab:* 500 mg ext-rel
▶ *dirithromycin* (C)(G) 500 mg daily x 7 days
Pediatric: <12 years: not recommended; ≥12 years: same as adult
    Dynabac *Tab:* 250 mg
▶ *doxycycline* (D)(G) 100 mg bid x 10 days
Pediatric: <8 years: not recommended; ≥8 years, <100 lb: 2 mg/lb on first day in 2 divided doses, followed by 1 mg/lb/day in 1-2 divided doses; ≥8 years, ≥100 lb: same as adult; *see page 561 for dose by weight*
    Actilate *Tab:* 75, 150**mg
    Adoxa *Tab:* 50, 75, 100, 150 mg ent-coat
    Doryx *Tab:* 75, 100, 150 mg del-rel
    Monodox *Cap:* 50, 75, 100 mg
    Oracea *Cap:* 40 mg del-rel
    Vibramycin *Cap:* 50, 100 mg; *Syr:* 50 mg/5 ml (raspberry; sulfites); *Oral susp:* 25 mg/5 ml (raspberry-apple)
    Vibra-Tab *Tab:* 100 mg film-coat
Comment: *doxycycline* is contraindicated <8 years-of-age, in pregnancy, and lactation (discolors developing tooth enamel). A side effect may be photo-sensitivity (photophobia). Do not give with antacids, calcium supplements, milk or other dairy, or within two hours of taking another drug.
▶ *erythromycin ethylsuccinate* (B)(G) 400 mg qid x 7 days
Pediatric: 30-50 mg/kg/day in 4 divided doses x 7 days; may double dose with severe infection; max 100 mg/kg/day; *see page 563 for dose by weight*
    EryPed *Oral susp:* 200 mg/5 ml (100, 200 ml) (fruit); 400 mg/5 ml (60, 100, 200 ml) (banana); *Oral drops:* 200, 400 mg/5 ml (50 ml) (fruit); *Chew tab:* 200 mg wafer (fruit)
    E.E.S. *Oral susp:* 200, 400 mg/5 ml (100 ml) (fruit)
    E.E.S. Granules *Oral susp:* 200 mg/5 ml (100, 200 ml) (cherry)
    E.E.S. 400 Tablets *Tab:* 400 mg
Comment: *erythromycin* may increase INR with concomitant *warfarin*, as well as increase serum level of *digoxin*, benzodiazepines and statins.
▶ *gemifloxacin* (C) 320 mg daily x 5 days
Pediatric: <18 years: not recommended
    Factive *Tab:* 320*mg
Comment: *gemifloxacin* is contraindicated <18 years-of-age, and during pregnancy and lactation. Risk of tendonitis or tendon rupture, especially 60 years-of-age and older.
▶ *levofloxacin* (C) *Uncomplicated:* 500 mg daily x 7 days; *Complicated:* 750 mg daily x 7 days
Pediatric: <18 years: not recommended
    Levaquin *Tab:* 250, 500, 750 mg

Comment: *levofloxacin* is contraindicated <18 years-of-age, and during pregnancy and lactation. Risk of tendonitis or tendon rupture, especially 60 years-of-age and older.

▷ *loracarbef* (B) 200-400 mg bid x 7 days
Pediatric: 30 mg/kg/day in 2 divided doses x 7 days; ≥12 years: same as adult; *see page 570 for dose by weight*
  Lorabid *Pulvule:* 200, 400 mg; *Oral susp:* 100 mg/5 ml (50, 100 ml); 200 mg/5 ml (50, 75, 100 ml) (strawberry bubble gum)

▷ *moxifloxacin* (C)(G) 400 mg daily x 5 days
Pediatric: <18 years: not recommended
  Avelox *Tab:* 400 mg; IV soln: 400 mg/250 ml (latex-free, preservative-free)

Comment: *moxifloxacin* is contraindicated <18 years-of-age and during pregnancy and lactation. Risk of tendonitis or tendon rupture, especially 60 years-of-age and older.

▷ *ofloxacin* (C)(G) 400 mg bid x 10 days
Pediatric: <18 years: not recommended
  Floxin *Tab:* 200, 300, 400 mg

Comment: *ofloxacin* is contraindicated <18 years-of-age and during pregnancy and lactation. Risk of tendonitis or tendon rupture, especially 60 years-of-age and older.

▷ *telithromycin* (C) 2 x 400 mg tabs in a singe dose daily x 5 days
Pediatric: <18 years: not recommended
  Ketek *Tab:* 400 mg

▷ *tetracycline* (D)(G) 250-500 mg qid x 7 days
Pediatric: <8 years: not recommended; ≥8 years, <100 lb: 25-50 mg/kg/day in 2-4 divided doses x 7 days; ≥8 years, ≥100 lb: same as adult; *see page 574 for dose by weight*
  Achromycin V *Cap:* 250, 500 mg
  Sumycin *Tab:* 250, 500 mg; *Cap:* 250, 500 mg; *Oral susp:* 125 mg/5 ml (100, 200 ml) (fruit) (sulfites)

Comment: *tetracycline* is contraindicated <8 years-of-age, in pregnancy, and lactation (discolors developing tooth enamel). A side effect may be photo-sensitivity (photophobia). Do not give with antacids, calcium supplements, milk or other dairy, or within two hours of taking another drug.

▷ *trimethoprim/sulfamethoxazole* (D)(G) bid x 10 days
Pediatric: <2 months: not recommended; ≥2 months: 40 mg/kg/day of *sulfamethoxazole* in 2 divided doses bid x 10 days; ≥12 years: same as adult; *see page 579 for dose by weight*
  Bactrim, Septra 2 tabs bid x 10 days
    Tab: trim 80 mg/*sulfa* 400 mg*
  Bactrim DS, Septra DS 1 tab bid x 10 days
    Tab: trim 160 mg/*sulfa* 800 mg*
  Bactrim Pediatric Suspension, Septra Pediatric Suspension
    Oral susp: trim 40 mg/*sulfa* 200 mg per 5 ml (100 ml) (cherry) (alcohol 0.3%)

Comment: *trimethoprim/sulfamethoxazole* is not recommended in pregnancy or lactation. *CrCl 15-30 mL/min:* reduce dose by 1/2; *CrCl <15 mL/min:* not recommended

BRONCHITIS: CHRONIC CHRONIC OBSTRUCTIVE PULMONARY DISEASE (COPD)

Oral Beta₂-Agonists (Bronchodilators) *see Asthma page* 35
Inhaled Corticosteroids *see Asthma page* 29
Parenteral Corticosteroids *see page* 499
Oral Corticosteroids *see page* 497
Inhaled Beta₂-Agonists (Bronchodilators) *see Asthma page* 29

LONG-ACTING INHALED BETA2-AGONIST (LABA)

▷ *indacaterol* (C) inhale contents of one 75 mcg cap daily
 Pediatric: not established
  Arcapta Neohaler *Neohaler Device/Cap:* 75 mcg pwdr for inhalation (5 blister cards, 6 caps/card)
 Comment: Remove cap from blister cap immediately before use. For oral inhalation with **Neohaler** device only. *indacaterol* is indicated for the long-term maintenance treatment of bronchoconstriction in patients with COPD. Not indicated for treating asthma, for primary treatment of acute symptoms, or for acute deterioration of COPD.

▷ *indacaterol/glycopyrrolate* (C) inhale the contents of one cap twice daily
 Pediatric: not established
  Utibron Neohaler *Neohaler Device/Cap: inda* 27.5 mcg/*glyco* 15.6 mcg pwdr for inhalation (1, 10 blister cards, 6 caps/card)

▷ *olodaterol* (C)
 Pediatric: not established
  Striverdi Respimat 12 mcg q 12 hours
   Inhal soln: 2.5 mcg/cartridge (metered actuation) (40 g, 60 metered actuations) (benzalkonium chloride)

▷ *salmeterol* (C)(G) 1 inhalation q 12 hours
 Serevent Diskus
  Pediatric: <4 years: not recommended; ≥4 years: same as adult
   Diskus (pwdr): 50 mcg/actuation (60 doses/disk)

INHALED ANTICHOLINERGICS

▷ *ipratropium bromide* (B)(G)
 Pediatric: not recommended
  Atrovent 2 inhalations qid; max 12 inhalations/day
   Inhaler: 14 g (200 inh)
  Atrovent Inhalation Solution 500 mcg by nebulizer tid-qid
   Inhal soln: 0.02% (2.5 ml)
 Comment: *ipatropium bromide* is contraindicated with severe hypersensitivity to milk proteins.

▷ *umeclidinium* (C) 1 inhalation once daily at the same time each day
 Pediatric: not established
  Incruse Ellipta *Inhal pwdr:* 62.5 mcg/inhalation (30 doses) (lactose)

Comment: **Incruse Ellipta** is contraindicated with allergy to *atropine* or its derivatives.

INHALED LONG-ACTING ANTI-CHOLINERGICS (LAA) (ANTIMUSCARINICS)

Comment: Inhaled LAAs are for prophylaxis and chronic treatment, only. Not for primary (rescue) treatment of acute attack. Avoid getting powder in eyes. Caution with narrow-angle glaucoma, BPH, bladder neck obstruction, and pregnancy. Contraindicated with allergy to atropine or its derivatives (e.g., *ipratropium*). Avoid other anticholinergic agents.

▷ *aclidinium bromide* (C) 1 inhalation twice daily using inhaler
   Pediatric: not recommended
      Tudorza Pressair *Inhal device:* 400 mcg/actuation (60 doses per inhalation device)

▷ *tiotropium (as bromide monohydrate)* (C) 1 inhalation daily using inhaler; do not swallow caps
   Pediatric: not recommended
      Spiriva HandiHaler *Inhal device:* 18 mcg/cap (5, 30, 90 caps w. inhalation device)

ANTI-CHOLINERGIC/INHALED LONG-ACTING BETA2-AGONIST (LABA)

▷ *ipratropium/albuterol* (C) 1 inhalation qid; max 6 inhalations/day
   Pediatric: not established
      Combivent Respimat *Inhal soln:* ipra 20 mcg/alb 100 mcg per inhalation (4 g, 120 inhal)
      Comment: **Combivent Respimat** is contraindicted with *atropine* allergy.

▷ *tiotropium/olodaterol* (C) 2 inhalations once daily at the same time each day; max 2 inhalations/day
   Pediatric: not established
      Stiolto Respimat *Inhal soln:* tio 2.5 mcg/olo 2.5 mcg per actuation (4 g, 60 inh) (benzalkonium chloride)
      Comment: **Stiolto Respimat** is not for treating asthma, for relief of acute bronchospasm, or acutely deteriorating COPD.

▷ *umeclidinium/vilanterol* (C) 1 inhalation once daily at the same time each day
   Pediatric: not established
      Anoro Ellipta *Inhal soln:* ume 62.5 mcg/vila 25 mcg per inhalation (30 doses)
      Comment: **Anoro Ellipta** is contraindicted with severe hypersensitivity to milk proteins.

CORTICOSTEROID/INHALED LONG-ACTING BETA AGONIST (LABA)

▷ *fluticasone furoate/vilanterol* (C) 1 inhalation 100/25 once daily at the same time each day
   Pediatric: <17 years: not established
      Breo Ellipta 100/25 *Inhal pwdr:* flu 100 mcg/vil 25 mcg dry pwdr per inhalation (30 doses)
      Breo Ellipta 200/25 *Inhal pwdr:* flu 200 mcg/vil 25 mcg dry pwdr per inhalation (30 doses)
      Comment: **Breo Ellipta** is contraindicated with severe hypersensitivity to milk proteins.

METHYLXANTHINES

Comment: Check serum theophylline level just before 5th dose is administered.
Therapeutic theophylline level: 10-20 mcg/ml.

▷ *theophylline* (C)(G)
>
> **Theo-24** initially 300-400 mg once daily at HS; after 3 days, increase to 400-600 mg once daily at HS; max 600 mg/day
>
>> *Pediatric:* <45 kg: initially 12-14 mg/kg/day; max 300 mg/day; increase after 3 days to 16 mg/kg/day to max 400 mg; after 3 more days increase to 30 mg/kg/day to max 600 mg/day; ≥45 kg: same as adult
>>
>> *Cap:* 100, 200, 300, 400 mg ext-rel
>
> **Theo-Dur** initially 150 mg bid; increase to 200 mg bid after 3 days; then increase to 300 mg bid after 3 more days
>
>> *Pediatric:* <6 years: not recommended; ≥6-15 years: initially 12-14 mg/kg/day in 2 divided doses; max 300 mg/day; then increase to 16 mg/kg in 2 divided doses; max 400 mg/day; then to 20 mg/kg/day in 2 divided doses; max 600 mg/day
>>
>> *Tab:* 100, 200, 300 mg ext-rel
>
> **Theolair-SR** *Tab:* 200, 250, 300, 500 mg sust-rel
>
>> *Pediatric:* not recommended
>
> **Uniphyl** 400-600 mg daily with meals
>
>> *Pediatric:* not recommended
>>
>> *Tab:* 400*, 600*mg cont-rel

METHYLXANTHINE/EXPECTORANT COMBINATION

▷ *dyphylline/guaifenesin* (C)
>
> **Lufyllin GG** 1 tab qid <u>or</u> 15-30 ml qid
>
>> *Tab:* dyphy 200 mg/*guaif* 200 mg; *Elix:* dyphy 100 mg/*guaif* 100 mg per 15 ml

SELECTIVE PHOSPHODIESTERASE 4 (PDE4) INHIBITOR

▷ *roflumilast (C)*
>
> *Pediatric:* not recommended
>
>> **Daliresp** 500 mcg once daily
>>
>> *Tab:* 500 mcg
>
> Comment: *roflumilast* is indicated to reduce the risk of COPD exacerbations in severe COPD patients with chronic bronchitis and a history of exacerbations.

⬤ BULIMIA NERVOSA

SELECTIVE SEROTONIN REUPTAKE INHIBITOR (SSRI)

▷ *fluoxetine* (C)(G)
>
> **Prozac** initially 20 mg daily; may increase after 1 week; doses >20 mg/day may be divided into AM and noon doses; usual daily dose 60 mg; max 80 mg/day
>
>> *Pediatric:* <8 years: not recommended; 8-17 years: initially 10-20 mg/day; start lower weight children at 10 mg/day; if starting at 10 mg daily, may increase after 1 week to 20 mg daily
>>
>> *Cap:* 10, 20, 40 mg; *Tab:* 30*, 60*mg; *Oral soln:* 20 mg/5 ml (4 oz) (mint)
>
> **Prozac Weekly** following daily *fluoxetine* therapy at 20 mg/day for 13 weeks, may initiate **Prozac Weekly** 7 days after the last 20 mg *fluoxetine* dose

Pediatric: not recommended
Cap: 90 mg ent-coat del-rel pellets

 BURN: MINOR

▷ *silver sulfadiazine* (C)(G) apply topically to burn 1-2 x daily
Pediatric: not recommended
   Silvadene *Crm:* 1% (20, 50, 85, 400, 1000 g jar; 20 g tube)
   Comment: *silver sulfadiazine* is contradicted in sulfa allergy.

TOPICAL/TRANSDERMAL ANESTHETICS

Comment: *lidocaine* should not be applied to non-intact skin.
▷ *lidocaine* burn gel (B)(G)
Pediatric: not recommended
▷ *lidocaine* cream (B)
Pediatric: not recommended
   LidaMantle *Crm:* 3% (1, 2 oz)
   Lidoderm *Crm:* 3% (85 g)
▷ *lidocaine* lotion (B)
Pediatric: not recommended
   LidaMantle *Lotn:* 3% (177 ml)
▷ *lidocaine* 5% patch (B)(G) apply up to 3 patches at one time for up to 12 hours/24 hour period (12 hours on/12 hours off); patches may be cut into smaller sizes before removal of the release liner; do not re-use
Pediatric: not recommended
   Lidoderm *Patch:* 5% (10x14 cm; 30/carton)
▷ *lidocaine* 2.5%/*prilocaine* 2.5%
   Emla Cream (B) (5, 30 g)

BURSITIS

Acetaminophen for IV Infusion *see Pain page 296*
Oral Prescription NSAIDs *see page 489*
Other Oral Analgesics *see Pain page 298*
Topical/Transdermal NSAIDs *see Pain page 297*
Parenteral Corticosteroids *see page 499*
Oral Corticosteroids *see page 497*
Topical Analgesic and Anesthetic Agents *see page 487*

CANDIDIASIS: ORAL (THRUSH)

ORAL ANTIFUNGALS

▷ *clotrimazole* (C) *Prophylaxis:* 1 troche dissolved in mouth tid; *Treatment:* 1 troche dissolved in mouth 5 times/day x 10-14 days

Pediatric: <3 years: not recommended; ≥3 years: same as adult
> **Mycelex Troches** *Troches:* 10 mg

▶ *fluconazole* (C) 200 mg x 1 dose first day; then 100 mg once daily x 13 days
Pediatric: >2 weeks: 6 mg/kg x 1 day; then 3 mg/kg/day for at least 3 weeks; *see page 566 for dose by weight*
> **Diflucan** *Tab:* 50, 100, 150, 200 mg; *Oral susp:* 10, 40 mg/ml (35 ml) (orange)

▶ *gentian violet* (NR)(G) apply to oral mucosa with a cotton swab tid x 3 days

▶ *itraconazole* (C) 200 mg daily x 7-14 days
Pediatric: 5 mg/kg daily x 7-14 days; max 200 mg/day; *see page 569 for dose by weight*
> **Sporanox** *Oral soln:* 10 mg/ml (150 ml) (cherry-caramel)

▶ *miconazole* (C) One buccal tab once daily x 14 days; apply to upper gum region; hold in place 30 seconds; do not crush, chew, or swallow
Pediatric: <16 years: not recommended; ≥16 years: same as adult
> **Oravig** *Buccal tab:* 50 mg (14/pck)

▶ *nystatin* (C)(G)
> **Mycostatin** 1-2 pastilles dissolved slowly in mouth 4-5 times/day x 10-14 days; max 14 days
> *Pediatric:* same as adult
> *Pastille:* 200,000 units/pastille (30 pastilles/pck)
> **Mycostatin Suspension** 4-6 ml qid swish and swallow
> *Pediatric: Infants:* 1 ml in each cheek qid after feedings; *Older children:* same as adult
> *Oral susp:* 100,000 units/ml (60 ml w. dropper)

INVASIVE INFECTION

▶ *posaconazole* (D) take with food; 100 mg bid on day one; then 100 mg once daily x 13 days; refractory, 400 mg bid
Pediatric: <13 years: not recommended; ≥13 years: same as adult
> **Noxafil** *Oral susp:* 40 mg/ml (105 ml) (cherry)
> **Comment:** **Noxafil** is indicated as prophylaxis for invasive aspergillus and candida infections in patients >13-years-old who are at high risk due to being severely compromised.

CANDIDIASIS: SKIN

TOPICAL ANTIFUNGALS

▶ *butenafine* (B) apply bid x 1 week or once daily x 4 weeks
Pediatric: <12 years: not recommended; ≥12 years: same as adult
> **Lotrimin Ultra** (C)(OTC) *Crm:* 1% (12, 24 g)
> **Mentax** *Crm:* 1% (15, 30 g)
Comment: *butenafine* is a benzylamine, not an azole. Fungicidal activity continues for at least 5 weeks after the last application.

▶ *ciclopirox* (B)
> **Loprox Cream** apply bid; max 4 weeks
> *Pediatric:* <10 years: not recommended; ≥10 years: same as adult
> *Crm:* 0.77% (15, 30, 90 g)

> Loprox Lotion apply bid; max 4 weeks
>> *Pediatric:* <10 years: not recommended; ≥10 years: same as adult
>> *Lotn:* 0.77% (30, 60 ml)
> Loprox Gel apply bid; max 4 weeks
>> *Pediatric:* <16 years: not recommended; ≥16 years: same as adult
>> *Gel:* 0.77% (30, 45 g)
▷ *clotrimazole* (B) apply bid x 7 days
  Pediatric: same as adult
  Lotrimin *Crm:* 1% (15, 30, 45 g)
  Lotrimin AF (OTC) *Crm:* 1% (12 g); *Lotn:* 1% (10 ml); *Soln:* 1% (10 ml)
▷ *econazole* (C) apply bid x 14 days
  Spectazole *Crm:* 1% (15, 30, 85 g)
▷ *ketoconazole* (C) apply once daily x 14 days
  Nizoral Cream *Crm:* 2% (15, 30, 60 g)
▷ *miconazole* 2% (C) apply once daily x 2 weeks
  Pediatric: same as adult
  Lotrimin AF Spray Liquid (OTC) *Spray liq:* 2% (113 g) (alcohol 17%)
  Lotrimin AF Spray Powder (OTC) *Spray pwdr:* 2% (90 g) (alcohol 10%)
  Monistat-Derm *Crm:* 2% (1, 3 oz); *Spray liq:* 2% (3.5 oz); *Spray pwdr:* 2% (3 oz)
▷ *nystatin* (C)
  Nystop Powder dust affected skin freely bid-tid
  Pwdr: nystatin 100,000 U/g (15 g)

ORAL ANTIFUNGALS

▷ *amphotericin b* (B) apply tid-qid x 7-14 days
  Fungizone *Oral susp:* 100 mg/ml (24 ml w. dropper)
▷ *ketoconazole* (C) 400 mg once daily x 1-2 weeks
  Pediatric: <2 years: not recommended; ≥2 years: 3.3-6.6 mg/kg once daily
  Nizoral *Tab:* 200 mg

INVASIVE INFECTION

▷ *posaconazole* (D) take with food; 100 mg bid on day one; then 100 mg once daily x 13 days; refractory, 400 mg bid x 13 days
  Pediatric: <13 years: not recommended; ≥13 years: same as adult
  Noxafil *Oral susp:* 40 mg/ml (105 ml) (cherry)
  Comment: Noxafil is indicated as prophylaxis for invasive aspergillus and candida infections in patients >13 years old who are at high risk due to being severely compromised.

⬤ CANDIDIASIS: VULVOVAGINAL (MONILIASIS)

PROPHYLAXIS

▷ *acetic acid/oxyquinolone* (C) one full applicator intravaginally bid for up to 30 days
  Pediatric: not recommended
  Relagard *Gel:* acetic acid 0.9%/*oxyquin* 0.025% (50 g tube w. applicator)

Comment: The following treatment regimens for vulvovaginal candidiasis (VVC) are published in the **2015 CDC Sexually Transmitted Diseases Treatment Guidelines**. Treatment regimens are presented by generic drug name first, followed by information about brands and dose forms. Complicated VVC (recurrent, severe, non-albicans, or women with uncontrolled diabetes, debilitation, or immunosuppression) may require more intensive treatment and/or longer duration of treatment. VVC frequently occurs during pregnancy. Only topical azole therapies, applied for 7 days, are recommended during pregnancy.

ORAL Rx AGENT

▷ *fluconazole* 150 mg in a single dose; complicated VVC, 150 mg x 3 doses on days 1, 4, 7 or weekly x 6 months

Rx INTRAVAGINAL AGENTS

Regimen 1

▷ *butoconazole* 2% cream (bioadhesive product) 5 g intravaginally in a single dose

Regimen 2

▷ *nystatin* 100,000-unit vaginal tablet once daily x 14 days

Regimen 3

▷ *terconazole* 0.4% cream 5 g intravaginally once daily x 7 days

Regimen 4

▷ *terconazole* 0.8% cream 5 g intravaginally once daily x 3 days

Regimen 5

▷ *terconazole* 80 mg vaginal suppository intravaginally once daily x 3 days

OTC INTRAVAGINAL AGENTS

Regimen 1

▷ *butoconazole* 2% cream 5 g intravaginally once daily x 3 days

Regimen 2

▷ *clotrimazole* 1% cream intravaginally once daily x 7-14 days

Regimen 3

▷ *clotrimazole* 2% cream intravaginally once daily x 3 days

Regimen 4

▷ *miconazole* 2% cream intravaginally once daily x 7 days

Regimen 5

▷ *miconazole* 4% cream intravaginally once daily x 3 days

Regimen 6

▷ *miconazole* 100 mg vaginal suppository intravaginally once daily x 7 days

Regimen 7

▷ *miconazole* 200 mg vaginal suppository intravaginally once daily x 3 days

Regimen 8

▷ *miconazole* 1,200 mg vaginal suppository intravaginally in a single application

Regimen 9

▷ *tioconazole* 6.5% ointment 5 g intravaginally in a single application

DRUG BRANDS AND DOSE FORMS

▷ *butoconazole* cream 2% (C)
   Gynazole-12% Vaginal Cream *Prefilled vag applicator:* 5 g
   Femstat-3 Vaginal Cream (OTC) *Vag crm:* 2% (20 g w. 3 applicators); *Prefilled vag applicator:* 5 g (3/pck)
▷ *clotrimazole* (B)(OTC)
   Gyne-Lotrimin Vaginal Cream (OTC) *Vag crm:* 1% (45 g w. applicator)
   Gyne-Lotrimin Vaginal Suppository (OTC) *Vag supp:* 100 mg (7/pck)
   Gyne-Lotrimin 3 Vaginal Suppository (OTC) *Vag supp:* 200 mg (3/pck)
   Gyne-Lotrimin Combination Pack (OTC) *Combination pck:* 7-100 mg supp with 7 g 1% cream
   Gyne-Lotrimin 3 Combination Pack (OTC) *Combination pck:* 200 mg supp (7/pck) plus 1% cream (7 g)
   Mycelex-G Vaginal Cream *Vag crm:* 1% (45, 90 g w. applicator)
   Mycelex-G Vaginal Tab 1 *Tab:* 500 mg (1/pck)
   Mycelex Twin Pack *Twin pck:* 500 mg tab (7/pck) with 1% crm (7 g)
   Mycelex-7 Vaginal Cream (OTC) *Vag crm:* 1% (45 g w. applicator)
   Mycelex-7 Vaginal Inserts (OTC) *Vag insert:* 100 mg insert (7/pck)
   Mycelex-7 Combination Pack (OTC) *Combination pck:* 100 mg inserts (7/pck) plus 1% crm (7 g)
▷ *fluconazole* (C)
   Diflucan *Tab:* 50, 100, 150, 200 mg; *Oral susp:* 10, 40 mg/ml (35 ml) (orange)
▷ *miconazole* (B)
   Monistat-3 Combination Pack (OTC) *Combination pck:* 200 mg supp (3/pck) plus 2% crm (9 g)
   Monistat-7 Combination Pack (OTC) *Combination pck:* 100 mg supp (7/pck) plus 2% crm (9 g)
   Monistat-7 Vaginal Cream (OTC) *Vag crm:* 2% (45 g w. applicator)
   Monistat-7 Vaginal Suppositories (OTC) *Vag supp:* 100 mg supp (7/pck)
   Monistat-3 Vaginal Suppositories (OTC) *Vag supp:* 200 mg supp (3/pck)
▷ *nystatin* (C)
   Mycostatin *Vag tab:* 100,000 U (1/pck)

▷ *terconazole* (C)
 Terazol-3 Vaginal Cream *Vag crm:* 0.8% (20 g w. applicator)
 Terazol-3 Vaginal Suppositories *Vag supp:* 80 mg supp (3/pck)
 Terazol-7 Vaginal Cream *Vag crm:* 0.4% (45 g w. applicator)
▷ *tioconazole* (C)
 1-Day (OTC) *Vag oint:* 6.5% (prefilled applicator x 1)
 Monistat 1 Vaginal Ointment (OTC) *Vag oint:* 6.5% (prefilled applicator x 1)
 Vagistat-1 Vaginal Ointment (OTC) *Vag oint:* 6.5% (prefilled applicator x 1)

INVASIVE INFECTION

▷ *posaconazole* (D) take with food; 100 mg bid on day 1; then 100 mg once daily x 13
 days; refractory, 400 mg bid
 Pediatric: <13 years: not recommended; ≥13 years: same as adult
 Noxafil *Oral susp:* 40 mg/ml (105 ml) (cherry)
 Comment: **Noxafil** is indicated as prophylaxis for invasive aspergillus and
 candida infections in patients >13-years-old who are at high risk due to being
 severely compromised.

 CARPAL TUNNEL SYNDROME (CTS)

Acetaminophen for IV Infusion *see Pain page 296*
Oral Prescription NSAIDs *see page 489*
Other Oral Analgesics *see Pain page 298*
Topical/Transdermal NSAIDs *see Pain page 297*
Parenteral Corticosteroids *see page 499*
Oral Corticosteroids *see page 497*
Topical Analgesic and Anesthetic Agents *see page 487*

 CAT SCRATCH FEVER (BARTONELLA INFECTION)

Comment: Cat scratch fever is usually self-limited. Treatment should be limited to
severe <u>or</u> debilitating cases.

ANTI-INFECTIVES

▷ *azithromycin* (B)(G) 500 mg x 1 dose on day 1, then 250 mg daily on days 2-5 <u>or</u> 500
 mg daily x 3 days <u>or</u> **Zmax** 2 g in a single dose
 Pediatric: 12 mg/kg/day x 5 days; max 500 mg/day; *see page 548 for dose by weight*
 Zithromax *Tab:* 250, 500, 600 mg; *Oral susp:* 100 mg/5 ml (15 ml); 200 mg/5 ml
 (15, 22.5, 30 ml) (cherry); *Pkt:* 1 g for reconstitution (cherry-banana)
 Zithromax Tri-pak *Tab:* 3 x 500 mg tabs/pck
 Zithromax Z-pak *Tab:* 6 x 250 mg tabs/pck
 Zmax *Oral susp:* 2 g ext-rel for reconstitution (cherry-banana) (148 mg Na⁺)
▷ *doxycycline* (D)(G) 100 mg daily bid
 Pediatric: <8 years: not recommended; >8 years, <100 lb: 2 mg/lb on first day in
 2 divided doses, followed by 1 mg/lb/day in 1-2 divided doses; ≥8 years, >100 lb:
 same as adult; *see page 561 for dose by weight*

Actilate *Tab:* 75, 150**mg
Adoxa *Tab:* 50, 75, 100, 150 mg ent-coat
Doryx *Tab:* 75, 100, 150 mg del-rel
Monodox *Cap:* 50, 75, 100 mg
Oracea *Cap:* 40 mg del-rel
Vibramycin *Cap:* 50, 100 mg; *Syr:* 50 mg/5 ml (raspberry; sulfites); *Oral susp:* 25 mg/5 ml (raspberry-apple)
Vibra-Tab *Tab:* 100 mg film-coat

Comment: *doxycycline* is contraindicated <8 years-of-age, in pregnancy, and lactation (discolors developing tooth enamel). A side effect may be photo-sensitivity (photophobia). Do not give with antacids, calcium supplements, milk or other dairy, or within two hours of taking another drug.

➤ *erythromycin base* **(B)(G)** 500-1000 mg qid x 4 weeks
Pediatric: <45 kg: 30-50 mg in 2-4 divided doses x 4 weeks; ≥45 kg: same as adult
Ery-Tab *Tab:* 250, 333, 500 mg ent-coat
PCE *Tab:* 333, 500 mg

Comment: *erythromycin* may increase INR with concomitant *warfarin*, as well as increase serum level of *digoxin*, benzodiazepines and statins.

➤ *erythromycin ethylsuccinate* **(B)(G)** 400 mg qid x 4 weeks
Pediatric: 30-50 mg/kg/day in 4 divided doses x 4 weeks; may double dose with severe infection; max 100 mg/kg/day; *see page 563 for dose by weight*
EryPed *Oral susp:* 200 mg/5 ml (100, 200 ml) (fruit); 400 mg/5 ml (60, 100, 200 ml) (banana); *Oral drops:* 200, 400 mg/5 ml (50 ml) (fruit); Chew tab: 200 mg wafer (fruit)
E.E.S. *Oral susp:* 200, 400 mg/5 ml (100 ml) (fruit)
E.E.S. Granules *Oral susp:* 200 mg/5 ml (100, 200 ml) (cherry)
E.E.S. 400 Tablets *Tab:* 400 mg

Comment: *erythromycin* may increase INR with concomitant *warfarin*, as well as increase serum level of *digoxin*, benzodiazepines and statins.

➤ *trimethoprim/sulfamethoxazole* **(D)(G)** bid x 10 days
Pediatric: <2 months: not recommended; ≥2 months: 40 mg/kg/day of *sulfamethox-azole* in 2 divided doses bid x 10 days; *see page 576 for dose by weight*
Bactrim, Septra 2 tabs bid x 10 days
Tab: trim 80 mg/*sulfa* 400 mg*
Bactrim DS, Septra DS 1 tab bid x 10 days
Tab: trim 160 mg/*sulfa* 800 mg*
Bactrim Pediatric Suspension, Septra Pediatric Suspension
Oral susp: trim 40 mg/sulfa 200 mg per 5 ml (100 ml) (cherry) (alcohol 0.3%)

Comment: *trimethoprim/sulfamethoxazole* is not recommended in pregnancy or lactation. *CrCl 15-30 mL/min:* reduce dose by 1/2; *CrCl <15 mL/min:* not recommended

 CELLULITIS

Comment: Duration of treatment should be 10-30 days. Obtain culture from site. Consider blood cultures.

ANTI-INFECTIVES

▷ *amoxicillin* (B)(G) 500-875 mg bid or 250-500 mg tid x 10 days
  Pediatric: <40 kg (88 lb): 20-40 mg/kg/day in 3 divided doses x 10 days or 25-45 mg/kg/day in 2 divided doses x 10 days; ≥40 kg: same as adult; *see page 543 for dose by weight*
  Amoxil *Cap:* 250, 500 mg; *Tab:* 875*mg; *Chew tab:* 125, 200, 250, 400 mg (cherry-banana-peppermint) (phenylalanine); *Oral susp:* 125, 250 mg/5 ml (80, 100, 150 ml) (strawberry); 200, 400 mg/5 ml (50, 75, 100 ml) (bubble gum); *Oral drops:* 50 mg/ml (30 ml) (bubble gum)
  Moxatag *Tab:* 775 mg ext-rel
  Trimox *Tab:* 125, 250 mg; *Cap:* 250, 500 mg; *Oral susp:* 125, 250 mg/5 ml (80, 100, 150 ml) (raspberry-strawberry)
▷ *amoxicillin/clavulanate* (B)(G) 500 mg tid or 875 mg bid x 10 days
  Augmentin *Tab:* 250, 500, 875 mg; *Chew tab:* 125, 250 mg (lemon-lime); 200, 400 mg (cherry-banana) (phenylalanine); *Oral susp:* 125 mg/5 ml (banana), 250 mg/5 ml (75, 100, 150 ml) (orange); 200, 400 mg/5 ml (50, 75, 100 ml) (orange) (phenylalanine)
    Pediatric: 40-45 mg/kg/day divided tid x 10 days or 90 mg/kg/day divided bid x 10 days *see page 545 for dose by weight*
  Augmentin ES-600 *Oral susp:* 600 mg/5 ml (50, 75, 100, 125, 150, 200 ml) (strawberry cream) (phenylalanine) every 12 hours
    Pediatric: <3 months: not recommended; ≥3 months, <40 kg: 90 mg/kg/day in 2 divided doses; ≥40 kg: not recommended
  Augmentin XR 2 tabs q 12 hours x 7-10 days
    Pediatric: <16 years: use other forms; ≥16 years: same as adult
    Tab: 1000*mg ext-rel
▷ *azithromycin* (B)(G) 500 mg x 1 dose on day 1, then 250 mg daily on days 2-5 or 500 mg daily x 3 days or **Zmax** 2 g in a single dose
  Pediatric: 12 mg/kg/day x 5 days; max 500 mg/day; *see page 548 for dose by weight*
  Zithromax *Tab:* 250, 500, 600 mg; *Oral susp:* 100 mg/5 ml (15 ml); 200 mg/5 ml (15, 22.5, 30 ml) (cherry); *Pkt:* 1 g for reconstitution (cherry-banana)
  Zithromax Tri-pak *Tab:* 3 x 500 mg tabs/pck
  Zithromax Z-pak *Tab:* 6 x 250 mg tabs/pck
  Zmax *Oral susp:* 2 g ext-rel for reconstitution (cherry-banana) (148 mg Na⁺)
▷ *cefaclor* (B)(G) 250-500 mg q 8 hours x 10 days; max 2 g/day
  Pediatric: <1 month: not recommended; 20-40 mg/kg bid or q 12 hours x 10 days; max 1 g/day; *see page 549 for dose by weight*
  Tab: 500 mg; *Cap:* 250, 500 mg; *Susp:* 125 mg/5 ml (75, 150 ml) (strawberry); 187 mg/5 ml (50, 100 ml) (strawberry); 250 mg/5 ml (75, 150 ml) (strawberry); 375 mg/5 ml (50, 100 ml) (strawberry)
  CefaclorRExtended Release
    Pediatric: <16 years: ext-rel not recommended; ≥16years: same as adult
    Tab: 375, 500 mg ext-rel
▷ *cefpodoxime proxetil* (B) 400 mg bid x 7-14 days
  Pediatric: <2 months: not recommended; ≥2 months-12 years: 10 mg/kg/day (max 400 mg/ dose) or 5 mg/kg/day bid (max 200 mg/dose) x 7-14 days; >12 years: same as adult; *see page 553 for dose by weight*
  Vantin *Tab:* 100, 200 mg; *Oral susp:* 50, 100 mg/5 ml (50, 75, 100 mg) (lemon cream)

▷ *cefprozil* (B) 500 mg q 12 hours x 10 days
  Pediatric: <2 years: not recommended; 2-12 years: 15 mg/kg q 12 hours x 10 days;
  >12 years: same as adult; *see page 554 for dose by weight*
    Cefzil *Tab:* 250, 500 mg; *Oral susp:* 125, 250 mg/5 ml (50, 75, 100 ml) (bubble
    gum) (phenylalanine)
▷ *ceftaroline fosamil* (B) administer 600 mg once every 12 hours, by IV infusion over
  5-60 minutes, x 5-14 days
  Pediatric: <18 years: not established
    Teflaro *Vial:* 400, 600 mg pwdr for reconstitution, single-use (10/carton)
    Comment: **Teflaro** is indicated for the treatment of adults with acute bacterial
    skin and skin structures infection (ABSSSI).
▷ *ceftriaxone* (B)(G) 1-2 g daily x 5-14 days IM; max 4 g daily
  Pediatric: 50-75 mg/kg IM in 1-2 divided doses x 5-14 days; max 2 g/day
    Rocephin *Vial:* 250, 500 mg; 1, 2 g
▷ *cefuroxime axetil* (B)(G) 250-500 mg bid x 10 days
  Pediatric: <3 months: not recommended; ≥3 months: 30 mg/kg/day in 2 divided
  doses x 10 days; *see page 556 for dose by weight*
    Ceftin *Tab:* 250, 500 mg; *Oral susp:* 125, 250 mg/5 ml (50, 100 ml) (tutti-frutti)
▷ *cephalexin* (B)(G) 500 mg bid x 10 days
  Pediatric: 25-50 mg/kg/day in 4 divided doses x 10 days; *see page 557 for dose by
  weight*
    Keflex *Cap:* 250, 333, 500, 750 mg; *Oral susp:* 125, 250 mg/5 ml (100, 200 ml)
    (strawberry)
▷ *clarithromycin* (C)(G) 500 mg q 12 hours <u>or</u> 500 mg ext-rel once daily x 10 days
  Pediatric: <6 months: not recommended; ≥6 months: 7.5 mg/kg bid x 10 days; *see
  page 558 for dose by weight*
    Biaxin *Tab:* 250, 500 mg
    Biaxin Oral Suspension *Oral susp:* 125, 250 mg/5 ml (50, 100 ml) (fruit-punch)
    Biaxin XL *Tab:* 500 mg ext-rel
▷ *dalbavancin* (C) 1000 mg administered once as a single dose via IV infusion over
  30 minutes <u>or</u> initially 1,000 mg once, followed by 500 mg 1 week later; infuse over
  30 minutes; *CrCl <30 mL/min:* not receiving dialysis: initially 750 mg, followed by
  375 mg 1 week later
  Pediatric: <18 years: not established
    Dalvance *Vial:* 500 mg pwdr for reconstitution, single-use (preservative-free)
    Comment: **Dalvance** is indicated for the treatment of adults with acute bacterial
    skin and skin structures infection (ABSSSI) caused by gram positive bacteria.
▷ *dicloxacillin* (B)(G) 500 mg q 6 hours x 10 days
  Pediatric: 12.5-25 mg/kg/day in 4 divided doses x 10 days; *see page 560 for dose by
  weight*
    Dynapen *Cap:* 125, 250, 500 mg; *Oral susp:* 62.5 mg/5 ml (80, 100, 200 ml)
▷ *dirithromycin* (C)(G) 500 mg once daily x 5-7 days
  Pediatric: <12 years: not recommended; ≥12 years: same as adult
    Dynabac *Tab:* 250 mg
▷ *erythromycin base* (B)(G) 250 mg qid <u>or</u> 333 mg tid <u>or</u> 500 mg bid x 7-10 days; then
  taper to lowest effective dose
  Pediatric: <45 kg: 30-50 mg in 2-4 divided doses x 7-10 days; ≥45 kg: same as adult
    Ery-Tab *Tab:* 250, 333, 500 mg ent-coat
    PCE *Tab:* 333, 500 mg

Comment: *erythromycin* may increase INR with concomitant **warfarin**, as well as increase serum level of *digoxin*, benzodiazepines and statins.

▷ *erythromycin ethylsuccinate* (B)(G) 400 mg qid x 7-10 days
Pediatric: 30-50 mg/kg/day in 4 divided doses x 7-10 days; may double dose with severe infection; max 100 mg/kg/day; *see page 563 for dose by weight*
    EryPed *Oral susp:* 200 mg/5 ml (100, 200 ml) (fruit); 400 mg/5 ml (60, 100, 200 ml) (banana); *Oral drops:* 200, 400 mg/5 ml (50 ml) (fruit); *Chew tab:* 200 mg wafer (fruit)
    E.E.S. *Oral susp:* 200, 400 mg/5 ml (100 ml) (fruit)
    E.E.S. Granules *Oral susp:* 200 mg/5 ml (100, 200 ml) (cherry)
    E.E.S. 400 Tablets *Tab:* 400 mg

Comment: *erythromycin* may increase INR with concomitant **warfarin**, as well as increase serum level of *digoxin*, benzodiazepines and statins.

▷ *linezolid* (C)(G) 600 mg q 12 hours x 10-14 days
Pediatric: <5 years: 10 mg/kg q 8 hours x 10-14 days; 5-11 years: 10 mg/kg q 12 hours x 10-14 days; >11years: same as adult
    Zyvox *Tab:* 400, 600 mg; *Oral susp:* 100 mg/5 ml (150 ml) (orange) (phenylalanine)

Comment: *linezolid* is indicated to treat susceptible vancomycin-resistant *E. faecium* infections of skin and skin structures, including diabetic foot without osteomyelitis.

▷ *loracarbef* (B) 200 mg bid x 10 days
Pediatric: 15 mg/kg/day in 2 divided doses x 10 days; *see page 570 for dose by weight*
    Lorabid *Pulvule:* 200, 400 mg; *Oral susp:* 100 mg/5 ml (50, 100 ml); 200 mg/5 ml (50, 75, 100 ml) (strawberry bubble gum)

▷ *moxifloxacin* (C)(G) 400 mg once daily x 5 days
Pediatric: <18 years: recommended
    Avelox *Tab:* 400 mg; *IV soln:* 400 mg/250 mg (latex-free, presservative-free)

Comment: *moxifloxacin* is contraindicated <18 years of age and during pregnancy and lactation. Risk of tendonitis or tendon rupture, especially 60 years-of-age and older.

▷ *oritavancin* (C) administer 1,200 mg as a single dose by IV infusion over 3 hours
Pediatric: <18 years: not established
    Orbactiv *Vial:* 400 mg pwdr for reconstitution, single-use (10/carton) (mannitol; preservative-free)

Comment: **Orbactiv** is indicated for the treatment of adults with acute bacterial skin and skin structures infection (ABSSSI).

▷ *penicillin V potassium* (B) 250-500 mg q 6 hours x 5-7 days
Pediatric: >12 years: same as adult; *see page 572 for dose by weight*
    Pen-Vee K *Tab:* 250, 500 mg; *Oral soln:* 125 mg/5 ml (100, 200 ml); 250 mg/5 ml (100, 150, 200 ml)

▷ *tedizolid phosphate* (C) administer 200 mg once daily x 6 days, via PO <u>or</u> IV infusion over 1 hour
Pediatric: <18 years: not established
    Sivextro *Tab:* 200 mg (6/blister pck)

Comment: **Sivextro** is indicated for the treatment of adults with acute bacterial skin and skin structures infection (ABSSSI).

▷ *tigecycline* (D)(G) 100 mg as a single dose; then 50 mg q 12 hours x 5-14 days; with severe hepatic impairment (Child Pugh C), 100 mg as a single dose; then 25 mg q 12 hours
Pediatric: <18 years: not recommended
    Tygacil *Vial:* 50 mg pwdr for reconstitution and IV infusion (preservative-free)

CERUMEN IMPACTION

OTIC ANALGESIC

▷ *antipyrine/benzocaine/zinc acetate dihydrate* otic (C) fill ear canal with solution; then moisten cotton plug with solution and insert into meatus; may repeat every 1-2 hours prn
Pediatric: same as adult
   Otozin *Otic soln:* antipyr 5.4%/benz 1%/zinc1% per ml (10 ml w. dropper)

CERUMINOLYTICS

▷ *triethanolamine* (NR)(OTC)(G) fill ear canal and insert cotton plug for 15-30 minutes before irrigating with warm water
   Cerumenex *Soln:* 10% (6, 12 ml)
▷ *carbamide peroxide* (NR)(OTC)(G) instill 5-10 drops in ear canal; keep drops in ear several minutes; then irrigate with warm water; repeat bid for up to 4 days
   Debrox *Soln:* 15, 30 ml squeeze bottle w. applicator

OTIC ANALGESIC/ANESTHETIC/ANTIBACTERIAL COMBINATION

▷ *acetic acid/antipyrine/benzocaine/u-policosanol 410* otic (C) fill ear canal with solution; then moisten cotton plug with solution and insert into meatus; may repeat every 1-2 hours prn
Pediatric: same as adult
   Auralgan Otic *Otic soln:* acet acid 0.01%/antipyr 5.4%/benz 1.4%/u-poly 0.01% per ml (14 ml w. dropper)

CHANCROID

ANTI-INFECTIVES

▷ *azithromycin* (B)(G) 500 mg x 1 dose on day 1, then 250 mg daily on days 2-5 or 500 mg daily x 3 days or **Zmax** 2 g in a single dose
Pediatric: 12 mg/kg/day x 5 days; max 500 mg/day; *see page 548 for dose by weight*
   Zithromax *Tab:* 250, 500, 600 mg; *Oral susp:* 100 mg/5 ml (15 ml); 200 mg/5 ml (15, 22.5, 30 ml) (cherry); *Pkt:* 1 g for reconstitution (cherry-banana)
   Zithromax Tri-pak *Tab:* 3 x 500 mg tabs/pck
   Zithromax Z-pak *Tab:* 6 x 250 mg tabs/pck
   Zmax *Oral susp:* 2 g ext-rel for reconstitution (cherry-banana) (148 mg Na$^+$)
▷ *ceftriaxone* (B)(G) 250 mg IM in a single dose
Pediatric: <45 kg: 125 mg IM in a single dose; ≥45 kg: same as adult
   Rocephin *Vial:* 250, 500 mg; 1, 2 g
▷ *ciprofloxacin* (C) 500 mg bid x 3 days
Pediatric: <18 years: not recommended
   Cipro *Tab:* 250, 500, 750 mg; *Oral susp:* 250, 500 mg/5 ml (100 ml) (strawberry)
   Cipro XR *Tab:* 500, 1000 mg ext-rel
   ProQuin XR *Tab:* 500 mg ext-rel

Comment: *ciprofloxacin* is contraindicated <18 years-of-age, and during pregnancy and lactation. Risk of tendonitis or tendon rupture, especially 60 years-of-age and older.

▷ *erythromycin base* (B)(G) 500 mg qid x 7 days
  Pediatric: 30-50 mg/kg/day divided bid-qid; max 100 mg/kg/day
    Ery-Tab *Tab:* 250, 333, 500 mg ent-coat
    PCE *Tab:* 333, 500 mg
  Comment: *erythromycin* may increase INR with concomitant *warfarin*, as well as increase serum level of *digoxin*, benzodiazepines and statins.

▷ *erythromycin ethylsuccinate* (B)(G) 400 mg qid x 7 days
  Pediatric: 30-50 mg/kg/day in 4 divided doses x 7 days; may double dose with severe infection; max 100 mg/kg/day; *see page 563 for dose by weight*
    EryPed *Oral susp:* 200 mg/5 ml (100, 200 ml) (fruit); 400 mg/5 ml (60, 100, 200 ml) (banana); *Oral drops:* 200, 400 mg/5 ml (50 ml) (fruit); *Chew tab:* 200 mg wafer (fruit)
    E.E.S. *Oral susp:* 200, 400 mg/5 ml (100 ml) (fruit)
    E.E.S. Granules *Oral susp:* 200 mg/5 ml (100, 200 ml) (cherry)
    E.E.S. 400 Tablets *Tab:* 400 mg
  Comment: *erythromycin* may increase INR with concomitant *warfarin*, as well as increase serum level of *digoxin*, benzodiazepines and statins.

 CHICKENPOX (VARICELLA)

PROPHYLAXIS

▷ *Varicella virus* vaccine, live, attenuated (C)
    Varivax 0.5 ml SC; repeat 4-8 weeks later
      Pediatric: <12 months: not recommended; 12 months-12 years: 1 dose of 0.5 ml SC; repeat 4-6 weeks later
      Vial: 1350 PFU/0.5 ml single-dose w. diluent (preservative-free)
    Comment: Administer **Varivax** SC in the deltoid for adults and children.

TREATMENT

Antipyretics *see Fever page 143*

ORAL ANTIPRURITICS

▷ *diphenhydramine* (B)(OTC)(G) 25-50 mg q 6-8 hours; max 100 mg/day
  Pediatric: <2 years: not recommended; 2-6 years: 6.25 mg q 4-6 hours; max 37.5 mg/day; >6-12 years: 12.5-25 mg q 4-6 hours; max 150 mg/day; >12 years: same as adult
    Benadryl (OTC) *Chew tab:* 12.5 mg (grape; phenylalanine); *Liq:* 12.5 mg/5 ml (4, 8 oz); *Cap:* 25 mg; *Tab:* 25 mg; *dye-free soft gel:* 25 mg; *Dye-free liq:* 12.5 mg/5 ml (4, 8 oz)

▷ *hydroxyzine* (C)(G) 50-100 mg qid; max 600 mg/day
  Pediatric: <6 years: 50 mg/day divided qid; ≥6 years: 50-100 mg/day divided qid
    AtaraxR *Tab:* 10, 25, 50, 100 mg; *Syr:* 10 mg/5 ml (alcohol 0.5%)
    VistarilR *Cap:* 25, 50, 100 mg; *Oral susp:* 25 mg/5 ml (4 oz) (lemon)

ANTIVIRALS

▷ *acyclovir* (B)(G) 800 mg qid x 5 days
   Pediatric: <2 years: not recommended; ≥2 years, <40 kg: 20 mg/kg qid x 5 days;
   ≥2 years, >40 kg: 800 mg qid x 5 days; *see page 541 for dose by weight*
     Zovirax *Cap:* 200 mg; *Tab:* 400, 800 mg
     Zovirax Oral Suspension *Oral susp:* 200 mg/5 ml (banana)

◯ CHLAMYDIA TRACHOMATIS

Comment: The following treatment regimens for *C. trachomatis* are published in
the **2015 CDC Sexually Transmitted Diseases Treatment Guidelines**. Treatment
regimens are presented by generic drug name first, followed by information about
brands and dose forms. Treat all sexual contacts. Patients who are HIV-positive
should receive the same treatment as those who are HIV-negative. Sexual abuse must
be considered a cause of chlamydial infection in preadolescent children, although
perinatally transmitted *C. trachomatis* infections of the nasopharynx, urogenital tract,
and rectum may persist for >1 year.

RECOMMENDED REGIMENS: ADOLESCENT AND ADULT, NON-PREGNANT
Regimen 1

▷ *azithromycin* 1 g in a single dose

Regimen 2

▷ *doxycycline* 100 mg bid x 7 days

ALTERNATIVE REGIMENS: ADOLESCENT AND ADULT, NON-PREGNANT
Regimen 1

▷ *erythromycin base* 500 mg qid x 7 days

Regimen 2

▷ *erythromycin ethylsuccinate* 800 mg qid x 7 days

Regimen 3

▷ *levofloxacin* 500 mg once daily x 7 days

Regimen 4

▷ *ofloxacin* 300 mg bid x 7 days

RECOMMENDED REGIMENS: PREGNANCY
Regimen 1

▷ *azithromycin* 1 g in a single dose

Regimen 2

▷ *amoxicillin* 500 mg tid x 7 days

ALTERNATE REGIMENS: PREGNANCY
Regimen 1

▷ *erythromycin base* 500 mg qid x 7 days

Regimen 2

▷ *erythromycin base* 250 mg qid x 14 days

Regimen 3

▷ *erythromycin ethylsuccinate* 800 mg qid x 7 days

Regimen 4

▷ *erythromycin ethylsuccinate* 400 mg qid x 14 days

ALTERNATE REGIMENS: CHILDREN (>8 YEARS)
Regimen 1

▷ *azithromycin* 1 g in a single dose

Regimen 2

▷ *doxycycline* 100 mg bid x 7 days

ALTERNATE REGIMEN: CHILDREN (>45 KG; <8 YEARS)
Regimen 1

▷ *azithromycin* 1 g in a single dose

ALTERNATE REGIMENS: INFANTS
Regimen 1

▷ *erythromycin base* 50 mg/kg/day in divided doses qid x 14 days

Regimen 2

▷ *erythromycin ethylsuccinate* 50 mg/kg/day divided qid x 14 days

DRUG BRANDS AND DOSE FORMS

▷ *azithromycin* **(B)(G)** 500 mg x 1 dose on day 1, then 250 mg daily on days 2-5 or 500 mg daily x 3 days or **Zmax** 2 g in a single dose
  Pediatric: 12 mg/kg/day x 5 days; max 500 mg/day; *see page* 548 *for dose by weight*
    Zithromax *Tab:* 250, 500, 600 mg; *Oral susp:* 100 mg/5 ml (15 ml); 200 mg/5 ml (15, 22.5, 30 ml) (cherry); *Pkt:* 1 g for reconstitution (cherry-banana)
    Zithromax Tri-pak *Tab:* 3 x 500 mg tabs/pck

> **Zithromax Z-pak** *Tab:* 6 x 250 mg tabs/pck
> **Zmax** *Oral susp:* 2 g ext-rel for reconstitution (cherry-banana) (148 mg Na$^+$)

▶ *doxycycline* (D)(G)
> **Actilate** *Tab:* 75, 150**mg
> **Adoxa** *Tab:* 50, 75, 100, 150 mg ent-coat
> **Doryx** *Tab:* 75, 100, 150 mg del-rel
> **Monodox** *Cap:* 50, 75, 100 mg
> **Oracea** *Cap:* 40 mg del-rel
> **Vibramycin** *Cap:* 50, 100 mg; *Syr:* 50 mg/5 ml (raspberry; sulfites); *Oral susp:* 25 mg/5 ml (raspberry-apple)
> **Vibra-Tab** *Tab:* 100 mg film-coat

Comment: *doxycycline* is contraindicated <8 years-of-age, in pregnancy, and lactation (discolors developing tooth enamel). A side effect may be photo-sensitivity (photophobia). Do not give with antacids, calcium supplements, milk or other dairy, or within two hours of taking another drug.

▶ *erythromycin base* (B)(G)
> **Ery-Tab** *Tab:* 250, 333, 500 mg ent-coat
> **PCE** *Tab:* 333, 500 mg

Comment: *erythromycin* may increase INR with concomitant *warfarin*, as well as increase serum level of *digoxin*, benzodiazepines and statins.

▶ *erythromycin ethylsuccinate* (B)(G)
> **EryPed** *Oral susp:* 200 mg/5 ml (100, 200 ml) (fruit); 400 mg/5 ml (60, 100, 200 ml) (banana); *Oral drops:* 200, 400 mg/5 ml (50 ml) (fruit); *Chew tab:* 200 mg wafer (fruit)
> **E.E.S.** *Oral susp:* 200, 400 mg/5 ml (100 ml) (fruit)
> **E.E.S. Granules** *Oral susp:* 200 mg/5 ml (100, 200 ml) (cherry)
> **E.E.S. 400 Tablets** *Tab:* 400 mg

Comment: *erythromycin* may increase INR with concomitant *warfarin*, as well as increase serum level of *digoxin*, benzodiazepines and statins.

▶ *levofloxacin* (C)
> **Levaquin** *Tab:* 250, 500, 750 mg

Comment: *levofloxacin* is contraindicated <18 years-of-age, and during pregnancy and lactation. Risk of tendonitis or tendon rupture, especially 60 years-of-age and older.

▶ *ofloxacin* (C)(G)
> **Floxin** *Tab:* 200, 300, 400 mg

Comment: *ofloxacin* is contraindicated <18 years-of-age, and during pregnancy and lactation. Risk of tendonitis or tendon rupture, especially 60 years-of-age and older.

⬤ CHOLELITHIASIS

▶ *ursodiol* (B) 8-10 mg/kg/day in 2-3 divided doses
Pediatric: not recommended
> **Actigall** *Cap:* 300 mg
> Comment: **Actigall** is indicated for the dissolution of radiolucent, noncalciferous, gallstones <20 mm in diameter and for prevention of gallstones during rapid weight loss.

◯ CHOLERA (*VIBRIO CHOLERAE*)

Comment: June 10, 2016, the FDA approved the first vaccine for the prevention of cholera caused by serogroup O1 (the most predominant cause of cholera globally [WHO]) in adults age 18-64 years traveling to cholera-affected areas. https://www .drugs.com/newdrugs/fda-approves-vaxchora-cholera-vaccine-live-oral-prevent-cholera-travelers-4396.html. Vaxchora (R) is the only FDA approved vaccine for the prevention of cholera. The bacterium *Vibrio cholerae* is acquired by ingesting contaminated water or food and causes nausea, vomiting, and watery diarrhea that may be mild to severe. Profuse fluid loss may cause life-threatening dehydration if antibiotics and fluid replacement are not initiated promptly.

VACCINE PROPHYLAXIS

▷ *Vibrio cholerae* vaccine

Vaxchora reconstitute the buffer component in 100 ml purified bottled water; then add the active component (lyophilized V. cholerae CVD 103-HgR); total dose after reconstitution is 100 ml; instruct the patient to avoid eating or drink-ing fluids for 60 minutes before and after ingestion of the dose

Comment: Vaxchora is a live, attenuated vaccine that is taken as a single oral dose at least 10 days before travel to a cholera-affected area and at least 10 days before starting antimalarial prophylaxis. Diminished immune response when taken concomitantly with *chloroquine*. Avoid concomitant administration with systemic antibiotics since these agents may be active against the vaccine strain. Do not administer to patients who have received an oral or parental antibiotic within 14 days prior to vaccination. Vaxchora may be shed in the stool of recipients for at least 7 days. There is potential for transmission of the vaccine strain to non-vaccinated and immunocompromised close contacts. The Centers for Disease Control and Prevention and several health professional organizations state that vaccines given to a nursing mother do not affect the safety of breastfeeding for mothers or infants and that breastfeeding is not a contraindication to cholera vaccine. Vaxchora is not absorbed systemically, and maternal use is not expected to result in fetal exposure to the drug. The Vaxchora pregnancy exposure registry for reporting adverse events is 800-533-5899. There are 0 disease interactions, but at least 165 drug-drug interactions with Vaxchora (see mfr literature).

TREATMENT

Comment: The first line treatment for *V. cholerae* is oral rehydration therapy (ORT) and intravenous fluid replacement as indicated. Antibiotic therapy may shorten the duration and severity of symptoms, but is optional in other than severe cases. Although *doxycycline* is contraindicated in pregnancy and in children under 7 years-of-age, the benefits may outweigh the risks (WHO, CDC, UNICEF). Although *ciprofloxacin* is contraindicated in children under 18 years-of-age, the benefits may outweigh the risks (WHO, CDC, UNICEF). Cholera is not transmitted from person to person, but rather the fecal-oral route. Therefore, chemoprophylaxis is not usually required with strict hand hygiene and sanitation measures, and avoidance of contaminated food and water. Drugs and dosages for chemoprophylaxis are the same as for treatment.

ADULTS 15 YEARS AND OLDER, NON-PREGNANT WOMEN
Regimen 1

▷ *doxycycline* (D)(G) 300 mg in a single dose
    Actilate *Tab:* 75, 150**mg
    Adoxa *Tab:* 50, 75, 100, 150 mg ent-coat
    Doryx *Tab:* 75, 100, 150 mg del-rel
    Monodox *Cap:* 50, 75, 100 mg
    Oracea *Cap:* 40 mg del-rel
    Vibramycin *Cap:* 50, 100 mg
    Vibra-Tab *Tab:* 100 mg film-coat

Regimen 2

▷ *azithromycin* (B) 1000 mg in a single dose
    Zithromax *Tab:* 250, 500, 600 mg
    Zmax *Oral susp:* 2 g ext-rel for reconstitution (cherry-banana) (148 mg Na^+)
    or
▷ *ciprofloxacin* (C)(G) 1000 mg in a single dose
    Cipro *Tab:* 250, 500, 750 mg;
    Cipro XR *Tab:* 500, 1000 mg ext-rel
    ProQuin XR *Tab:* 500 mg ext-rel

PREGNANT WOMEN, 15 YEARS AND OLDER

▷ *azithromycin* (B) 1000 mg in a single dose
    Zithromax *Tab:* 250, 500, 600 mg
    Zmax *Oral susp:* 2 g ext-rel for reconstitution (cherry-banana) (148 mg Na^+)
    or
▷ *erythromycin* (B)(G) 500 mg q 6 hours x 3 days
    E.E.S. 400 Tablets *Tab:* 400 mg
    Ery-Tab *Tab:* 250, 333, 500 mg ent-coat
    PCE *Tab:* 333, 500 mg

CHILDREN 3-15 YEARS WHO CAN SWALLOW TABLETS
Regimen 1

▷ *erythromycin* (B)(G) 12.5 mg/kg q 6 hours x 3 days
    E.E.S. 400 Tablets *Tab:* 400 mg
    Ery-Tab *Tab:* 250, 333, 500 mg ent-coat
    PCE *Tab:* 333, 500 mg
    or
▷ *azithromycin* (B) 20 mg/kg in a single dose; max 1 g
    Zithromax *Tab:* 250, 500, 600 mg
    Zmax *Oral susp:* 2 g ext-rel for reconstitution (cherry-banana) (148 mg Na^+)

Regimen 2

▷ *ciprofloxacin* (D)(G) 20 mg/kg in a single dose
    Cipro *Tab:* 250, 500, 750 mg;
    Cipro XR *Tab:* 500, 1000 mg ext-rel

    ProQuin XR *Tab:* 500 mg ext-rel
      or
▷ *doxycycline* (D)(G) 2-4 mg/kg in a single dose
    Actilate *Tab:* 75, 150**mg
    Adoxa *Tab:* 50, 75, 100, 150 mg ent-coat
    Doryx *Tab:* 75, 100, 150 mg del-rel
    Monodox *Cap:* 50, 75, 100 mg
    Oracea *Cap:* 40 mg del-rel
    Vibramycin *Cap:* 50, 100 mg
    Vibra-Tab *Tab:* 100 mg film-coat

CHILDREN UNDER 3 YEARS

Regimen 1

▷ *erythromycin ethylsuccinate* (B)(G) 12.5 mg/kg q 6 hours x 3 days; use suspension
    E.E.S. *Oral susp:* 200, 400 mg/5 ml (100 ml) (fruit)
    E.E.S. Granules *Oral susp:* 200 mg/5 ml (100, 200 ml) (cherry, fruit); *Chew tab:* 200 mg wafer (fruit)
    EryPed *Oral susp:* 200 mg/5 ml (100, 200 ml) (fruit); 400 mg/5 ml (60, 100, 200 ml) (banana); *Oral drops:* 200, 400 mg/5 ml (50 ml) (fruit); *Chew tab:* 200 mg wafer (fruit)
      or
▷ *azithromycin* (B) 20 mg/kg in a single dose; max 1 g; use suspension
    Zithromax *Tab:* 250, 500, 600 mg; *Oral susp:* 100 mg/5 ml (15 ml); 200 mg/5 ml (15, 22.5, 30 ml) (cherry)
    Zmax *Oral susp:* 2 g ext-rel for reconstitution (cherry-banana) (148 mg Na$^+$)

Regimen 2

▷ *ciprofloxacin* (C)(G) 20 mg/kg in a single dose; use suspension
    Cipro *Oral susp:* 250, 500 mg/5 ml (100 ml) (strawberry)
      or
▷ *doxycycline* (D)(G) 2-4 mg/kg in a single dose; use suspension or syrup
    Vibramycin *Syr:* 50 mg/5 ml (raspberry; sulfites); *Oral susp:* 25 mg/5 ml (raspberry-apple)

◯ COLIC: INFANTILE

▷ *hyoscyamine* (C)(G)
    Levsin Drops
      Pediatric: 3-4 kg: 4 drops q 4 hours prn; max 24 drops/day; 5 kg: 5 drops q 4 hours prn; max 30 drops/day; 7 kg: 6 drops q 4 hours prn; max 36 drops/day; 10 kg: 8 drops q 4 hours prn; max 40 drops/day; *Oral drops:* 0.125 mg/ml (15 ml) (orange) (alcohol 5%)
▷ *simethicone* (C) 0.3 ml qid pc and HS
    Mylicon Drops (OTC) *Oral drops:* 40 mg/0.6 ml (30 ml)

COMMON COLD (VIRAL UPPER RESPIRATORY INFECTION [URI])

Oral Drugs for Allergy, Cough, and Cold *see page* 524
Oral Decongestants *see page* 524
Oral Expectorants *see page* 524
Oral Antitussives *see page* 524
Oral Antipyretic-Analgesics *see Fever page* 143

NASAL SALINE DROPS/SPRAYS

Comment: Homemade saline nose drops: 1/4 tsp salt added to 8 oz boiled water, then cool water.
▷ *saline* nasal spray (NR)(G)
Afrin Saline Mist w. Eucalyptol and Menthol (OTC) 2-6 sprays in each nostril prn
Pediatric: 1 month-2 years: 1-2 sprays in each nostril prn; >2-12 years: 1-4 sprays in each nostril prn; >12 years: same as adult
Squeeze bottle: 45 ml
Afrin Moisturizing Saline Mist (OTC) 2-6 sprays in each nostril prn
Pediatric: 1 month-2 years: 1-2 sprays in each nostril prn; 2-12 years: 1-4 sprays in each nostril prn; >12 years: same as adult
Squeeze bottle: 45 ml
Ocean Mist (OTC) 2-6 sprays in each nostril prn
Pediatric: 1 month-2 years: 1-2 sprays in each nostril prn; >2-12 years: 1-4 sprays in each nostril prn; >12 years: same as adult
Squeeze bottle: saline 0.65% (45 ml) (alcohol-free)
Pediamist (OTC) 2-6 sprays in each nostril prn
Pediatric: 1 month-2 years: 1-2 sprays in each nostril prn; >2-12 years: 1-4 sprays in each nostril prn; >12 years: same as adult
Squeeze bottle: saline 0.5% (15 ml) (alcohol-free)

NASAL SYMPATHOMIMETICS

▷ *oxymetazoline* (C)(OTC) 2-3 drops <u>or</u> sprays in each nostril q 10-12 hours prn; max 2 doses/day; max duration 5 days
Pediatric: <6 years: not recommended; ≥6 years: same as adult
4-hour formulation: 2-3 drops <u>or</u> sprays q 4 hours prn; max duration 5 days
Pediatric: not recommended
Afrin 12-Hour Extra Moisturizing Nasal Spray
Afrin 12-Hour Nasal spray Pump Mist
Afrin 12-Hour Original Nasal spray
Afrin 12-Hour Original Nose Drops
Afrin 12-Hour Severe Congestion Nasal Spray
Afrin 12-Hour Sinus Nasal Spray
Nasal spray: 0.05% (45 ml); *Nasal drops:* 0.05% (45 ml)
Afrin 4-Hour Nasal Spray
Neo-Synephrine 12 Hour Nasal Spray
Neo-Synephrine 12 Hour Extra Moisturizing Nasal Spray
Nasal spray: 0.05% (15 ml)

▷ *phenylephrine* (C)
    Afrin Allergy Nasal Spray (OTC) 2-3 sprays in each nostril q 4 hours prn; max
    duration 5 days
        Pediatric: <12 years: not recommended; ≥12 years: same as adult
        Nasal spray: 0.5% (15 ml)
    Afrin Nasal Decongestant Childrens Pump Mist (OTC)
        Pediatric: <6 years: not recommended; ≥6 years: 2-3 sprays in each nostril
        q 4 hours prn; max duration 5 days
        Nasal spray: 0.25% (15 ml)
    Neo-Synephrine Extra Strength (OTC) 2-3 sprays <u>or</u> drops in each nostril
    q 4 hours prn; max duration 5 days
        Pediatric: <12 years: not recommended; ≥12 years: same as adult
        Nasal spray: 0.1% (15 ml); *Nasal drops:* 0.1% (15 ml)
    Neo-Synephrine Mild Formula (OTC) 2-3 sprays <u>or</u> drops in each nostril
    q 4 hours prn; max duration 5 days
        Pediatric: <6 years: not recommended; ≥6 years: same as adult
        Nasal spray: 0.25% (15 ml)
    Neo-Synephrine Regular Strength (OTC) 2-3 sprays <u>or</u> drops in each nostril q 4
    hours prn; max duration 5 days
        Pediatric: <12 years: not recommended; ≥12 years: same as adult
        Nasal spray: 0.5% (15 ml); *Nasal drops:* 0.5% (15 ml)
▷ *tetrahydrozoline* (C)
    Tyzine 2-4 drops <u>or</u> 3-4 sprays in each nostril q 3-8 hours prn; max duration
    5 days
        Pediatric: <6 years: not recommended; ≥6 years: same as adult
        Nasal spray: 0.1% (15 ml); *Nasal drops:* 0.1% (30 ml)
    Tyzine Pediatric Nasal Drops 2-3 sprays <u>or</u> drops in each nostril q 3-6 hours prn
        Nasal drops: 0.05% (15 ml)

CONJUNCTIVITIS: ALLERGIC

Oral Prescription Drugs for the Management of Allergy, Cough, and Cold Symptoms
page 524

OPHTHALMIC CORTICOSTEROIDS

Comment: Concomitant contact lens wear is contraindicated during therapy. Ophthalmic
steroids are contraindicated with ocular, fungal, mycobacterial, viral (except herpes
zoster), and untreated bacterial infection. Ophthalmic steroids may mask <u>or</u> exacerbate
infection, and may increase intraocular pressure, optic nerve damage, cataract formation,
<u>or</u> corneal perforation. Limit ophthalmic steroid use to 2-3 days if possible; usual max 2
weeks. With prolonged or frequent use, there is risk of corneal and scleral thinning and
cataract formation.
▷ *dexamethasone* (C) initially 1-2 drops hourly during the day and q 2 hours at night;
    then prolong dosing interval to 4-6 hours as condition improves
    Pediatric: not recommended
    Maxidex *Ophth susp:* 0.1% (5, 15 ml) (benzalkonium chloride)
▷ *dexamethasone phosphate* (C) initially 1-2 drops hourly during the day and q 2 hours
    at night; then 1 drop q 4-8 hours <u>or</u> more as condition improves
    Pediatric: not recommended

Decadron *Ophth soln:* 0.1% (5 ml) (sulfites)
▷ *fluorometholone* (C) 1 drop bid-qid <u>or</u> 1/2 inch of ointment once daily-tid; may increase dose frequency during initial 24-48 hours
Pediatric: <2 years: not recommended; ≥2 years: same as adult
    FML *Ophth susp:* 0.1% (5, 10, 15 ml) (benzalkonium chloride)
    FML Forte *Ophth susp:* 0.25% (5, 10, 15 ml) (benzalkonium chloride)
    FML S.O.P. Ointment *Ophth oint:* 0.1% (3.5 g)
▷ *fluorometholone acetate* (C) initially 2 drops q 2 hours during the first 24-48 hours; then 1-2 drops qid as condition improves
Pediatric: not recommended
    Flarex *Ophth susp:* 0.1% (2.5, 5 10 ml) (benzalkonium chloride)
▷ *loteprednol etabonate* (C)
Pediatric: not recommended
    Alrex 1 drop qid
      Ophth susp: 0.2% (5, 10 ml) (benzalkonium chloride)
    Lotemax 1-2 drops qid
      Ophth susp: 0.5% (5, 10, 15 ml) (benzalkonium chloride)
▷ *medrysone* (C) 1 drop up to q 4 hours
Pediatric: not recommended
    HMS *Ophth susp:* 1% (5, 10 ml) (benzalkonium chloride)
▷ *rimexolone* (C) initially 1-2 drops hourly while awake x 1 week; then 1 drop q 2 hours while awake x 1 week; then taper as condition improves
Pediatric: not recommended
    Vexol *Ophth susp:* 0.1% (5, 10 ml) (benzalkonium chloride)
▷ *prednisolone acetate* (C)
Pediatric: not recommended
    Econopred 2 drops qid
      Ophth susp: 0.125% (5, 10 ml)
    Econopred Plus 2 drops qid
      Ophth susp: 1% (5, 10 ml)
    Pred Forte initially 2 drops hourly x 24-48 hours; then 1-2 drops bid-qid
      Ophth susp: 1% (1, 5, 10, 15 ml) (benzalkonium chloride, sulfites)
    Pred Mild initially 2 drops hourly x 24-48 hours; then 1-2 drops bid-qid
      Ophth susp: 0.12% (5, 10 ml) (benzalkonium chloride)
▷ *prednisolone sodium phosphate* (C) initially 1-2 drops hourly during the day and q 2 hours at night; then 1 drop q 4 hours; then 1 drop tid-qid as condition improves
Pediatric: not recommended
    Inflamase Forte *Ophth soln:* 1% (5, 10, 15 ml) (benzalkonium chloride)
    Inflamase Mild *Ophth soln:* 1/8% (5, 10 ml) (benzalkonium chloride)

OPHTHALMIC H₁ ANTAGONISTS (ANTIHISTAMINES)

Comment: May insert contact lens 10 minutes after administration of ophthalmic antihistamine.
▷ *emedastine* (C) 1 drop qid prn
Pediatric: <3 years: not recommended; ≥3 years: same as adult
    Emadine *Ophth soln:* 0.05% (5 ml) (benzalkonium chloride)
▷ *levocabastine* (C) 1 drop qid prn
Pediatric: not recommended
    Livostin *Ophth susp:* 0.05% (2.5, 5, 10 ml) (benzalkonium chloride)

OPHTHALMIC MAST CELL STABILIZERS

Comment: Concomitant contact lens wear is contraindicated during treatment.
▷ *cromolyn sodium* (B) 1-2 drops 4-6 x/day at regular intervals
　　Pediatric: <4 years: not recommended; ≥4 years: same as adult
　　　Crolom *Ophth soln:* 4% (10 ml) (benzalkonium chloride)
▷ *lodoxamide tromethamine* (B) 1-2 drops qid up to 3 months
　　Pediatric: <2 years: not recommended; ≥2 years: same as adult
　　　Alomide *Ophth soln:* 1% (10 ml) (benzalkonium chloride)
▷ *nedocromil* (B) 1-2 drops bid
　　Pediatric: <3 years: not recommended; ≥3 years: same as adult
　　　Alocril *Ophth soln:* 2% (5 ml) (benzalkonium chloride)
▷ *pemirolast potassium* (C) 1-2 drops qid
　　Pediatric: <3 years: not recommended; ≥3 years: same as adult
　　　Alamast *Ophth soln:* 0.1% (10 ml) (lauralkonium chloride)

OPHTHALMIC ANTIHISTAMINE/MAST CELL STABILIZER COMBINATIONS

▷ *alcaftadine* (B) 1 drop each eye daily
　　Pediatric: <2 years: not recommended; ≥2 years: same as adult
　　　Lastacaft *Ophth soln:* 0.25% (6 ml) (benzalkonium chloride)
　　Comment: May insert contact lens 10 minutes after ophthalmic administration.
▷ *azelastine* (C) 1 drop each eye bid
　　Pediatric: <3 years: not recommended; ≥3 years: same as adult
　　　Optivar *Ophth soln:* 0.05% (6 ml) (benzalkonium chloride)
　　Comment: May insert contact lens 10 minutes after ophthalmic administration.
▷ *bepotastine besilate* (C) 1 drop each eye bid
　　Pediatric: <2 years: not recommended; ≥2 years: same as adult
　　　Bepreve *Ophth soln:* 1.5% (10 ml) (benzalkonium chloride)
　　Comment: May insert contact lens 10 minutes after ophthalmic administration.
▷ *epinastine* (C)(G) 1 drop each eye bid
　　Pediatric: <3 years: not recommended; ≥3 years: same as adult
　　　Elestat *Ophth soln:* 0.05% (5 ml) (benzalkonium chloride)
▷ *ketotifen fumarate* (C) 1 drop each eye q 8-12 hours
　　Pediatric: <3 years: not recommended; ≥3 years: same as adult
　　　Alaway (OTC) *Ophth soln:* 0.025% (10 ml) (benzalkonium chloride)
　　　Claritin Eye (OTC) *Ophth soln:* 0.025% (5 ml) (benzalkonium chloride)
　　　Refresh Eye Itch Relief (OTC) *Ophth soln:* 0.025% (5 ml) (benzalkonium chloride)
　　　Zaditor (OTC) *Ophth soln:* 0.025% (5 ml) (benzalkonium chloride)
　　　Zyrtec Itchy Eye (OTC) *Ophth soln:* 0.025% (5 ml) (benzalkonium chloride)
▷ *olopatadine* (C) 1 drop each eye bid
　　Pediatric: <3 years: not recommended; ≥3 years: same as adult
　　　Pataday (G) *Ophth soln:* 0.2% (2.5 ml) (benzalkonium chloride)
　　　Patanol *Ophth soln:* 0.1% (5 ml) (benzalkonium chloride)
　　　Pazeo *Ophth soln:* 0.7% (2.5 ml) (benzalkonium chloride)
　　Comment: May insert contact lens 10 minutes after administration.

OPHTHALMIC VASOCONSTRICTORS

Comment: Concomitant contact lens wear is contraindicated during treatment.

▷ *naphazoline* (C) 1-2 drops each eye qid prn
  Pediatric: not recommended
    Vasocon-A *Ophth soln:* 0.1% (15 ml) (benzalkonium chloride)
▷ *oxymetazoline* (NR)(OTC) 1-2 drops each eye qid prn
  Pediatric: <6 years: not recommended; ≥6 years: same as adult
    Visine L-R *Ophth soln:* 0.025% (15, 30 ml)
▷ *tetrahydrozoline* (NR)(OTC)(G) 1-2 drops each eye qid prn
  Pediatric: <6 years: not recommended; ≥6 years: same as adult
    Visine *Ophth soln:* 0.05% (15, 22.5, 30 ml)

OPHTHALMIC VASOCONSTRICTOR/MOISTURIZER COMBINATION

Comment: Concomitant contact lens wear is contraindicated during treatment.
▷ *tetrahydrozoline/polyethylene glycol 400/povidone/dextran 70* (NR)(OTC) 1-2
  drops each eye qid prn
  Pediatric: <6 years: not recommended; ≥6 years: same as adult
    Advanced Relief Visine *Ophth soln: tetra* 0.025%/*poly* 1%/*pov* 1%/*dex* 0.1% (15,
    30 ml)

OPHTHALMIC VASOCONSTRICTOR/ASTRINGENT COMBINATION

Comment: Concomitant contact lens wear is contraindicated during treatment.
▷ *tetrahydrozoline/zinc sulfate* (NR)(OTC) 1-2 drops each eye qid prn
  Pediatric: <6 years: not recommended; ≥6 years: same as adult
    Visine AC *Ophth soln: tetra* 0.025%/*zinc* 0.05% (15, 30 ml)

OPHTHALMIC VASOCONSTRICTOR/ANTI-HISTAMINE COMBINATIONS

Comment: Concomitant contact lens wear is contraindicated during treatment.
▷ *naphazoline/pheniramine* (C) 1-2 drops each eye qid
  Pediatric: <6 years: not recommended; ≥6 years: same as adult
    Naphcon-A (OTC) *Ophth soln: naph* 0.025%/*phen* 0.3% (15 ml) (benzalkonium
    chloride)

OPHTHALMIC NSAIDs

Comment: Concomitant contact lens wear is contraindicated during treatment.
▷ *diclofenac* (B) 1 drop affected eye(s) qid
  Pediatric: not recommended
    Voltaren Ophthalmic Solution *Ophth soln:* 0.1% (2.5, 5 ml)
▷ *ketorolac tromethamine* (C) 1 drop affected eye(s) qid; max x 4 days
  Pediatric: <3 years: not recommended; ≥3 years: same as adult
    Acular *Ophth soln:* 0.5% (3, 5, 10 ml) (benzalkonium chloride)
    Acular LS *Ophth soln:* 0.4% (5 ml) (benzalkonium chloride)
    Acular PF *Ophth soln:* 0.5% (0.4 ml; 12 single-use vials/carton) (preserva-
    tive-free)
▷ *nepafenac* (C) 1 drop affected eye(s) tid
  Pediatric: <10 years: not recommended; ≥10 years: same as adult
    Nevanac Ophthalmic Suspension *Ophth susp:* 0.1% (3 ml) (benzalkonium
    chloride)

◯ CONJUNCTIVITIS/BLEPHAROCONJUNCTIVITIS: BACTERIAL

OPHTHALMIC ANTI-INFECTIVES

▷ *azithromycin* ophthalmic solution (B) 1 drop to affected eye(s) bid x 2 days; then 1 drop once daily for the next 5 days
Pediatric: <1 year: not recommended; ≥1 year: same as adult
   AzaSite Ophthalmic Solution *Ophth susp:* 1% (2.5 ml) (benzalkonium chloride)

▷ *bacitracin* ophthalmic ointment (C)(G) apply 1/2 inch ribbon to the lower conjunctival sac of affected eye(s) 1-3 x daily x 7 days
Pediatric: same as adult
   Bacitracin Ophthalmic Ointment *Ophth oint:* 500 units/g (3.5 g)

▷ *besifloxacin* ophthalmic solution (C) 1 drop to affected eye(s) tid x 7 days
Pediatric: <1 year: not recommended; ≥1 year: same as adult
   Besivance Ophthalmic Solution *Ophth susp:* 0.6% (5 ml) (benzalkonium chloride)

▷ *ciprofloxacin* ophthalmic ointment (C) apply 1/2 inch ribbon to the lower conjunctival sac of affected eye(s) tid x 2 days; then bid x 5 days
Pediatric: <2 years: not recommended; ≥2 years: same as adult
   Ciloxan Ophthalmic Ointment *Ophth oint:* 0.3% (3.5 g)

▷ *ciprofloxacin* ophthalmic solution (C) 1-2 drops to affected eye(s) q 2 hours while awake x 2 days; then, q 4 hours while awake x 5 days
Pediatric: <1 years: not recommended; ≥1 year: same as adult
   Ciloxan Ophthalmic Solution *Ophth soln:* 0.3% (2.5, 5, 10 ml) (benzalkonium chloride)

▷ *erythromycin* ophthalmic ointment (B) apply 1/2 inch ribbon to the lower conjunctival sac of affected eye(s) up to 6 x /day
Pediatric: same as adult
   Ilotycin Ophthalmic Ointment *Ophth oint:* 5 mg/g (1/8 oz)

▷ *gatifloxacin* ophthalmic solution (C)
Pediatric: <1 years: not recommended; ≥1 year: same as adult
   Zymar Ophthalmic Solution initially 1 drop to affected eye(s) q 2 hours while awake up to 8 times/day for 2 days; then 1 drop qid while awake x 5 more days
      Ophth soln: 0.3% (5 ml) (benzalkonium chloride)
   Zymaxid Ophthalmic Solution initially 1 drop to affected eye(s) q 2 hours while awake up to 8 times/day on day 1; then 1 drop bid-qid while awake on days 2-7
      Ophth soln: 0.5% (2.5 ml) (benzalkonium chloride)

▷ *gentamicin sulfate* ophthalmic ointment (C)(G) apply 1/2 inch ribbon to the lower conjunctival sac of affected eye(s) bid-tid
Pediatric: same as adult
   Garamycin Ophthalmic Ointment *Ophth oint:* 3 mg/g (3.5 g) (preservative-free formulation available)
   Genoptic Ophthalmic Ointment *Ophth oint:* 3 mg/g (3.5 g)
   Gentacidin Ophthalmic Ointment *Ophth oint:* 3 mg/g (3.5 g)

▷ *gentamicin sulfate* ophthalmic solution (C)(G) 1-2 drops to affected eye(s) q 4 hours x 7-14 days; max 2 drops q 1 h
Pediatric: same as adult
   Garamycin Ophthalmic Solution *Ophth soln:* 0.3% (5 ml) (benzalkonium chloride)
   Genoptic Ophthalmic Solution *Ophth soln:* 0.3% (3, 5 ml)

▷ *levofloxacin* ophthalmic solution (C) 1-2 drops to affected eye(s) q 2 hours while awake on days 1 and 2 (max 8 times/day); then 1-2 drops q 4 hours while awake on days 3-7; max 4 x /day
  Pediatric: <1 years: not recommended; ≥1 years: same as adult
    Quixin Ophthalmic Solution *Ophth soln:* 0.5% (2.5, 5 ml) (benzalkonium chloride)

▷ *moxifloxacin* ophthalmic solution (C) 1 drop to affected eye(s) tid x 7 days
  Pediatric: <1 years: not recommended; ≥1 year: same as adult
    Moxeza Ophthalmic Solution (G) *Ophth soln:* 0.5% (3 ml)
    Vigamox Ophthalmic Solution *Ophth soln:* 0.5% (3 ml)

▷ *ofloxacin* ophthalmic solution (C) 1-2 drops to affected eye(s) q 2-4 hours x 2 days; then qid x 5 days
  Pediatric: <1 years: not recommended; ≥1 year: same as adult
    Ocuflox Ophthalmic Solution *Ophth soln:* 0.3% (5, 10 ml) (benzalkonium chloride)

▷ *sulfacetamide* ophthalmic solution and ointment (C)
    Bleph-10 Ophthalmic Solution 1-2 drops to affected eye(s) q 2-3 hours x 7-10 days
      Pediatric: <2 months: not recommended; ≥2 months: 1-2 drops q 2-3 hours during the day x 7-10 days
      Ophth soln: 10% (2.5, 5, 15 ml) (benzalkonium chloride)
    Bleph-10 Ophthalmic Ointment apply 1/2 inch ribbon to the lower conjunctival sac of affected eye(s) q 3-4 hours and HS x 7-10 days
      Pediatric: <2 years: not recommended; ≥2 years: same as adult
      Ophth oint: 10% (3.5 g) (phenylmercuric acetate)
    Cetamide Ophthalmic Solution initially 1-2 drops to affected eye(s) q 2-3 hours; then increase dosing interval as condition improves
      Pediatric: <2 years: not recommended; ≥2 years: same as adult
      Ophth soln: 15% (5, 15 ml)
    Isopto Cetamide Ophthalmic Ointment initially 1/2 inch ribbon in lower conjunctival sac of affected eye(s) q 3-4 hours; then increase dosing interval as condition improves
      Pediatric: <2 years: not recommended; ≥2 years: same as adult
      Ophth oint: 10% (3.5 g)
    Isopto Cetamide Ophthalmic Solution initially 1-2 drops to affected eye(s) q 2-3 hours; then increase dosing interval as condition improves
      Pediatric: <2 years: not recommended; ≥2 years: same as adult
      Ophth soln: 15% (5, 15 ml)

▷ *tobramycin* (B)
    Tobrex Ophthalmic Solution 1-2 drops to affected eye(s) q 4 hours
      Pediatric: same as adult
      Ophth soln: 0.3% (5 ml) (benzalkonium chloride)
    Tobrex Ophthalmic Ointment apply 1/2 inch ribbon to the lower conjunctival sac of affected eye(s) bid-tid
      Pediatric: same as adult
      Ophth oint: 0.3% (3.5 g) (chlorobutanol)

OPHTHALMIC ANTI-INFECTIVE COMBINATIONS

▷ *polymyxin B sulfate/bacitracin* ophthalmic ointment (C) apply 1/2 inch ribbon to the lower conjunctival sac of affected eye(s) q 3-4 hours x 7-10 days
  Pediatric: same as adult

Polysporin Ophthalmic Ointment *Ophth oint: poly b* 10,000 U/*bac* 500 U (3.75 g)

▷ *polymyxin B sulfate/bacitracin zinc/neomycin sulfate* ophthalmic ointment (C) apply 1/2 inch ribbon to the lower conjunctival sac of affected eye(s) q 3-4 hours x 7-10 days
Pediatric: same as adult

Neosporin Ophthalmic Ointment *Ophth oint: poly b* 10,000 U/*bac* 400 U/*neo* 3.5 mg/g (3.75 g)

▷ *polymyxin B sulfate/gramicidin/neomycin* ophthalmic solution (C) 1-2 drops to affected eye(s) q 1 hour x 2-3 doses; then 1-2 drops bid-qid x 7-10 days
Pediatric: not recommended

Neosporin Ophthalmic Solution *Ophth soln: poly b* 10,000 U/*gram* 0.025 mg/ *neo* 1.7 mg/g (10 ml)

▷ *trimethoprim/polymyxin B sulfate* ophthalmic solution (C) 1 drop to affected eye(s) q 3 hours x 7-10 days; max 6 doses/day
Pediatric: <2 years: not recommended; ≥2 years: same as adult

Polytrim *Ophth soln: trim* 1 mg/*poly b* 10,000 U/ml (10 ml) (benzalkonium chloride)

OPHTHALMIC ANTI-INFECTIVE/STEROID COMBINATIONS

Comment: Ophthalmic corticosteroids are contraindicated after removal of a corneal foreign body, epithelial herpes simplex keratitis, *varicella*, other viral infections of the cornea or conjunctiva, fungal ocular infections, and mycobacterial ocular infections. Limit ophthalmic steroid use to 2-3 days if possible; usual max 2 weeks. With prolonged or frequent use, there is risk of corneal and scleral thinning and cataract formation.

▷ *gentamicin sulfate/prednisolone acetate* ophthalmic suspension (C)
Pediatric: not recommended

Pred-G Ophthalmic Suspension 1 drop to affected eye(s) bid-qid; max 20 ml/ therapeutic course
Ophth susp: gent 0.3%/*pred* 1%/ml (2, 5, 10 ml) (benzalkonium chloride)

Pred-G Ophthalmic Ointment apply 1/2 inch ribbon to the lower conjunctival sac of affected eye(s) once daily-tid; max 8 g/therapeutic course
Ophth oint: gent 0.3%/*pred* 0.6%/g (3.5 g)

▷ *neomycin sulfate/polymyxin B sulfate/dexamethasone* ophthalmic suspension (C)
Pediatric: not recommended

Maxitrol Ophthalmic Suspension 1-2 drops to affected eye(s) q 1 hour (severe infection) or qid (mild to moderate infection)
Ophth susp: neo 0.35%/*poly b* 10,000 U/*dexa* 1%/ml (5 ml) (benzalkonium chloride)

Maxitrol Ophthalmic Ointment apply 1/2 inch ribbon to the lower conjunctival sac of affected eye(s) q 1 hour (severe infection) or qid (mild to moderate infection)
Ophth oint: neo 0.35%/*poly b* 10,000 U/*dexa* 0.1%/g (3.5 g)

▷ *neomycin sulfate/polymyxin B sulfate/prednisolone acetate ophthalmic suspension* (C)
Pediatric: not recommended

Poly-Pred Ophthalmic Suspension 1-2 drops to affected eye(s) q 3-4 hours; more often as necessary; max 20 ml/therapeutic course.
Ophth susp: neo 0.35%/*poly b* 10,000 U/*pred* 0.5%/ml (10 ml)

▷ *polymyxin B sulfate/neomycin sulfate/hydrocortisone* ophthalmic suspension (C)

Pediatric: not recommended

> **Cortisporin Ophthalmic Suspension** 1-2 drops to affected eye(s) tid-qid; more often if necessary; max 20 ml/therapeutic course
>
> *Ophth susp: poly b* 10,000 U/*neo* 0.35%/*hydro* 1%/ml (7.5 ml) (thimerosal)

▶ *polymyxin B sulfate/neomycin sulfate/bacitracin zinc/hydrocortisone* ophthalmic ointment (C)

Pediatric: not recommended

> **Cortisporin Ophthalmic Ointment** apply 1/2 inch ribbon to the lower conjunctival sac of affected eye(s) tid-qid; more often if necessary; max 8 g/therapeutic course
>
> *Ophth oint: poly b* 10,000 U/*neo* 0.35%/*bac* 400 U/*hydro* 1%/g (3.5 g)

▶ *sulfacetamide sodium/fluorometholone* suspension (C) 1 drop to affected eye(s) qid; max 20 ml/therapeutic course

Pediatric: not recommended

> **FML-S** *Ophth susp: sulfa* 10%/*fluoro* 0.1%/ml (5, 10, 15 ml) (benzalkonium chloride)

▶ *sulfacetamide sodium/prednisolone acetate* ophthalmic suspension and ointment (C)

Pediatric: <6 years: not recommended; ≥6 years: same as adult

> **Blephamide Liquifilm** 2 drops to affected eye(s) qid and HS
>
> *Ophth susp: sulfa* 10%/*pred* 0.2%/ml (5, 10 ml) (benzalkonium chloride)
>
> **Blephamide S.O.P. Ophthalmic Ointment** apply 1/2 inch ribbon to the lower conjunctival sac of affected eye(s) tid-qid
>
> *Ophth oint: sulfa* 10%/*pred* 0.2%/g (3.5 g) (benzalkonium chloride)

▶ *sulfacetamide sodium/prednisolone sodium phosphate* ophthalmic solution (C) 2 drops to affected eye(s) q 4 hours

Pediatric: <6 years: not recommended; ≥6 years: same as adult

> **Vasocidin Ophthalmic Solution** *Ophth soln: sulfa* 10%/*pred* 0.25%/ml (5, 10 ml)

▶ *tobramycin/dexamethasone* ophthalmic solution and ointment (C)

> **TobraDex Ophthalmic Solution** 1-2 drops to affected eye(s) q 2-6 hours x 24-48 hours; then 4-6 hours; reduce frequency of dose as condition improves; max 20 ml per therapeutic course
>
> *Pediatric:* >2 years: not recommended; >2 years: 1-2 drops q 4-6 hours; may start with 1-2 drops q 2 hours first 1-2 days
>
> *Ophth susp: tobra* 0.3%/*dexa* 0.1%/ml (2.5, 5 ml) (benzalkonium chloride)
>
> **TobraDex Ophthalmic Ointment** apply 1/2 inch ribbon to the lower conjunctival sac of affected eye(s) tid-qid; may use at HS in conjunction with daytime drops; max 8 g/therapeutic course
>
> *Pediatric:* <2 years: not recommended; >2 years: apply 1/2 inch ribbon to lower conjunctival sac tid-qid
>
> *Ophth oint: tobra* 0.3%/*dexa* 0.1%/g (3.5 g) (chlorobutanol chloride)
>
> **TobraDex ST** 1-2 drops to affected eye(s) q 2-6 hours x 24-48 hours; then 4-6 hours; reduce frequency of dose as condition improves; max 20 ml per therapeutic course
>
> *Pediatric:* not recommended
>
> *Ophth susp: tobra* 0.3%/*dexa* 0.05%/ml (2.5, 5, 10 ml) (benzalkonium chloride)

▶ *tobramycin/loteprednol etabonate* ophthalmic suspension (C)

Pediatric: not recommended

> **Zylet** 1-2 drops to affected eye(s) q 1-2 hours first 24-48 hours; reduce frequency of dose to q 4-6 hours as condition improves; max 20 ml per therapeutic course
>
> *Ophth susp: tobra* 0.3%/*lote etab* 0.5%/ml (2.5, 5, 10 ml) (benzalkonium chloride)

⬤ CONJUNCTIVITIS: CHLAMYDIAL

Comment: A chlamydial etiology should be considered for all infants aged ≤30 days that have conjunctivitis, especially if the mother has a history of chlamydia infection. Topical antibiotic therapy alone is inadequate for treatment for ophthalmia neonatorum caused by chlamydia and is unnecessary when systemic treatment is administered.

ANTI-INFECTIVES

▷ *amoxicillin* (B)(G) 500 mg tid x 7 days
Pediatric: <40 kg (88 lb): 20-40 mg/kg/day in 3 divided doses x 7 days >40 kg: same as adult; *see page 543 for dose by weight*
   Amoxil *Cap:* 250, 500 mg; *Tab:* 875*mg; *Chew tab:* 125, 200, 250, 400 mg (cherry-banana-peppermint) (phenylalanine); *Oral susp:* 125, 250 mg/5 ml (80, 100, 150 ml) (strawberry); 200, 400 mg/5 ml (50, 75, 100 ml) (bubble gum); *Oral drops:* 50 mg/ml (30 ml) (bubble gum)

RECOMMENDED 1ST LINE REGIMEN

▷ *erythromycin base* (B)(G) 250 mg qid x 14 days <u>or</u> 500 mg qid x 7 days
Pediatric: <45 kg: 50 mg/kg/day in 4 divided doses x 14 days; ≥45 kg: same as adult
   Ery-Tab *Tab:* 250, 333, 500 mg ent-coat
   PCE *Tab:* 333, 500 mg
Comment: *erythromycin* may increase INR with concomitant *warfarin*, as well as increase serum level of *digoxin*, benzodiazepines and statins.
▷ *erythromycin ethylsuccinate* (B)(G) 400 mg qid x 14 days <u>or</u> 800 mg qid x 7 days
Pediatric: 50 mg/kg/day in 4 divided doses x 7 days; max 100 mg/kg/day; *see page 563 for dose by weight*
   EryPed *Oral susp:* 200 mg/5 ml (100, 200 ml) (fruit); 400 mg/5 ml (60, 100, 200 ml) (banana); *Oral drops:* 200, 400 mg/5 ml (50 ml) (fruit); *Chew tab:* 200 mg wafer (fruit)
   E.E.S. *Oral susp:* 200, 400 mg/5 ml (100 ml) (fruit)
   E.E.S. Granules *Oral susp:* 200 mg/5 ml (100, 200 ml) (cherry)
   E.E.S. 400 Tablets *Tab:* 400 mg
Comment: *erythromycin* may increase INR with concomitant *warfarin*, as well as increase serum level of *digoxin*, benzodiazepines and statins.

ALTERNATE REGIMEN

▷ *azithromycin* (B) 500 mg x 1 dose on day 1; then 250 mg once daily on days; 2-5 <u>or</u> 500 mg daily x 3 days <u>or</u> 2 g in a single dose
Pediatric: 20 mg/kg in a single dose once daily x 3 days
   Zithromax *Tab:* 250, 500, 600 mg; *Oral susp:* 100 mg/5 ml (15 ml); 200 mg/5 ml (15, 22.5, 30 ml) (cherry); *Pkt:* 1 g for reconstitution (cherry-banana)
   Zithromax Tri-pak *Tab:* 3 x 500 mg tabs/pck
   Zithromax Z-pak *Tab:* 6 x 250 mg tabs/pck
   Zmax *Oral susp:* 2 g ext-rel for reconstitution (cherry-banana) (148 mg Na⁺)

CONJUNCTIVITIS: FUNGAL

▶ **natamycin** ophthalmic suspension **(C)** 1 drop q 1-2 hours x 3-4 days; then 1 drop every 6 hours; treat for 14-21 days; withdraw dose gradually at 4- to -7-day intervals
Pediatric: <1 year: not recommended; ≥1 year: same as adult
  Natacyn Ophthalmic Suspension *Ophth susp:* 0.5% (15 ml) (benzalkonium chloride)

CONJUNCTIVITIS: GONOCOCCAL

RECOMMENDED REGIMENS

Regimen 1

▶ **ceftriaxone (B)(G)** 250 mg IM x 1 dose
Pediatric: <45 kg: 50 mg/kg IM x 1 dose; max 125 mg IM
  Rocephin *Vial:* 250, 500 mg; 1, 2 g

Regimen 2

▶ **erythromycin base (B)(G)** 250 mg qid x 10-14 days
Pediatric: <45 kg: 50 mg/kg/day in 4 divided doses x 10-14 days; ≥45 kg: same as adult
  Ery-Tab *Tab:* 250, 333, 500 mg ent-coat
  PCE *Tab:* 333, 500 mg
Comment: *erythromycin* may increase INR with concomitant *warfarin*, as well as increase serum level of *digoxin*, benzodiazepines and statins.
▶ **erythromycin ethylsuccinate (B)(G)** 400 mg qid x 14 days or 800 mg qid x 7 days
Pediatric: 50 mg/kg/day in 4 divided doses x 7 days; max 100 mg/kg/day; *see page 563 for dose by weight*
  EryPed *Oral susp:* 200 mg/5 ml (100, 200 ml) (fruit); 400 mg/5 ml (60, 100, 200 ml) (banana); *Oral drops:* 200, 400 mg/5 ml (50 ml) (fruit); *Chew tab:* 200 mg wafer (fruit)
  E.E.S. *Oral susp:* 200, 400 mg/5 ml (100 ml) (fruit)
  E.E.S. Granules *Oral susp:* 200 mg/5 ml (100, 200 ml) (cherry)
  E.E.S. 400 Tablets *Tab:* 400 mg
Comment: *erythromycin* may increase INR with concomitant *warfarin*, as well as increase serum level of *digoxin*, benzodiazepines and statins.

ALTERNATE REGIMEN

▶ **azithromycin (B)** 500 mg x 1 dose on day 1; then 250 mg once daily on days; 2-5 or 500 mg daily x 3 days or 2 g in a single dose
Pediatric: not recommended for bronchitis in children
  Zithromax *Tab:* 250, 500, 600 mg; *Oral susp:* 100 mg/5 ml (15 ml); 200 mg/5 ml (15, 22.5, 30 ml) (cherry); *Pkt:* 1 g for reconstitution (cherry-banana)
  Zithromax Tri-pak *Tab:* 3 x 500 mg tabs/pck
  Zithromax Z-pak *Tab:* 6 x 250 mg tabs/pck
  Zmax *Oral susp:* 2 g ext-rel for reconstitution (cherry-banana) (148 mg Na$^+$)

◯ CONJUNCTIVITIS: VIRAL

Comment: For prevention of secondary bacterial infection, see agents listed under bacterial conjunctivitis. Ophthalmic corticosteroids are contraindicated with herpes simplex, keratitis, *Varicella*, and other viral infections of the cornea.

▷ *trifluridine* ophthalmic suspension (C) 1 drop q 2 hours while awake; max 9 drops/day; after re-epithelialization, 1 drop q 4 h x 7 days (at least 5 drops/day); max 21 days of therapy
   Pediatric: <6 years: not recommended; ≥6 years: same as adult
   Viroptic Ophthalmic Solution *Ophth soln:* 1% (7.5 ml) (thimerosal)

◯ CONSTIPATION

CHRONIC IDIOPATHIC CONSTIPATION (CIC)

▷ *lubiprostone (chloride channel activator [GI motility enhancer])* (C) 1 cap bid with food
   Pediatric: not recommended
   Amitiza *Cap:* 24 mcg
▷ *linaclotide (guanylate cyclase-c agonist)* (C) 290 mcg once daily; take on an empty stomach at least 30 minutes before the first meal of the day; swallow whole
   Pediatric: <6 years: not recommended; 6-17 years: avoid
   Linzess *Cap:* 145, 290 mcg

BULK-FORMING AGENTS

▷ *calcium polycarbophil* (C)
   FiberCon (OTC) 2 tabs once daily to qid
      Pediatric: <6 years: not recommended; 6-12 years: 1 tab daily to qid
      Cplt: 625 mg
   Konsyl Fiber Tablets (OTC) *Tab:* 625 mg
▷ *methylcellulose*
   Citrucel 1 heaping tbsp in 8 oz cold water tid
      Pediatric: <6 years: not recommended; 6-12 years: 1/2 adult dose
      Oral pwdr: 16, 24, 30 oz and single-dose pkts (orange)
   Citrucel Sugar-Free 1 heaping tblsp in 8 oz cold water tid
      Pediatric: <6 years: not recommended; 6-12 years: 1/2 adult dose
      Oral pwdr: 16, 24, 30 oz and single-dose pkts (orange) (sugar-free, phenylalanine)
▷ *psyllium husk* (B)
   Pediatric: <6 years: not recommended; 6-12 years: 1/2 adult dose in 8 oz liquid tid
   Metamucil (OTC) wafer or cap or 1 pkt or 1 rounded tsp (1 rounded tblsp for sugar-containing form) in 8 oz liquid tid
      Cap: psyllium husk 5.2 g (100, 150/carton); *Wafer: psyllium husk* 3.4 g/rounded tsp (24/carton) (apple crisp, cinnamon spice); *Plain and flavored pwdr:* 3.4 g/rounded tsp (15, 20, 24, 29, 30, 36, 44, 48 oz); *Efferv sugar-free flav pkts:* 3.4 g/pkt (30/pkt) (phenylalanine)
▷ *psyllium* hydrophilic mucilloid (B) 2 rounded tsp in 8 oz water qid
   Pediatric: <6 years: not recommended; 6-12 years: 1 rounded tsp in 8 oz liquid tid
   Konsyl (OTC) *Pwdr:* 6 g/rounded tsp (10.6, 15.9 oz); *Pwdr pkt:* 6 g/rounded tsp (30/carton)

Konsyl-D (OTC) *Pwdr:* 3.4 g/rounded tsp (11.5, 17.59 oz); *Pwdr pkt:* 3.4 g/rounded tsp (30/carton)
Konsyl Easy Mix Formula (OTC) *Pwdr:* 3.4 g/rounded tsp (8 oz) (sugar-free, low sodium)
Konsyl Orange (OTC) *Pwdr:* 3.4 g/rounded tsp (19 oz); *Pwdr pkt:* 3.4 g/rounded tsp (30/carton)
Konsyl Orange SF (OTC) *Pwdr:* 3.5 g/rounded tsp (15 oz) (phenylalanine); *Pwdr pkt:* 3.5 g/rounded tsp (30/carton) (phenylalanine)

STOOL SOFTENERS

▷ *docusate sodium* (OTC) 50-200 mg/day
   Pediatric: <3 years: 10-40 mg/day; 3-6 years: 20-60 mg/day; >6 years: 40-120 mg/day
      Cap: 50, 100 mg; *Liq:* 10 mg/ml (30 ml w. dropper); *Syr:* 20 mg/5 ml (8 oz) (alcohol ≤1%)
   Dialose 1 tab q HS
      Pediatric: <6 years: not recommended; ≥6 years: same as adult
      Tab: 100 mg
   Surfak (OTC) 240 mg/day
      Pediatric: not recommended
      Cap: 240 mg

OSMOTIC LAXATIVES

▷ *lactulose* (B)(G) take 10-20 g dissolved in 4 oz water once daily prn; max 40 g/day
   Pediatric: not recommended
      Kristalose *Crystals for oral soln:* 10, 20 g single-dose pkts (30/carton)
▷ *magnesium citrate* (B)(G) 1 full bottle (120-300 ml) once daily prn
   Pediatric: <2 years: not recommended; 2-6 years: 4-12 ml once daily prn; ≥6-12 years: 50-100 ml once daily prn
      Citrate of Magnesia (OTC) *Oral soln:* 300 ml
▷ *magnesium hydroxide* (B) 30-60 ml/day in a single or divided doses prn
   Pediatric: 2-5 years: 5-15 ml/day in a single or divided doses; 6-11 years: 15-30 ml/day in a single or divided doses; ≥12 years: same as adult
      Milk of Magnesia *Liq:* 390 mg/5 ml (10, 15, 20, 30, 100, 120, 180, 360, 720 ml)
▷ *polyethylene glycol (PEG)* (C)(OTC)(G) 1 tblsp (17 g) dissolved in 4-8 oz water per day for up to max 7 days; may need 2-4 days for results
   Pediatric: ≤17: not recommended
      GlycoLax Powder for Oral Solution *Oral pwdr:* 7, 14, 30, and 45 dose bottles w. 17 g dosing cup (gluten-free, sugar-free); 17 g single-dose pkts (20/carton)
      MiraLAX Powder for Oral Solution *Oral pwdr:* 7, 14, 30, and 45 dose bottles w. 17 g dosing cup (gluten-free, sugar-free)
      Polyethylene Glycol 3350 Powder for Oral Solution (G) *Oral pwdr:* 3350 g w. dosing cup; 17 g/scoop
Comment: *PEG* is an osmotic indicated for occasional constipation without affecting glucose and electrolyte levels. Contraindicated with suspected or known bowel obstruction.

STIMULANTS

▷ *bisacodyl* (B) 2-3 tabs or 1 suppository bid prn
      Dulcolax, Gentlax *Tab:* 5 mg; *Rectal supp:* 10 mg

Pediatric: <12 years: 1/2 suppository once daily prn; 6-12 years: 1 tablet <u>or</u>
1/2 suppository once daily prn; >12 years: same as adult

Senokot (OTC) initially 2-4 tabs <u>or</u> 1 level tsp at HS prn; max 4 tabs <u>or</u> 2 tsp bid
Pediatric: <2 years: not recommended; 2-6 years: 1/4 tab <u>or</u> 1/2 tsp once daily
prn; max 1 tab <u>or</u> 1/2 tsp bid; 6-12 years: 1 tab <u>or</u> 1/2 tsp once daily prn; max
2 tabs <u>or</u> 1 tsp once daily
Tab: 8.6*mg; *Granules:* 15 mg/tsp (2, 6, 12 oz) (cocoa)

Senokot Syrup (OTC) initially 10-15 ml at HS prn; max 15 ml bid
Pediatric: use Childrens Syrup
Syr: 8.8 mg/5 ml (2, 8 oz) (chocolate) (alcohol-free)

Senokot Childrens Syrup (OTC)
Pediatric: <2 years: not recommended; 2-6 years: 2.5-3.75 ml once daily prn;
max 3.75 ml bid prn; ≥6-12 years: 5-7.5 ml once daily prn; max 7.5 ml bid
Syr: 8.8 mg/5 ml (2.5 oz) (chocolate) (alcohol-free)

Senokot Xtra (OTC) 1 tab at HS prn; max 2 tabs bid
Pediatric: <2 years: not recommended; 2-6 years: use Childrens Syrup; 6-12
years: 1/2 tab once daily at HS; max 1 tab bid
Tab: 17*mg

BULK FORMING AGENT/STIMULANT COMBINATIONS

▷ *psyllium/senna* (B)
Perdiem (OTC) 1-2 rounded tsp swallowed with 8 oz cool liquid daily bid
Pediatric: <7 years: not recommended; 7-11 years: 1 rounded tsp swallowed
with 8 oz cool liquid once daily-bid; ≥12 years: same as adult
Canister: 8.8, 14 oz; *Individual pkt:* 6 g (6/pck)

SennaPrompt (OTC) initially 2-5 caps bid
Pediatric: not recommended
Cap: psyl 500 mg/*senna* 9 mg

STOOL SOFTENER/STIMULANT COMBINATIONS

▷ *docusate/casanthranol* (C)
Doxidan (OTC) 1-3 caps/day; max 1 week
Pediatric: <2 years: not recommended; ≥2 years: 1 cap/day
Cap: doc 60 mg/*cas* 30 mg

Peri-Colace (OTC) 1-2 caps <u>or</u> 15-30 ml q HS; max 2 caps <u>or</u> 30 ml bid <u>or</u> 3 caps
q HS
Pediatric: 5-15 ml q HS
Cap: doc 100 mg/*cas* 30 mg; *Syr: doc* 60 mg/*cas* 30 mg per 15 ml (8, 16 oz)

▷ *docusate/senna* concentrate (C)
Senokot S (OTC) 2 tabs q HS; max 4 tabs bid
Pediatric: <2 years: not recommended; 2-6 years: 1/2 tab daily; max 1 tab bid;
>6-12 years: 1 tab daily; max 2 tabs bid
Tab: doc 50 mg/*senna* 8.6 mg

ENEMAS AND OTHER AGENTS

▷ *sodium biphosphate/sodium phosphate* enema (C)(OTC)
Fleets Adult 59-118 ml rectally
Pediatric: <2 years: not recommended; ≥2-12 years: 59 ml rectally

    Enema: Na biphos 19 g/Na phos 7 g (59, 118 ml w. applicator)
   Fleets Pediatric 59 ml
    Pediatric: rectally
    Enema: na biphos 19 g/*na phos* 7 g (59 ml w. applicator)
▷ *glycerin* suppositories (C)(OTC)
  Pediatric: <6 years: 1 pediatric suppository; ≥6 years: 1 adult suppository

CORNEAL EDEMA

▷ *sodium chloride* (NR)(G)
  Pediatric: same as adult
    Various (OTC) 1-2 drops or 1 inch ribbon q 3-4 hours prn; reduce frequency as edema subsides
     Ophth soln: 2, 5% (15, 30 ml); *Ophth oint:* 5% (3.5 g)

CORNEAL ULCERATION

ANTIBACTERIAL OPHTHALMIC SOLUTION/OINTMENT

see Conjunctivitis/Blepharoconjunctivitis: Bacterial page 89

COSTOCHONDRITIS (CHEST WALL SYNDROME)

Acetaminophen for IV Infusion *see Pain page 296*
Oral Prescription NSAIDs *see page 489*
Other Oral Analgesics *see Pain page 298*
Topical/Transdermal NSAIDs *see Pain page 297*
Parenteral Corticosteroids *see page 499*
Oral Corticosteroids *see page 497*
Topical Analgesic and Anesthetic Agents *see page 487*

CRAMPS: ABDOMINAL, INTESTINAL

ANTISPASMODIC/ANTICHOLINERGIC COMBINATIONS

▷ *dicyclomine* (B)(G) initially 20 mg bid-qid; may increase to 40 mg qid PO; usual IM dose 80 mg/day divided qid; do not use IM route for more than 1-2 days
  Pediatric: not recommended
    Bentyl *Tab:* 20 mg; *Cap:* 10 mg; *Syr:* 10 mg/5 ml (16 oz); *Vial:* 10 mg/ml (10 ml); *Amp:* 10 mg/ml (2 ml)
▷ *methscopolamine bromide* (B) 1 tab q 6 hours prn
  Pediatric: not recommended
    Pamine *Tab:* 2.5 mg
    Pamine Forte *Tab:* 5 mg

ANTICHOLINERGICS

▷ *hyoscyamine* (C)(G)

Anaspaz 1-2 tabs q 4 hours prn; max 12 tabs/day
Pediatric: <2 years: not recommended; 2-12 years: 0.0625-0.125 mg q 4 hours prn; max 0.75 mg/day; ≥12 years: same as adult
Tab: 0.125*mg

Levbid 1-2 tabs q 12 hours prn; max 4 tabs/day
Pediatric: <12 years: not recommended; ≥12 years: same as adult
Tab: 0.375*mg ext-rel

Levsin 1-2 tabs q 4 hours prn; max 12 tabs/day
Pediatric: <6 years: not recommended; ≥6-12 years: 1 tab q 4 hours prn
Tab: 0.125*mg

Levsinex SL 1-2 tabs q 4 hours SL or PO; max 12 tabs/day
Pediatric: 2-12 years: 1 tab SL or PO q 4 hours; max 6 tabs/day
Tab: 0.125 mg sublingual

Levsinex Timecaps 1-2 caps q 12 hours; may adjust to 1 cap q 8 hours
Pediatric: 2-12 years: 1 cap q 12 hours; max 2 caps/day
Cap: 0.375 mg time-rel

NuLev dissolve 1-2 tabs on tongue, with or without water, q 4 hours prn; max 12 tabs/day
Pediatric: <2 years: not recommended; 2-12 years: dissolve 1 tab on tongue, with or without water, q 4 hours prn; max 6 tabs/day; >12 years: same as adult
ODT: 0.125 mg (mint) (phenylalanine)

▷ *simethicone* (C)(G) 0.3 ml qid pc and HS

Mylicon Drops (OTC) *Oral drops:* 40 mg/0.6 ml (30 ml)

▷ *phenobarbital/hyoscyamine/atropine/scopolamine* (C)(IV)(G)

Donnatal 1-2 tabs ac and HS
Pediatric: not recommended
Tab: pheno 16.2 mg/*hyo* 0.1037 mg/*atro* 0.0194 mg/*scop* 0.0065 mg

Donnatal Elixir 1-2 tsp ac and HS
Pediatric: 20 lb: 1 ml q 4 hours or 1.5 ml q 6 hours; 30 lb: 1.5 ml q 4 hours or 2 ml q 6 hours; 50 lb: 1/2 tsp q 4 hours or 3/4 tsp q 6 hours; 75 lb: 3/4 tsp q 4 hours or 1 tsp q 6 hours; 100 lb: 1 tsp q 4 hours or 1 tsp q 6 hours
Elix: pheno 16.2 mg/*hyo* 0.1037 mg/*atro* 0.0194 mg/*scop* 0.0065 mg per 5 ml (4, 16 oz)

Donnatal Extentabs 1 tab q 12 hours
Pediatric: not recommended
Tab: pheno 48.6 mg/*hyo* 0.3111 mg/*atro* 0.0582 mg/*scop* 0.0195 mg ext-rel

ANTICHOLINERGIC/SEDATIVE COMBINATION

▷ *chlordiazepoxide/clidinium* (D)(IV) 1-2 caps ac and HS; max 8 caps/day
Pediatric: not recommended
Librax *Cap:* chlor 5 mg/clid 2.5 mg

CROHN'S DISEASE

Comment: Standard treatment regimen for active disease (flare) is: antibiotic, antispasmodic, and bowel rest; progress to clear liquids; then progress to high-fiber diet.

Parenteral Corticosteroids *see page* 499
Oral Corticosteroids *see page* 497

▷ *azathioprine* (D)(G)

Imuran *Tab:* 50*mg; *Injectable:* 100 mg
Comment: Imuran is usually administered on a daily basis. The initial dose should be approximately 1.0 mg/kg (50 to 100 mg) as a single dose or divided bid. Dose may be increased beginning at 6-8 weeks, and thereafter at 4-week intervals, if there are no serious toxicities and if initial response is unsatisfactory. Dose increments should be 0.5 mg/kg/day, up to max 2.5 mg/kg per day. Therapeutic response usually occurs after 6-8 weeks of treatment. An adequate trial should be a minimum of 12 weeks. Patients not improved after 12 weeks can be considered refractory. **Imuran** may be continued long-term in patients with clinical response, but patients should be monitored carefully, and gradual dosage reduction should be attempted to reduce risk of toxicities. Maintenance therapy should be at the lowest effective dose, and the dose given can be lowered decrementally with changes of 0.5 mg/kg or approximately 25 mg daily every 4 weeks while other therapy is kept constant. The optimum duration of maintenance **Imuran** has not been determined. **Imuran** can be discontinued abruptly, but delayed effects are possible.

▷ *infliximab (tumor necrosis factor-alpha blocker)* (B) administer 5 mg/kg/dose by IV infusion over at least 2 h; *Fistulizing disease:* initial dose; repeat dose at 2 weeks and 6 weeks (total 3 doses); then repeat dose every 8 weeks; *Maintenance:* usually 5 mg/kg/dose every 8 weeks; may increase to 10 mg/kg/dose
Pediatric: not recommended

Remicade *Vial:* 100 mg pwdr for IV infusion single-use (preservative-free)

▷ *mesalamine* (B)

Asacol 800 mg tid x 6 weeks; maintenance 1.6 g/day in divided doses; swallow whole, do not crush or chew
Pediatric: not recommended
Tab: 400 mg del-rel
Comment: 2 **Asacol** 400 mg tabs are not bioequivalent to 1 **Asacol HD** 800 mg tab.

Asacol HD 1600 mg tid x 6 weeks; swallow whole, do not crush or chew
Pediatric: not recommended
Tab: 800 mg del-rel
Comment: 1 **Asacol HD** 800 mg tab is not bioequivalent to 2 **Asacol** 400 mg tabs

Canasa 1 g qid for up to 8 weeks
Rectal supp: 1 g del-rel (30, 42/pck)

Delzicol *Treatment:* 800 mg tid x 6 weeks; maintenance 1.6 g/day in 2-4 divided doses daily; swallow whole; do not crush or chew
Pediatric: <5 years: not established; > years: same as adult
Cap: 400 mg del-rel
Comment: 2 **Delzicol** 400 mg caps are not bioequivalent to 1 *mesalamine* 800 mg del-rel tab

Lialda 2.4-4.8 g daily in a single dose for up to 8 weeks; swallow whole, do not crush or chew
Pediatric: <18 years: not recommended
Tab: 1.2 g del-rel

Pentasa 1 g qid for up to 8 weeks; swallow whole, do not crush or chew
Pediatric: not recommended

Cap: 250 mg cont-rel
Rowasa Enema 4 g rectally by enema q HS; retain for 8 hours x 3-6 weeks
    Enema: 4 g/60 ml (7, 14, 28/pck; kit, 7, 14, 28/pck w. wipes)
Rowasa Suppository 1 suppository rectally bid x 3-6 weeks; retain for 1-3 hours
or longer
    Rectal supp: 500 mg
Sulfite-Free Rowasa Rectal Suspension 4 g rectally by enema q HS; retain for
8 hours x 3-6 weeks
    Enema: 4 g/60 ml (7, 14, 28/pck; kit, 7, 14, 28/pck w. wipes)

▷ *olsalazine* (C)
    Dipentum 1 g/day in 2 divided doses; max 2 g/day
        Cap: 250 mg
Comment: Indicated in persons who cannot tolerate *sulfasalazine*.

▷ *sulfasalazine* (B)(G)
    Azulfidine initially 1-2 g/day; increase to 3-4 g/day in divided doses pc until
    clinical symptoms controlled; maintenance 2 g/day; max 4 g/day
        Tab: 500*mg
        Pediatric: <2 years: not recommended; 2-16 years: initially 40-60 mg/kg/day
        in 3-6 divided doses; max 2 g/day
    Azulfidine EN initially 500 mg in the PM x 7 days; then 500 mg bid x 7 days;
    then 500 mg in the AM and 1 g in the PM x 7 days; then 1 g bid; max 4 g/day
        Pediatric: not recommended
        Tab: 500 mg ent-coat
Comment: sulfasalazine

▷ *vedolizumab* (B) administer by IV infusion over 30 minutes; 300 mg at weeks 0, 2, 6;
then once every 8 weeks
Pediatric: not established
    Entyvio
        Vial: 300 mg (20 ml) single dose, pwdr for IV infusion after reconstitution
        (preservative-free)

▷ *budesonide micronized* (C)
Pediatric: not recommended
    Entocort EC *Treatment* 9 mg once daily in the AM for up to 8 weeks; may repeat
    an 8-week course; *Maintenance of remission*: 6 mg once daily for up to 3 months
        Cap: 3 mg ent-coat ext-rel granules
    Comment: Taper other systemic steroids when transferring to **Entocort EC**. When
    glucocorticosteroids are used chronically, systemic effects such as hypercorticism
    and adrenal suppression may occur. Glucocorticosteroids can reduce the response
    of the hypothalamus-pituitary-adrenal (HPA) axis to stress. In situations where
    patients are subject to surgery or other stress situations, supplementation with a
    systemic glucocorticosteroid is recommended. General precautions concerning
    glucocorticoids should be followed.

ORAL ANTI-INFECTIVES

▷ *metronidazole* (**not for use in 1st; B in 2nd, 3rd**)(G) 500 mg tid or 750 mg bid; max
8 weeks
Pediatric: 35-50 mg/kg/day in 3 divided doses x 10 days
    Flagyl *Tab:* 250*, 500*mg
    Flagyl 375 *Cap:* 375 mg

Flagyl ER *Tab:* 750 mg ext-rel
Comment: Alcohol is contraindicated during treatment with oral *metronidazole*
and for 72 hours after therapy due to a possible *disulfiram*-like reaction (nausea,
vomiting, flushing, headache).

TUMOR NECROSIS FACTOR (TNF) BLOCKER

▷ *adalimumab* (B) 40 mg SC once every other week; may increase to once weekly without MTX; administer in abdomen or thigh; rotate sites
Pediatric: <2 years, <10 kg: not recommended; 10-<15 kg: 10 mg every other week;
15-<30 kg: 20 mg every other week; ≥30 kg: 40 mg every other week; 2-17 years,
supervise first dose
Humira *Prefilled syringe:* 20 mg/0.4 ml; 40 mg/0.8 ml single-dose (2/pck; 2, 6/
starter pck) (preservative-free)
Comment: May use with methotrexate (MTX), DMARDS, glucocorticoids, salicylates,
NSAIDs, or analgesics.
▷ *certolzumab* (B) 400 mg SC (2 x 200 mg inj at two different sites on day 1); then,
400 mg SC at weeks 2 and 4; maintenance 400 mg SC every 4 weeks; administer in
abdomen or thigh; rotate sites
Pediatric: not recommended
Cimzia *Vial:* 200 mg (2/pck); *Prefilled syringe:* 200 mg/ml single-dose (2/pck; 2,
6/starter pck) (preservative-free)
▷ *infliximab* (B) administer by IV infusion over 2 hours; 5 mg/kg weeks 0, 2, 6; then
once every 8 weeks
Pediatric: <6 years: not recommended; ≥6 years: same as adult
Remicade
Vial: 100 mg pwdr for reconstitution for IV infusion (preservative-free)
▷ *vedolizumab* (B) administer by IV infusion over 30 minutes; 300 mg at weeks 0, 2, 6;
then 300 mg once every 8 weeks
Pediatric: not established
Entyvio
Vial: 300 mg (20 ml) single dose, pwdr for IV infusion after reconstitution
(preservative-free)

INTEGRIN RECEPTOR ANTAGONIST (IMMUNOMODULATOR)

▷ *natalzumab* (C) administer by IV infusion over 1 hour; monitor during and for 1
hour postinfusion; 300 mg every 4 weeks; discontinue after 12 weeks if no therapeutic response, or if unable to taper off chronic concomitant steroids within 6 months;
may continue aminosalicylates
Pediatric: not established
Tysarbi
Vial: 300 mg single-dose, soln after dilution for IV infusion
(preservative-free)

⊙ CRYPTOSPORIDIUM PARVUM

▷ *nitazoxanide* (B) 500 mg by mouth q 12 hours x 3 days
Pediatric: 12-47 months: 5 ml q 12 hours x 3 days; 4-11 years: 10 ml q 12 hours x 3
days; ≥12 years: same as adult

Alinia *Oral susp:* 100 mg/5 ml (60 ml)
Comment: Alinia is an antiprotozoal for the treatment of diarrhea due to *G. lamblia* or *C. parvum*.

CYSTIC FIBROSIS

▷ *acetylcysteine* (B)(G) administer via face mask, mouth piece, tracheostomy T-piece, mist tent, or croupette; routine tracheostomy care, 1 to 2 ml of a 10% to 20% solution may be administered by direct instillation into the tracheostomy every 1 to 4 hours
Pediatric: same as adult
Mucomyst *Vial:* 10, 20% (4, 10, 30 ml) soln for inhalation
Comment: Mucomyst is a mucolytic. For inhalation, the 10% concentration may be used undiluted; the 20% concentration should be diluted with sterile water or normal saline (either for injection or inhalation).

▷ *lumacaftor/ivacaftor* (B) 2 tabs q 12 hours; reduce dose with moderate to severe hepatic impairment
Pediatric: <12 years: not established
Orkambi *Tab: luma* 200 mg/*iva* 125 mg film-coat

DEEP VEIN THROMBOSIS (DVT)

Anticoagulation Therapy *see page* 515

DEHYDRATION

ORAL REHYDRATION AND ELECTROLYTE REPLACEMENT THERAPY

▷ *oral electrolyte replacement* (NR)(OTC)(G)
KaoLectrolyte 1 pkt dissolved in 8 oz water q 3-4 hours
Pediatric: not indicated <2 years *Pkt: sod* 12 mEq/*pot* 5 mEq/*chlor* 10 mEq/*citrate* 7 mEq/*dextrose* 5 g/*calories* 22 per 6.2 g
Pedialyte
Pediatric: <2 years: as desired and as tolerated; >2 years: 1-2 liters/day
Oral soln: dextrose 20 g/*fructose* 5 g/*sodium* 25 mEq/*potassium* 20 mEq/*chloride* 35 mEq/*citrate* 30 mEq/*calories* 100 per liter (8 oz, 1 L)
Pedialyte Freezer Pops
Pediatric: as desired and as tolerated
Pops: dextrose 1.6 g/*sodium* 2.8 mEq/*potassium* 1.25 mEq/*chloride* 2.2 mEq/*citrate* 1.88 mEq/*calories* 6.25 per 62.5 ml (2.1 fl oz) pop

DEMENTIA

Comment: Underlying cause should be explored, accurately diagnosed, and addressed. All antipsychotic agents are associated with increased risk of mortality in elderly patients with dementia-related psychosis (Black Box Warning.) APA recommends that non-emergency antipsychotic medication should only be used for the treatment of agitation or psychosis in patients with dementia when symptoms are severe, are dangerous and/or cause significant distress to the patient. APA recommends that before nonemergency treatment with an antipsychotic is initiated in patients with dementia, the potential risks and benefits are discussed with the patient and the patient's surrogate decision maker with input from family or others involved with the patient.

Alzheimer's Disease *see page* 11
Antidepressants *see Depression page* 105
Hypnotics/Sedatives *see Insomnia page* 233

ANTIPSYCHOTICS

▷ *haloperidol* (C)(G) 0.5-1 mg q HS
  Haldol *Tab:* 0.5, 1, 2, 5, 10, 20 mg
▷ *mesoridazine* (C) initially 25 mg tid; max 300 mg/day
  Serentil *Tab:* 10, 25, 50, 100 mg; *Conc:* 25 mg/ml (118 ml)
▷ *olanzapine* (C) initially 2.5-10 mg daily; increase to 10 mg/day within a few days; then by 5 mg/day at weekly intervals; max 20 mg/day
  Zyprexa *Tab:* 2.5, 5, 7.5, 10 mg
  Zyprexa Zydis *ODT:* 5, 10, 15, 20 mg (phenylalanine)
▷ *quetiapine fumarate* (C)
  SeroQUEL initially 25 mg bid, titrate q 2nd or 3rd day in increments of 25-50 mg bid-tid; usual maintenance 400-600 mg/day in 2-3 divided doses
    Tab: 25, 50, 100, 200, 300, 400 mg
  SeroQUEL XR administer once daily in the PM; *Day 1:* 50 mg; *Day 2:* 100 mg; *Day 3:* 200 mg; *Day 4:* 300 mg; usual range 400-600 mg/day
    Tab: 50, 150, 200, 300, 400 mg ext-rel
▷ *risperidone* (C) 0.5 mg bid x 1 day; adjust in increments of 0.5 mg bid; usual range 0.5-5 mg/day
  Risperdal *Tab:* 1, 2, 3, 4 mg; *Oral soln:* 1 mg/ml (100 ml)
  Risperdal M-Tab *Tab:* 0.5, 1, 2 mg
▷ *thioridazine* (C)(G) 10-25 mg bid
  Mellaril *Tab:* 10, 15, 25, 50, 100, 150, 200 mg; *Oral susp:* 25 mg/5 ml, 100 mg/5 ml; *Oral conc:* 30 mg/ml, 100 mg/ml (4 oz)

◯ DENTAL ABSCESS

▷ *amoxicillin/clavulanate* (B)(G) 500 mg tid or 875 mg bid x 10 days
  Augmentin *Tab:* 250, 500, 875 mg; *Chew tab:* 125, 250 mg (lemon-lime); 200, 400 mg (cherry-banana) (phenylalanine); *Oral susp:* 125 mg/5 ml (banana), 250 mg/5 ml (75, 100, 150 ml) (orange); 200, 400 mg/5 ml (50, 75, 100 ml) (orange) (phenylalanine)
    Pediatric: 40-45 mg/kg/day divided tid x 10 days or 90 mg/kg/day divided bid x 10 days *see page* 545 *for dose by weight*
  Augmentin ES-600 *Oral susp:* 600 mg/5 ml (50, 75, 100, 125, 150, 200 ml) (strawberry cream) (phenylalanine) every 12 hours
    Pediatric: <3 months: not recommended; ≥3 months, <40 kg: 90 mg/kg/day in 2 divided doses; ≥40 kg: not recommended
  Augmentin XR 2 tabs q 12 hours x 7-10 days
    Pediatric: <16 years: use other forms; ≥16 years: same as adult
    Tab: 1000*mg ext-rel

▶ *clindamycin* (B) (administer with fluoroquinolone in adults and TMP-SMX in children) 300 mg qid x 10 days
Pediatric: 8-16 mg/kg/day in 3-4 divided doses x 10 days
    Cleocin (G) *Cap:* 75 (tartrazine), 150 (tartrazine), 300 mg
    Cleocin Pediatric Granules (G) *Oral susp:* 75 mg/5 ml (100 ml) (cherry)

▶ *erythromycin base* (B)(G) 500 mg q 6 hours x 10 days
Pediatric: 30-40 mg/kg/day in 3-4 divided doses x 10 days
    Ery-Tab *Tab:* 250, 333, 500 mg ent-coat
    PCE *Tab:* 333, 500 mg
Comment: *erythromycin* may increase INR with concomitant *warfarin*, as well as increase serum level of *digoxin*, benzodiazepines and statins.

▶ *erythromycin ethylsuccinate* (B)(G) 400 mg qid x 7 days
Pediatric: 30-50 mg/kg/day in 4 divided doses x 7 days; may double dose with severe infection; max 100 mg/kg/day; *see page 563 for dose by weight*
    EryPed *Oral susp:* 200 mg/5 ml (100, 200 ml) (fruit); 400 mg/5 ml (60, 100, 200 ml) (banana); *Oral drops:* 200, 400 mg/5 ml (50 ml) (fruit); *Chew tab:* 200 mg wafer (fruit)
    E.E.S. *Oral susp:* 200, 400 mg/5 ml (100 ml) (fruit)
    E.E.S. Granules *Oral susp:* 200 mg/5 ml (100, 200 ml) (cherry)
    E.E.S. 400 Tablets *Tab:* 400 mg
Comment: *erythromycin* may increase INR with concomitant *warfarin*, as well as increase serum level of *digoxin*, benzodiazepines and statins.

▶ *penicillin V potassium* (B) 250-500 mg q 6 hours x 5-7 days
Pediatric: 25-50 mg/kg/day divided q 6 hours x 5-7 days; >12 years: same as adult; *see page 572 for dose by weight*
    Pen-Vee K *Tab:* 250, 500 mg; *Oral soln:* 125 mg/5 ml (100, 200 ml); 250 mg/5 ml (100, 150, 200 ml)

◉ DENTURE IRRITATION

DEBRIDING AGENT/CLEANSER

▶ *carbamide peroxide 10%* (NR)(OTC) apply 10 drops to affected area; swish x 2-3 minutes, then spit; do not rinse; repeat treatment qid
Pediatric: with adult supervision only
    Gly-Oxide *Liq:* 10% (15, 60 ml, squeeze bottle w. applicator)

◉ DEPRESSION, MAJOR DEPRESSIVE DISORDER (MDD)

Comment: Abrupt withdrawal or interruption of treatment with an antidepressant medication is sometimes associated with an antidepressant discontinuation syndrome which may be mediated by gradually tapering the drug over a period of two weeks or longer, depending on the dose strength and length of treatment. Common symptoms of antidepressant withdrawal include flu-like symptoms, insomnia, nausea, imbalance, sensory disturbances, and hyperarousal. These medications include SSRIs, TCAs, MAOIs, and atypical agents such as *venlafaxine* (Effexor), *mirtazapine* (Remeron), trazodone (Desyrel), and duloxetine (Cymbalta). Common symptoms of the serotonin discontinuation syndrome include flu-like symptoms (nausea, vomiting, diarrhea, headaches, sweating), sleep disturbances (insomnia, nightmares, constant sleepiness), mood disturbances (dysphoria, anxiety, agitation), cognitive disturbances (mental confusion, hyperarousal), sensory and movement disturbances (imbalance, tremors, vertigo, dizziness, electric-shock-like sensations in the brain, often described by sufferers as "brain zaps."

SELECTIVE SEROTONIN REUPTAKE INHIBITORS (SSRIs)

Comment: Co-administration of SSRIs with TCAs requires extreme caution. Concomitant use of MAOIs and SSRIs is absolutely contraindicated. Avoid St. John's wort and other serotonergic agents. A potentially fatal adverse event is *serotonin syndrome*, caused by serotonin excess. Milder symptoms require HCP intervention to avert severe symptoms which can be rapidly fatal without urgent/emergent medical care. Symptoms include restlessness, agitation, confusion, tachycardia, hypertension, dilated pupils, muscle twitching, muscle rigidity, loss of muscle coordination, diaphoresis, diarrhea, headache, shivering, piloerection, hyperpyrexia, cardiac arrhythmias, seizures, loss of consciousness, coma, death. Common symptoms of the *serotonin discontinuation syndrome* include flu-like symptoms (nausea, vomiting, diarrhea, headaches, sweating), sleep disturbances (insomnia, nightmares, constant sleepiness), mood disturbances (dysphoria, anxiety, agitation), cognitive disturbances (mental confusion, hyperarousal, hallucinations), sensory and movement disturbances (imbalance, tremors, vertigo, dizziness, electric-shock-like sensations in the brain, often described by sufferers as "brain zaps."

➤ *citalopram* (C)(G) initially 20 mg daily; may increase after one week to 40 mg; max 40 mg
  Pediatric: not recommended
      Celexa *Tab:* 10, 20, 40mg; *Oral soln:* 10 mg/5 ml (120 ml) (pepper mint) (sugar-free, alcohol-free, parabens)
➤ *escitalopram* (C)(G) initially 10 mg daily; may increase to 20 mg daily after 1 week; elderly or hepatic impairment, 10 mg once daily
  Pediatric: <12 years: not recommended; 12-17 years: initially 10 mg daily; may increase to 20 mg daily after 3 weeks
      Lexapro *Tab:* 5, 10*, 20*mg
      Lexapro Oral Solution *Oral soln:* 1 mg/ml (240 ml) (peppermint) (parabens)
➤ *fluoxetine* (C)(G)
      Prozac initially 20 mg daily; may increase after 1 week; doses >20 mg/day should be divided into AM and noon doses; max 80 mg/day
          Pediatric: <8 years: not recommended; 8-17 years: initially 10 mg/day; may increase after 1 week to 20 mg/day; range 20-60 mg/day; range for lower weight children, 20-30 mg/day
          Cap: 10, 20, 40 mg; *Tab:* 30*, 60*mg; *Oral soln:* 20 mg/5 ml (4 oz) (mint)
      Prozac Weekly following daily fluoxetine therapy at 20 mg/day for 13 weeks, may initiate **Prozac Weekly** 7 days after the last 20 mg fluoxetine dose
          Pediatric: not recommended
          Cap: 90 mg ent-coat del-rel pellets
➤ *levomilnacipran* (C) swallow whole; initially 20 mg once daily for 2 days; then increase to 40 mg once daily; may increase dose in 40 mg increments at intervals of ≥2 days; max 120 mg once daily; *CrCl 30-59 mL/min:* max 80 mg once daily; *CrCl 15-29 mL/min:* max 40 mg once daily

Fetzima
> *Pediatric:* not recommended
> *Cap:* 20, 40, 80, 120 mg ext-rel

▷ *paroxetine maleate* (D)(G)
> *Pediatric:* not recommended
>> **Paxil** initially 20 mg daily in AM; may increase by 10 mg/day at weekly intervals as needed; max 60 mg/day
>>> *Tab:* 10*, 20*, 30, 40 mg
>> **Paxil CR** initially 25 mg daily in AM; may increase by 12.5 mg at weekly intervals as needed; max 62.5 mg/day
>>> *Tab:* 12.5, 25, 37.5 mg cont-rel ent-coat
>> **Paxil Suspension** initially 20 mg daily in AM; may increase by 10 mg/day at weekly intervals as needed; max 60 mg/day
>>> *Oral susp:* 10 mg/5 ml (250 ml) (orange)

▷ *sertraline* (C)(G) initially 50 mg daily; increase at 1 week intervals if needed; max 200 mg daily; dilute oral concentrate immediately prior to administration in 4 oz water, ginger ale, lemon/lime soda, lemonade, <u>or</u> orange juice
> *Pediatric:* <6 years: not recommended; 6-12 years: initially 25 mg daily; max 200 mg/day; 13-17 years: initially 50 mg daily; max 200 mg/day
>> **Zoloft** *Tab:* 25*, 50*, 100*mg; *Oral conc:* 20 mg per ml (60 ml) (alcohol 12%)

SEROTONIN AND NOREPINEPHRINE REUPTAKE INHIBITORS (SNRIs)

▷ *desvenlafaxine* (C)(G) swallow whole; initially 50 mg once daily; max 120 mg/day
> *Pediatric:* not recommended
>> **Pristiq** *Tab:* 50, 100 mg ext-rel

▷ *duloxetine* (C)(G) swallow whole; initially 30 mg once daily x 1 week; then, increase to 60 mg once daily; max 120 mg/day
> *Pediatric:* not recommended
>> **Cymbalta** *Cap:* 20, 30, 40, 60 mg del-rel

▷ *venlafaxine* (C)(G)
>> **Effexor** initially 75 mg/day in 2-3 divided doses; may increase at 4 day intervals in 75 mg increments to 150 mg/day; max 225 mg/day
>>> *Pediatric:* <18 years: not recommended
>>> *Tab:* 37.5, 75, 150, 225 mg
>> **Effexor XR** initially 75 mg q AM; may start at 37.5 mg daily x 4-7 days, then increase by increments of up to 75 mg/day at intervals of at least 4 days; usual max 375 mg/day
>>> *Pediatric:* not recommended
>>> *Tab/Cap:* 37.5, 75, 150 mg ext-rel

▷ *vortioxetine* (C) initially 10 mg once daily; max 30 mg/day
> *Pediatric:* <18 years: not restablished
>> **Brintellix** *Tab:* 5, 10, 15, 20 mg

SELECTIVE SEROTONIN REUPTAKE INHIBITOR (SSRI)/5-HT-14 RECEPTOR PARTIAL AGONIST COMBINATION

▷ *vilazodone* (C) take with food; initially 10 mg once daily x 7 days; then, 20 mg once daily x 7 days; then, 40 mg once daily
> *Pediatric:* <18 years: not restablished
>> **Viibryd** *Tab:* 10, 20, 40 mg

THIENOBENZODIAZEPINE/SSRI COMBINATION

▷ *olanzapine/fluoxetine* (C) initially one 6/25 cap in the PM; titrate; max one 18/75 cap once daily in the PM
Pediatric: <10 years: not established; <10 years: same as adult
    Symbyax
        Cap: Symbyax **3/25**: *olan* 3 mg/*fluo* 25 mg
               Symbyax **6/25**: *olan* 6 mg/*fluo* 25 mg
               Symbyax **6/50**: *olan* 6 mg/*fluo* 50 mg
               Symbyax **12/25**: *olan* 12 mg/*fluo* 25 mg
               Symbyax **12/50**: *olan* 12 mg/*fluo* 50 mg
    Comment: **Symbyax** is a thienobenzodiazepine-SSRI indicated for the treatment of depressive episodes associated with bipolar depression disorder and treatment resistant depression (TRD).

TRICYCLIC ANTIDEPRESSANTS (TCAs)

Comment: Co-administration of TCAs with SSRIs requires extreme caution.
▷ *amitriptyline* (C)(G) initially 75 mg/day in divided doses <u>or</u> 50-100 mg in a single dose at HS; max 300 mg/day
Pediatric: not recommended
    Tab: 10, 25, 50, 75, 100, 150 mg
▷ *amoxapine* (C) initially 50 mg bid-tid; after 1 week may increase to 100 mg bid-tid; usual effective dose 200-300 mg/day; if total dose exceeds 300 mg/day, give in divided doses (max 400 mg/day); may give as a single bedtime dose (max 300 mg q HS)
Pediatric: not recommended
    Tab: 25, 50, 100, 150 mg
▷ *desipramine* (C)(G) 100-200 mg/day in single <u>or</u> divided doses; max 300 mg/day
Pediatric: not recommended
    Norpramin *Tab:* 10, 25, 50, 75, 100, 150 mg
▷ *doxepin* (C)(G) 75 mg/day; max 150 mg/day
Pediatric: not recommended
    Cap: 10, 25, 50, 75, 100, 150 mg; *Oral conc:* 10 mg/ml (4 oz w. dropper)
▷ *imipramine* (C)(G)
Pediatric: not recommended
    Tofranil initially 75 mg daily (max 200 mg); adolescents initially 30-40 mg daily (max 100 mg/day); if maintenance dose exceeds 75 mg daily, may switch to **Tofranil PM** for divided <u>or</u> bedtime dose
        Tab: 10, 25, 50 mg
    Tofranil PM initially 75 mg daily 1 hour before HS; max 200 mg
        Cap: 75, 100, 125, 150 mg
    Tofranil Injection 50 mg IM; lower dose for adolescents; switch to oral form as soon as possible
        Amp: 25 mg/2 ml (2 ml)
▷ *nortriptyline* (D)(G) initially 25 mg tid-qid; max 150 mg/day
Pediatric: not recommended
    Pamelor *Cap:* 10, 25, 50, 75 mg; *Oral soln:* 10 mg/5 ml (16 oz)
▷ *protriptyline* (C) initially 5 mg tid; usual dose 15-40 mg/day in 3-4 divided doses; max 60 mg/day
Pediatric: <12 years: not recommended

      Vivactyl *Tab:* 5, 10 mg
▷ *trimipramine* (C) initially 75 mg/day in divided doses; max 200 mg/day
    Pediatric: not recommended
      Surmontil *Cap:* 25, 50, 100 mg

AMINOKETONES

▷ *bupropion HBr* (C)(G)
    Pediatric: not established
      Aplenzin initially 100 mg bid for at least 3 days; may increase to 375 or 400
      mg/day after several weeks; then after at least 3 more days, 450 mg in 4 divided
      doses; max 450 mg/day, 174 mg/single-dose
        Tab: 174, 348, 522 mg
      Forfivo XL do not use for initial treatment; use immediate-release bupropion
      forms for initial titration; switch to **Forfivo XL** 450 mg once daily when total
      dose/day reaches 450 mg; may switch to **Forfivo XL** when total dose/day reach-
      es 300 mg for 2 weeks and patient needs 450 mg/day to reach therapeutic target;
      swallow whole, do not crush or chew
        Tab: 450 mg ext-rel
▷ *bupropion HCl* (C)(G)
    Pediatric: <18 years: not recommended
      Wellbutrin initially 100 mg bid for at least 3 days; may increase to 375 or 400
      mg/day after several weeks; then after at least 3 more days, 450 mg in 4 divided
      doses; max 450 mg/day, 150 mg/single-dose
        Tab: 75, 100 mg
      Wellbutrin SR initially 150 mg in AM for at least 3 days; increase to 150 mg bid
      if well tolerated; usual dose 300 mg/day; max 400 mg/day
        Tab: 100, 150 mg sust-rel
      Wellbutrin XL initially 150 mg in AM for at least 3 days; increase to 150 mg bid
      if well tolerated; usual dose 300 mg/day; max 450 mg/day
        Tab: 150, 300 mg sust-rel

MONOAMINE OXIDASE INHIBITORS (MAOIs)

Comment: Many drug and food interactions with this class of drugs, use cautiously.
Should be reserved for refractory depression that has not responded to other classes of
antidepressants. Concomitant use of MAOIs and SSRIs is an absolute contraindication.
See mfr literature for drug and food interactions.
▷ *isocarcatronazid* (C)(G) initially 10 mg bid; increase by 10 mg every 2-4 days up to
    40 mg/day; may increase by 20 mg/week to max 60 mg/day divided bid-qid
      Marplan
        Pediatric: <16 years: not recommended; ≥16 years: same as adult
        Tab: 10 mg
▷ *phenelzine* (C)(G) initially 15 mg tid; max 90 mg/day
      Nardil
        Pediatric: <16 years: not recommended; ≥16 years: same as adult
        Tab: 15 mg
▷ *selegiline* (C) initially 10 mg tid; max 60 mg/day
      Emsam *Transdermal patch:* 6 mg/24 h, 9 mg/24 h, 12 mg/24 h
      Comment: With the **Emsam** transdermal patch 6 mg/24 h dose, the dietary
      restrictions commonly required when using nonselective MAOIs are not necessary.

▷ *tranylcypromine* (C) initially 10 mg tid; may increase in 10 mg/day every 1-3 weeks; max 60 mg/day
    Parnate *Tab:* 10 mg

TETRACYCLICS

▷ *maprotiline* (B)(G) initially 75 mg/day for 2 weeks then change gradually as needed in 25 mg increments; max 225 mg/day
    Pediatric: <18 years: not recommended
        Ludiomil *Tab:* 25, 50, 75 mg
▷ *mirtazapine* (C) initially 15 mg q HS; increase at intervals of 1-2 weeks; usual range 15-45 mg/day; max 45 mg/day
    Pediatric: not recommended
        Remeron *Tab:* 15*, 30*, 45*mg
        Remeron SolTab *ODT:* 15, 30, 45 mg (orange) (phenylalanine)
▷ *chlordiazepoxide/amitriptyline* (C)(IV)
    Pediatric: not recommended
        Limbitrol 3-4 tabs in divided doses
            Tab: chlor 5 mg/*amit* 12.5 mg
        Limbitrol DS 3-4 tabs in divided doses; max 6 tabs/day
            Tab: chlor 10 mg/*amit* 25 mg
▷ *trazodone* (C)(G) initially 150 mg/day in divided doses with food; increase by 50 mg/day q 3-4 days; max 400 mg/day in divided doses
    Pediatric: <18 years: not recommended
        Oleptro *Tab:* 50, 100*, 150*, 200, 250, 300 mg

ATYPICAL ANTIPSYCHOTICS

▷ *aripiprazole* (C) initially 15 mg daily; may increase to max 30 mg/day
    Pediatric: <10 years: not recommended; 10-17 years: initially 2 mg/day for 2 days; then, increase to 5 mg/day for 2 days; then, increase to target dose of 10 mg/day; may increase by 5 mg/day at 1 week intervals as needed to max 30 mg/day
        Abilify *Tab:* 2, 5, 10, 15, 20, 30 mg
        Abilify Discmelt *Tab:* 15 mg orally disintegrating (vanilla) (phenylalanine)
        Abilify Maintena *Vial:* 300, 400 mg ext-rel pwdr for IM injection after reconstitution; 300, 400 mg single-dose prefilled dual-chamber syringes w. supplies
        Comment: **Abilify** is indicated for acute and maintenance treatment of manic <u>or</u> mixed episodes in bipolar I disorder, as monotherapy <u>or</u> as an adjunct to *lithium* <u>or</u> *valproate*, as adjunct to antidepressants for major depressive disorder (MDD), and for irritability associated with autistic disorder.
▷ *brexpiprazole* (C) initially 0.5 <u>or</u> 1 mg once daily; titrate weekly up to target 2 mg/day; max 3 mg/day; moderate-severe hepatic impairment, renal impairment, <u>or</u> ESRD, max 2 mg/day
    Pediatric: not established
        Rexulti *Tab:* 0.25, 0.5, 1, 2, 3, 4 mg

 DERMATITIS: ATOPIC (ECZEMA)

Oral Antihistamines: *see* **Oral Drugs for Allergy, Cough, and Cold** *see page* 524
Parenteral Corticosteroids *see page* 499

Oral Corticosteroids *see page* 497
Topical Steroids (For other topical steroids, *see* **Topical Corticosteroids** *page* 494)
Comment: Topical steroids should be applied sparingly and for the shortest time
necessary. Do not use in the diaper area. Do not use an occlusive dressing. Systemic
absorption of topical corticosteroids can induce reversible hypothalamic-pituitary-
adrenal (HPA) axis suppression with the potential for clinical glucocorticoid
insufficiency.

▷ *desonide* 0.05% topical gel (C) apply sparingly bid-tid; max 4 weeks
   Pediatric: <3 months: not recommended; ≥3 months: same as adult
     Desonate *Gel:* 0.05% (60 g) (89% purified water; fragrance-free, surfactant-free,
     alcohol-free)

MOISTURIZING AGENTS

    Aquaphor Healing Ointment (OTC) *Oint:* 1.75, 3.5, 14 oz (alcohol)
    Eucerin Daily Sun Defense (OTC) *Lotn:* 6 oz (fragrance-free)
    Comment: **Eucerin Daily Sun Defense** is a moisturizer with SPF-15 sunscreen.
    Eucerin Facial Lotion (OTC) *Lotn:* 4 oz
    Eucerin Light Lotion (OTC) *Lotn:* 8 oz
    Eucerin Lotion (OTC) *Lotn:* 8, 16 oz
    Eucerin Original Creme (OTC) *Crm:* 2, 4, 16 oz (alcohol)
    Eucerin Plus Creme (OTC) *Crm:* 4 oz
    Eucerin Plus Lotion (OTC) *Lotn:* 6, 12 oz
    Eucerin Protective Lotion (OTC) *Lotn:* 4 oz (alcohol)
    Comment: **Eucerin Protective Lotion** is a moisturizer with SPF-25 sunscreen.
    Lac-Hydrin Cream (OTC) *Crm:* 280, 385 g
    Lac-Hydrin Lotion (OTC) *Lotn:* 25, 400 g
    Lubriderm Dry Skin Scented (OTC) *Lotn:* 6, 10, 16, 32 oz
    Lubriderm Dry Skin Unscented (OTC) *Lotn:* 3.3, 6, 10, 16 oz (fragrance-free)
    Lubriderm Sensitive Skin Lotion (OTC) *Lotn:* 3.3, 6, 10, 16 oz (lanolin-free)
    Lubriderm Dry Skin (OTC) *Lotn (scented):* 2.5, 6, 10, 16 oz;
     Lotn (fragrance-free): 1, 2.5, 6, 10, 16 oz
    Lubriderm Bath 1-2 capfuls in bath <u>or</u> rub onto wet skin as needed, then rinse
     Oil: 8 oz
    Moisturel apply as needed
     Crm: 4, 16 oz; *Lotn:* 8, 12 oz; *Clnsr:* 8.75 oz

OATMEAL COLLOIDS

    Aveeno (OTC) add to bath as needed
     Regular: 1.5 oz (8/pck); *Moisturizing:* 0.75 oz (8/pck)
    Aveeno Oil (OTC) add to bath as needed
     Oil: 8 oz
    Aveeno Moisturizing (OTC) apply as needed
     Lotn: 2.5, 8, 12 oz; *Crm:* 4 oz
    Aveeno Cleansing Bar (OTC) *Bar:* 3 oz
    Aveeno Gentle Skin Cleanser (OTC) *Liq clnsr:* 6 oz

TOPICAL OIL

▷ *fluocinolone acetamide* 0.01% topical oil (C)
   Pediatric: <6 years: not recommended; ≥6 years: apply sparingly bid for up to 4 weeks

Derma-Smoothe/FS Topical Oil apply sparingly tid
Topical oil: 0.01% (4 oz) (peanut oil)

TOPICAL ANALGESICS

➤ *capsaicin* cream (B)(G) apply tid-qid prn
Pediatric: <2 years: not recommended; ≥2 years: apply sparingly tid-qid prn
Axsain *Crm:* 0.075% (1, 2 oz)
Capsin (OTC) *Lotn:* 0.025, 0,075% (59 ml)
Capzasin-P (OTC) *Crm:* 0.025% (1.5 oz); *Lotn:* 0.025% (2 oz)
Capzasin-HP (OTC) *Crm:* 0.075% (1.5 oz); *Lotn:* 0.075% (2 oz)
Dolorac *Crm:* 0.025% (28 g)
Double Cap (OTC) *Crm:* 0.05% (2 oz)
R-Gel *Gel:* 0.025% (15, 30 g)
Zostrix (OTC) *Crm:* 0.025% (0.7, 1.5, 3 oz)
Zostrix HP (OTC) *Emol crm:* 0.075% (1, 2 oz)
Comment: Provides some relief by 1-2 weeks; optimal benefit may take 4-6 weeks.
Avoid contact with mucous membranes.
➤ *doxepin* (B) cream apply to affected area qid at intervals of at least 3-4 hours;
max 8 days
Pediatric: not recommended
Prudoxin *Crm:* 5% (45 g)
Zonalon *Crm:* 5% (30, 45 g)
➤ *pimecrolimus* 1% cream (C) apply to affected area bid; do not occlude
Pediatric: <2 years: not recommended; ≥2 years: same as adult
Elidel *Crm:* 1% (30, 60, 100 g)
Comment: *pimecrolimus* is indicated for short-term and intermittent long-term
use. Discontinue use when resolution occurs. Contraindicated if the patient is
immunosuppressed. Change to the 0.1% preparation or if secondary bacterial
infection is present.
➤ *tacrolimus* (C) apply to affected area bid; do not occlude or apply to wet skin; continue for 1 week after clearing
Pediatric: <2 years: not recommended; 2-15 years: use 0.03% strength; apply to
affected area bid; continue for 1 week after clearing; >15 years: same as adult
Protopic *Oint:* 0.03, 0.1% (30, 60, 100 g)

TOPICAL ANESTHETIC

➤ *lidocaine* (B) apply to affected area bid-tid prn
Pediatric: reduce dosage commensurate with age, body weight, and physical condition
Lidoderm *Crm:* 3% (85 g)

 DERMATITIS: CONTACT

PROPHYLAXIS

➤ *bentoquatam* (NR) apply as a wet film to exposed skin at least 15 minutes prior to
possible contact; reapply at least q 4 hours; remove with soap and water
Pediatric: <6 years: not recommended; ≥6 years: same as adult

IvyBlock (OTC) *Soln:* 120 ml
Comment: Provides protection against genus rhus (poison ivy, oak, and sumac).

TREATMENT

Oatmeal Colloids

Aveeno (OTC) add to bath as needed
Regular: 1.5 oz (8/pck); *Moisturizing:* 0.75 oz (8/pck)
Aveeno Oil (OTC) add to bath as needed
Oil: 8 oz
Aveeno Moisturizing (OTC) apply as needed
Lotn: 2.5, 8, 12 oz; *Crm:* 4 oz
Aveeno Cleansing Bar (OTC) *Bar:* 3 oz
Aveeno Gentle Skin Cleanser (OTC) *Liq clnsr:* 6 oz
Oral Drugs for Allergy, Cough, and Cold *see page* 524
Topical Corticosteroids *see page* 494
Parenteral Corticosteroids *see page* 499
Oral Corticosteroids *see page* 497

DERMATITIS: SEBORRHEIC

ANTIFUNGAL SHAMPOOS AND TOPICAL AGENTS

▷ *chloroxine* shampoo (C) massage onto wet scalp; wait 3 minutes, rinse, repeat, and rinse thoroughly; use twice weekly
Pediatric: not recommended

Capitrol Shampoo *Shampoo:* 2% (4 oz)

▷ *ciclopirox* (B) apply gel once daily <u>or</u> apply cream <u>or</u> lotion twice daily, x 4 weeks <u>or</u> shampoo twice weekly; massage shampoo onto wet scalp; wait 3 minutes, rinse, repeat, and rinse thoroughly; shampoo twice weekly

Loprox Cream
Pediatric: <10 years: not recommended; ≥10 years: same as adult
Crm: 0.77% (15, 30, 90 g)

Loprox Gel
Pediatric: <16 years: not recommended; ≥16 years: same as adult
Gel: 0.77% (30, 45 g)

Loprox Lotion
Pediatric: <10 years: not recommended; ≥10 years: same as adult
Lotn: 0.77% (30, 60 ml)

Loprox Shampoo *Shampoo:* 1% (120 ml)

▷ *coal tar* (C)(G)
Pediatric: same as adult

Scytera (OTC) apply once daily-qid; use lowest effective dose
Foam: 2%

T/Gel Shampoo Extra Strength (OTC) use every other day; max 4 x/week; massage into wet scalp for 5 minutes; rinse; repeat *Shampoo:* 1%

T/Gel Shampoo Original Formula (OTC) use every other day; max 7 x/week; massage into wet scalp for 5 minutes; rinse; repeat
Shampoo: 0.5%

T/Gel Shampoo Stubborn Itch Control (OTC) use every other day; max 7 x/week; massage into wet scalp for 5 minutes; rinse; repeat
> *Shampoo:* 0.5%

▶ *fluocinolone acetamide* (C)
Derma-Smoothe/FS Shampoo apply up to 1 oz to scalp daily, lather, and leave on x 5 minutes, then rinse twice
> *Pediatric:* not recommended
> *Shampoo:* 0.01% (4 oz)

Derma-Smoothe/FS Topical Oil *fluocinolone acetamide* 0.01% topical oil (C) apply sparingly tid; for scalp psoriasis wet or dampen hair or scalp, then apply a thin film, massage well, cover with a shower cap and leave on for at least 4 hours or overnight, then wash hair with regular shampoo and rinse
> *Pediatric:* <6 years: not recommended; ≥6 years: apply sparingly bid for up to 4 weeks
> *Topical oil:* 0.01% (4 oz) (peanut oil)

▶ *ketoconazole* (C) apply cream or gel once daily x 4 week or apply up to 1 oz shampoo to scalp daily, lather, leave on x 5 minutes, then rinse twice
Pediatric: not recommended
Nizoral Cream *Crm:* 2% (15, 30, 60 g)
Nizoral Shampoo *Shampoo:* 2% (4 oz)
Xolegel *Gel:* 2% (45 g)
Xolegel Duo *Kit:* **Xolegel** *Gel:* 2% (45 g) + **Xolex** *Shampoo:* 2% (4 oz)

▶ *selenium sulfide* (C) massage cream into scalp twice weekly x 2 weeks or massage into wet scalp, wait 2-3 minutes, rinse; repeat twice weekly x 2 weeks; may continue treatment with lotion of shampoo 1-2 x weekly as needed
Pediatric: not recommended
Exsel Shampoo *Shampoo:* 2.5% (4 oz)
Selsun Rx *Lotn:* 2.5% (4 oz)
Selsun Shampoo *Shampoo:* 1% (120, 210, 240, 330 ml); 2.5% (120 ml)

▶ *sodium sulfacetamide/sulfur* (C)
Clinia Emollient Cream apply daily tid
> *Emol crm:* sod sulfa 10%/sulfur 5% (10 oz)
Clinia Foaming Wash wash 1-2 x /daily
> *Wash:* sod sulfa 10%/sulfur 5% (6, 12 oz)
Rosula Gel apply daily tid
> *Gel:* sod sulfa 10%/sulfur 5% (45 ml)
Rosula Lotion apply daily tid
> *Lotn:* sod sulfa 10%/sulfur 5% (45 ml) (alcohol-free)
Rosula Wash wash bid
> *Clnsr:* sod sulfa 10%/sulfur 5% (335 ml)

TOPICAL STEROID

▶ *betamethasone valerate* 0.12% foam (C)(G) apply twice daily in AM and PM; invert can and dispense a small amount of foam onto a clean saucer or other cool surface (do not apply directly to hand) and massage a small amount into affected area until foam disappears
Pediatric: not recommended
Luxiq Foam: 100 g
Other Topical Corticosteroids *see page* 494

◯ DIABETIC PERIPHERAL NEUROPATHY

NUTRITIONAL SUPPLEMENT

▷ *L-methylfolate calcium (as metafolin)/pyridoxyl 5-phosphate/methyl-cobalamin* **(NR)** 1 cap twice daily <u>or</u> 2 caps once daily
Pediatric: not recommended
   Metanx *Cap: meta* 3 mg/*pyr* 35 mg/*methyl* 2 mg
   Comment: **Metanx** is indicated as adjunct treatment for patients with endothelial cell dysfunction, who have loss of protective sensation and neuropathic pain associated with diabetic peripheral neuropathy.
Acetaminophen for IV Infusion *see Pain page* 296

ORAL ANALGESICS

▷ *acetaminophen* **(B)(G)** *see Fever page* 143
▷ *aspirin* **(D)(G)** *see Fever page* 145
   Comment: *aspirin*-containing medications are contraindicated with history of allergic-type reaction to *aspirin*, children and adolescents with *Varicella* <u>or</u> other viral illness, and 3rd trimester pregnancy.
▷ *tramadol* **(C)(IV)(G)**
   Rybix ODT initially 100 mg once daily; may increase by 100 mg every 5 days; max 300 mg/day; *CrCl <30 mL/min <u>or</u> severe hepatic impairment*: not recommended; *Cirrhosis*: max 50 mg q 12 hours
      Pediatric: <17 years: not recommended
      ODT: 50 mg (mint) (phenylalanine)
   Ryzolt initially 100 mg once daily; may increase by 100 mg every 5 days; max 300 mg/day; *CrCl <30 mL/min <u>or</u> severe hepatic impairment*: not recommended
      Pediatric: <16 years: not recommended; ≥16 years: same as adult
      Tab: 100, 200, 300 mg ext-rel
   Ultram 50-100 mg q 4-6 hours prn; max 400 mg/day; *CrCl <30 mL/min*, max 100 mg q 12 hours; cirrhosis, max 50 mg q 12 hours
      Pediatric: <16 years: not recommended
      Tab: 50*mg
   Ultram ER initially 100 mg once daily; may increase by 100 mg every 5 days; max 300 mg/day; *CrCl <30 mL/min <u>or</u> severe hepatic impairment*: not recommended
      Pediatric: <18 years: not recommended
      Tab: 100, 200, 300 mg ext-rel
▷ *tramadol/acetaminophen* **(C)(IV)(G)** 2 tabs q 4-6 hours; max 8 tabs/day x 5 days; *CrCl <30 mL/min:* max 2 tabs q 12 hours; max 4 tabs/day x 5 days
   Pediatric: <16 years: not recommended
   Ultracet *Tab: tram* 37.5/*acet* 325 mg
Other Oral Analgesics *see Pain page* 296

TOPICAL ANALGESICS

▷ *capsaicin* cream **(B)(G)** apply tid-qid after lesions have healed
   Pediatric: <2 years: not recommended; ≥2 years: same as adult
      Axsain *Crm:* 0.075% (1, 2 oz)

Capsin *Lotn:* 0.025, 0.075% (59 ml)
Capsaicin-P (OTC) *Crm:* 0.025% (1.5 oz); *Lotn:* 0.025% (2 oz)
Capsaicin-HP (OTC) *Crm:* 0.075% (1.5 oz); *Lotn:* 0.075% (2 oz); *Crm:* 0.025% (45, 90 g)
Dolorac *Crm:* 0.025% (28 g)
Double Cap (OTC) *Crm:* 0.05% (2 oz)
R-Gel *Gel:* 0.025% (15, 30 g)
Zostrix (OTC) *Crm:* 0.025% (0.7, 1.5, 3 oz)
Zostrix HP *Emol crm:* 0.075% (1, 2 oz)

▷ *capsaicin* 8% patch **(B)** apply up to 4 patches for one 60-minute application to clean dry skin; may prep area with topical anesthetic; wear nonlatex gloves; patches may be cut to size/shape; treatment may be repeated every 3 months
Pediatric: <18 years: not recommended
  Qutenza *Patch:* 8% 1640 mcg/cm (179 mg) (1 or 2 patches w. 1-50 g tube cleansing gel/carton)

▷ *lidocaine* 5% patch **(B)(G)** apply up to 3 patches at one time for up to 12 hours/24-hour period (12 hours on/12 hours off); patches may be cut into smaller sizes before removal of the release liner; do not re-use
Pediatric: not recommended
  Lidoderm *Patch:* 5% 10x14 cm (30 patches/carton)

ANTICONVULSANTS

Gamma Aminobutyric Acid Analog

▷ *gabapentin* **(C)**
Pediatric: <3 years: not recommended; 3-12 years: initially 10-15 mg/kg/day in 3 divided doses; max 12 hours between doses; titrate over 3 days; 3-4 years: titrate to 40 mg/kg/day; 5-12 years: titrate to 25-35 mg/kg/day; max 50 mg/kg/day
  Gralise (C) initially 300 mg on Day 1; then 600 mg on Day 2; then 900 mg on Days 3-6; then 1200 mg on Days 7-10; then 1500 mg on Days 11-14; titrate up to 1800 mg on Day 15; take entire dose once daily with the evening meal; do not crush, split, or chew
    Tab: 300, 600 mg
  Neurontin (G) *Tab:* 600*, 800* mg; *Cap:* 100, 300, 400 mg; *Oral soln:* 250 mg/5 ml (480 ml) (strawberry-anise)
▷ *gabapentin enacarbil* **(C)** 600 mg once daily at about 5:00 PM; if dose not taken at recommended time, next dose should be taken the following day; swallow whole; take with food; *CrCl 30-59 mL/min:* 600 mg on Day 1, Day 3, and every day thereafter; *CrCl <30 mL/min:* or on hemodialysis: not recommended
Pediatric: not recommended
  Horizant *Tab:* 300, 600 mg ext-rel
Comment: Avoid abrupt cessation of *gabapentin* and *gabapentin enacarbil*. To discontinue, withdraw gradually over 1 week or longer.
▷ *pregabalin* (*GABA analog*) **(C)(V)** initially 50 mg tid; may titrate to 100 mg tid within one week; max 600 mg divided tid; discontinue over 1 week
Pediatric: <18 years: not recommended
  Lyrica *Cap:* 25, 50, 75, 100, 150, 200, 225, 300 mg; *Oral soln:* 20 mg/ml

TRICYCLIC ANTIDEPRESSANTS (TCAs)

Comment: Co-administration of TCAs with SSRIs requires extreme caution.

▷ *amitriptyline* (C)(G) titrate to achieve pain relief; max 300 mg/day
   Pediatric: not recommended
      Tab: 10, 25, 50, 75, 100, 150 mg

▷ *amoxapine* (C) titrate to achieve pain relief; if total dose exceeds 300 mg/day, give
   in divided doses; max 400 mg/day
   Pediatric: not recommended
      Tab: 25, 50, 100, 150 mg

▷ *desipramine* (C)(G) titrate to achieve pain relief; max 300 mg/day
   Pediatric: not recommended
      Norpramin *Tab:* 10, 25, 50, 75, 100, 150 mg

▷ *doxepin* (C)(G) titrate to achieve pain relief; max 150 mg/day
   Pediatric: not recommended
      Cap: 10, 25, 50, 75, 100, 150 mg; *Oral conc:* 10 mg/ml (4 oz w. dropper)

▷ *imipramine* (C)(G)
   Pediatric: not recommended
      Tofranil titrate to achieve pain relief; max 200 mg/day; adolescents max 100
      mg/day; if maintenance dose exceeds 75 mg/day, may switch to **Tofranil PM** at
      bedtime
         Tab: 10, 25, 50 mg
      Tofranil PM titrate to achieve pain relief; initially 75 mg at HS; max 200 mg at HS
         Cap: 75, 100, 125, 150 mg
      Tofranil Injection 50 mg IM; lower dose for adolescents; switch to oral form as
      soon as possible
         Amp: 25 mg/2 ml (2 ml)

▷ *nortriptyline* (D)(G) titrate to achieve pain relief; initially 10-25 mg tid-qid; max
   150 mg/day; lower doses for elderly and adolescents
   Pediatric: not recommended
      Pamelor titrate to achieve pain relief; max 150 mg/day
         Cap: 10, 25, 50, 75 mg; *Oral soln:* 10 mg/5 ml (16 oz)

▷ *protriptyline* (C) titrate to achieve pain relief; initially 5 mg tid; max 60 mg/day
   Pediatric: <12 years: not recommended
      Vivactyl *Tab:* 5, 10 mg

▷ *trimipramine* (C) titrate to achieve pain relief; max 200 mg/day
   Pediatric: not recommended
      Surmontil *Cap:* 25, 50, 100 mg

◯ DIAPER RASH

Topical Corticosteroids *see page* 494
Comment: Low to intermediate potency topical corticosteroids are indicated if
inflammation is present.

PROTECTIVE BARRIERS

▷ *aloe/vitamin E/zinc oxide* (NR) ointment apply at each diaper change after thoroughly cleansing skin
      Balmex *Oint:* 2, 4 oz tube; 16 oz jar

➤ *vitamin A&D* **(NR)** **(G)** ointment apply at each diaper change after thoroughly cleansing skin
    A&D Ointment *Oint:* 1.5, 4 oz
➤ *zinc oxide* **(NR)(G)** cream and ointment apply at each diaper change after thoroughly cleansing the skin
    A&D Ointment with Zinc Oxide *Oint:* 10% (1.5, 4 oz)
    Desitin *Oint:* 40% (1, 2, 4, 9 oz)
    Desitin Cream *Crm:* 10% (2, 4 oz)

TOPICAL ANTIFUNGALS

Comment: Use if caused by *Candida albicans.*
➤ *butenafine* **(B)(G)** apply bid x 1 week or once daily x 4 weeks
    Pediatric: <12 years: not recommended
    Lotrimin Ultra (C)(OTC) *Crm:* 1% (12, 24 g)
    Mentax *Crm:* 1% (15, 30 g)
    Comment: *butenafine* is a benzylamine, not an azole. Fungicidal activity continues for at least 5 weeks after last application.
➤ *clotrimazole* **(B)** apply to affected area bid x 7 days
    Pediatric: same as adult
    Lotrimin (OTC) *Crm:* 1% (15, 30, 45 g)
    Lotrimin AF (OTC) *Crm:* 1% (12 g); *Lotn:* 1% (10 ml); *Soln:* 1% (10 ml)
➤ *econazole* **(C)** apply bid x 7 days
    Spectazole *Crm:* 1% (15, 30, 85 g)
➤ *ketoconazole* **(C)(G)**
    Nizoral Cream *Crm:* 2% (15, 30, 60 g)
➤ *miconazole* 2% **(C)(G)** apply bid x 7 days
    Pediatric: same as adult
    Lotrimin AF Spray Liquid (OTC) *Spray liq:* 2% (113 g) (alcohol 17%)
    Lotrimin AF Spray Powder (OTC) *Spray pwdr:* 2% (90 g) (alcohol 10%)
    Monistat-Derm *Crm:* 2% (1, 3 oz); *Spray liq:* 2% (3.5 oz); *Spray pwdr:* 2% (3 oz)
➤ *nystatin* **(C)(G)** apply bid x 7 days
    Mycostatin *Crm:* 100,000 U/g (15, 30 g)

COMBINATION AGENT

➤ *clotrimazole/betamethasone* **(C)(G)** cream apply bid x 7 days
    Lotrisone *Crm:* 15, 45 g

 DIARRHEA: ACUTE

➤ *attapulgite* **(C)**
    Donnagel (OTC) 30 ml after each loose stool; max 7 doses/day x 2 days
        Pediatric: <3 years: not recommended; 3-6 years: 7.5 ml; >6-12 years: 15 ml; >12 years: same as adult
        Liq: 600 mg/15 ml (120, 240 ml)

Donnagel Chewable Tab (OTC) 2 tabs after each loose stool; max 14 tabs/day
Pediatric: <3 years: not recommended; 3-6 years: 1/2 tab after each loose stool; max 7 doses /day; >6-12 years: 1 tab after each loose stool; max 7 tabs/day
Chew tab: 600 mg

Kaopectate (OTC) 30 ml after each loose stool; max 7 doses/day x 2 days
Pediatric: <3 years: not recommended; 3-6 years: 7.5 ml after each loose stool; >6-12 years: 15 ml after each loose stool; >12 years: same as adult
Liq: 600 mg/15 ml (120, 240 ml)

▷ *bismuth subsalicylate* (C; D in 3rd)(G)

Pepto-Bismol (OTC) 2 tabs or 30 ml q 30-60 minutes as needed; max 8 doses/day
Pediatric: <3 years (14-18 lb): 2.5 ml q 4 hours; max 6 doses/day; <3 years (18-28 lb): 5 ml q 4 hours; max 6 doses/day; 3-6 years: 1/3 tab or 5 ml q 30-60 minutes; max 8 doses/day; >6-9 years: 2/3 tab or 10 ml q 30-60 minutes; max 8 doses/day; >9-12 years: 1 tab or 15 ml q 30-60 minutes; max 8 doses/day
Chew tab: 262 mg; *Liq:* 262 mg/15 ml (4, 8, 12, 16 oz)

Pepto-Bismol Maximum Strength (OTC) 30 ml q 60 minutes; max 4 doses/day
Pediatric: <3 years: not recommended; 3-6 years: 5 ml q 60 minutes; max 4 doses/day; >6-9 years: 10 ml q 60 minutes; max 4 doses/day; >9-12 years: 15 ml q 60 minutes; max 4 doses/day
Liq: 525 mg/15 ml (4, 8, 12, 16 oz)

Comment: *aspirin*-containing medications are contraindicated with history of allergic-type reaction to *aspirin*, children and adolescents with *Varicella* or other viral illness, and 3rd trimester pregnancy.

▷ *calcium polycarbophil* (C)
Pediatric: <6 years: not recommended; 6-12 years: 1 tab daily qid; >12 years: same as adult

Fibercon (OTC) 2 tabs daily qid
Cplt: 625 mg

▷ *crofelmer* (C) 2 tabs once daily; swallow whole with or without food; do not crush or chew
Pediatric: not established

Fulyzaq
Tab: 125 mg del-rel

Comment: *crofelmer* is indicated for the symptomatic relief of non-infectious diarrhea in adult patients with HIV/AIDS on antiretroviral therapy.

▷ *difenoxin/atropine* (C)
Pediatric: <2 years: not recommended; ≥2 years: same as adult

Motofen 2 tabs, then 1 tab after each loose stool or 1 tab q 3-4 hours as needed; max 8 tab/day x 2 days
Tab: dif 1 mg/*atro* 0.025 mg

▷ *diphenoxylate/atropine* (C)(V)(G)
Pediatric: <2 years: not recommended; 2-12 years: initially 0.3-0.4 mg/kg/day in 4 divided doses; >12 years: same as adult

Lomotil 2 tabs or 10 ml qid until diarrhea is controlled
Tab: diphen 2.5 mg/*atrop* 0.025 mg; *Liq:* diphen 2.5 mg/*atrop* 0.025 mg per 5 ml (2 oz)

▷ *loperamide* (B)(OTC)(G)
Imodium 4 mg initially, then 2 mg after each loose stool; max 16 mg/day x 2 days

Pediatric: <5 years: not recommended; ≥5 years: same as adult
Cap: 2 mg

Imodium A-D 4 mg initially, then 2 mg after each loose stool; usual max 8 mg/day x 2 days
Pediatric: <2 years: not recommended; 2-5 years (24-47 lb): 1 mg up to tid x 2 days; 6-8 years (48-59 lb): 2 mg initially, then 1 mg after after each loose stool; max 4 mg/day x 2 days; 9-11 years (60-95 lb): 2 mg initially, then 1 mg after each loose stool; max 6 mg/day x 2 days
Cplt: 2 mg; *Liq:* 1 mg/5 ml (2, 4 oz) (cherry-mint) (alcohol 0.5%)

➤ *loperamide/simethicone* (B)(OTC)(G)
Imodium Advanced 2 tabs chewed after loose stool, then 1 after the next loose stool; max 4 tabs/day
Pediatric: 6-8 years: chew 1 tab after loose stool, then chew 1/2 tab after next loose stool; 9-11 years: chew 1 tab after loose stool, then chew 1/2 tab after next loose stool; max 3 tabs/day; ≥12 years: same as adult
Chew tab: *loper* 2 mg/*simeth* 125 mg (vanilla-mint)

ORAL REHYDRATION AND ELECTROLYTE REPLACEMENT THERAPY

➤ *oral electrolyte replacement* (NR)(OTC)
CeraLyte 50 dissolve in 8 oz water
Pediatric: <4 years: not indicated; ≥4 years, same as adult
Pkt: *sodium* 50 mEq/*potassium* 20 mEq/*chloride* 40 mEq/*citrate* 30 mEq/*rice syrup solids* 40 g/*calories* 190 per liter (mixed berry) (gluten-free)
CeraLyte 70 dissolved in 8 oz water
Pediatric: <4 years: not indicated; ≥4 years: same as adult
Pkt: *sodium* 70 mEq/*potassium* 20 mEq/*chloride* 60 mEq/*citrate* 30 mEq/*rice syrup solids* 40 g/*calories* 165 per liter (natural or lemon) (gluten-free)
KaoLectrolyte 1 pkt dissolved in 8 oz water q 3-4 hours
Pediatric: <2 years: not indicated; ≥2 years: same as adult
Pkt: *sod* 12 mEq/*pot* 5 mEq/*chlor* 10 mEq/*citrate* 7 mEq/*dextrose* 5 g/calories 22 per 6.2 g
Pedialyte
Pediatric: <2 years: as desired and as tolerated; ≥2 years: 1-2 L/day
Oral soln: *dextrose* 20 g/*fructose* 5 g/*sodium* 25 mEq/*potassium* 20 mEq/*chloride* 35 mEq/*citrate* 30 mEq/*calories* 100 per liter (8 oz, 1 L)
Pedialyte Freezer Pops
Pediatric: as desired and as tolerated
Pops: *dextrose* 1.6 g/*sodium* 2.8 mEq/*potassium* 1.25 mEq/*chloride* 2.2 mEq/*citrate* 1.88 mEq/*calories* 6.25 per 6.25 ml pop (8 oz, 1 L)

◯ DIARRHEA: CHRONIC

➤ *cholestyramine* (C)
Questran Powder for Oral Suspension initially 1 pkt or scoop daily; usual maintenance 2-4 pkts or scoops daily in 2 doses; max 6 pkts or scoops daily
Oral pwdr: 9 g pkts; 9 g equal 4 g *anhydrous cholestyramine resin* (60/pck); *Bulk can:* 378 g w. scoop

Questran Light initially 1 pkt or scoop daily; usual maintenance 2-4 pkts or scoops daily in 2 doses

Light: 5 g pkts; 5 g equals 4 g *anhydrous cholestyramine resin* (60/pck); *Bulk can:* 210 g w. scoop

Comment: Use *cholestyramine* only if diarrhea is due to bile salt malabsorption.

▶ *crofelmer* (C) 2 tabs daily; swallow whole with or without food; do not crush or chew
Pediatric: not recommended

Fulyzaq

Tab: 125 mg del-rel

Comment: *crofelmer* is indicated for the symptomatic relief of non-infectious diarrhea in adult patients with HIV/AIDS on antiretroviral therapy.

▶ *difenoxin/atropine* (C)
Pediatric: <2 years: not recommended; ≥2 years: same as adult

Motofen 2 tabs, then 1 tab after each loose stool or 1 tab q 3-4 hours prn; max 8 tab/day x 2 days

Tab: dif 1 mg/atrop 0.025 mg

▶ *diphenoxylate/atropine* (B)(V)(G)
Pediatric: <2 years: not recommended; 2-12 years: initially 0.3-0.4 mg/kg/day in 4 divided doses; >12 years: same as adult

Lomotil 5-20 mg/day in divided doses

Tab: diphen 2.5 mg/atrop 0.025 mg; *Liq:* diphen 2.5 mg/atrop 0.025 mg per 5 ml (2 oz w. dropper)

▶ *attapulgite* (C)(G)

Donnagel (OTC) 30 ml after each loose stool; max 7 doses/day

Pediatric: <2 years: not recommended; 2-6 years: 7.5 ml after each loose stool; >6 years: same as adult

Liq: 600 mg/15 ml (120, 240 ml)

Donnagel Chewable Tab 2 tabs after each loose stool; max 14 tabs/day

Pediatric: <3 years: not recommended; 3-6 years: 1/2 tab after each stool; max 7 doses/day; >6-12 years: 1 tab after each loose stool; max 7 tabs/day; >12 years: same as adult

▶ *loperamide* (B)(OTC)(G)

Imodium (OTC) 4-16 mg/day in divided doses

Pediatric: <5 years: not recommended; ≥5 years: same as adult

Cap: 2 mg

Imodium A-D (OTC) 4-16 mg/day in divided doses

Pediatric: <2 years: not recommended; 2-5 years (24-47 lb): 1 mg up to tid x 2 days; 6-8 years (48-59 lb): 2 mg initially, then 1 mg after after each loose stool; max 4 mg/day x 2 days; 9-11 years (60-95 lb): 2 mg initially, then 1 mg after each loose stool; max 6 mg/day x 2 days; ≥12 years: same as adult

Cplt: 2 mg; *Liq:* 1 mg/5 ml (2, 4 oz)

▶ *loperamide/simethicone* (B)(OTC)(G)

Imodium Advanced 2 tabs chewed after loose stool, then 1 after the next loose stool; max 4 tabs/day

Pediatric: 6-8 years: chew 1 tab after loose stool, then chew 1/2 tab after next loose stool; 9-11 years: chew 1 tab after loose stool, then chew 1/2 tab after next loose stool; max 3 tabs/ day

Chew tab: loper 2 mg/simeth 125 mg

DIARRHEA: TRAVELERS

▷ *ciprofloxacin* (C) 500 mg bid x 3 days
Pediatric: <18 years: not recommended
    Cipro (G) *Tab:* 250, 500, 750 mg; *Oral susp:* 250, 500 mg/5 ml (100 ml) (strawberry)
    Cipro XR *Tab:* 500, 1000 mg ext-rel
    ProQuin XR *Tab:* 500 mg ext-rel
    Comment: *ciprofloxacin* is contraindicated <18 years-of-age, and during pregnancy and lactation. Risk of tendonitis or tendon rupture, especially 60 years-of-age and older.
▷ *rifaximin* (C) 200 mg tid x 3 days; discontinue if diarrhea worsens <u>or</u> persists more than 24 hours; not for use if diarrhea is accompanied by fever <u>or</u> blood in the stool <u>or</u> if causative organism other than *E. coli* is suspected.
Pediatric: <12 years: not recommended; ≥12 years: same as adult
    Xifaxan *Tab:* 200 mg
▷ *trimethoprim/sulfamethoxazole* (C)(G) bid x 10 days
Pediatric: <2 months: not recommended; >2 months: 40 mg/kg/day of *sulfamethoxazole* in 2 divided doses x 10 days; *see page 576 for dose by weight*
    Bactrim, Septra 2 tabs bid x 10 days
    Tab: trim 80 mg/*sulfa* 400 mg*
    Bactrim DS, Septra DS 1 tab bid x 10 days
    Tab: trim 160 mg/*sulfa* 800 mg*
    Bactrim Pediatric Suspension, Septra Pediatric Suspension
    Oral susp: trim 40 mg/*sulfa* 200 mg per 5 ml (100 ml) (cherry) (alcohol 0.3%)
    Comment: *trimethoprim/sulfamethoxazole* is not recommended in pregnancy <u>or</u> lactation. *CrCl 15-30 mL/min:* reduce dose by 1/2; *CrCl <15 mL/min:* not recommended

DIGITALIS TOXICITY

Comment: The digitalis therapeutic index is narrow, 0.8-1.2 ng/mL. Whether acute <u>or</u> chronic toxicity, the patient should be treated in the emergency department <u>and/or</u> admitted to in-patient service for continued monitoring and care. Signs and symptoms of digitalis toxicity include: loss of appetite, nausea, vomiting, abdominal pain, diarrhea, visiual disturbances (diplopia, blurred, <u>or</u> yellow vision, yellow-green halos around lights and other visual images, spots, blind spots), decreased urine output, generalized edema, orthopnea, confusion, delerium, decreased consciousness, potentially lethal cardiac arrhythmias (ranging from ventricular tachycardia (VT) and ventricular fibrillation (VF) to sino-atrial heart block AVB). Treatment measures include repeated doses of charcoal via NG tube administered after gastric lavage for acute ingestion (methods to induce vomiting are usually discouraged because vomiting can worsen bradyarrhythmias), digitalis binders. Monitoring includes: serial ECGs, serum digitalis level, chemistries, potassium (hyperkalemia), magnesium (hypomagnesemia), BUN and creatinine.

DIGOXIN BINDER

▷ *digoxin (immune fab [ovine])*(B)
    Digibind contents of one vial of **Digibind** neutralizes 0.5 mg digoxin; dose based on amount of *digoxin* <u>or</u> *digitoxin* to be neutralized; see mfr literature

Pediatric: see mfr literature
Vial: 38 mg

Digifab dose is based on amount of digoxin or digitoxin to be neutralized (see mfr literature for dosage; contents of 1 vial neutralizes 0.5 mg digoxin.
Pediatric: see mfr literature
Vial: 40 mg for IV injection after reconstitution (preservative-free)

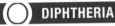

DIPHTHERIA

Prophylaxis *see Childhood Immunizations page* 466

POSTEXPOSURE PROPHYLAXIS FOR NON-IMMUNIZED PERSONS

▷ *erythromycin base* (B)(G) 500 mg qid x 14 days
Pediatric: <45 kg: 50 mg/kg/day in 4 divided doses x 14 days; ≥45 kg: same as adult
Ery-Tab *Tab:* 250, 333, 500 mg ent-coat
PCE *Tab:* 333, 500 mg
Comment: *erythromycin* may increase INR with concomitant *warfarin*, as well as increase serum level of *digoxin*, benzodiazepines and statins.

▷ *erythromycin ethylsuccinate* (B)(G) 400 mg qid x 14 days
Pediatric: 30-50 mg/kg/day in 4 divided doses x 14 days; may double dose with severe infection; max 100 mg/kg/day; *see page 563 for dose by weight*
EryPed *Oral susp:* 200 mg/5 ml (100, 200 ml) (fruit); 400 mg/5 ml (60, 100, 200 ml) (banana); *Oral drops:* 200, 400 mg/5 ml (50 ml) (fruit); *Chew tab:* 200 mg wafer (fruit)
E.E.S. *Oral susp:* 200, 400 mg/5 ml (100 ml) (fruit)
E.E.S. Granules *Oral susp:* 200 mg/5 ml (100, 200 ml) (cherry)
E.E.S. 400 Tablets *Tab:* 400 mg
Comment: *erythromycin* may increase INR with concomitant *warfarin*, as well as increase serum level of *digoxin*, benzodiazepines and statins.

▷ *Immunization Series*
see Childhood Immunizations page 466

POSTEXPOSURE PROPHYLAXIS FOR IMMUNIZED PERSONS

▷ *Diphtheria* immunization booster

DIVERTICULITIS

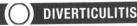

▷ *amoxicillin* (B)(G) 500 mg q 8 hours or 875 mg q 12 hours x 7 days
Amoxil *Cap:* 250, 500 mg; *Tab:* 875*mg; *Chew tab:* 125, 200, 250, 400 mg (cherry-banana-peppermint) (phenylalanine); *Oral susp:* 125, 250 mg/5 ml (80, 100, 150 ml) (strawberry); 200, 400 mg/5 ml (50, 75, 100 ml) (bubble gum); *Oral drops:* 50 mg/ml (30 ml) (bubble gum)
Moxatag *Tab:* 775 mg ext-rel

Trimox *Tab:* 125, 250 mg; *Cap:* 250, 500 mg; *Oral susp:* 125, 250 mg/5 ml (80, 100, 150 ml) (raspberry-strawberry)

▶ *amoxicillin/clavulanate* (B)(G) 500 mg tid or 875 mg bid x 10 days

Augmentin *Tab:* 250, 500, 875 mg; *Chew tab:* 125, 250 mg (lemon-lime); 200, 400 mg (cherry-banana) (phenylalanine); *Oral susp:* 125 mg/5 ml (banana), 250 mg/5 ml (75, 100, 150 ml) (orange); 200, 400 mg/5 ml (50, 75, 100 ml) (orange) (phenylalanine)

Pediatric: 40-45 mg/kg/day divided tid x 10 days or 90 mg/kg/day divided bid x 10 days *see pages 545-546 for dose by weight*

Augmentin ES-600 *Oral susp:* 600 mg/5 ml (50, 75, 100, 125, 150, 200 ml) (strawberry cream) (phenylalanine) every 12 hours

Pediatric: <3 months: not recommended; ≥3 months, <40 kg: 90 mg/kg/day in 2 divided doses; ≥40 kg: not recommended

Augmentin XR 2 tabs q 12 hours x 7-10 days

Pediatric: <16 years: use other forms; ≥16 years: same as adult

Tab: 1000*mg ext-rel

▶ *ciprofloxacin* (C) 500 mg bid x 7 days

Cipro (G) *Tab:* 250, 500, 750 mg; *Oral susp:* 250, 500 mg/5 ml (100 ml) (strawberry)

Cipro XR *Tab:* 500, 1000 mg ext-rel

ProQuin XR *Tab:* 500 mg ext-rel

Comment: *ciprofloxacin* is contraindicated <18 years-of-age, and during pregnancy and lactation. Risk of tendonitis or tendon rupture, especially 60 years-of-age and older.

▶ *metronidazole* (not for use in 1st; B in 2nd, 3rd)(G) 250-500 mg q 8 hours or 750 mg q 12 hours x 7 days

Flagyl *Tab:* 250*, 500*mg

Flagyl 375 *Cap:* 375 mg

Flagyl ER *Tab:* 750 mg ext-rel

Comment: Alcohol is contraindicated during treatment with oral *metronidazole* and for 72 hours after therapy due to a possible *disulfiram*-like reaction (nausea, vomiting, flushing, headache).

▶ *trimethoprim/sulfamethoxazole* (D)(G) bid x 7 days

Bactrim, Septra 2 tabs bid x 7 days

Tab: trim 80 mg/*sulfa* 400 mg*

Bactrim DS, Septra DS 1 tab bid x 7 days

Tab: trim 160 mg/*sulfa* 800 mg*

Bactrim Pediatric Suspension, Septra Pediatric Suspension 20 ml bid x 7 days

Oral susp: trim 40 mg/sulfa 200 mg per 5 ml (100 ml) (cherry) (alcohol 0.3%)

Comment: *trimethoprim/sulfamethoxazole* is not recommended in pregnancy or lactation. *CrCl 15-30 mL/min:* reduce dose by 1/2; *CrCl <15 mL/min:* not recommended

 DIVERTICULOSIS

BULK-PRODUCING AGENTS

see Constipation page 95

DRY EYE SYNDROME

OPHTHALMIC IMMUNOMODULATOR/ANTI-INFLAMMATORY

▷ *cyclosporine* (C) 1 drop q 12 hours
  Pediatric: <16 years: not recommended
    Restasis *Ophth emul:* 0.05% (0.4 ml) (preservative-free)
Comment: Ophthalmic Immunomodulators are contraindicated with active ocular infection. Allow at least 15 minutes between doses of artificial tears. May re-insert contact lenses 15 minutes after treatment.

OCULAR LUBRICANTS

Comment: Remove contact lens prior to using an ocular lubricant.
▷ *dextran 70/hypromellose* (NR) 1-2 drops prn
  Pediatric: same as adult
    Bion Tears (OTC) *Ophth soln:* single-use containers (28/pck) (preservative-free)
▷ *hydroxypropyl cellulose* (NR) apply 1/2 inch ribbon <u>or</u> 1 insert in each inferior cul-de-sac 1-2 times/day prn
  Pediatric: same as adult
    Lacrisert *Ophth inserts:* 5 mg (60/pck) (preservative-free)
    Hypotears Ophthalmic Ointment (OTC) *Ophth oint:* 1% (3.5 g)
    (preservative-free)
Comment: Place insert in the inferior cul-de-sac of the eye, beneath the base of the tarsus, not in apposition to the cornea nor beneath the eyelid at the level of the tarsal plate.
▷ *hydroxypropyl methylcellulose* (NR) 1-2 drops prn
  Pediatric: same as adult
    GenTeal Mild, GenTeal Moderate (OTC) *Ophth soln:* (15 ml) (perborate)
    GenTeal Severe (OTC) *Ophth soln:* (15 ml) (carbopol 980, perborate)
▷ *petrolatum/mineral oil* (NR) apply 1/2 inch ribbon prn
  Pediatric: same as adult
    Hypotears Ophthalmic Ointment (OTC) *Ophth oint:* 1% (3.5 g) (benzalkonium chloride, alcohol 1%)
    Hypotears PF Ophthalmic Ointment (OTC) *Ophth oint:* 1% (3.5 g) (preservative-free, alcohol 1%)
    Lacri-Lube (OTC) *Ophth oint:* 1% (3.5, 7 g)
    Lacri-Lube NP (OTC) *Ophth oint:* 1% (0.7 g, 24/pck) (preservative-free)
▷ *petrolatum/lanolin/mineral oil* (NR) apply 1/4 inch ribbon prn
  Pediatric: same as adult
    Duratears Naturale (OTC) *Ophth oint:* 3.5 g (preservative-free)
▷ *polyethylene glycol/glycerin/hydroxypropyl methylcellulose* (NR) 1-2 drops prn
  Pediatric: same as adult
    Visine Tears (OTC) *Ophth soln:* 1% (15, 30 ml)
▷ *polyethylene glycol* 400 0.4%/*propylene glycol* 0.3% (NR) 1-2 drops prn
  Pediatric: same as adult
    Systane (OTC) *Ophth soln:* (15, 30, 40 ml) (polyquaternium-1, zinc chloride); *Vial:* 0.01 oz (28) (preservative-free)
    Systane Ultra (OTC) *Ophth soln:* (10, 20 ml) (aminomethylpropanol, polyquaternium-1, sorbitol (zinc chloride); *Vial:* 0.01 oz (24) (preservative-free)

▷ *polyvinyl alcohol* (NR) 1-2 drops prn
  Pediatric: same as adult
    Hypotears (OTC) *Ophth soln:* 1% (15, 30 ml)
    Hypotears PF (OTC) 1-2 drops q 3-4 hours prn
      Ophth soln: 1% (0.02 oz single-use containers, 30/pck) (preservative-free)
▷ *propylene glycol* 0.6% (NR) 1-2 drops prn
  Pediatric: same as adult
    Systane Balance (OTC) *Ophth soln:* (10 ml) (polyquaternium-1)

DYSHIDROSIS

Topical Corticosteroids *see page 494*
Comment: Intermediate to high potency ophthalmic steroid treatment is indicated for dyshidrosis.

DYSFUNCTIONAL UTERINE BLEEDING (DUB)

▷ *medroxyprogesterone acetate* (X) 10 mg daily x 10-13 days
  Provera *Tab:* 2.5, 5, 10 mg
▷ *Oral contraceptives* (X) with 35 mcg estrogen equivalent
see **Combined Oral Contraceptives** *page 474*
Oral Prescription NSAIDs *see page 489*
Other Oral Analgesics *see* **Pain** *page 298*

DYSLIPIDEMIA (HYPERCHOLESTEROLEMIA, HYPERLIPIDEMIA, MIXED DYSLIPIDEMIA)

OMEGA 3-ACID ETHYL ESTERS

▷ *omega 3-acid ethyl esters* (C)(G) 2 g bid or 4 g once daily
  Pediatric: <18 years: not recommended
    Lovaza *Soft gel cap:* 1 g (α-tocopherol 4 mg/cap)

MICROSOMAL TRIGLYCERIDE-TRANSFER PROTEIN (MTP) INHIBITOR

▷ *lomitapide mesylate* (X) 10 mg daily
  Pediatric: not established
    Juxtapid *Cap:* 5, 10, 20 mg
    Comment: **Juxtapid** is an adjunct to low-fat diet and other lipid-lowering treatments, including LDL apheresis where available, to reduce LDL-C, total cholesterol, apoB, and non-HDL-C in patients with homozygous familial hypercholesterolemia (HoFH); not for patients with hypercholesterolemia who do not have HoFH.

OLIGONUCLEOTIDE INHIBITOR OF APO B-100 SYNTHESIS

▷ *mipomersen* (B) administer 200 mg SC once weekly, on the same day, in the upper arm, abdomen, or thigh; administer 1st injection under appropriate professional supervision
  Pediatric: not established

Kynamro *Vial/Prefilled syringe:* 200 mg mg/ml soln for SC inj single-use vial (preservative-free)
Comment: **Kynamro** is an adjunct to low-fat diet and other lipid-lowering treatments, to reduce LDL-C, apo-B, total cholesterol (TC), non-HDL-C in patients with homozygous familial hypercholesterolemia (HoFH).

CHOLESTEROL ABSORPTION INHIBITOR

▷ *ezetimibe* (C)(G) 10 mg daily
    Pediatric: <10 years: not recommended; ≥10 years: same as adult
    Zetia *Tab:* 10 mg
Comment: *ezetimibe* is contraindicated with concomitant statins in liver disease, persistent elevations in serum transaminase, pregnancy, and nursing mothers. Concomitant fibrates are not recommended. Potentiated by *fenofibrate, gemfibrozil,* and possibly *cyclosporine.* Separate dosing of bile acid sequestrants is required; take *ezetimibe* at least 2 hours before or 4 hours after.

PROPROTEIN CONVERTASE SUBTILISIN KEXIN TYPE 9 (PCSK9) INHIBITOR

Comment: PCSK9 inhibitors are an adjunct to maximally tolerated statin therapy in persons who require additional lowering of LDL-C.
▷ *alirocumab* (NR)
    Pediatric: not established
    Praluent administer SC in the upper outer arm, abdomen, or thigh; initially 75 mg SC once every 2 weeks; measure LDL 4-8 weeks after initiation or titration; if inadequate response, may increase to 150 mg SC every 2 weeks
        Soln for SC inj: 75, 150 mg/ml single-use prefilled syringe (preservative-free)
    Comment: Although **Praluent**, does not have an assigned pregnancy category, it is contraindicated in the 2nd and 3rd trimester of pregnancy.
▷ *evolocumab* (NR)
    Pediatric: HeFH, primary hyperlipidemia: not established; HoFH: <13 years: not established; >13 years: same as adult
    Repatha administer SC in the upper outer arm, elbow, or thigh; measure LDL 4-8 weeks after initiation; *HeFH or primary hyperlipidemia:* 140 mg SC once every 2 weeks or 420 mg once monthly; *HoFH:* 420 mg once monthly
        Soln for SC inj: single-use prefilled syringe; 140 mg/syringe; single-use pre-filled SureClick autoinjector (140 mg/syringe preservative-free)
    Comment: To administer 420 mg of **Repatha**, administer 150 mg SC x 3 within 30 minutes. Although **Repatha**, does not have an assigned pregnancy category, it is contraindicated in pregnancy.

HMG-COA REDUCTASE INHIBITORS (STATINS)

Comment: The statins decrease total cholesterol, LDL-C, TG, and apo-B, and increase HDL-C. Before initiating and at 4-6 weeks, 3 months, and 6 months of therapy, check fasting lipid profile and LFTs. Side effects include myopathy and increased liver enzymes. Relative contraindications include concomitant use of cyclosporine, a macrolide antibiotic, various oral antifungal agents, and CYP-450 inhibitors. An absolute contraindication is active or chronic liver disease.
▷ *atorvastatin* (X)(G) initially 10 mg daily; usual range 10-80 mg/day
    Pediatric: <10 years: not recommended; ≥10 years (female post-menarche): same as adult

       Lipitor *Tab:* 10, 20, 40, 80 mg

▷ *fluvastatin* **(X)(G)** initially 20-40 mg q HS; usual range 20-80 mg/day
    Pediatric: <18 years: not recommended
        Lescol *Cap:* 20, 40 mg
        Lescol XL *Tab:* 80 mg ext-rel

▷ *lovastatin* **(X)**
        Mevacor initially 20 mg daily at evening meal; may increase at 4-week intervals; max 80 mg/day in single or divided doses; if concomitant fibrates, niacin, or CrCl <30 mL/min, usual max 20 mg/day
          Pediatric: <10 years: not recommended; 10-17 years: initially 10-20 mg daily at evening meal; may increase at 4-week intervals; max 40 mg daily
          Tab: 10, 20, 40 mg
        Altoprev initially 20 mg daily at evening meal; may increase at 4-week intervals; max 60 mg/day; if concomitant fibrates, or *niacin*; >1 g/day, usual max 40 mg/day; if concomitant cyclosporine, *amiodarone*, or *verapamil*, or CrCl <30 mL/min, usual max 20 mg/day
          Pediatric: <20 years: not recommended
          Tab: 10, 20, 40, 60 mg ext-rel

▷ *pitavastatin* **(X)** initially 2 mg q HS; may increase to 4 mg after 4 weeks; max 4 mg/day; if concomitant *erythromycin* or CrCl <60 ml/min; 1 mg/day with usual max 2 mg/day; if concomitant rifampin, max 2 mg once daily
    Pediatric: not established
        Livalo *Tab:* 1, 2, 4 mg

▷ *pravastatin* **(X)** initially 10-20 mg q HS; usual range 10-40 mg/day; may start at 40 mg/day
    Pediatric: <8 years: not recommended; 8-13 years: 20 mg daily; 14-18 years: 40 mg daily
        Pravachol *Tab:* 10, 20, 40, 80 mg

▷ *rosuvastatin* **(X)(G)** initially 10-20 mg q HS; usual range 5-40 mg/day; adjust at 4-week intervals
    Pediatric: <10 years: not recommended; 10-17 years: 5-20 mg/day; max 20 mg/day
        Crestor *Tab:* 5, 10, 20, 40 mg

▷ *simvastatin* **(X)** initially 20 mg q PM; usual range 5-80 mg/day; adjust at 4-week intervals
    Pediatric: <10 years: not recommended; ≥10 years (female postmenarche): same as adult
        Zocor *Tab:* 5, 10, 20, 40, 80 mg

CHOLESTEROL ABSORPTION INHIBITOR/HMG-COA REDUCTASE INHIBITOR COMBINATION

▷ *ezetimibe/simvastatin* **(X)(G)** Take once daily in the PM; may start at 10/40; swallow whole
    Pediatric: <17 years: not recommended
    Tab: **Vytorin 10/10** *ezet* 10 mg/*simva* 10 mg
        Vytorin 10/20 *ezet* 10 mg/*simva* 20 mg
        Vytorin 10/40 *ezet* 10 mg/*simva* 40 mg
        Vytorin 10/80 *ezet* 10 mg/*simva* 80 mg

ISOBUTYRIC ACID DERIVATIVES AND FIBRATE

Comment: These agents decrease total cholesterol, LDL-C, and TG; increase HDL-C. They are indicated when the primary problem is very high TG level. Side effects include epigastric discomfort, dyspepsia, abdominal pain, cholelithiasis, myopathy, and neutropenia. Before initiating, and at 4-6 weeks, 3 months, and 6 months of therapy, check fasting CBC, lipid profile, LFT, and serum creatinine. Absolute contraindications include severe renal disease and severe hepatic disease.

ISOBUTYRIC ACID DERIVATIVES

➢ *gemfibrozil* (C)(G) 600 mg bid 30 minutes before AM and PM meal
   Pediatric: not recommended
     Lopid *Tab:* 600*mg

FIBRATES (FIBRIC ACID DERIVATIVES)

➢ *fenofibrate* (C) take with meals; adjust at 4- to 8-week intervals; discontinue if inadequate response after 2 months; lowest dose or contraindicated with renal impairment and the elderly
   Pediatric: not recommended
     Antara (G) 43-130 mg daily; max 130 mg/day
       Cap: 43, 87, 130 mg
     FibriCor 30-105 mg daily; max 105 mg/day
       Tab: 30, 105 mg
     TriCor (G) 48-145 mg daily; max 145 mg/day
       Tab: 48, 145 mg
     TriLipix (G) 45-135 mg daily; max 135 mg/day
       Cap: 45, 135 mg del-rel
     Lipofen (G) 50-150 mg daily; max 150 mg/day
       Cap: 50, 150 mg
     Lofibra 67-200 mg daily; max 200 mg/day
       Tab: 67, 134, 200 mg

NICOTINIC ACID DERIVATIVES

Comment: Nicotinic acid derivatives decrease total cholesterol, LDL-C, and TG; increase HDL-C. Before initiating and at 4-6 weeks, 3 months, and 6 months of therapy, check fasting lipid profile, LFT, glucose, and uric acid. Side effects include hyperglycemia, upper GI distress, hyperuricemia, hepatotoxicity, and significant transient skin flushing. Take with food and take *aspirin* 325 mg 30 minutes before dose to decrease flushing. Relative contraindications include diabetes, hyperuricemia (gout), and PUD and absolute contraindications include severe gout and chronic liver disease.

➢ *niacin* (C)
     Niaspan (G) 375 mg daily for 1st week, then 500 mg daily for 2nd week, then 750 mg daily for 3rd week, then 1 g daily for weeks 4-7; may increase by 500 mg q 4 weeks; usual range 1-2 g/day; max 2 g/day
       Pediatric: <21 years: not recommended
       Tab: 500, 750, 1000 mg ext-rel
     Slo-Niacin one 250 or 500 mg tab q AM or HS or one-half 750 mg tab q AM or HS
       Pediatric: not recommended
       Tab: 250, 500, 750 mg cont-rel

BILE ACID SEQUESTRANTS

Comment: Bile acid sequestrants decrease total cholesterol, LDL-C, and increase HDL-C, but have no effect on triglycerides. A relative contraindication is TG ≥200 mg/dL and an absolute contraindication is TG ≥400 mg/dL. Before initiating and at 4-6 weeks, 3 months, and 6 months of therapy, check fasting lipid profile. Side effects include sandy taste in mouth, abdominal gas, abdominal cramping, and constipation. These agents decrease the absorption of many other drugs.

▷ *cholestyramine* (C)

Pediatric: see mfr literature

Questran Powder for Oral Suspension initially 1 pkt or scoop daily; usual maintenance 2-4 pkts or scoops daily in 2 divided doses; max 6 pkts or scoops daily

Pwdr: 9 g pkts; 9 g equals 4 g anhydrous *cholestyramine* resin for reconstitution (60/pck); *Bulk can:* 378 g w. scoop

Questran Light initially 1 pkt or scoop daily; usual maintenance 2-4 pkts or scoops daily in 2 doses

Light: 5 g pkts; 5 g equals 4 g anhydrous *cholestyramine* resin (60/pck): *Bulk can:* 210 g w. scoop

▷ *colesevelam* (B)

Monotherapy: 3 tabs bid or 6 tabs once daily or one 1.875 g pkt bid or one 3.75 g pkt once daily

Pediatric: not recommended

WelChol *Tab:* 625 mg; *Pwdr for oral susp:* 1.875 g pwdr pkts (60/carton); 3.75 g pwdr pkts (30/carton) (citrus; phenylalanine)

Comment: **WelChol** is indicated as adjunctive therapy to improve glycemic control in adults with type 2 diabetes. It can be added to metformin, sulfonylureas, or insulin alone or in combination with other antidiabetic agents

▷ *colestipol* (C)

Pediatric: not recommended

Colestid tabs: 2-16 g daily in a single or divided doses; granules: 5-30 g daily in a single or divided dose

Tabs: 1 g (120); *Granules:* unflavored: 5 g pkt (30, 90/carton); unflavored bulk: 300, 500 g w. scoop; orange-flavored: 7.5 g pkt (60/carton) (aspartame); orange-flavored bulk: 450 g w. scoop (aspartame) flavored: 7.5 g pkt; flavored bulk: 450 g w. scoop

Colestid Tab initially 2 g bid; increase by 2 g bid at 1-2-month intervals; usual maintenance 2-16 g/day

Tab: 1 g

Comment: *colestipol* lowers LDL and total cholesterol.

ANTILIPID COMBINATIONS

Nicotinic Acid Derivative/HMG-CoA Reductase Inhibitors

▷ *niacin/lovastatin* (X)

Pediatric: <18 years: not recommended

Advicor swallow whole at bedtime with a low-fat snack; may pretreat with aspirin; start at lowest niacin dose; may titrate niacin by no more than 500 mg/day every 4 weeks; max 2000/40 daily

Tab: **Advicor 500/20** *nia* 500 mg ext-rel/*lova* 20 mg

Advicor 750/20 *nia* 750 mg ext-rel/*lova* 20 mg

Advicor 1000/20 *nia* 1000 mg ext-rel/*lova* 20 mg
Advicor 1000/40 *nia* 1000 mg ext-rel/*lova* 40 mg

▷ *niacin/simvastatin* (X)
 Pediatric: <18 years: not recommended
  Simcor swallow whole at bedtime with a low-fat snack; may pretreat with
  aspirin; start at lowest *niacin* dose; may titrate *niacin* by no more than 500 mg/
  day every 4 weeks; max 2000/40 daily
   Tab: **Simcor 500/20** *nia* 500 mg ext-rel/*simva* 20 mg
     Simcor 750/20 *nia* 750 mg ext-rel/*simva* 20 mg
     Simcor 1000/20 *nia* 1000 mg ext-rel/*simva* 20 mg
     Simcor 500/40 *nia* 500 mg ext-rel/*simva* 40 mg
     Simcor 1000/40 *nia* 1000 mg ext-rel/*simva* 40 mg

ANTIHYPERTENSIVE/ANTILIPID COMBINATIONS

Calcium Channel Blocker/HMG-CoA Reductase Inhibitor (Statin) Combinations

▷ *amlodipine/atorvastatin* (X)(G)
  Caduet select according to blood pressure and lipid values; titrate amlodipine over 7-14 days; titrate atorvastatin according to monitored lipid values; max amlodipine 10 mg/day and max atorvastatin 80 mg/day; refer to
  contraindications and precautions for CCB and statin therapy
   Pediatric: <10 years: not recommended; ≥10 years (female, post-menarche):
   same as adult
   Tab: **Caduet 5/10** amlo 5 mg/ator 10 mg
     Caduet 5/20 *amlo* 5 mg/*ator* 20 mg
     Caduet 5/40 *amlo* 5 mg/*ator* 40 mg
     Caduet 5/80 *amlo* 5 mg/*ator* 80 mg
     Caduet 10/10 *amlo* 10 mg/*ator* 10 mg
     Caduet 10/20 *amlo* 10 mg/*ator* 20 mg
     Caduet 10/40 *amlo* 10 mg/*ator* 40 mg
     Caduet 10/80 *amlo* 10 mg/*ator* 80 mg

 DYSMENORRHEA: PRIMARY

Acetaminophen for IV Infusion *see Pain page 296*
Oral Prescription NSAIDs *see page 489*
Other Oral Analgesics *see Pain page 298*

BENZENEACETIC ACID DERIVATIVE

▷ *diclofenac* (C) 50-100 mg once; then 50 tid
 Pediatric: <14 years: not recommended; ≥14 years: same as adult
  Cataflam *Tab:* 50 mg
  Voltaren *Tab:* 25, 50, 75 mg ent-coat
  Voltaren-XR *Tab:* 100 mg ext-rel
 Comment: *diclofenac* is contraindicated with *aspirin* allergy and late (≥30 weeks)
 pregnancy.

FENAMATE

▷ *mefenamic acid* (C) 500 mg once; then 250 mg q 6 hours for up to 2-3 days; take with food
  Pediatric: <14 years: not recommended
    Ponstel *Cap:* 250 mg
Comment: Avoid *aspirin* with a fenamate.

COX-2 INHIBITORS

Comment: Cox-2 inhibitors are contraindicated with history of asthma, urticaria, and allergic-type reactions to *aspirin*, other NSAIDs, and sulfonamides, 3rd trimester of pregnancy, and coronary artery bypass graft (CABG) surgery.
▷ *celecoxib* (C)(G) 400 mg x 1 dose; then 200 mg more on 1st day if needed; then 400 mg daily-bid; max 800 mg/day
  Pediatric: <18 years: not recommended
    Celebrex *Cap:* 50, 100, 200, 400 mg
▷ *meloxicam* (C)(G) initially 7.5 mg once daily; max 15 mg once daily
  Pediatric: <2 years: not recommended; ≥2 years: 0.125 mg/kg; max 7.5 mg once daily
    Mobic *Tab:* 7.5, 15 mg; *Oral susp:* 7.5 mg/5 ml (100 ml) (raspberry)
    Vivlodex *Cap:* 5, 10 mg
Combined Oral Contraceptives see page 474

DYSPAREUNIA
POSTMENOPAUSAL PAINFUL INTERCOURSE

Comment: Vulvar and vaginal atrophy due to menopause can cause painful intercourse.
Oral Hormonal and Transdermal Therapy see *Menopause* page 254

NONHORMONAL THERAPY

▷ *ospemifene*
    Osphena *Tab:* 60 mg

VAGINAL PREPARATIONS (WITHOUT UTERUS)

Comment: Vaginal preparations provide relief from vaginal and urinary symptoms only (i.e., atrophic vaginitis, dyspareunia, dysuria, and urinary frequency).
▷ *estradiol* (X)(G)
    Vagifem Tabs insert one 10 mcg or 25 mcg vaginal tablet once daily x 2 weeks; then twice weekly x 2 weeks (e.g., tues/fri); consider the addition of a progestin
    Vag tab: 10, 25 mcg (8, 18/blister pck with applicator)

EDEMA

THIAZIDE DIURETICS

▷ *chlorthalidone* (B)(G) initially 30-60 mg daily or 60 mg on alternate days; max 90-120 mg/day
    Thalitone *Tab:* 15 mg

▶ *chlorothiazide* (B)(G) 0.5-1 g/day in a single or divided doses; max 2 g/day
  Pediatric: <6 months: up to 15 mg/lb/day in 2 divided doses; ≥6 months: 10 mg/lb/day in 2 divided doses; max 375 mg/day
    Diuril *Tab:* 250*, 500*mg; *Oral susp:* 250 mg/5 ml (237 ml)
▶ *hydrochlorothiazide* (B)(G)
  Pediatric: not recommended
    Esidrix 25-200 mg daily
      Tab: 25, 50, 100 mg
    Microzide 12.5 mg daily; usual max 50 mg/day
      Cap: 12.5 mg
▶ *hydroflumethiazide* (B) 50-200 mg/day in a single or 2 divided doses
  Pediatric: not recommended
    Saluron *Tab:* 50 mg
▶ *methyclothiazide/deserpidine* (B) initially 2.5 mg daily; max 5 mg daily
  Pediatric: not recommended
    Enduronyl *Tab: methy* 5 mg/*deser* 0.25 mg*
    Enduronyl Forte *Tab: methy* 5 mg/*deser* 0.5 mg*
▶ *polythiazide* (C) 1-4 mg daily
  Pediatric: not recommended
    Renese *Tab:* 1, 2, 4 mg

POTASSIUM-SPARING DIURETICS

▶ *amiloride* (B)(G) initially 5 mg; may increase to 10 mg; max 20 mg
  Pediatric: not recommended
    Tab: 5 mg
▶ *spironolactone* (D)(G) initially 25-200 mg in a single or divided doses; titrate at 2-week intervals
  Pediatric: not recommended
    Aldactone *Tab:* 25, 50*, 100*mg
▶ *triamterene* (B) 100 mg bid; max 300 mg
  Pediatric: not recommended
    Dyrenium *Cap:* 50, 100 mg

LOOP DIURETICS

▶ *bumetanide* (C)(G) 0.5-2 mg daily; *Tab:* 5 mg; may repeat at 4-5 hour intervals; max 10 mg/day
  Pediatric: <18 years: not recommended
    Tab: 1* mg
  Comment: *bumetanide* is contraindicated with sulfa drug allergy.
▶ *ethacrynic acid* (B) initially 50-100 mg once daily-bid; max 400 mg/day
  Pediatric: Infants: not recommended; ≥1 month: initially 25 mg/day; then adjust dose in 25 mg increments
    Edecrin *Tab:* 25, 50 mg
▶ *ethacrynate sodium* (B)(G) for IV injection
    Sodium Edecrin *Vial:* 50 mg single-dose
    Comment: **Sodium Edecrin** is more potent than more commonly used loop and thiazide diuretics.
▶ *furosemide* (C)(G) initially 20-80 mg as a single dose
  Pediatric: not recommended

Lasix *Tab:* 20, 40*, 80 mg; *Oral soln:* 10 mg/ml (2, 4 oz w. dropper)
Comment: *furosemide* is contraindicated with sulfa drug allergy.
▷ *torsemide* (B) 5 mg daily; may increase to 10 mg daily
Pediatric: not recommended
Demadex *Tab:* 5*, 10*, 20*, 100*mg

OTHER DIURETICS

▷ *indapamide* (B) initially 1.25 mg daily; may titrate every 4 weeks if needed; max
5 mg/day
Pediatric: not recommended
Lozol *Tab:* 1.25, 2.5 mg
Comment: *indapamide* is contraindicated with sulfa drug allergy.
▷ *metolazone* (B)
Pediatric: not recommended
Mykrox initially 0.5 mg q AM; max 1 mg/day
Tab: 0.5 mg
Zaroxolyn 2.5-5 mg once daily
Tab: 2.5, 5, 10 mg
Comment: *metolazone* is contraindicated with sulfa drug allergy.

DIURETIC COMBINATIONS

▷ *amiloride/hydrochlorothiazide* (B)(G) initially 1 tab daily; may increase to 2 tabs/day
in a single or divided doses
Pediatric: not recommended
Moduretic *Tab: amil* 5 mg/*hydro* 50 mg*
▷ *spironolactone/hydrochlorothiazide* (D)(G) usual maintenance is 100 mg each of
spironolactone and hydrochlorothiazide daily, in a single dose or in divided doses;
range 25-200 mg of each component daily depending on the response to the initial
titration
Pediatric: not recommended
Aldactazide 25
Tab: spiro 25 mg/*hydro* 25 mg
Aldactazide 50
Tab: spiro 50 mg/*hydro* 50 mg
▷ *triamterene/hydrochlorothiazide* (C)(G)
Pediatric: not recommended
Dyazide 1-2 caps once daily
Cap: triam 37.5 mg/*hydro* 25 mg
Maxzide 1 tab once daily
Tab: triam 75 mg/*hydro* 50 mg*
Maxzide-25 1-2 tabs once daily
Tab: triam 37.5 mg/*hydro* 25 mg*

 EMPHYSEMA

Inhaled Corticosteroids *see* **Asthma** *page* 34
Parenteral Corticosteroids *see page* 499
Oral Corticosteroids *see page* 497

Inhaled Beta Agonists (Bronchodilators) *see Asthma page* 31
Oral Beta-Agonists (Bronchodilators) *see Asthma page* 35

LONG-ACTING INHALED BETA AGONIST (LABA)

▷ *indacaterol* (C)
>> **Arcapta Neohaler** inhale contents of one 75 mcg cap once daily
>>> *Neohaler Device/Cap:* 75 mcg (5 blister cards, 6 caps/card)
>> Comment: Remove cap from blister cap immediately before use. For oral
>> inhalation with neohaler device only. **Arcapta Neohaler** is indicated for the long-
>> term maintenance treatment of bronchoconstriction in persons with COPD. It is
>> not indicated for treating asthma, for primary treatment of acute symptoms, <u>or</u>
>> for acute deterioration of COPD.
▷ *olodaterol* (C)
> *Pediatric:* not established
>> **Striverdi Respimat** 12 mcg q 12 hours
>>> *Inhal soln:* 2.5 mcg/cartridge (metered actuation) (40 g, 60 metered actuations)
>>> (benzalkonium chloride)

CORTICOSTEROID/INHALED LONG-ACTING BETA-AGONIST (LABA)

▷ *fluticasone furoate/vilanterol* (C) 1 inhalation 100/25 <u>or</u> 200/25 once daily at the
same time each day
> *Pediatric:* <17 years: not established
>> **Breo Ellipta 100/25** *Inhal pwdr: flu* 100 mcg/*vil* 25 mcg dry pwdr per inhal
>> (30 doses)
>> **Breo Ellipta 200/25** *Inhal pwdr: flu* 200 mcg/*vil* 25 mcg dry pwdr per inhal
>> (30 doses)
>> Comment: **Breo Ellipta** is contraindicated with severe hypersensitivity to milk
>> proteins.

INHALED ANTICHOLINERGICS (ANTIMUSCARINICS)

▷ *ipratropium* (B)(G)
>> **Atrovent** 2 inhalations qid; max 12 inhalations/day
>>> *Inhaler:* 14 g (200 inh)
>> **Atrovent Inhaled Solution** 500 mcg by nebulizer tid to qid
>>> *Inhal soln:* 0.02%; 500 mcg (2.5 ml)

INHALED LONG-ACTING ANTICHOLINERGICS (ANTIMUSCARINICS)

Comment: Inhales LAA's are indicated for prophylaxis and chronic treatment, only.
Not for primary (rescue) treatment of acute attack. Avoid getting powder in eyes.
Caution with narrow-angle glaucoma, BPH, bladder neck obstruction, and pregnancy.
Contraindicated with allergy to atropine <u>or</u> its derivatives (e.g., *ipratropium*). Avoid
other anticholinergic agents.
▷ *aclidinium bromide* (C) 1 inhalation twice daily using inhaler
> *Pediatric:* not recommended
>> **Tudorza Pressair** *Inhal device:* 400 mcg/actuation (60 doses per inhalation
>> device)

INHALED LONG-ACTING ANTICHOLINERGICS

▶ *glycopyrrolate* (C) inhale the contents of 1 capsule 2 x/day at the same times of day, AM and PM, using the neohaler; do not swallow caps
Pediatric: not established
> **Seebri Neohaler** *Inhal cap:* 15.6 mcg (60/blister pck) dry pwdr for inhalation w. 1 Neohaler device (lactose)

▶ *tiotropium (as bromide monohydrate)* (C) 2 inhalations once daily using inhalation device; do not swallow caps
Pediatric: <12 years: not recommended; ≥12 years: same as adult
> **Spiriva HandiHaler** *Inhal device:* 18 mcg/cap pwdr for inhalation (5, 30, 90 caps w. inhalation device)
> **Spiriva Respimat** *Inhal device:* 1.25, 2.5 mcg/actuation cartridge w. inhalation device (4 g, 60 metered actuations) (benzylkonian chloride)

Comment: *tiotropium is f*or prophylaxis and chronic treatment, only. Not for primary (rescue) treatment of acute attack. Avoid getting powder in eyes. Caution with narrow-angle glaucoma, BPH, bladder neck obstruction, and pregnancy. Contraindicated with allergy to *atropine* or its derivatives (e.g., *ipratropium*).

▶ *umeclidinium* (C) one inhalation once daily at the same time each day
Pediatric: not established
> **Incruse Ellipta** *Inhal pwdr:* 62.5 mcg/inhalation (30 doses) (lactose)

Comment: **Incruse Ellipta** is contraindicated with allergy to atropine or its derivatives.

INHALED BRONCHODILATOR/ANTICHOLINERGIC COMBINATION

▶ *ipratropium/albuterol* (C)
> **Combivent MDI** 2 inhalations qid; max 12 inhalations/day
> *Inhaler:* 14.7 g (200 inh)

INHALED ANTICHOLINERGIC/LONG-ACTING BETA AGONIST (LABA) COMBINATIONS

▶ *indacaterol/glycopyrrolate* (C)
> **Utibron Neohaler** inhale the contents of 1 capsule 2 x/day at the same times of day, AM and PM, using the neohaler; do not swallow caps
> *Inhal cap: indac* 27.5 mcg/*glycop* 15.6 mcg per cap (60/blister pck) dry pwdr for inhalation w. 1 Neohaler device (lactose)

▶ *ipratropium/albuterol* (C) 1 inhalation once daily; max 6 inhalations/day
> **Combivent Respimat** *Inhal soln: ipra* 20 mcg/*alb* 100 mcg per inhal (4 g, 120 inhal)
> Comment: When the labeled number of metered actuations (120) has been dispensed from the **Combivent Respimat** inhaler, the locking mechanism engages and no more actuations can be dispensed. **Combivent Respimat** is contraindicted with atropine allergy.

▶ *tiotropium/olodaterol* (C) 2 inhalations once daily at the same time each day; max 2 inhalations/day
> **Stiolto Respimat** *Inhal soln: tio* 2.5 mcg/*olo* 2.5 mcg per actuation (4 g, 60 inh) (benzalkonium chloride)
> Comment: **Stiolto Respimat** is not for treating asthma, for relief of acute bronchospasm, or acutely deteriorating COPD.

▶ *umeclidinium/vilanterol* (C) 1 inhalation once daily at the same time each day
> **Anoro Ellipta** *Inhal soln: ume* 62.5 mcg/*vila* 25 mcg per inhal (30 doses)
> Comment: **Anoro Ellipta** is contraindicated with severe hypersensitivity to milk proteins.

METHYLXANTHINES

see Asthma page 28

METHYLXANTHINE/EXPECTORANT COMBINATION

▷ *dyphylline/guaifenesin* (C)
  Pediatric: not recommended
      Lufyllin GG 1 tab qid
          Tab: dyph 200 mg/*guaif* 200 mg
      Lufyllin GG Elixir 30 ml qid
          Elix: dyph 100 mg/*guaif* 100 mg per 15 ml (16 oz)

OTHER METHYLXANTHINE COMBINATION

▷ *theophylline/potassium iodide/ephedrine/phenobarbital* (X)(II) 1 tab tid-qid prn; add
  an additional dose q HS as needed
  Pediatric: <6 years: not recommended; ≥6-12 years: 1/2 tab tid
      Quadrinal *Tab:* theo 130 mg/*pot iod* 320 mg/*ephed* 24 mg/*phenol* 24 mg

 ENCOPRESIS

INITIAL BOWEL EVACUATION

▷ *mineral oil* (C) 1 oz x 1 day
▷ *bisacodyl* (B)
  Pediatric: <12 years: 1/2 suppository daily pen
      Dulcolax *Rectal supp:* 10 mg
▷ *glycerin* suppository
  Pediatric: <6 years: 1 pediatric suppository; ≥6 years: 1 adult suppository

MAINTENANCE

▷ *mineral oil* (C) 5-15 ml once daily
▷ *multivitamin* (A) 1 daily
  Comment: Mineral oil can inhibit absorption of fat-soluble vitamins.

ENDOMETRIOSIS

Acetaminophen for IV Infusion *see Pain page 296*
Oral Prescription NSAIDs *see page 489*
Other Oral Analgesics *see Pain page 298*
Contraceptives *see page 474*
▷ *medroxyprogesterone* (X) 30 mg daily
      Provera *Tab:* 2.5, 5, 10 mg
▷ *medroxyprogesterone acetate* injectable (X) 100-400 mg IM monthly
      Depo-Provera Injectable: 300 mg/ml (2.5, 10 ml)
▷ *norethindrone acetate* (X) initially 5 mg daily x 2 weeks; then increase by 2.5 mg/day
  every 2 weeks up to 15 mg/day maintenance dose; then continue for 6 to 9 months
  unless breakthrough bleeding is intolerable
      Aygestin *Tab:* 5*mg

GONADOTROPIN-RELEASING HORMONE ANALOGS

▷ *goserelin (GnRH analogue)* implant (X) implant SC into upper abdominal wall; 1 SC implant q 28 days for up to 6 months; re-treatment not recommended
Pediatric: <18 years: not recommended
Zoladex SC implant in syringe: 3.6 mg

▷ *leuprolide acetate (GnRH analogue)* (X)
Pediatric: <18 years: not recommended
Lupron Depot 3.75 mg 3.75 mg SC monthly for up to 6 months; may repeat one 6-month cycle
Syringe: 3.75 mg (single-dose depo susp for SC injection)
Lupron Depot-3 Month 22.5 mg SC q 3 months (84 days); max 2 injections
Syringe: 22.5 mg (single-dose depo susp for IM injection)
Comment: Do not split doses.

▷ *nafarelin acetate* (X) 1 spray (200 mcg) into one nostril q AM, then 1 spray (200 mcg) into the other nostril q PM x 6 months; if no response after 2 months, may increase to 2 sprays (400 mcg) bid
Synarel *Nasal spray:* 2 mg/ml (10 ml)
Comment: Start on 3rd or 4th day of menstrual period or after a negative pregnancy test.

OTHER AGENTS

▷ *danazol* (X) initially 400 mg bid; gradual downward titration of dosage may be considered dependent upon patient response; mild cases may respond to 100-200 mg bid
Danocrine *Cap:* 50, 100, 200 mg

⬤ ENURESIS: PRIMARY, NOCTURNAL

VASOPRESSIN

▷ *desmopressin acetate* (B)
DDAVP usual dosage 0.1-1.2 mg/day in 2-3 divided doses; 0.2 mg q HS prn for nocturnal enuresis
Pediatric: <6 years: not recommended
Tab: 0.1*, 0.2*mg
DDAVP Rhinal Tube
Pediatric: <6 years: not recommended; ≥6 years: 10 mcg or 0.1 ml of soln each nostril (20 mcg total dose) q HS prn; max 40 mcg total dose
Nasal spray: 10 mcg/actuation (5 ml, 50 sprays); *Rhinal tube:* 0.1 mg/ml (2.5 ml)

TRICYCLIC ANTIDEPRESSANT(TCA)

▷ *imipramine* (C)(G)
Pediatric: <6 years: not recommended; 6-12 years: 25 mg 1 hour before bedtime; after 1 week, may increase to 50 mg; max 50 mg; >12 years: 25 mg 1 hour before bedtime; after 1 week, may increase to 50 mg; max 75 mg; *Early night bedwetters:* administer 25 mg in the afternoon and repeat at bedtime; max 2.5 mg/kg/day
Comment: If drug response favorable, consider gradual tapering and attempting drug-free periods.
Tofranil initially 75 mg daily (max 200 mg); if maintenance dose exceeds 75 mg daily, may switch to **Tofranil PM** for divided or bedtime dose
Tab: 10, 25, 50 mg

Tofranil PM initially 75 mg 1 hour before HS; max 200 mg
   Cap: 75, 100, 125, 150 mg

EPICONDYLITIS

Acetaminophen for IV Infusion *see Pain page* 296
Oral Prescription NSAIDs *see page* 489
Other Oral Analgesics *see Pain page* 298
Topical/Transdermal NSAIDs *see Pain page* 297
Parenteral Corticosteroids *see page* 499
Oral Corticosteroids *see page* 497
Topical Analgesic and Anesthetic Agents *see page* 487

EPIDIDYMITIS

Comment: The following treatment regimens for epididymitis are published in the **2015 CDC Transmitted Diseases Treatment Guidelines**. Treatment regimens are presented by generic drug name first, followed by information about brands and dose forms. Empiric treatment requires concomitant treatment of chlamydia. Treat all sexual contacts. Patients who are HIV-positive should receive the same treatment as those who are HIV-negative.

RECOMMENDED REGIMEN

Regimen 1

▷ *ceftriaxone* (B)(G) 250 mg IM in a single dose
   plus
▷ *doxycycline* (D)(G) 100 mg bid x 10 days

RECOMMENDED REGIMENS: LIKELY CAUSED BY ENTERIC ORGANISMS

Regimen 1

▷ *levofloxacin* (C) 500 mg daily x 10 days

Regimen 2

▷ *ofloxacin* (C)(G) 300 mg bid x 10 day

DRUG BRANDS AND DOSE FORMS

▷ *ceftriaxone* (B)(G)
   Rocephin *Vial:* 250, 500 mg; 1, 2 g
▷ *doxycycline* (D)(G)
   Actilate *Tab:* 75, 150**mg
   Adoxa *Tab:* 50, 75, 100, 150 mg ent-coat
   Doryx *Tab:* 75, 100, 150 mg del-rel
   Monodox *Cap:* 50, 75, 100 mg
   Oracea *Cap:* 40 mg del-rel
   Vibramycin *Cap:* 50, 100 mg; *Syr:* 50 mg/5 ml (raspberry-apple) (sulfites); *Oral susp:* 25 mg/5 ml (raspberry)

Vibra-Tab *Tab:* 100 mg film-coat
Comment: *doxycycline* is contraindicated <8 years-of-age, in pregnancy, and lactation (discolors developing tooth enamel). A side effect may be photo-sensitivity (photophobia). Do not give with antacids, calcium supplements, milk or other dairy, or within two hours of taking another drug.

▷ *levofloxacin* (C)
Levaquin *Tab:* 250, 500, 750 mg; *Oral soln:* 25 mg/ml (480 ml) (benzyl alcohol)
Comment: *levofloxacin* is contraindicated <18 years-of-age, and during pregnancy and lactation. Risk of tendonitis or tendon rupture, especially 60 years-of-age and older.

▷ *ofloxacin* (C)(G)
Floxin *Tab:* 200, 300, 400 mg
Comment: *ofloxacin* is contraindicated <18 years-of-age, and during pregnancy and lactation. Risk of tendonitis or tendon rupture, especially 60 years-of-age and older.

◯ ERECTILE DYSFUNCTION (ED)

Comment: Due to a degree of cardiac risk with sexual activity, consider cardiovascular status of patient before instituting therapeutic measures for erectile dysfunction.

PHOSPHODIESTERASE TYPE 5 (PDE5) INHIBITORS, CGMP-SPECIFIC

Comment: Oral PDE5 inhibitors (**Cialis**, **Levitra**, **Staxyn**, **Viagra**) are contraindicated in patients taking nitrates. Caution with history of recent MI, stroke, life-threatening arrhythmia, hypotension, hypertension, cardiac failure, unstable angina, retinitis pigmentosa, CYP3A4 inhibitors (e.g., *cimetidine*, the azoles, *erythromycin*, grapefruit juice), protease inhibitors (e.g., *ritonavir*), CYP3A4 inducers (e.g., *rifampin*, *carbamazepine*, *phenytoin*, *phenobarbital*), alcohol, antihypertensive agents. Side effects include headache, flushing, nasal congestion, rhinitis, dyspepsia, and diarrhea. Use with caution in patients with anatomical deformation of the penis (e.g., angulation, cavernosal fibrosis, or Peyronie's disease) or in patients who have conditions, which may predispose them to priapism (e.g., sickle cell anemia, multiple myeloma, or leukemia). In the event of an erection that persists longer than 4 hours, the patient should seek immediate medical assistance. If priapism (painful erection greater than 6 hours in duration) is not treated immediately, penile tissue damage and permanent loss of potency could result.

▷ *avanafil* (B) initially 100 mg taken 30 min prior to sexual activity; may decrease to 50 mg or increase to 200 mg based on response; max one administration/day
Stendra *Tab:* 50, 100, 200 mg

▷ *sildenafil citrate* (B)(G) one dose about 1 hour (range 30 min-4 hrs) before sexual activity; usual initial dose 50 mg; may decrease to 25 mg or increase to max 100 mg/dose based on response; max one administration/day
Viagra *Tab:* 25, 50, 100 mg

▷ *tadalafil* (B) initially 10 mg prior to sexual activity up to once daily; may decrease to 5 mg or increase to 20 mg based on response; max one administration/day; effect may last 36 hours
Cialis *Tab:* 2.5, 5, 10, 20 mg

▷ *vardenafil* (B) initially 10 mg taken 60 min prior to sexual activity; may decrease to 5 mg or increase to 20 mg based on response; max one administration/day
Levitra *Tab:* 2.5, 5, 10, 20 mg film-coat
Comment: **Levitra** is not interchangeable with **Staxyn**.

➤ *vardenafil (as HCl)* (B) dissolve 1 tab on tongue 60 min prior to sexual activity, max once daily
    Staxyn *Tab:* 10 mg orally disintegrating (peppermint) (phenylalanine)
    Comment: Staxyn is not interchangeable with **Levitra**.
➤ *alprostadil* (X) *urethral suppository* initially 125 or 250 mcg inserted in the urethra after urination; adjust dose in stepwise manner on separate occasions; max two administrations/ day
    Muse *Urethral supp:* 125, 250, 500, 1000 mcg
    Comment: Contraindicated with urethral stricture, balanitis, severe hypospadias and curvature, urethritis, predisposition to venous thrombosis, hyperviscosity syndrome. Extreme caution with anticoagulant therapy (e.g., warfarin, heparin). Potential for hypotension and/or syncope.
➤ *alprostadil* (X) *injection* inject over 5-10 seconds into the dorsal lateral aspect of the proximal third of the penis; avoid visible veins; rotate injection sites and sides; if no initial response, may give next higher dose within 1 hour; if partial response, give next higher dose after 24 hours; max 60 mcg and 3 self-injections/week; allow at least 24 hours between doses; reduce dose if erection lasts >1 hour.
    Caverject *Vial:* 5, 10, 20, 40 mcg/vial (pwdr for reconstitution w. diluent)
    Caverject Impulse *Cartridge:* 10, 20 mcg (2 cartridge starter and refill pcks)
    Edex *Vial:* 5, 10, 20, 40 mcg (6/pck); *Syringe:* 5, 10, 20, 40 mcg (4/pck); *Cartridge:* 10, 20, 40 mcg (2 cartridge starter and refill pcks)
    Comment: Determine dose of injectable prostaglandins in the office. Contraindicated with predisposition to priapism, penile angulation, cavernosal fibrosis, Peyronies disease, penile implant. Extreme caution with anticoagulant therapy (e.g., *warfarin*, *heparin*).

⃝ ERYSIPELAS

Comment: Erysipelas is most commonly due to GABHS (Group A beta-hemolytic Strept).

TREATMENT OF CHOICE

➤ *penicillin V potassium* (B) 250-500 mg q 6 hours x 10 days
    Pediatric: 25-50 mg/kg/day divided q 6 hours x 10 days; *see page 572 for dose by weight*
    Pen-Vee K *Tab:* 250, 500 mg; *Oral soln:* 125 mg/5 ml (100, 200 ml); 250 mg/5 ml (100, 150, 200 ml)

TREATMENT IF PENICILLIN ALLERGIC

➤ *erythromycin base* (B)(G) 250 mg q 6 hours x 10 days
    Pediatric: 30-40 mg/kg/day divided q 6 hours x 10 days; >40 kg: same as adult
    Ery-Tab *Tab:* 250, 333, 500 mg ent-coat
    PCE *Tab:* 333, 500 mg
    Comment: *erythromycin* may increase INR with concomitant *warfarin*, as well as increase serum level of *digoxin*, benzodiazepines and statins.
➤ *erythromycin ethylsuccinate* (B)(G) 400 mg qid x 7 days
    Pediatric: 30-50 mg/kg/day in 4 divided doses x 7 days; may double dose with severe infection; max 100 mg/kg/day; *see page 563 for dose by weight*

EryPed *Oral susp:* 200 mg/5 ml (100, 200 ml) (fruit); 400 mg/5 ml (60, 100, 200 ml) (banana); *Oral drops:* 200, 400 mg/5 ml (50 ml) (fruit); *Chew tab:* 200 mg wafer (fruit)
E.E.S. *Oral susp:* 200, 400 mg/5 ml (100 ml) (fruit)
E.E.S. Granules *Oral susp:* 200 mg/5 ml (100, 200 ml) (cherry)
E.E.S. 400 Tablets *Tab:* 400 mg
Comment: *erythromycin* may increase INR with concomitant *warfarin*, as well as increase serum level of *digoxin*, benzodiazepines and statins.

ESOPHAGITIS, EROSIVE

Antacids *see* **GERD** *page* 150
H₂ Antagonists *see* **GERD** *page* 152
Proton Pump Inhibitors *see* **GERD** *page* 152
▷ *sucralfate* (B)(G) *Active ulcer:* 1 g qid; *Maintenance:* 1 g bid
    Carafate *Tab:* 1*g; *Oral susp:* 1 g/10 ml (14 oz)

EYE PAIN

Acetaminophen for IV Infusion *see* **Pain** *page* 296

OPHTHALMIC NSAIDs

Comment: Concomitant contact lens wear is contraindicated during therapy. Etiology of eye pain must be known prior to use of these agents
▷ *diclofenac* (B) 1 drop affected eye qid
    Pediatric: not recommended
        Voltaren Ophthalmic Solution *Ophth soln:* 0.1% (2.5, 5 ml)
▷ *ketorolac tromethamine* (C) 1 drop affected eye qid for up to 4 days
    Pediatric: <3 years: not recommended; ≥3 years: same as adult
        Acular *Ophth soln:* 0.5% (3, 5, 10 ml; benzalkonium chloride)
        Acular LS *Ophth soln:* 0.4% (5 ml; benzalkonium chloride)
        Acular PF *Ophth soln:* 0.5% (0.4 ml; 12 single-use vials/carton) (preservative-free)
▷ *nepafenac* (C) 1 drop affected eye tid
    Pediatric: <10 years: not recommended; ≥10 years: same as adult
        Nevanac Ophthalmic Suspension *Ophth susp:* 0.1% (3 ml) (benzalkonium chloride)

OPHTHALMIC STEROIDS

Comment: Contraindications: ocular fungal, viral, or mycobacterial infections. Effectiveness of treatment should be assessed after 2 days. The corticosteroid should be tapered and treatment concluded within 14 days if possible due to risk of corneal and/ or scleral thinning with prolonged use.
▷ *difluprednate* (C) 1 drop affected eye qid; *Post-op Pain:* beginning 24 hours after surgery, 1 drop affected eye qid; continue for 2 weeks post-op; then bid x 1 week; then taper until resolved

Pediatric: not recommended
> **Durezol Ophthalmic Solution** *Ophth emul:* 0.05% (5 ml)

▷ *etabonate* **(C)** 1 drop affected eye qid
Pediatric: not recommended
> **Alrex Ophthalmic Solution** *Ophth emul:* 0.2% (5 ml) (benzylkonium chloride)

⬤ FACIAL HAIR, EXCESSIVE/UNWANTED

TOPICAL HAIR GROWTH RETARDANT

▷ *eflornithine* 13.9% cream **(C)** apply a thin layer to affected areas of face and under the chin bid at least 8 hours apart; rub in thoroughly; do not wash treated area for at least 4 hours following application
Pediatric: not recommended
> **Vaniqa** *Crm:* 13.9% (30, 60 g)
> **Comment:** After **Vaniqa** dries, may apply cosmetics <u>or</u> sunscreen. Hair removal techniques may be continued as needed.

⬤ FECAL ODOR

▷ *bismuth subgallate powder* **(B)(OTC)** 1-2 tabs tid with meals
> **Devron** *Chew tab:* 200 mg; *Cap:* 200 mg
> **Comment:** **Devron** is an internal (oral) deodorant for control of odors from ileostomy <u>or</u> colostomy drainage <u>or</u> fecal incontinence.

⬤ FEVER (PYREXIA)

ACETAMINOPHEN FOR IV INFUSION

▷ *acetaminophen* injectable **(B)** administer by IV infusion over 15 minutes; 1000 mg q 6 hours prn <u>or</u> 650 mg q 4 hours prn; max 4,000 mg/day
Pediatric: <2 years: not recommended; 2-13 years <50 kg: 15 mg/kg q 6 hours prn <u>or</u> 12.5 mg/kg q 4 hours prn; max 750 mg single-dose; max 75 mg/kg per day
> **Ofirmev** *Vial:* 10 mg/ml (100 ml) (preservative-free)
> **Comment:** The **Ofirmev** vial is intended for single-use. If any portion is withdrawn from the vial, use within 6 hours. Discard the unused portion. For pediatric patients, withdraw the intended dose and administer via syringe pump. Do not ad-mix **Ofirmev** with any other drugs. **Ofirmev** is physically incompatable with diazepam and chlorpromazine hydrochloride.

▷ *acetaminophen* **(B)(G)**
> **Children's Tylenol (OTC)** 10-20 mg/kg q 4-6 hours prn
> > *Oral susp:* 80 mg/tsp
> > > 4-11 months (12-17 lb): 1/2 tsp q 4 hours prn; 12-23 months (18-23 lb): 3/4 tsp q 4 hours prn; 2-3 years (24-35 lb): 1 tsp q 4 hours prn; 4-5 years (36-47 lb): 1 tsp q 4 hours prn; 6-8 years (48-59 lb): 2 tsp q 4 hours

prn; 9-10 years (60-71 lb): 2 tsp q 4 hours prn; 11 years (72-95 lb): 3 tsp q 4 hours prn; All: max 5 doses/day
Elix: 160 mg/5 ml (2, 4 oz)
Chew tab: 80 mg
2-3 years (24-35 lb): 2 tabs q 4 hours prn; 4-5 years (36-47 lb): 3 tabs q 4 hours prn; 6-8 years (48-59 lb): 4 tabs q 4 hours prn; 9-10 years (60-71 lb): 5 tabs q 4 hours prn; 11 years (72-95 lb): 6 tabs q 4 hours prn; All: max 5 doses/day
Junior Strength:
6-8 years: 2 tabs q 4 hours prn; 9-10 years: 2 tabs q 4 hours prn; 11 years: 3 tabs q 4 hours prn; 12 years: 4 tabs q 4 hours prn; All: max 5 doses/day
Chew tab: 160 mg
Junior cplt: 160 mg
Infant's Drops and Suspension: 80 mg/0.8 ml (1/2, 1 oz)
<3 months: 0.4 ml q 4 hours prn; 4-11 months: 0.8 ml q 4 hours prn; 12-23 months: 1.2 ml q 4 hours prn; 2-3 years (24-35 lb): 1.6 ml q 4 hours prn; 4-5 years (36-47 lb): 2.4 ml q 4 hours prn; All: max 5 doses/day
Extra Strength Tylenol (OTC) 1 g q 4-6 hours prn; max 4 g/day
Pediatric: not recommended
Tab/Cplt/Gel tab/Gel cap: 500 mg; *Liq:* 500 mg/15 ml (8 oz)
FeverAll Extra Strength Tylenol (OTC)
Pediatric: <3 months: not recommended; 3-36 months: 80 mg q 4 hours prn; 3-6 years: 120 mg q 4 hours prn; ≥6 years: 325 mg q 4 hours prn; *Rectal supp:* 80, 120, 325 mg (6/carton)
Maximum Strength Tylenol Sore Throat (OTC) 500-1000 mg q 4-6 hours prn
Pediatric: not recommended
Liq: 1000 mg/30 ml (8 oz)
Tylenol (OTC) 650 mg q 4-6 hours; max 4 g/day
Pediatric: <6 years: not recommended; 6-11 years: 325 mg q 4-6 hours prn; max 1.625 g/day; ≥12 years: same as adult
▶ *aspirin* (D)(G)
Bayer (OTC) 325-650 mg q 4 hours prn; max: 5 doses/day
Pediatric: not recommended
Tab/Cplt: 325 mg ext-rel
Extra Strength Bayer (OTC) 500 mg-1 g q 4-6 hours prn; max 4 g/day
Pediatric: not recommended
Cplt: 500 mg
Extended-Release Bayer 8 Hour (OTC) 650-1300 mg q 8 hours prn
Pediatric: not recommended
Cplt: 650 mg ext-rel
Comment: *aspirin*-containing medications are contraindicated with history of allergic-type reaction to *aspirin*, children and adolescents with *Varicella* or other viral illness, and 3rd trimester pregnancy.
▶ *aspirin/caffeine* (D)(G)
Anacin (OTC) 800 mg q 4 hours prn; max 4 g/day
Pediatric: <6 years: not recommended; 6-12 years: 400 mg q 4 hours prn; max 2 g/day; ≥12 years: same as adult

> *Tab/Cplt:* 400 mg
> **Anacin Maximum Strength (OTC)** 1 g tid-qid
>> *Pediatric:* not recommended
>> *Tab:* 500 mg

Comment: *aspirin*-containing medications are contraindicated with history of allergic-type reaction to aspirin, children and adolescents with *Varicella* or other viral illness, and 3rd trimester pregnancy.

▷ *aspirin/antacid* (D)(G)
> **Extra Strength Bayer Plus (OTC)** 500 mg-1 g q 4-6 hours prn; usual max 4 g/day
>> *Pediatric:* not recommended
>> *Cplt:* 500 mg *aspirin* with *calcium carbonate*
> **Bufferin (OTC)** 650 mg q 4 hours; max 3.9 mg/day
>> *Pediatric:* not recommended
>> *Tab:* 325 mg *aspirin* with *calcium carbonate*, *magnesium carbonate*, and *magnesium oxide*

Comment: *aspirin*-containing medications are contraindicated with history of allergic-type reaction to *aspirin*, children and adolescents with *Varicella* or other viral illness, and 3rd trimester pregnancy.

▷ *ibuprofen* (B; not for use in 3rd)(G)
Comment: *ibuprofen* is contraindicated in children <6 months-of-age.
> **Children's Advil (OTC), ElixSure IB (OTC), Motrin (OTC), PediaCare (OTC), PediaProfen (OTC)**
>> *Pediatric:* 5-10 mg/kg q 6-8 hours; max 40 mg/kg/day; <24 lb (<2 years): individualize; 24-35 lb (2-3 years): 5 ml q 6-8 hours prn; 36-47 lb (4-5 years): 7.5 ml q 6-8 hours prn; 48-59 lb (6-8 years): 10 ml or 2 tabs q 6-8 hours prn; 60-71 lb (9-10 years): 12.5 ml or 2 tabs q 6-8 hours prn; 72-95 lb (11 years): 15 ml or 3 tabs q 6-8 hours prn
>> *Oral susp:* 100 mg/5 ml (2, 4 oz) (berry); *Junior tabs:* 100 mg
> **Children's Motrin Drops (OTC), PediaCare Drops (OTC)**
>> *Pediatric:* <24 lb (<2 years): individualize; 24-35 lb (2-3 years): 2.5 ml q 6-8 hours prn; *Oral drops:* 50 mg/1.25 ml (15 ml; berry)
> **Children's Motrin Chewables and Caplets (OTC)**
>> *Pediatric:* 48-59 lb (6-8 years): 200 mg q 6-8 hours prn; 60-71 lb (9-10 years): 250 mg q 6-8 hours prn; 72-95 lb (11 years): 300 mg q 6-8 hours prn; ≥12 years: same as adult
>> *Chew tab:* 100*mg (citrus; phenylalanine)
>> *Cplt:* 100 mg
> **Motrin (OTC)** 400 mg q 6 hours prn
>> *Pediatric:* <6 months: not recommended; >6 months, fever <102.5: 5 mg/kg q 6-8 hours prn; >6 months, fever >102.5: 10 mg/kg q 6-8 hours prn
>> All: max 40 mg/kg/day
>> *Tab:* 400 mg; *Cplt:* 100*mg; *Chew tab:* 50*, 100*mg (citrus; phenylalanine); *Oral susp:* 100 mg/5 ml (4, 16 oz) (berry); *Oral drops:* 40 mg/ml (15 ml) (berry)
> **Advil (OTC), Motrin IB (OTC), Nuprin (OTC)** 200-400 mg q 4-6 hours; max 1.2 g/day
>> *Pediatric:* not recommended
>> *Tab/Cplt/Gel cap:* 200 mg

▷ *naproxen* (B)(G)
> *Pediatric:* <2 years: not recommended; ≥2 years: 2.5-5 mg/kg bid-tid; max: 15 mg/kg/day
>> **Aleve** (OTC) 400 mg x 1 dose; then 200 mg q 8-12 hours prn; max 10 days
>>> *Tab/Cplt/Gel cap:* 200 mg
>> **Anaprox** 550 mg x 1 dose; then 550 mg q 12 hours or 275 mg q 6-8 hours prn; max 1.375 g first day and 1.1 g/day thereafter
>>> *Tab:* 275 mg
>> **Anaprox DS** 1 tab bid
>>> *Tab:* 550 mg
>> **EC-Naprosyn** 375 or 500 mg bid prn; may increase dose up to max 1500 mg/day as tolerated
>>> *Tab:* 375, 500 mg del-rel
>> **Naprelan** 1 g daily or 1.5 g daily for limited time; max 1 g/day thereafter
>>> *Tab:* 375, 500 mg
>> **Naprosyn** initially 500 mg, then 500 mg q 12 hours or 250 mg q 6-8 hours prn; max 1.25 g first day and 1 g/day thereafter
>>> *Tab:* 250, 375, 500 mg; *Oral susp:* 125 mg/5 ml (473 ml) (pineapple-orange)

 ## FIBROCYSTIC BREAST DISEASE

Contraceptives *see page 474*
▷ *spironolactone* (D)(G) 10 mg bid premenstrually
> **Aldactone** *Tab:* 25, 50*, 100*mg
▷ *vitamin E* (A) 400-600 IU daily
▷ *vitamin B6* (A) 50-100 mg daily
▷ *danazol* (X) 50-200 mg bid x 2-6 months
> **Danocrine** *Cap:* 50, 100, 200 mg
Comment: Start on 3rd or 4th day of menstrual period or after a negative pregnancy test.

 ## FIBROMYALGIA

Acetaminophen for IV Infusion *see Pain page 296*
Oral Prescription NSAIDs *see page 489*
Other Oral Analgesics *see Pain page 298*
Topical/Transdermal NSAIDs *see Pain page 297*
Parenteral Corticosteroids *see page 499*
Oral Corticosteroids *see page 497*
Topical Analgesic and Anesthetic Agents *see page 487*

SEROTONIN AND NOREPINEPHRINE REUPTAKE INHIBITORS (SNRIs)

▷ *duloxetine* (C)(G) swallow whole; initially 30 mg once daily x 1 week; then increase to 60 mg once daily; max 120 mg/day
> *Pediatric:* not recommended
>> **Cymbalta**
>>> *Cap:* 20, 30, 60 mg ent-coat pellets

▷ *milnacipran* (C) *Day 1:* 12.5 mg once; *Days 2-3:* 12.5 mg bid; *Days 4-7:* 25 mg bid; max 100 mg bid
  Pediatric: <17 years: not recommended
    Savella
      Tab: 12.5, 25, 50, 100 mg

GAMMA-AMINOBUTYRIC ACID ANALOG

▷ *gabapentin* (C)
  Pediatric: not applicable
▷ *Gralise* initially 300 mg on Day 1; then 600 mg on Day 2; then 900 mg on Days 3-6; then 1200 mg on Days 7-10; then 1500 mg on Days 11-14; titrate up to 1800 mg on Day 15; take entire dose once daily with the evening meal; do not crush, split, or chew
    Tab: 300, 600 mg
      Neurontin (G) 100 mg daily x 1 day; then 100 mg bid x 1 day; then 100 mg tid continuously or 300 mg bid; max 900 mg tid
        Tab: 600*, 800* mg; *Cap:* 100, 300, 400 mg; *Oral soln:* 250 mg/5 ml (480 ml) (strawberry-anise)
▷ *gabapentin enacarbil* (C) 600 mg once daily at about 5:00 PM; if dose not taken at recommended time, next dose should be taken the following day; swallow whole; take with food; *CrCl 30-59 mL/min:* 600 mg on Day 1, Day 3, and every day thereafter; *CrCl <30 mL/min:* or on hemodialysis: not recommended
  Pediatric: not recommended
    Horizant *Tab:* 300, 600 mg ext-rel
    Comment: Avoid abrupt cessation of *gabapentin* and *gabapentin* enacarbil. To discontinue, withdraw gradually over 1 week or longer.

α₂-DELTA LIGAND

▷ *pregabalin (GABA analog)* (C)(V) initially 50 mg tid; may titrate to 100 mg tid within one week; max 600 mg divided tid; discontinue over one week
  Pediatric: <18 years: not recommended
    Lyrica *Cap:* 25, 50, 75, 100, 150, 200, 225, 300 mg; *Oral soln:* 20 mg/ml

OTHER AGENTS

▷ *amitriptyline* (C)(G) 20 mg q HS; may increase gradually to max 50 mg q HS
  Pediatric: not recommended
    Tab: 10, 25, 50, 75, 100, 150 mg
▷ *cyclobenzaprine* (B)(G) 10 mg tid; usual range 20-40 mg/day in divided doses; max 60 mg/day x 2-3 weeks or 15 mg ext-rel once daily; max 30 mg ext-rel/day x 2-3 weeks
  Pediatric: <15 years: not recommended
    Amrix *Cap:* 15, 30 mg ext-rel
    Fexmid *Tab:* 7.5 mg
    Flexeril *Tab:* 5, 10 mg
▷ *flurazepam* (X)(IV)(G) 15 mg q HS; may increase to 30 mg q HS
    Dalmane *Cap:* 15, 30 mg
▷ *trazodone* (C)(G) 50 mg q HS
    Desyrel *Tab:* 50, 100, 150, 300 mg
▷ *triazolam* (X)(IV)(G) 0.125 mg q HS, may increase gradually to 0.5 mg
    Halcion *Tab:* 0.125, 0.25* mg

▷ *zolpidem* (B)(IV)(G) 5 mg q HS, may increase to 10 mg
  Ambien *Tab:* 5, 10 mg

FIFTH DISEASE (ERYTHEMA INFECTIOSUM)

Antipyretics *see Fever page 143*

FLATULENCE

▷ *simethicone* (C)(G)
  Gas-X (OTC) 2-4 tabs pc and HS prn
    Tab: 40, 80, 125 mg; *Cap:* 125 mg
  Mylicon (OTC) 2-4 tabs pc and HS prn
    Tab: 40, 80, 125 mg; *Cap:* 125 mg
  Phazyme-95 1-2 tabs with each meal and HS prn
    Tab: 95 mg
  Phazyme Infant Oral Drops
    Pediatric: <2 years: 0.3 ml qid pc and HS prn; 2-12 years: 0.6 ml qid pc and
    HS prn; >12 years: 1.2 ml qid pc and HS prn;
    Oral drops: 40 mg/0.6 ml (15, 30 ml w. calibrated dropper) (orange)
    (alcohol-free)
  Maximum Strength Phazyme 1-2 caps with each meal and HS prn
    Cap: 125 mg

FLUORIDATION, WATER, <0.6 PPM

▷ *fluoride* (NR)(G)
  Luride
    Pediatric: Water fluoridation 0.3-0.6 ppm: <3 years: use drops; 3-6 years: 0.25 mg
    daily; 7-16 years: 0.5 mg daily; *Water fluoridation <0.3 ppm:* <3 years: use drops;
    6 months-3 years: 0.25 mg daily; 4-6 years: 0.5 mg daily; 7-16 years: 1 mg daily
    Chew tab: 0.25, 0.5, 1 mg (sugar-free)
  Luride Drops
    Pediatric: Water fluoridation 0.3-0.6 ppm: 6 months-3 years: 0.25 ml once
    daily; 4-6 years: 0.5 ml once daily; 7-16 years: 1 ml once daily; *Water fluori-
    dation <0.3 ppm:* 6 months-3 years: 0.5 ml once daily; 4-6 years: 1 ml once
    daily; 7-16 years: 2 ml daily
    Oral drops: 0.5 mg/ml (50 ml) (sugar-free)

COMBINATION AGENTS

▷ *fluoride/vitamin a/vitamin d/vitamin c* (NR)(G)
  Pediatric: Water fluoridation 0.3-0.6 ppm: <3 years: not recommended; 3-6 years:
  0.25 mg fluoride/day; 7-16 years: 0.5 mg fluoride/day; *Water fluoridation <0.3 ppm:*

<6 months: not recommended; 6 months-3 years: 0.25 mg fluoride/day; 4-6 years: 0.5 mg fluoride/day; 7-16 years: 1 mg fluoride/day

Tri-Vi-Flor Drops
Oral drops: fluoride 0.25 mg/*vit a* 1500 u/*vit d* 400 u/*vit c* 35 mg per ml (50 ml)
Oral drops: fluoride 0.5 mg/*vit a* 1500 u/*vit d* 400 u/*vit c* 35 mg per ml (50 ml)

▷ *fluoride/vitamin a/vitamin d/vitamin c/iron* (NR)
Pediatric: Water fluoridation 0.3-0.6 ppm: <3 years: not recommended; 3-6 years: 0.25 mg fluoride/day; 7-16 years: 0.5 mg fluoride/day; *Water fluoridation <0.3 ppm:* <6 months: not recommended; 6 months-3 years: 0.25 mg fluoride/day; 4-6 years: 0.5 mg fluoride/day; 7-16 years: 1 mg fluoride/day

Tri-Vi-Flor w. Iron Drops
Oral drops: fluoride 0.25 mg/*vit a* 1500 u/*vit d* 400 u/*vit c* 35 mg/*iron* 10 mg per ml (50 ml)

FOLLICULITIS BARBAE

TOPICAL AGENTS

▷ *benzoyl peroxide* (B) 5% apply once daily after shaving
Pediatric: same as adult
see Acne Vulgaris for benzoyl peroxide preparations page 4

▷ *clindamycin* topical (B) apply bid
Pediatric: same as adult
Cleocin T *Pad:* 1% (60/pck; alcohol 50%); *Lotn:* 1% (60 ml); *Gel:* 1% (30, 60 g); *Soln w. applicator:* 1% (30, 60 ml) (alcohol 50%)
Clindagel *Gel:* 1% (42, 77 g)
Clindets *Pad:* 1% (60/pck)
Evoclin *Foam:* 1% (50, 100 g) (alcohol)

▷ *clindamycin/benzoyl peroxide* topical (C)
Pediatric: <12 years: not recommended; ≥12 years: same as adult
Acanya apply once daily-bid
Gel: clin 1.2%/*benz* 2.5% (50 g)
BenzaClin apply bid
Gel: clin 1%/*benz* 5% (25, 50 g)
Duac apply daily in the evening
Gel: clin 1%/*benz* 5% (45 g)

▷ *dapsone* topical (C) apply bid
Pediatric: <12 years: not recommended; ≥12 years: same as adult
Aczone *Gel:* 5% (30 g)

▷ *hydrocortisone* 1% (C)(OTC)(G) apply q HS
Pediatric: same as adult
see Topical Corticosteroids page 494

▷ *tazarotene* (X) apply daily at HS
Pediatric: not recommended
Avage Cream *Crm:* 0.1% (30 g)
Tazorac Cream *Crm:* 0.05, 0.1% (15, 30, 60 g)
Tazorac Gel *Gel:* 0.05, 0.1% (30, 100 g)

▷ *tretinoin* (C) apply q HS
Pediatric: <12 years: not recommended

Avita *Crm/Gel:* 0.025% (20, 45 g)
Renova *Crm:* 0.02% (40 g); 0.05% (40, 60 g)
Retin-A Cream *Crm:* 0.025, 0.05, 0.1% (20, 45 g)
Retin-A Gel *Gel:* 0.01, 0.025% (15, 45 g) (alcohol 90%)
Retin-A Liquid *Liq:* 0.05% (28 ml) (alcohol 55%)
Retin-A Micro *Microspheres:* 0.04, 0.1% (20, 45 g)

FOREIGN BODY: ESOPHAGUS

➤ *glucagon* (B) 0.02 mg/kg IV or IM with serial x-rays; max 1 mg
    Glucagon (rDNA origin or beef/pork derived)
      Vial: 1 mg/ml w. diluent
Comment: *glucagon* facilitates passage of foreign body from esophagus into stomach.

FOREIGN BODY: EYE

➤ *proparacaine* (NR) 1-2 drops to anesthetize surface of eye; then flush with normal saline
    Ophthaine *Ophth soln:* 0.5% (15 ml)
Comment: *proparacaine* facilitates the search, location, and removal of foreign body and examination of the cornea.

GASTRITIS

Antacids *see GERD page* 150
H2 Antagonists *see GERD page* 152

GASTROESOPHAGEAL REFLUX DISEASE (GERD)

Comment: Precipitators of gastric reflux include narcotics, benzodiazepines, calcium antagonists, alcohol, nicotine, chocolate, and peppermint.

ANTACIDS

Comment: Antacids with *aluminum hydroxide* may potentiate constipation. Antacids with *magnesium hydroxide* may potentiate diarrhea.
➤ *aluminum hydroxide* (C)
    ALTernaGEL (OTC) 5-10 ml between meals and HS prn; max 90 ml/day
      Pediatric: not recommended
      Liq: 500 mg/5 ml (5, 12 oz)
    Amphojel (OTC) 10 ml 5-6 times/day between meals and HS prn; max 60 ml/day
      Pediatric: not recommended
      Oral susp: 320 mg/5 ml (12 oz)
    Amphojel Tab (OTC) 600 mg 5-6 times/day between meals and HS prn; max 3.6 g/day
      Pediatric: not recommended
      Tab: 300, 600 mg

▷ *aluminum hydroxide/magnesium hydroxide* (C)(OTC)(G)
    Maalox 10-20 ml qid and HS prn
      Pediatric: not recommended
      Oral susp: alum 225 mg/*mag* 200 mg per 5 ml (5, 12, 26 oz) (mint, lemon, cherry)
    Maalox Therapeutic Concentrate 10-20 ml qid pc and HS prn
      Pediatric: not recommended
      Oral susp: alum 600 mg/*mag* 300 mg per 5 ml (12 oz) (mint)
▷ *aluminum hydroxide/magnesium hydroxide/simethicone* (C)(OTC)(G)
    Maalox Plus 10-20 ml qid pc and HS prn
      Pediatric: not recommended
      Tab: alum 200 mg/*mag* 200 mg/*sim* 25 mg
    Extra Strength Maalox Plus 10-20 ml qid pc and HS prn
      Pediatric: not recommended
      Tab: alum 350 mg/*mag* 350 mg/*sim* 30 mg
      Oral susp: alum 500 mg/*mag* 450 mg/*sim* 40 mg per 5 ml (5, 12, 26 oz)
    Extra Strength Maalox Plus Tab 1-3 tabs qid pc and HS prn
      Pediatric: not recommended
      Tab: alum 350 mg/*mag* 350 mg/*sim* 30 mg
    Mylanta 10-20 ml between meals and HS prn
      Pediatric: not recommended
      Liq: alum 200 mg/*mag* 200 mg/*sim* 20 mg per 5 ml (5, 12, 24 oz)
    Mylanta Double Strength 10-20 ml between meals and HS prn
      Pediatric: not recommended
      Liq: alum 700 mg/*mag* 400 mg/*sim* 40 mg per 5 ml (5, 12, 24 oz)
▷ *aluminum hydroxide/magnesium carbonate* (C)(OTC)(G)
    Maalox HRF 10-20 ml qid pc and HS prn
      Pediatric: not recommended
      Oral susp: alum 280 mg/*mag* 350 mg per 10 ml (10 oz)
▷ *aluminum hydroxide/magnesium trisilicate* (C)(G)
    Gaviscon chew 2-4 tabs qid pc and HS prn
      Pediatric: not recommended
      Tab: alum 80 mg/*mag* 20 mg
    Gaviscon Liquid 15-30 ml qid pc and HS prn
      Pediatric: not recommended
      Liq: alum 95 mg/*mag* 359 mg per 15 ml (6, 12 oz)
    Gaviscon Extra Strength 2-4 tabs qid pc and HS prn
      Pediatric: not recommended
      Tab: alum 160 mg/*mag* 105 mg
    Gaviscon Extra Strength Liquid 10-20 ml qid prn
      Pediatric: not recommended
      Liq: alum 508 mg/*mag* 475 mg per 10 ml (12 oz)
▷ *aluminum hydroxide/magnesium hydroxide/simethicone* (C)(OTC)(G)
    Maalox Maximum Strength 10-20 ml qid prn; max 60 ml/day
      Pediatric: not recommended
      Oral susp: alum 500 mg/*mag* 450 mg/*sim* 40 mg per 5 ml (5, 12, 26 oz) (mint, cherry)
▷ *calcium carbonate* (C)(OTC)(G)
    Children's Mylanta Tab
      Pediatric: <2 years: not recommended; 2-5 years (24-47 lb): 1 tab as needed up to tid; 6-11 years (48-95 lb): 2 tabs as needed up to tid

   Tab: 400 mg
Children's Mylanta
   Pediatric: <2 years: not recommended; 2-5 years (24-47 lb): 1 tab as needed
   up to tid; 6-11 years (48-95 lb): 2 tabs as needed up to tid
   Liq: 400 mg/5 ml (4 oz)
Maalox Tab chew 2-4 tabs prn; max 12 tabs/day
   Pediatric: not recommended
   Chew tab: 600 mg (wild berry, lemon, wintergreen) (phenylalanine)
Maalox Maximum Strength Tab 1-2 tabs prn; max 8 tabs/day
   Pediatric: not recommended
   Tab: 1 g (wild berry, lemon, wintergreen; phenylalanine)
Rolaids Extra Strength 1-2 tabs dissolved in mouth <u>or</u> chewed q 1 hour prn;
max 8 tabs/day
   Tab: 1000 mg
Tums 1-2 tabs dissolved in mouth <u>or</u> chewed q 1 hour prn; max 16 tabs/day
   Tab: 500 mg
Tums E-X 1-2 tabs dissolved in mouth <u>or</u> chewed q 1 hour prn; max 16 tabs/day
   Tab: 750 mg

▷ *calcium carbonate/magnesium hydroxide* (C)
   Mylanta Tab 2-4 tabs between meals and HS prn
      Pediatric: not recommended
      Tab: calib 350 mg/*mag* 150 mg
   Mylanta DS Tab 2-4 tabs between meals and HS prn
      Pediatric: not recommended
      Tab: calib 700 mg/*mag* 300 mg
   Rolaids Sodium-Free 1-2 tabs dissolved in mouth <u>or</u> chewed q 1 hour as needed
      Tab: calib 317 mg/*mag* 64 mg
▷ *calcium carbonate/magnesium carbonate* (C)
   Mylanta Gel Caps (OTC) 2-4 caps prn
      Gel cap: calib 550 mg/*mag* 125 mg
▷ *dihydroxyaluminum* (NR)
   Rolaids (OTC) 1-2 tabs dissolved in mouth <u>or</u> chewed q 1 hour prn; max
   24 tabs/day
      Tab: 334 mg

H2 ANTAGONISTS

▷ *cimetidine* (B)(OTC)(G) 800 mg bid <u>or</u> 400 mg qid; max 12 weeks
   Pediatric: <16 years: not recommended; ≥16 years: same as adult
      Tagamet 800 mg bid or 400 mg qid; max 12 weeks
         Tab: 200, 300, 400*, 800*mg
      Tagamet HB *Prophylaxis:* 1 tab ac; *Treatment:* 1 tab bid
         Tab: 200 mg
      Tagamet HB Oral Suspension *Prophylaxis:* 1-3 tsp ac; *Treatment:* 1 tsp bid
         Oral susp: 200 mg/20 ml (12 oz)
      Tagamet Liquid *Liq:* 300 mg/5 ml (mint-peach) (alcohol 2.8%)
▷ *famotidine* (B)(OTC)(G)
   Pediatric: 0.5 mg/kg/day q HS prn <u>or</u> in 2 divided doses; max 40 mg/day
      Maximum Strength Pepcid AC 1 tab ac
         Tab: 20 mg

Pepcid 20-40 mg bid; max 6 weeks
   Tab: 20 mg; *Tab:* 40 mg; *Oral susp:* 40 mg/5 ml (50 ml)
Pepcid AC 1 tab ac; max 2 doses/day
   Tab/Rapid dissolving tab: 10 mg
Pepcid Complete (OTC) 1 tab ac; max 2 doses/day
   Tab: fam 10 mg/*CaCO2* 800 mg/*mg hydroxide* 165 mg
Pepcid RPD *Tab:* 20, 40 mg rapid dissolv
▷ *nizatidine* (B)(OTC)(G) 150 mg bid <u>or</u> 300 mg once daily
Pediatric: not recommended
   Axid *Cap:* 150, 300 mg; *Oral soln:* 15 mg/ml (480 ml) (bubble gum)
▷ *ranitidine* (B)(OTC)(G)
Pediatric: <1 month: not recommended; 1 month to 16 years: 2-4 mg/kg/day in 2
divided doses; max 300 mg/day; *Duodenal/Gastric Ulcer:* 2-4 mg/kg/day divided
bid; max 300 mg/day; *Erosive Esophagitis:* 5-10 mg/kg/day divided bid; max 300
mg/day; 20 lb, 9 kg: 0.6 ml; 30 lb, 13.6 kg: 0.9 ml; 40 lb, 18.2 kg: 1.2 ml; 50 lb, 22.7
kg: 1.5 ml; 60 lb, 27.3 kg: 1.8 ml; 70 lb, 31.8 kg: 2.1 ml
   Zantac 150 mg bid <u>or</u> 300 mg q HS
      Tab: 150, 300 mg
   Zantac 75 1 tab ac
      Tab: 75 mg
   Zantac EFFERdose dissolve 25 mg tab in 5 ml water and dissolve 150 mg tab in
   6-8 oz water
      Efferdose: 25, 150 mg effervescent
   Zantac Syrup *Syr:* 15 mg/ml (peppermint) (alcohol 7.5%)
▷ *ranitidine bismuth citrate* (C) 400 mg bid
Pediatric: not recommended
   Tritec *Tab:* 400 mg

PROTON PUMP INHIBITORS

▷ *dexlansoprazole* (B) 30-60 mg daily for up to 4 weeks
Pediatric: <18 years: not recommended
   Dexilant *Cap:* 30, 60 mg ent-coat del-rel granules; may open and sprinkle on
   applesauce; do not crush <u>or</u> chew granules
   Dexilant SoluTab *Tab:* 30 mg del-rel orally disint
▷ *esomeprazole* (B)(OTC)(G) 20-40 mg once daily; max 8 weeks; take 1 hour before
food; swallow whole <u>or</u> mix granules with food <u>or</u> juice and take immediately; do not
crush <u>or</u> chew granules
Pediatric: <1 month: not established; 1 month-<1 year, 3-5 kg: 2.5 mg; 5-7.5 kg: 5
mg; >7.5-12 kg: 10 mg; 1-11 years, <20 kg: 10 mg; ≥20 kg: 10-20 mg; 12-17 years:
20 mg; max 8 weeks
   Nexium *Cap:* 20, 40 mg ent-coat del-rel pellets
   Nexium for Oral Suspension *Oral susp:* 10, 20, 40 mg ent-coat del-rel granules/
   pkt; mix in 2 tblsp water and drink immediately; 30 pkt/carton
▷ *lansoprazole* (B)(OTC)(G) 15-30 mg daily for up to 8 weeks; may repeat course; take
before eating
Pediatric: <1 year: not recommended; 1-11 years, <30 kg: 15 mg once daily;
>11 years: same as adult
   Prevacid *Cap:* 15, 30 mg ent-coat del-rel granules; swallow whole <u>or</u> mix granules with food <u>or</u> juice and take immediately; do not crush <u>or</u> chew granules;
   follow with water

Prevacid for Oral Suspension *Oral susp:* 15, 30 mg ent-coat del-rel granules/pkt; mix in 2 tblsp water and drink immediately; 30 pkt/carton (strawberry)
Prevacid SoluTab *ODT:* 15, 30 mg (strawberry) (phenylalanine)
Prevacid 24HR 15 mg ent-coat del-rel granules; swallow whole <u>or</u> mix granules with food <u>or</u> juice and take immediately; do not crush <u>or</u> chew granules; follow with water

▶ *omeprazole* (C)(OTC)(G) 20-40 mg daily for 14 days; may repeat course in 4 months; take before eating; swallow whole or mix granules with applesauce and take immediately; do not crush or chew granules; follow with water
Pediatric: <1 year: not recommended; 5- <10 kg: 5 mg daily; 10- <20 kg: 10 mg daily; ≥20 kg: same as adult
   Prilosec *Cap:* 10, 20, 40 mg ent-coat del-rel granules
      Pediatric: <1 year: not recommended; 5-<10 kg: 5 mg daily; 10-<20 kg: 10 mg daily; ≥20 kg: same as adult
   Prilosec OTC *Tab:* 20 mg del-rel (regular, wildberry)
      Pediatric: <18 years: not recommended

▶ *pantoprazole* (B) 40 mg daily
Pediatric: not recommended
   Protonix (G)
      Tab: 40 mg ent-coat del-rel
   Protonix for Oral Suspension *Oral susp:* 40 mg ent-coat del-rel granules/pkt; mix in 1 tsp apple juice for 5 seconds <u>or</u> sprinkle on 1 tsp apple sauce, and swallow immediately; do not mix in water <u>or</u> any other liquid <u>or</u> food; take approximately 30 minutes prior to a meal; 30 pkt/carton

▶ *rabeprazole* (B)(OTC)(G) *Tab:* 20 mg daily after breakfast; do not crush <u>or</u> chew; *Cap:* open cap and sprinkle contents on a small amount of soft food <u>or</u> liquid
Pediatric: <1 year: not recommended; 1-11 years, <15 kg: 5 mg once daily for up to 12 weeks; ≥12 years, ≥15 kg: same as adult
   AcipHex *Tab:* 20 mg ent-coat del-rel
   AcipHex Sprinkle *Cap:* 5, 10 mg del-rel

PROTON PUMP INHIBITORS/SODIUM BICARBONATE COMBINATION

▶ *omeprazole/na bicarbonate* (B) 20 mg daily; do not crush <u>or</u> chew; max 8 weeks
Pediatric: <18 years: not recommended
   Zegerid *Cap:* omep 20 mg/*na bicarb* 1100 mg; *omep* 40 mg/*na bicarb* 1100 mg
   Zegerid OTC (OTC) *Cap:* omep 20 mg/*na bicarb* 1100 mg
   Zegerid for Oral Suspension *Pwdr for oral susp:* omep 20 mg/*na bicarb* 1680 mg; *omep* 40 mg/*na bicarb* 1680 mg (30 pkt/carton)

PROMOTILITY AGENT

▶ *metoclopramide* (B)(G) 10-15 mg qid 30 minutes ac and HS prn; up to 20 mg prior to provoking situation; max 12 weeks per therapeutic course
Pediatric: <18 years: not recommended
   Metozolv ODT *ODT:* 5, 10 mg (mint)
   Reglan *Tab:* 5*, 10 mg; *Syr:* 5 mg/5 ml
   Reglan ODT *ODT:* 5, 10 mg (orange)
Comment: *metoclopropamide* is contraindicated when stimulation of GI motility may be dangerous. Observe for tardive dyskinesia and Parkinsonism. Avoid concomitant drugs which may cause an extrapyramidal reaction (e.g., phenothiazines, *haloperidol*).

GIARDIASIS (GIARDIA LAMBLIA)

▷ *metronidazole* (not for use in 1st; B in 2nd, 3rd)(G) 250 mg tid x 5-10 days
  Pediatric: 35-50 mg/kg/day in 3 divided doses x 10 days
    Flagyl *Tab:* 250*, 500*mg
    Flagyl 375 *Cap:* 375 mg
    Flagyl ER *Tab:* 750 mg ext-rel
  Comment: Alcohol is contraindicated during treatment with oral *metronidazole*
  and for 72 hours after therapy due to a possible *disulfiram*-like reaction (nausea,
  vomiting, flushing, headache).
▷ *tinidazole* (not for use in 1st; B in 2nd, 3rd) 2 g in a single dose; take with food
  Pediatric: <3 years: not recommended; ≥3 years: 50 mg/kg daily in a single dose;
  take with food; max 2 g
    Tindamax *Tab:* 250*, 500*mg
  Comment: Alcohol is contraindicated during treatment with oral *tinidazole* and for
  72 hours after therapy due to a possible *disulfiram*-like reaction (nausea, vomiting,
  flushing, headache).
▷ *nitazoxanide* (B) 500 mg q 12 hours x 3 days; take with food
  Pediatric: <1 year: not recommended; 1-3 years; 100 mg q 12 hours x 3 days; 4-11
  years: 200 mg q 12 hours x 3 days; ≥12 years: same as adult
    Alinia *Tab:* 500 mg; *Oral susp:* 100 mg/5 ml (60 ml)
    Comment: **Alinia** is an antiprotozoal for the treatment of diarrhea due to *G.
    lamblia* or *C. parvum*.

GINGIVITIS/PERIODONTITIS

ANTI-INFECTIVE ORAL RINSES

Comment: Oral treatments should be preceded by brushing and flossing the teeth.
Avoid foods and liquids for 2-3 hours after a treatment.
▷ *chlorhexidine gluconate* (B)(G) swish 15 ml undiluted for 30 seconds bid; do not
  swallow; do not rinse mouth after treatment.
    Peridex, PerioGard *Oral soln:* 0.12% (480 ml)

GLAUCOMA: OPEN ANGLE

Comment: Other ophthalmic medications should not be administered within 5-10
minutes of administering an ophthalmic antiglaucoma medication. Contact lenses
should be removed prior to instillation of antiglaucoma medications and may
be replaced 15 minutes later. Interactions with ophthalmic anti-glaucoma agents
include MAOIs, CNS depressants, beta-blockers, tricyclic antidepressants, and
hypoglycemics.

OPHTHALMIC ALPHA-2-AGONISTS

Comment: Ophthalmic alpha-2-agonists are contraindicated with concomitant
MAOI use. Cautious use with CNS depressants, beta-blockers (ocular and systemic),
antihypertensives, cardiac glycosides, and tricyclic antidepressants.

▷ *apraclonidine* ophthalmic solution **(C)** 1-2 drops affected eye tid
  Pediatric: not recommended
    Iopidine *Ophth soln:* 0.5% (5 ml) (benzalkonium chloride)
▷ *brimonidine tartrate* ophthalmic solution **(B)** 1 drop affected eye q 8 hours
  Pediatric: <2 years: not recommended; ≥2 years: 1 drop affected eye q 8 hours
    Alphagan P *Ophth soln:* 0.1, 0.15% (5, 10, 15 ml) (purite)

OPHTHALMIC CARBONIC ANHYDRASE INHIBITORS

Comment: Ophthalmic carbonic anhydrase inhibitors are contraindicated in patients with sulfa allergy.
▷ *brinzolamide* ophthalmic suspension **(C)** 1 drop affected eye tid
  Pediatric: not recommended
    Azopt *Ophth susp:* 1% (2.5, 5, 10, 15 ml) (benzalkonium chloride)
▷ *dorzolamide* ophthalmic solution **(C)(G)** 1 drop affected eye tid
  Pediatric: same as adult
    Trusopt *Ophth soln:* 2% (10 ml) (benzalkonium chloride)

OPHTHALMIC ALPHA-2 ADRENERGIC RECEPTOR AGONIST/CARBONIC ANHYDRASE INHIBITOR

▷ *brimonidine/brinzolamide* **(C)** 1 drop affected eye tid
  Pediatric: not recommended
    Simbrinza *Ophth soln: brim* 1% mg/*brinz* 0.2% per ml (10 ml)

OPHTHALMIC CHOLINERGICS (MIOTICS)

▷ *carbachol/hydroxypropyl methylcellulose* ophthalmic solution **(C)** 2 drops affected eye tid
  Pediatric: not recommended
    Isopto Carbachol *Ophth soln: carb* 0.75% or 2.25%/*hydroxy* 1% (15 ml); *carb* 1.5% or 3%/*hydroxy* 1% (15, 30 ml) (benzalkonium chloride)
▷ *pilocarpine* **(C)(G)**
  Pediatric: not recommended
    Isopto Carpine 2 drops affected eye tid-qid
      Ophth soln: 1, 2, 4% (15 ml) (benzalkonium chloride)
    Ocusert Pilo change ophthalmic insert once weekly
      Ophth inserts: 20 mcg/hr (8/pck)
    Pilocar Ophthalmic Solution 1-2 drops affected eye 1-6 times/day
      Ophth soln: 0.5, 1, 2, 3, 4, 6, 8% (15 ml)
    Pilopine HS apply 1/2 inch ribbon in lower conjunctival sac q HS
      Opth gel: 4% (4 g)

OPHTHALMIC CHOLINESTERASE INHIBITORS

▷ *demecarium bromide* ophthalmic solution **(X)** 1-2 drops affected eye q 12-48 hours
  Pediatric: not recommended
    Humorsol Ocumeter *Ophth soln:* 0.125, 0.25% (5 ml)
▷ *echothiophate iodide* ophthalmic solution **(C)** initially 1 drop of 0.03% affected eye bid; then increase strength as needed
  Pediatric: not recommended
    Phospholine Iodide *Ophth soln:* 0.03, 0.06, 0.125, 0.25% (5 ml)

OPHTHALMIC CARDIOSELECTIVE BETA-BLOCKERS

Comment: Ophthalmic beta-blockers are generally contraindicated in severe COPD, history of or current bronchial asthma, sinus bradycardia, 2nd or 3rd degree AV block.
▷ *betaxolol* ophthalmic solution (C)(G) 1-2 drops affected eye bid
  Pediatric: not recommended
      Betoptic *Ophth soln:* 0.5% (5, 10, 15 ml) (benzalkonium chloride)
      Betoptic S *Ophth soln:* 0.25% (2.5, 5, 10, 15 ml) (benzalkonium chloride)

OPHTHALMIC BETA-BLOCKERS (NONCARDIOSELECTIVE)

Comment: Ophthalmic beta-blockers are generally contraindicated in severe COPD, history of or current bronchial asthma, sinus bradycardia, 2nd or 3rd degree AV block.
▷ *carteolol* ophthalmic solution (C)(G) 1 drop affected eye bid
  Pediatric: not recommended
      Ocupress *Ophth soln:* 1% (5, 10, 15 ml) (benzalkonium chloride)
▷ *levobunolol* ophthalmic solution (C) 1-2 drops affected eye bid
  Pediatric: not recommended
      Betagan *Ophth soln:* 0.5% (5, 10, 15 ml) (benzalkonium chloride)
▷ *metipranolol* ophthalmic solution (C)(G) 1 drop affected eye bid
  Pediatric: not recommended
      OptiPranolol *Ophth soln:* 0.3% (5, 10 ml) (benzalkonium chloride)
▷ *timolol* ophthalmic solution and gel (C)(G)
  Pediatric: not recommended
      Betimol 1 drop affected eye bid
          Ophth soln: 0.25, 0.5% (5, 10, 15 ml) (benzalkonium chloride)
      Istalol 1 drop affected eye daily
          Ophth soln: 0.5% (2.5, 5 ml) (preservative-free)
      Timoptic 1 drop affected eye bid
          Ophth soln: 0.25, 0.5% (5, 10, 15 ml) (benzalkonium chloride)
      Timoptic Ocudose 1 drop bid
          Ophth soln: 0.25, 0.5% (0.2 ml/dose, 60 dose) (preservative-free)
      Timoptic-XE 1 drop affected eye bid
          Ophth gel: 0.25, 0.5% (2.5, 5 ml) (preservative-free)

OPHTHALMIC ALPHA-2 AGONIST/BETA-BLOCKER (NONCARDIOSELECTIVE) COMBINATION

Comment: Generally contraindicated in severe COPD, history of or current bronchial asthma, sinus bradycardia, 2nd or 3rd degree AV block.
▷ *brimonidine tartrate/timolol* ophthalmic solution (C) 1 drop affected eye bid
  Pediatric: <2 years: not recommended; ≥2 years: same as adult
      Combigan *Ophth soln: brimo* 0.2%/*timo* 0.5% (5, 10, 15 ml) (benzalkonium chloride)

OPHTHALMIC PROSTAMIDE ANALOGUES

▷ *bimatropost* ophthalmic solution (C) 1 drop q affected eye HS
  Pediatric: <16 years: not recommended; ≥16 years: same as adult
      Lumigan *Ophth soln:* 0.01, 0.03% (2.5, 5, 7.5 ml) (benzalkonium chloride)
▷ *latanoprost* ophthalmic solution (C) 1 drop affected eye q HS
  Pediatric: not recommended

Xalatan *Ophth soln:* 0.005% (2.5 ml) (benzalkonium chloride)
▷ **tafluprost** ophthalmic solution **(C)** 1 drop affected eye q HS
Pediatric: not recommended
Zioptan *Ophth soln:* 0.0015% (0.3 ml single-use, 30-60/carton) (preservative-free)
▷ **travoprost** ophthalmic solution **(C)(G)** 1 drop affected eye q HS
Pediatric: <16 years: not recommended; ≥16 years: same as adult
Travatan *Ophth soln:* 0.004% (2.5, 5 ml) (benzalkonium chloride)
Travatan Z *Ophth soln:* 0.004% (2.5, 5 ml) (boric acid, propylene glycol,
sorbitol, zinc chloride)

OPHTHALMIC SYMPATHOMIMETICS

Comment: Contraindicated in narrow-angle glaucoma. Use with caution in
cardiovascular disease, hypertension, hyperthyroidism, diabetes, and asthma.
▷ **dipivefrin** ophthalmic solution **(B)** 1 drop affected eye q 12 hours
Propine *Ophth soln:* 0.1% (5, 10, 15 ml) (benzalkonium chloride)

OPHTHALMIC CARBONIC ANHYDRASE INHIBITOR/NONCARDIOSELECTIVE OPHTHALMIC CARBONIC ANHYDRASE INHIBITOR/BETA-BLOCKER

▷ **dorzolamide/timolol** ophthalmic solution **(C)** 1 drop affected eye bid
Pediatric: not recommended
Cosopt *Ophth soln:* dorz 2%/tim 0.5% (10 ml) (benzalkonium chloride)
Cosopt PF *Ophth soln:* dorz 2%/tim 0.5% (10 ml) (preservative-free)

OPHTHALMIC SYNTHETIC DOCOSANOID

▷ **unoprostone isopropyl** ophthalmic solution **(C)** 1 drop affected eye bid
Pediatric: not recommended
Rescula *Ophth soln:* 0.15% (5 ml) (benzalkonium chloride)

ORAL CARBONIC ANHYDRASE INHIBITORS

▷ **acetazolamide (C)** 250-1000 mg/day in divided doses <u>or</u> 500 mg bid sust-rel tabs;
max 1 g/day
Pediatric: not recommended
Diamox *Tab:* 125*, 250*mg
Diamox Sequels *Tab:* 500 mg sust-rel
▷ **methazolamide (C)(G)** 50-100 mg bid-tid times daily
Pediatric: not recommended
Neptazane *Tab:* 25, 50 mg
Comment: Administer ophthalmic osmotic and miotic agents concomitantly.

 GONORRHEA (*NEISSERIA GONORRHOEAE*)

Comment: The following treatment regimens for *N. gonorrhoeae* are published in
the **2015 CDC Transmitted Diseases Treatment Guidelines**. Treatment regimens are
presented by generic drug name first, followed by information about brands and dose
forms. Empiric treatment requires concomitant treatment of chlamydia. Treat all sexual
contacts. Patients who are HIV-positive should receive the same treatment as those who

are HIV-negative. Sexual abuse must be considered a cause of gonococcal infection in preadolescent children.

RECOMMENDED REGIMENS: ADULT; UNCOMPLICATED INFECTIONS OF THE CERVIX, URETHRA, AND RECTUM

Regimen 1

▷ *ceftriaxone* 250 mg IM in a single dose
   plus
▷ *azithromycin* 1 g in a single dose

Regimen 2

▷ *ceftriaxone* 250 mg IM in a single dose
   plus
▷ *doxycycline* 100 mg bid x 7 days

RECOMMENDED REGIMENS: ADULT; UNCOMPLICATED INFECTIONS OF THE PHARYNX

Regimen 1

▷ *ceftriaxone* 250 mg IM in a single dose
   plus
▷ *azithromycin* 1 g in a single dose

Regimen 2

▷ *ceftriaxone* 250 mg IM in a single dose
   plus
▷ *doxycycline* 100 mg bid x 7 days

RECOMMENDED REGIMENS: CHILDREN >45 KG, >8 YEARS; UNCOMPLICATED INFECTIONS OF THE CERVIX, URETHRA, AND RECTUM

Regimen 1

▷ *ceftriaxone* 250 mg IM in a single dose
   plus
▷ *azithromycin* 1 g in a single dose

RECOMMENDED REGIMEN: CHILDREN >45 KG

Regimen 1

▷ *ceftriaxone* 250 mg IM in a single dose

RECOMMENDED REGIMEN: CHILDREN >45 KG WHO HAVE GONOCOCCAL BACTEREMIA OR ARTHRITIS

Regimen 1

▷ *ceftriaxone* 50 mg/kg IM or IV in a single dose daily x 7 days

RECOMMENDED REGIMENS: CHILDREN <45 KG, <8 YEARS; UNCOMPLICATED GONOCOCCAL VULVOVAGINITIS, CERVICITIS, URETHRITIS, PHARYNGITIS, <u>OR</u> PROCTITIS

Regimen 1

▷ *ceftriaxone* 250 mg IM in a single dose

RECOMMENDED REGIMEN: CHILDREN <45 KG, <8 YEARS WHO HAVE GONOCOCCAL BACTEREMIA <u>OR</u> ARTHRITIS

Regimen 1

▷ *ceftriaxone* 50 mg/kg (max dose 1 g) IM <u>or</u> IV in a single dose daily x 7 days

DRUG BRANDS AND DOSE FORMS

▷ *azithromycin* (B)
> **Zithromax** *Tab:* 250, 500, 600 mg; *Oral susp:* 100 mg/5 ml (15 ml); 200 mg/5 ml (15, 22.5, 30 ml) (cherry); *Pkt:* 1 g for reconstitution (cherry-banana)
> **Zithromax Tri-pak** *Tab:* 3 x 500 mg tabs/pck
> **Zithromax Z-pak** *Tab:* 6 x 250 mg tabs/pck
> **Zmax** *Oral susp:* 2 g ext-rel for reconstitution (cherry-banana) (148 mg Na⁺)

▷ *ceftriaxone* (B)(G)
> **Rocephin** *Vial:* 250, 500 mg; 1, 2 g

▷ *doxycycline* (D)(G)
> **Actilate** *Tab:* 75, 150** mg
> **Adoxa** *Tab:* 50, 75, 100, 150 mg ent-coat
> **Doryx** *Tab:* 75, 100, 150 mg del-rel
> **Monodox** *Cap:* 50, 75, 100 mg
> **Oracea** *Cap:* 40 mg del-rel
> **Vibramycin** *Cap:* 50, 100 mg; *Syr:* 50 mg/5 ml (raspberry) (sulfites); *Oral susp:* 25 mg/5 ml (raspberry-apple)
> **Vibra-Tab** *Tab:* 100 mg film-coat

ALTERNATIVE THERAPY

▷ *azithromycin* (B) 2 g x 1 dose
> *Pediatric:* not recommended for treatment of gonorrhea in children
> **Zithromax** *Tab:* 250, 500, 600 mg; *Oral susp:* 100 mg/5 ml (15 ml); 200 mg/5 ml (15, 22.5, 30 ml) (cherry); *Pkt:* 1 g for reconstitution (cherry-banana)
> **Zithromax Tri-pak** *Tab:* 3 x 500 mg tabs/pck
> **Zithromax Z-pak** *Tab:* 6 x 250 mg tabs/pck
> **Zmax** *Oral susp:* 2 g ext-rel for reconstitution (cherry-banana) (148 mg Na⁺)

▷ *cefotaxime* 500 mg IM x 1 dose
> **Claforan** *Vial:* 500 mg; 1, 2 g

▷ *cefotetan* 1 g IM x 1 dose
> *Pediatric:* not recommended
> **Cefotan** *Vial:* 1, 2 g

▷ *cefoxitin* (B) 2 g IM x 1 dose
> *Pediatric:* <3 months: not recommended
> **Mefoxin** *Vial:* 1, 2 g
> > *plus*

▷ *probenecid* (B)(G)
Benemid 1 g 30 minutes before *cefoxitin*
Pediatric: <2 years: not recommended; 2-14 years: 25 mg/kg 30 minutes
before *cefoxitin*; >14 years: same as adult
Tab: 500*mg; *Cap:* 500 mg
▷ *cefpodoxime proxetil* (B) 200 mg x 1 dose
Pediatric: <2 months: not recommended; 2 months-12 years: 10 mg/kg/day (max 400
mg/ dose) or 5 mg/kg/day bid (max 200 mg/dose)
Vantin *Tab:* 100, 200 mg; *Oral susp:* 50, 100 mg/5 ml (50, 75, 100 mg) (lemon creme)
▷ *ceftizoxime* (B) 1 g IM x 1 dose
Pediatric: <6 months: not recommended
Cefizox *Vial:* 500 mg; 1, 2, 10 g
▷ *cefuroxime axetil* (B)(G) 1000 mg x 1 dose
Pediatric: 30 mg/kg/day in 2 divided doses x 10 days
Ceftin *Tab:* 250, 500 mg; *Oral susp:* 125, 250 mg/5 ml (50, 100 ml) (tutti-frutti)
▷ *demeclocycline* (X) 600 mg initially, followed by 300 mg q 12 hours x 4 days (total 3 g)
Pediatric: <8 years: not recommended
Declomycin *Tab:* 300 mg
Comment: *demeclocycline* is contraindicated <8 years-of-age, in pregnancy,
and lactation (discolors developing tooth enamel). A side effect may be photo-
sensitivity (photophobia). Do not give with antacids, calcium supplements, milk or
other dairy, or within two hours of taking another drug.
▷ *enoxacin* (C) 400 mg x 1 dose
Pediatric: <18 years: not recommended
Penetrex *Tab:* 200, 400 mg
▷ *imipramine* (C) 400 mg x 1 dose
Pediatric: <18 years: not recommended
Maxaquin *Tab:* 400 mg
▷ *norfloxacin* (C) 800 mg x 1 dose
Pediatric: <18 years: not recommended
Noroxin *Tab:* 400 mg
▷ *spectinomycin* (B) 2 g IM x 1 dose
Pediatric: 40 mg/kg IM x 1 dose
Trobicin *Vial:* 2 g

GOUT

Pseudogout *see Pseudogout page 354*
Acetaminophen for IV Infusion *see Pain page 296*
Oral Prescription NSAIDs *see page 489*
Other Oral Analgesics *see Pain page 298*
Topical/Transdermal NSAIDs *see Pain page 297*
Parenteral Corticosteroids *see page 499*
Oral Corticosteroids *see page 497*

PEGYLATED URIC ACID SPECIFIC ENZYME

▷ *pegloticase* (C) premedicate with antihistamine and corticosteroid; 8 mg once every
2 weeks; administer IV infusion after dilution over at least 2 hours; observe at least
1 hour post-infusion

Pediatric: <18 years: not recommended
Krystexxa *Vial:* 8 mg/ml (1 ml) single-use pwdr for IV infusion after dilution
Comment: Slow rate, or stop and restart at lower rate, if infusion reaction occurs (e.g., **Krystexxa** is contraindicated with G6PD deficiency; screen patients of African or Mediterranean descent). **Krystexxa** is not for the treatment of asymptomatic hyperuricemia.

PROPHYLAXIS

▷ *allopurinol* (C)(G) initially 100 mg daily; increase by 100 mg weekly; max 800 mg/day and 300 mg/dose; usual range for mild symptoms 200-300 mg/day; for severe symptoms 400-600 mg/day; take with food
Pediatric: not recommended
Zyloprim *Tab:* 100*, 300*mg
Comment: Do not take concurrent with *colchicine*.

▷ *colchicine* (C)(G) 0.6-1.2 mg at first sign of attack; then 0.6 mg every hour or 1.2 mg every 2 hours until pain relief; then consider 0.6 mg/day or every other day for maintenance
Pediatric: not recommended
Colcrys *Tab:* 0.6 mg
Mitigare *Cap:* 0.6 mg
Comment: Do not take concurrent with *allopurinol*.

▷ *febuxostat* (C) initially 40 mg daily; after 2 weeks, may increase to 80 mg daily.
Pediatric: <18 years: not recommended
Uloric *Tab:* 40, 80 mg
Comment: Gout flare prophylaxis with *colchicine* or NSAID is recommended on initiation of *febuxostat* and up to 6 months.

URICOSURIC AGENT

▷ *probenecid* (C)(G) 250 mg bid x 1 week; maintenance 500 mg bid
Pediatric: not recommended
Tab: 500*mg; *Cap:* 500 mg
Comment: Avoid concomitant use of *probenecid* and salicylates.

URICOSURIC/ANTI-INFLAMMATORY COMBINATIONS

▷ *probenecid/colchicine* (NR)(G) 1 tab once daily x 1 week; then, 1 tab bid thereafter
Pediatric: not recommended
Tab: prob 500 mg/colch 0.5 mg
Comment: *probenecid/colchicine* is contraindicated in the treatment of acute gout attack, patients with blood dyscrasias, and patients with uric acid kidney stones. Concomitant salicylates antagonize the uricosuric effects.

▷ *sulfinpyrazone* (C) initially 200-400 mg bid; may gradually increase to 800 mg bid
Anturane *Cap:* 100, 200 mg
Comment: Goal is serum uric acid <6.5 mg/dL.

XANTHINE OXIDASE INHIBITOR

▷ *febuxostat* (C) 40 mg once daily x 2 weeks; if serum uric acid is not <6 mg/dL, may increase to 80 mg once daily

Pediatric: <18 years: not established
  Uloric *Tab:* 40, 80 mg

SELECTIVE URIC ACID REABSORPTION INHIBITOR (SURI)

▷ *lesinurad* (C) 200 mg once daily in combination with a xanthine oxidase inhibitor (XOI)
Pediatric: <18 years: not established
  Zurampic *Tab:* 200 mg
  Comment: **Zurampic** inhibits URATI, a urate transporter, which is responsible for the majority of renal absorption of uric acid and (OAT) 4, organic anion transporter, a uric acid transporter involved in diuretic-induced hyperuricemia. Do not use as monotherapy. Use in combination with an XOI, such as *allopurinol* or *febuxostat*, (to reduce the production of uric acid). Do not initiate if CrCl <45 mL/min, ESRD, dialysis, or kidney transplant.

 GOUTY ARTHRITIS

Acetaminophen for IV Infusion *see* **Pain** *page* 296
Oral Prescription NSAIDs *see page* 489
Other Oral Analgesics *see* **Pain** *page* 298
Topical/Transdermal NSAIDs *see* **Pain** *page* 297
Parenteral Corticosteroids *see page* 499
Oral Corticosteroids *see page* 497
Topical Analgesic and Anesthetic Agents *see page* 487

TOPICAL ANALGESICS

▷ *capsaicin* (B)(G) apply tid-qid prn to intact skin
Pediatric: <2 years: not recommended; ≥2 years: same as adult
  Axsain *Crm:* 0.075% (1, 2 oz)
  Capsin *Lotn:* 0.025, 0.075% (59 ml)
  Capzasin-P (OTC) *Crm:* 0.025% (1.5 oz); *Lotn:* 0.025% (2 oz)
  Dolorac *Crm:* 0.025% (28 g)
  Double Cap (OTC) *Crm:* 0.05% (2 oz)
  R-Gel *Gel:* 0.025% (15, 30 g)
  Zostrix (OTC) *Crm:* 0.025% (0.7, 1.5, 3 oz)
  Zostrix HP (OTC) *Emol crm:* 0.075% (1, 2 oz)
Comment: Provides some relief by 1-2 weeks; optimal benefit may take 4-6 weeks.

ORAL SALICYLATE

▷ *indomethacin* (C) initially 25 mg bid-tid; increase as needed at weekly intervals by 25-50 mg/day; max 200 mg/day
Pediatric: <14 years: usually not recommended; >2 years, if risk warranted: 1-2 mg/kg/day in divided doses; max 3-4 mg/kg/day (or 150-200 mg/day, whichever is less); <14 years, ER cap not recommended
Cap: 25, 50 mg; *Susp:* 25 mg/5 ml (pineapple-coconut, mint; alcohol 1%); *Supp:* 50 mg; *ER Cap:* 75 mg ext-rel

Comment: *indomethacin* is indicated only for acute painful flares. Administer with food and/or antacids. Use lowest effective dose for shortest duration.

NSAID PLUS PPI

➤ *esomeprazole/naproxen* (C; not for use in 3rd) 1 tab bid; use lowest effective dose for the shortest duration; swallow whole; take at least 30 minutes before a meal
Pediatric: <18 years: not recommended
  Vimovo *Tab:* nap 375 mg/*eso* 20 mg ext-rel; *nap* 500 mg/*eso* 20 mg ext-rel

COX-2 INHIBITORS

Comment: Cox-2 inhibitors are contraindicated with history of asthma, urticaria, and allergic-type reactions to *aspirin*, other NSAIDs, and sulfonamides, 3rd trimester of pregnancy, and coronary artery bypass graft (CABG) surgery.
➤ *celecoxib* (C)(G) 100-400 mg bid; max 800 mg/day
Pediatric: <18 years: not recommended
  Celebrex *Cap:* 50, 100, 200, 400 mg
➤ *meloxicam* (C)(G) initially 7.5 mg once daily; max 15 mg once daily
Pediatric: <2 years: not recommended; ≥2 years: 0.125 mg/kg; max 7.5 mg once daily
  Mobic *Tab:* 7.5, 15 mg; *Oral susp:* 7.5 mg/5 ml (100 ml) (raspberry)
  Vivlodex *Cap:* 5, 10 mg

 GRANULOMA INGUINALE (DONOVANOSIS)

Comment: The following treatment regimens are published in the **2015 CDC Sexually Transmitted Diseases Treatment Guidelines.** Treatment regimens are for adults only; consult a specialist for treatment of patients less than 18 years-of-age. Treatment regimens are presented by generic drug name first, followed by information about brands and dose forms. Persons who have sexual contact with a patient who has had granuloma inguinale within the past 60 days before onset of the patient's symptoms should be examined and offered therapy. Patients who are HIV-positive should receive the same treatment as those who are HIV-negative; however, the addition of a parenteral aminoglycoside (e.g., *gentamicin*) can also be considered.

RECOMMENDED REGIMEN

➤ *doxycycline* 100 mg bid x at least 3 weeks and until all lesions have completely healed

ALTERNATE REGIMENS

➤ *azithromycin* 1 g once weekly for at least 3 weeks and until all lesions have completely healed
➤ *ciprofloxacin* 750 mg bid x at least 3 weeks and until all lesions have completely healed
➤ *erythromycin base* 500 mg qid x 14 days or *erythromycin ethylsuccinate* 400 mg qid x 14 days
➤ *trimethoprim/sulfamethoxazole* 1 double-strength (160/800) dose bid x at least 3 weeks and until all lesions have completely healed

DRUG BRANDS AND DOSE FORMS

▷ *azithromycin* (B)
  Zithromax *Tab:* 250, 500, 600 mg; *Oral susp:* 100 mg/5 ml (15 ml); 200 mg/5 ml (15, 22.5, 30 ml) (cherry); *Pkt:* 1 g for reconstitution (cherry-banana)
  Zithromax Tri-pak *Tab:* 3 x 500 mg tabs/pck
  Zithromax Z-pak *Tab:* 6 x 250 mg tabs/pck
  Zmax *Oral susp:* 2 g ext-rel for reconstitution (cherry-banana) (148 mg Na⁺)

▷ *ciprofloxacin* (C)
  Cipro (G) *Tab:* 250, 500, 750 mg; *Oral susp:* 250, 500 mg/5 ml (100 ml) (strawberry)
  Cipro XR *Tab:* 500, 1000 mg ext-rel
  ProQuin XR *Tab:* 500 mg ext-rel
  Comment: *ciprofloxacin* is contraindicated <18 years-of-age, and during pregnancy and lactation. Risk of tendonitis or tendon rupture, especially 60 years-of-age and older.

▷ *doxycycline* (D)(G)
  Actilate *Tab:* 75, 150**mg
  Adoxa *Tab:* 50, 75, 100, 150 mg ent-coat
  Doryx *Tab:* 75, 100, 150 mg del-rel
  Monodox *Cap:* 50, 75, 100 mg
  Oracea *Cap:* 40 mg del-rel
  Vibramycin *Cap:* 50, 100 mg; *Syr:* 50 mg/5 ml (raspberry-apple) (sulfites); *Oral susp:* 25 mg/5 ml (raspberry-apple)
  Vibra-Tab *Tab:* 100 mg film-coat
  Comment: *doxycycline* is contraindicated <8 years-of-age, in pregnancy, and lactation (discolors developing tooth enamel). A side effect may be photosensitivity (photophobia). Do not give with antacids, calcium supplements, milk or other dairy, or within two hours of taking another drug.

▷ *erythromycin base* (B)(G)
  Ery-Tab *Tab:* 250, 333, 500 mg ent-coat
  PCE *Tab:* 333, 500 mg
  Comment: *erythromycin* may increase INR with concomitant *warfarin*, as well as increase serum level of *digoxin*, benzodiazepines and statins.

▷ *erythromycin ethylsuccinate* (B)(G)
  EryPed *Oral susp:* 200 mg/5 ml (100, 200 ml) (fruit); 400 mg/5 ml (60, 100, 200 ml) (banana); *Oral drops:* 200, 400 mg/5 ml (50 ml) (fruit); *Chew tab:* 200 mg wafer (fruit)
  E.E.S. *Oral susp:* 200, 400 mg/5 ml (100 ml) (fruit)
  E.E.S. Granules *Oral susp:* 200 mg/5 ml (100, 200 ml) (cherry)
  E.E.S. 400 Tablets *Tab:* 400 mg
  Comment: *erythromycin* may increase INR with concomitant *warfarin*, as well as increase serum level of *digoxin*, benzodiazepines and statins.

▷ *trimethoprim/sulfamethoxazole* (C)(G)
  Bactrim, Septra
    Tab: trim 80 mg/*sulfa* 400 mg*
  Bactrim DS, Septra DS
    Tab: trim 160 mg/*sulfa* 800 mg*
  Bactrim Pediatric Suspension, Septra Pediatric Suspension
    Oral susp: trim 40 mg/*sulfa* 200 mg per 5 ml (100 ml) (cherry) (alcohol 0.3%)

Comment: *trimethoprim/sulfamethoxazole* is not recommended in pregnancy or lactation. *CrCl 15-30 mL/min: reduce dose by 1/2; CrCl <15 mL/min: not recommended*

GROWTH FAILURE

Comment: Administer growth hormones by SC injection into thigh, buttocks, or abdomen. Rotate sites with each dose. Contraindicated in children with fused epiphyses or evidence of neoplasia.

▶ **mecasermin** (recombinant human insulin-like growth factor-1 [rhIGF-1])

Increlex (B) see mfr product literature

Vial: 10 mg/ml (benzyl alcohol)

Comment: **Increlex** is indicated for growth failure in children with severe primary IGF-1 deficiency (primary IGFD) or in those with growth hormone (GH) gene deletion who have developed neutralizing antibodies to GH.

▶ **somatropin** (rDNA origin)

Genotropin (B) initially not more than 0.04 mg/kg/week divided into 6-7 doses; may increase at 4-8 week intervals; max 0.08 mg/kg /week divided into 6-7 doses

Pediatric: usually 0.16-0.024 mg/kg/week divided into 6-7 doses

Intra-Mix Device: 1.5 mg (1.3 mg/ml after reconstitution), 5.8 mg (5 mg/ml after reconstitution) (two-chamber cartridge w. diluent); *Pen or Intra-Mix Device:* 5.8 mg (5 mg/ml after reconstitution), 13.8 mg (512 mg/ml after reconstitution) (two-chamber cartridge w. diluent)

Genotropin Miniquick (B) initially not more than 0.04 mg/kg/week divided into 6-7 doses; may increase at 4-8-week intervals; max 0.08 mg/kg/week divided into 6-7 doses

Pediatric: usually 0.16-0.024 mg/kg/week divided into 6-7 doses

MiniQuick: 0.2, 0.4, 0.6, 0.8, 1, 1.2, 1.4, 1.6, 1.8, 2 mg/0.25 ml (pwdr for SC injection after reconstitution) (2-chamber cartridge w. diluent)

Humatrope (C)

Pediatric: initially 0.18 mg/kg/week IM or SC divided into equal doses given either on 3 alternate days or 6 x/ week; max 0.3 mg/kg/week

Vial: 5 mg w. 5 ml diluent

Norditropin (C)

Pediatric: 0.024-0.034 mg/kg 6 to 7 times/week SC

Vial: 4 mg (12 IU), 8 mg (24 IU); *Cartridge for inj:* 5, 10, 15 mg/1.5 ml; *Flex-Pro prefilled pen:* 5, 10, 15 mg/1.5 ml

NordiFlex prefilled pen: 5, 10, 15 mg/1.5 ml; 30 mg/3 ml

Nutropin (C)

Pediatric: 0.7 mg/kg/week SC in divided daily doses

Vial: 5, 10 mg/vial w. diluent

Nutropin AQ (C)

<35 years: initially not more than 0.006 mg/kg SC daily; may increase to max 0.025 mg/kg SC daily; ≥35 years: initially not more than 0.006 mg/kg SC daily; may increase to max 0.0125 mg/kg SC daily

Pediatric: Prepubertal: up to 0.043 mg/kg SC daily; *Pubertal:* up to 0.1 mg/kg SC daily; *Turner Syndrome:* up to 0.0375 mg/kg/week divided into equal doses 3-7 times/week

Vial: 5 mg/ml (2 ml)

Nutropin Depot (C) 1.5 mg/kg SC monthly on same day each month; max 22.5 mg/inj; divide injection if >22.5 mg

Pediatric: same as adult

Vial: 13.5, 18, 22.5 mg/vial (pwdr for injection after reconstitution; single-use w. diluent and needle)

Omnitrope (B) 0.16-0.24 mg/kg/week SC divided 3-7 times/week

Vial: 5.8 mg

Omnitrope Pen 5 (B) 0.16-0.24 mg/kg/week SC divided 3-7 times/ week

Cartridge for inj: 5 mg/1.5 ml

Omnitrope Pen 10 (B) 0.16-0.24 mg/kg/week SC divided 3-7 times/week

Cartridge for inj: 10 mg/1.5 ml

Saizen (B) 0.18 mg/kg/week IM <u>or</u> SC divided 3-7 times/week

Vial: 5 mg (pwdr for SC injection w. diluent)

Serostem (B) 0.1 mg/kg SC once daily at HS; max 6 mg

Vial: 5, 4, 6, 8.8 mg (pwdr for SC injection w. diluent) (benzyl alcohol)

◯ HEADACHE: MIGRAINE/CLUSTER

ERGOTAMINE AGENTS

Comment: Do not use an ergotamine-type drug within 24 hours of any triptan <u>or</u> other 5-HT agonist.

▷ *dihydroxyergotamine mesylate* (X)

DHE 45 1 mg SC, IM, <u>or</u> IV; may repeat at 1 hour intervals; max 3 mg/day SC <u>or</u> IM/day; max 2 mg IV/day; max 6 mg/week

Pediatric: not recommended

Amp: 1 mg/ml (1 ml)

Migranal 1 spray in each nostril; may repeat 15 minutes later; max 6 sprays/day and 8 sprays/week

Pediatric: not recommended

Nasal spray: 4 mg/ml; 0.5 mg/spray (caffeine)

▷ *ergotamine* (X)(G) 1 tab SL at onset of attack; then q 30 minutes as needed; max 3 tabs/day and 5 tabs/week

Tab: 2 mg

▷ *ergotamine/caffeine* (X)(G)

Cafergot 2 tabs at onset of attack; then 1 tab every 1/2 hour if needed; max 6 tabs/attack and 10 tabs/week

Pediatric: not recommended

Tab: ergot 1 mg/caf 100 mg

Cafergot Suppository 1 suppository rectally at onset of headache; may repeat x 1 after 1 hour; max 2/attack, 5/week

Rectal supp: ergot 2 mg/caf 100 mg

5-HT RECEPTOR AGONISTS

Comment: Contraindications to 5-HT receptor agonists include cardiovascular disease, ischemic heart disease, cerebral vascular syndromes, peripheral vascular disease, uncontrolled hypertension, hemiplegic <u>or</u> basilar migraine. Do not use any triptan within 24 hours of ergot-type drugs <u>or</u> other 5-HT1A agonists, <u>or</u> within 2 weeks of taking an MAOI.

▷ *almotriptan* (C)(G) 6.25 or 12.5 mg; may repeat once after 2 hours; max 2 doses/day
    Pediatric: <12 years: not recommended; ≥12 years: same as adult
    Axert *Tab:* 6.25 mg (6/card), 12.5 mg (12/card)
Comment: *almotriptan* is indicated for patients 12-17 years-of-age with PMHx migraine headache lasting ≥4 hours untreated.

▷ *eletriptan* (C) 20 or 40 mg; may repeat once after 2 hours; max 80 mg/day
    Pediatric: <18 years: not recommended
    Relpax *Tab:* 20, 40 mg

▷ *frovatriptan* (C) 2.5 mg with fluids; may repeat once after 2 hours; max 7.5 mg/day
    Pediatric: <18 years: not recommended
    Frova *Tab:* 2.5 mg

▷ *naratriptan* (C) 1 or 2.5 mg with fluids; may repeat once after 4 hours; max 5 mg/day
    Pediatric: <18 years: not recommended
    Amerge *Tab:* 1, 2.5 mg

▷ *rizatriptan* (C) initially 5 or 10 mg; may repeat in 2 hours if needed; max 30 mg/day
    Pediatric: <18 years: not recommended
    Maxalt *Tab:* 5, 10 mg
    Maxalt-MLT *ODT:* 5, 10 mg (peppermint) (phenylalanine)

▷ *sumatriptan* (C)(G)
    Pediatric: <18 years: not recommended
    Alsuma 6 mg SC to the upper arm or lateral thigh only; may repeat after 1 hour if needed; max 2 doses/day
        Prefilled syringe: 6 mg/0.5 ml (2/pck with auto injector)
    Imitrex Injectable 4-6 mg SC; may repeat after 1 hour if needed; max 2 doses/day
        Prefilled syringe: 4, 6 mg/0.5 ml (2/pck with or without autoinjector)
    Imitrex Nasal Spray (G) 5-20 mg intranasally; may repeat once after 2 hours if needed; max 40 mg/day
        Nasal spray: 5, 20 mg/spray (single-dose)
    Imitrex Tab 25-200 mg x 1 dose; may be repeated at intervals of at least 2 hours if needed; max 200 mg/day
        Tab: 25, 50, 100 mg rapid-rel
    Imitrex STATdose Pen 6 mg/0.5 mg SC; may repeat once after 2 hours if needed; max 2 doses/day
        Prefilled needle-free autoinjector delivery system: 6 mg/0.5 ml (6/pck)
    Onzetra Xsail each disposable white nosepiece contains half a dose of medication (11 mg of sumatriptan). A full dose is 22 mg. Do not use more than 2 nosepieces per dose; attach the mouthpiece and one nasal piece; then press the white button on the delivery device to pierce the capsule in the nasal piece, then insert the nasal piece into one nostril and blow into the mouth piece to deliver the nasal powder in the contents of one capsule (11 mg); repeat in the opposite nostril for a total single 22 mg dose
        Cap: 11 mg nasal pwdr; *Kit:* nosepieces (2), capsules (2), reusable breath powered delivery device (1)
    Sumavel DosePro 6 mg SC to the upper arm or lateral thigh only; may repeat after 1 hour if needed; max 2 doses/day
        Prefilled needle-free delivery system: 6 mg/0.5 ml (6/pck)
    Zembrace SymTouch administer 3 mg SC at onset of headache; may repeat hourly; max 12 mg/24 hours
        Pediatric: <18 years: not recommended
        Autoinjector: 3 mg/0.5 ml (prefilled single-dose disposable autoinjector)

▷ *zolmitriptan* (C) initially 2.5 mg; may repeat after 2 hours if needed; max 10 mg/day
    Pediatric: <18 years: not recommended
        Zomig *Tab:* 2.5*, 5 mg
        Zomig Nasal Spray *Nasal spray:* 5 mg/spray (6 single dose/carton)
        Zomig-ZMT *ODT:* 2.5 mg (6 tabs), 5*mg (3 tabs) (orange) (phenylalanine)
Comment: Do not use any **triptan** within 24 hours of ergotamine-type drugs <u>or</u> other
5-HT agonists, <u>or</u> within 2 weeks of taking an MAOI.

5-HT IB/ID RECEPTOR AGONIST/NSAID COMBINATION

▷ *sumatriptan/naproxen* (C; D in 3rd)
    Pediatric: <18 years: not recommended
        Treximet initially 1 tab; may repeat after 2 hours; max 2 doses/day
            Tab: suma 85 mg/*naprox* 500 mg (9/blister card)
Comment: Do not use **sumatriptan** within 24 hours of ergot-type drugs <u>or</u> other
5-HT agonists, <u>or</u> within 2 weeks of taking an MAOI.

OTHER ANALGESICS

▷ *acetaminophen/aspirin/caffeine* (D)(G)
    Comment: *aspirin*-containing medications are contraindicated with history of
    allergic-type reaction to *aspirin*, children and adolescents with *Varicella* <u>or</u> other
    viral illness, and 3rd trimester pregnancy.
        Excedrin Migraine (OTC) 2 tabs q 6 hours prn; max 8 tabs/day x 2 days
            Pediatric: not recommended
            Tab: acet 250 mg/*asp* 250 mg/*caf* 65 mg
▷ *isometheptene mucate/dichloralphenazone/acetaminophen* (C)(IV)
        Midrin 2 caps initially; then 1 cap q 1 hour until relieved; max 5 caps/12 hours
            Pediatric: not recommended
            Cap: iso 65 mg/*dichlor* 100 mg/*acet* 325 mg

PROPHYLAXIS

▷ *topiramate* (D)(G) initially 25 mg daily in the PM and titrate up daily as tolerated;
    then 25 mg bid; then, 25 mg in the AM and 50 mg in the PM; then, 50 mg bid
    Pediatric: <12 years: not recommended
        Topamax *Tab:* 25, 50, 100, 200 mg
        Topamax Sprinkle Caps *Cap:* 15, 25 mg

BETA-BLOCKERS

▷ *atenolol* (D)(G) initially 25 mg bid; max 150 mg/day in divided doses
    Pediatric: not recommended
        Tenormin *Tab:* 25, 50, 100 mg
▷ *metoprolol succinate* (C)
    Pediatric: not recommended
        ToprolR-XL initially 25-100 mg in a single dose daily; increase weekly if need-
        ed; max 400 mg/day
            Tab: 25*, 50*, 100*, 200*mg ext-rel
▷ *metoprolol tartrate* (C)
    Pediatric: not recommended

Lopressor (G) initially 25-50 mg bid; increase weekly if needed; max 400 mg/day
Tab: 25, 37.5, 50, 75, 100 mg

▷ *nadolol* (C)(G) initially 20 mg daily; max 240 mg/day in divided doses
Pediatric: not recommended
Corgard *Tab:* 20*, 40*, 80*, 120*, 160*mg

▷ *propranolol* (C)(G)
Inderal initially 10 mg bid; usual range 160-320 mg/day in divided doses
Pediatric: not recommended
Tab: 10*, 20*, 40*, 60*, 80*mg
Inderal LA initially 80 mg daily in a single dose; increase q 3-7 days; usual range 120-160 mg/day; max 320 mg/day in a single dose
Pediatric: not recommended
Cap: 60, 80, 120, 160 mg sust-rel
InnoPran XL initially 80 mg q HS; max 120 mg/day
Cap: 80, 120 mg ext-rel

▷ *timolol* (C)(G) initially 5 mg bid; max 60 mg/day in divided doses
Pediatric: not recommended
Blocadren *Tab:* 5, 10*, 20*mg

CALCIUM ANTAGONISTS

▷ *diltiazem* (C)(G)
Cardizem initially 30 mg qid; may increase gradually every 1-2 days; max 360 mg/day in divided doses
Pediatric: not recommended
Tab: 30, 60, 90, 120 mg
Cardizem CD initially 120-180 mg once daily; adjust at 1- to 2-week intervals; max 480 mg/day
Pediatric: not recommended
Cap: 120, 180, 240, 300, 360 mg ext-rel
Cardizem LA initially 180-240 mg once daily; titrate at 2-week intervals; max 540 mg/day
Pediatric: not recommended
Tab: 120, 180, 240, 300, 360, 420 mg ext-rel
Cardizem SR initially 60-120 mg bid; adjust at 2-week intervals; max 360 mg/day
Pediatric: not recommended
Cap: 60, 90, 120 mg sust-rel

▷ *nifedipine* (C)(G)
Pediatric: not recommended
Adalat initially 10 mg tid; usual range 10-20 mg tid; max 180 mg/day
Cap: 10, 20 mg
Procardia initially 10 mg tid; titrate over 7-14 days: max 30 mg/dose and 180 mg/day in divided doses
Cap: 10, 20 mg
Procardia XL initially 30-60 mg daily; titrate over 7-14 days; max 90 mg/day in divided doses

▷ *verapamil* (C)(G)
Pediatric: not recommended
Calan 80-120 mg tid; increase daily or weekly if needed
Tab: 40, 80*, 120*mg

Covera HS initially 180 mg q HS; titrate in steps to 240 mg; then to 360 mg; then to 480 mg if needed
    Tab: 180, 240 mg ext-rel
Isoptin initially 80-120 mg tid
    Tab: 40, 80, 120 mg
Isoptin SR initially 120-180 mg in the AM; may increase to 240 mg in the AM; then, 180 mg q 12 hours or 240 mg in the AM and 120 mg in the PM; then, 240 mg q 12 hours
    Tab: 120, 180*, 240*mg sust-rel

Tricyclic Antidepressants (TCAs)

Comment: Co-administration of TCAs with SSRIs requires extreme caution.
▷ *amitriptyline* (C)(G) 10-20 mg q HS
    Pediatric: not recommended
    Tab: 10, 25, 50, 75, 100, 150 mg
▷ *doxepin* (C)(G) 10-200 mg q HS
    Pediatric: not recommended
    Cap: 10, 25, 50, 75, 100, 150 mg; *Oral conc:* 10 mg/ml (4 oz w. dropper)
▷ *imipramine* (C)(G) 10-200 mg q HS
    Tofranil 25-50 mg; max 200 mg/day; if maintenance dose exceeds 75 mg daily, may switch to **Tofranil PM**
        Pediatric: <6 years: not recommended; 6-12 years: initially 25 mg; >12 years: 50 mg max 2.5 mg/kg/day
        Tab: 10, 25, 50 mg
    Tofranil PM initially 75 mg once daily 1 hour before HS; max 200 mg
        Cap: 75, 100, 125, 150 mg
▷ *nortriptyline* (D)(G) 10-150 mg q HS
    Pediatric: not recommended
        Pamelor *Cap:* 10, 25, 50, 75 mg; *Oral soln:* 10 mg/5 ml (16 oz)

SSRI ANTIDEPRESSANTS

Comment: Co-administration of SSRIs with TCAs requires extreme caution. Concomitant use of MAOIs and SSRIs is absolutely contraindicated. Avoid other serotonergic drugs. A potentially fatal adverse event is Serotonin Syndrome, caused by serotonin excess. Milder symptoms require HCP intervention to avert severe symptoms which can be rapidly fatal without urgent/emergent medical care. Symptoms include restlessness, agitation, confusion, hallucinations, tachycardia, hypertension, dilated pupils, muscle twitching, muscle rigidity, loss of muscle coordination, diaphoresis, diarrhea, headache, shivering, piloerection, hyperpyrexia, cardiac arrhythmias, seizures, loss of consciousness, coma, death. Abrupt withdrawal or interruption of treatment with an antidepressant medication is sometimes associated with an Antidepressant Discontinuation Syndrome which may be mediated by gradually tapering the drug over a period of two weeks or longer, depending on the dose strength and length of treatment. Common symptoms of the Serotonin Discontinuation Syndrome include flu-like symptoms (nausea, vomiting, diarrhea, headaches, sweating), sleep disturbances (insomnia, nightmares, constant sleepiness), mood disturbances (dysphoria, anxiety, agitation), cognitive disturbances (mental confusion, hyperarousal), sensory and movement disturbances (imbalance, tremors, vertigo, dizziness, electric-shock-like sensations in the brain, often described by sufferers as "brain zaps."

▷ *fluoxetine* (C)(G)

Prozac initially 20 mg daily; may increase after 1 week; doses >20 mg/day may be divided into AM and noon doses; max 80 mg/day

Pediatric: <8 years: not recommended; 8-17 years: initially 10-20 mg/day; start lower weight children at 10 mg/day; if starting at 10 mg daily, may increase after 1 week to 20 mg once daily

Cap: 10, 20, 40 mg; *Tab:* 30*, 60*mg; *Oral soln:* 20 mg/5 ml (4 oz) (mint)

Prozac Weekly following daily fluoxetine therapy at 20 mg/day for 13 weeks, may initiate **Prozac Weekly** 7 days after the last 20 mg fluoxetine dose

Pediatric: not recommended

Cap: 90 mg ent-coat del-rel pellets

OTHER AGENTS

▷ *divalproex sodium* (D) *Delayed-release:* initially 250 mg bid; titrate weekly to usual max 500 mg bid; *Extended-release:* initially 500 mg once daily; may increase after one week to 1 g once daily

Pediatric: <10 years: not recommended; ≥10 years: same as adult

Depakene *Cap:* 250 mg del-rel; *syr:* 250 mg/5 ml (16 oz)

Depakote *Tab:* 125, 250, 500 mg del-rel

Depakote ER *Tab:* 250, 500 mg ext-rel

Depakote Sprinkle *Cap:* 125 mg del-rel

▷ *methysergide* (C) 4-8 mg daily in divided doses with food; max 8 mg/day; max 6 month treatment course; wean off over last 2-3 weeks of treatment course; separate treatment courses by 3-4 week drug-free interval

Sansert *Tab:* 2 mg

MAGNESIUM SUPPLEMENTS

▷ *magnesium* (B)

Slow-Mag 2 tabs daily

Tab: 64 mg (as chloride)/110 mg (as carbonate)

▷ *magnesium oxide* (B)

Mag-Ox 400 1-2 tabs daily

Tab: 400 mg

HEADACHE: TENSION (MUSCLE CONTRACTION HEADACHE)

Acetaminophen for IV Infusion *see Pain page 296*
Oral Prescription NSAIDs *see page 489*
Other Oral Analgesics *see Pain page 298*
Topical/Transdermal NSAIDs *see Pain page 297*
Parenteral Corticosteroids *see page 499*
Oral Corticosteroids *see page 497*
Topical Analgesic and Anesthetic Agents *see page 487*

TRICYCLIC ANTIDEPRESSANTS (TCAs)

Comment: Co-administration of TCAs with SSRIs requires extreme caution.

▷ *amitriptyline* (C)(G) 50-100 mg/day
   Pediatric: not recommended
   Tab: 10, 25, 50, 75, 100, 150 mg
▷ *desipramine* (C)(G) 50-100 mg bid
   Pediatric: not recommended
      Norpramin *Tab:* 10, 25, 50, 75, 100, 150 mg
▷ *imipramine* (C)(G)
   Pediatric: not recommended
      Tofranil initially 75 mg daily (max 200 mg); adolescents initially 30-40 mg daily
      (max 100 mg/day); if maintenance dose exceeds 75 mg daily, may switch to
      Tofranil PM for divided or bedtime dosing
        Tab: 10, 25, 50 mg
      Tofranil PM initially 75 mg once daily 1 hour before HS; max 200 mg
        Cap: 75, 100, 125, 150 mg
      Tofranil Injection 50 mg IM; lower dose for adolescents; switch to oral form as
      soon as possible
        Amp: 25 mg/2 ml (2 ml)
▷ *nortriptyline* (D)(G) 25-50 mg/day
   Pediatric: not recommended
      Pamelor *Cap:* 10, 25, 50, 75 mg; *Oral soln:* 10 mg/5 ml (16 oz)

ANALGESICS

▷ *butalbital/acetaminophen* (C)(G)
   Pediatric: <12 years: not recommended; ≥12 years: same as adult
      Phrenilin 1-2 tabs q 4 hours prn; max 6 tabs/day
        Tab: but 50 mg/*acet* 325 mg
      Phrenilin Forte 1 tab or cap q 4 hours prn; max 6 caps/day
        Cap/Tab: but 50 mg/*acet* 650 mg
▷ *butalbital/acetaminophen/caffeine* (C)(G)
   Pediatric: not recommended
      Fioricet 1-2 tabs q 4 hours prn; max 6/day
        Tab: but 50 mg/*acet* 325 mg/*caf* 40 mg
      Zebutal 1 cap q 4 hours prn; max 5/day
        Cap: but 50 mg/*acet* 500 mg/*caf* 40 mg
▷ *butalbital/acetaminophen/codeine/caffeine* (C)(III)(G)
   Pediatric: <12 years: not recommended
      Fioricet with Codeine 1-2 tabs at onset q 4 hours prn; max 6 tabs/day
        Tab: but 50 mg/*acet* 325 mg/*cod* 30 mg/*caf* 40 mg
▷ *butalbital/aspirin/caffeine* (C)(III)(G)
   Pediatric: <12 years: not recommended; ≥12 years: same as adult
      Fiorinal 1-2 tabs or caps q 4 hours prn; max 6 caps/tabs/day
        Tab/Cap: but 50 mg/*asa* 325 mg/*caf* 40 mg
▷ *butalbital/aspirin/codeine/caffeine* (C)(III)(G)
   Pediatric: <12 years: not recommended; ≥12 years: same as adult
      Fiorinal with Codeine 1-2 caps q 4 hours prn; max 6 caps/day
        Cap: but 50 mg/*asp* 325 mg/*cod* 30 mg/*caf* 40 mg
▷ *butorphanol* (C)(IV)(G) initially 1 spray in 1 nostril; may repeat after 60-90 minutes
   if needed; may repeat again in 3-4 hours
   Pediatric: <18 years: not recommended

Butorphanol Nasal Spray *Nasal spray:* 10 mg/ml, 1 mg/actuation (2.5 ml)
Stadol NS *Nasal spray:* 10 mg/ml, 1 mg/actuation (2.5 ml)
▷ *tramadol* (C)(IV)(G)
    Rybix ODT initially 100 mg once daily; may increase by 100 mg every 5 days;
    max 300 mg/day; *CrCl <30 mL/min* or *severe hepatic impairment:* not recom-
    mended; *Cirrhosis:* max 50 mg q 12 hours
      Pediatric: <17 years: not recommended
      ODT: 50 mg (mint) (phenylalanine)
    Ryzolt
      Pediatric: <16 years: not recommended; ≥16 years: same as adult
      Tab: 100, 200, 300 mg ext-rel
    Ultram
      Pediatric: <16 years: not recommended; ≥16 years: same as adult
      Tab: 50*mg
    Ultram ER
      Pediatric: <18 years: not recommended
      Tab: 100, 200, 300 mg ext-rel
▷ *tramadol/acetaminophen* (C)(IV)(G) 2 tabs q 4-6 hours prn; max 8 tabs/day; 5 days;
CrCl <30 mL/min: max 2 tabs q 12 hours; max 4 tabs/day x 5 days; *Cirrhosis or other
liver disease:* contraindicated
    Pediatric: <16 years: not recommended; ≥16 years: same as adult
    Ultracet *Tab:* tram 37.5/acet 325 mg

Other Oral Analgesics *see* **Pain** *page 298*

MAGNESIUM SUPPLEMENTS

▷ *magnesium* (B)
    Slow-Mag 2 tabs daily
      Tab: 64 mg (as chloride)/110 mg (as carbonate)
▷ *magnesium oxide* (B)
    Mag-Ox 400 1-2 tabs daily
      Tab: 400 mg

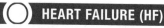

HEART FAILURE (HF)

ACE INHIBITORS (ACEIs)

▷ *captopril* (C; D in 2nd, 3rd)(G) initially 25 mg tid; after 1-2 weeks may increase to
50 mg tid; max 450 mg/day
Pediatric: not recommended
    Capoten *Tab:* 12.5*, 25*, 50*, 100*mg
▷ *enalapril* (C; D in 2nd, 3rd) initially 5 mg daily; usual dosage range 10-40 mg/day;
max 40 mg/day
Pediatric: not recommended
    Vasotec *Tab:* 2.5*, 5*, 10, 20 mg
▷ *fosinopril* (C; D in 2nd, 3rd) initially 10 mg daily, usual maintenance 20-40 mg/day
in a single or divided doses

Pediatric: <6 years, <50 kg: not recommended; 6-12 years, ≥50 kg: 5-10 mg daily; >12 years: same as adult

    Monopril *Tab:* 10*, 20, 40 mg

▷ *lisinopril* (C; D in 2nd, 3rd) initially 5 mg daily

Pediatric: not recommended

    Prinivil *Tab:* 2.5, 5*, 10, 20, 40 mg

    Zestril *Tab:* 2.5, 5, 10, 20, 40 mg

▷ *quinapril* (C; D in 2nd, 3rd) initially 5 mg bid; increase weekly to 10-20 mg bid

Pediatric: not recommended

    Accupril *Tab:* 5*, 10, 20, 40 mg

▷ *ramipril* (C; D in 2nd, 3rd) initially 2.5 mg bid; usual maintenance 5 mg bid

Pediatric: not recommended

    Altace *Tab/Cap:* 1.25, 2.5, 5, 10 mg

▷ *trandolapril* (C; D in 2nd, 3rd) initially 1 mg daily; titrate to dose of 4 mg daily as tolerated

Pediatric: not recommended

    Mavik *Tab:* 1*, 2, 4 mg

BETA-BLOCKERS (CARDIOSELECTIVE)

▷ *carvedilol* (C)

    Coreg initially 3.125 mg bid; may increase at 1-2 week intervals to 12.5 mg bid; usual max 50 mg bid

        Pediatric: <18 years: not recommended

        Tab: 3.125, 6.25, 12.5, 25 mg

    Coreg CR initially 10 mg once daily x 2 weeks; may double dose at 2 week intervals; max 80 mg once daily; may open caps and sprinkle on food

        Pediatric: <18 years: not recommended

        Cap: 10, 20, 40, 80 mg cont-rel

▷ *metoprolol succinate* (C)

Pediatric: not recommended

    Toprol-XL initially 12.5-25 mg in a single dose daily; increase weekly if needed; reduce if symptomatic bradycardia occurs; max 400 mg/day

        Tab: 25*, 50*, 100*, 200*mg ext-rel

▷ *metoprolol tartrate* (C)

Pediatric: not recommended

    Lopressor (G) initially 25-50 mg bid; increase weekly if needed; max 400 mg/day

        Tab: 25, 37.5, 50, 75, 100 mg

ANGIOTENSIN II RECEPTOR BLOCKERS (ARBs)

▷ *valsartan* (C; D in 2nd, 3rd) initially 40 mg bid; increase to 160 mg bid as tolerated or 320 mg daily after 2-4 weeks; usual range 80-320 mg/day

Pediatric: not recommended

    Diovan *Tab:* 40*, 80, 160, 320 mg

NEPRILYSIN INHIBITOR/ARB COMBINATION

▷ *sacubitril/valsartan* (D) initially 49/51 bid; double dose after 2-4 weeks; maintenance 97/103 bid; *eGFR <30 mL/min* or *moderate hepatic impairment:* initially 24/26 bid; double dose every 2-4 weeks to target maintenance 97/103 bid

Pediatric: not established

Entresto
Tab: **Entresto 24/26:** *sacu* 24 mg/*val* 26 mg
Entresto 49/51: *sacu* 49 mg/*val* 51 mg
Entresto 97/103: *sacu* 97 mg/*val* 103 mg

ALDOSTERONE RECEPTOR BLOCKER

▷ *eplerenone* (B) initially 25 mg once daily; titrate within 4 weeks to 50 mg once daily; adjust dose based on serum K⁺
Pediatric: not recommended
Inspra *Tab:* 25, 50 mg
Comment: **Inspra** is contraindicated with concomitant potent CYP3A4 inhibitors. Risk of hyperkalemia with concomitant ACEI or ARB. Monitor serum potassium at baseline, 1 week, and 1 month. Caution with serum *Cr >2 mg/dL* (male) or >1.8 mg/dL (female) and/or *CrCl <50 mL/min*, and DM with proteinuria.

THIAZIDE DIURETICS

Comment: Monitor hydration status, blood pressure, urine output, serum K⁺.
▷ *chlorothiazide* (C)(G) 0.5-1 g/day in single or divided doses; max 2g/day
Pediatric: <6 months: up to 15 mg/lb/day in 2 divided doses; ≥6 months: 10 mg/lb/day in 2 divided doses
Diuril *Tab:* 250*, 500*mg; *Oral susp:* 250 mg/5 ml (237 ml)
▷ *hydrochlorothiazide* (B)(G)
Pediatric: not recommended
Esidrix 25-100 mg once daily
Tab: 25, 50, 100 mg
Microzide 12.5 mg daily; usual max 50 mg/day
Cap: 12.5 mg
▷ *methyclothiazide/deserpidine* (B) initially 2.5 mg once daily; max 5 mg once daily
Pediatric: not recommended
Enduronyl *Tab:* *methy* 5 mg/*deser* 0.25 mg*
Enduronyl Forte *Tab:* *methy* 5 mg/*deser* 0.5 mg*
▷ *polythiazide* (C) 2-4 mg once daily
Pediatric: not recommended
Renese *Tab:* 1, 2, 4 mg

POTASSIUM-SPARING DIURETICS

Comment: Monitor hydration status, blood pressure, urine output, serum K⁺.
▷ *amiloride* (B) initially 5 mg once daily; may increase to 10 mg; max 20 mg
Pediatric: not recommended
Midamor *Tab:* 5 mg
▷ *spironolactone* (D)(G) initially 50-100 mg in a single or divided doses; titrate at 2 week intervals
Pediatric: not established
Aldactone *Tab:* 25, 50*, 100*mg

LOOP DIURETICS

Comment: Monitor hydration status, blood pressure, urine output, serum K⁺.

▷ *bumetanide* (C)(G) 0.5-2 mg as a single dose; may repeat at 4-5 hour intervals; max 10 mg/day
  Pediatric: <18 years: not recommended
    Bumex *Tab:* 0.5*, 1*, 2*mg
  Comment: *bumetanide* is contraindicated with sulfa drug allergy.
▷ *ethacrynic acid* (B) initially 50-200 mg once daily
  Pediatric: infants: not recommended; >1 month: initially 25 mg/day; then adjust dose in 25 mg increments
    Edecrin *Tab:* 25, 50 mg
▷ *furosemide* (C)(G) initially 40 mg bid
  Pediatric: not recommended
    Lasix *Tab:* 20, 40*, 80 mg; *Oral soln:* 10 mg/ml (2, 4 oz w. dropper)
  Comment: *furosemide* is contraindicated with sulfa drug allergy.
▷ *torsemide* (B) 5 mg once daily; may increase to 10 mg daily
  Pediatric: not recommended
    Demadex *Tab:* 5*, 10*, 20*, 100*mg

OTHER DIURETICS

Comment: Monitor hydration status, blood pressure, urine output, serum K⁺.
▷ *indapamide* (B) initially 1.25 mg once daily; may titrate dosage upward every 4 weeks if needed; max 5 mg/day
    Lozol *Tab:* 1.25, 2.5 mg
  Comment: *indapamide* is contraindicated with sulfa drug allergy.
▷ *metolazone* (B) 2.5-5 mg once daily
  Pediatric: not recommended
    Zaroxolyn *Tab:* 2.5, 5, 10 mg
  Comment: *metolazone* is contraindicated with sulfa drug allergy.

DIURETIC COMBINATIONS

Comment: Monitor hydration status, blood pressure, urine output, serum K⁺.
▷ *amiloride/hydrochlorothiazide* (B)(G) initially 1 tab once daily; may increase to 2 tabs/day in a single or divided doses
  Pediatric: not recommended
    Moduretic *Tab:* amil 5 mg/*hydro* 50 mg*
▷ *spironolactone/hydrochlorothiazide* (D)(G)
  Pediatric: not recommended
    Aldactazide 25 usual maintenance 50-100 mg in a single or divided doses
      Tab: spiro 25 mg/*hydro* 25 mg
    Aldactazide 50 usual maintenance 50-100 mg in a single or divided doses
      Tab: spiro 50 mg/*hydro* 50 mg
▷ *triamterene/hydrochlorothiazide* (C)(G)
  Pediatric: not recommended
    Dyazide 1-2 caps daily
      Cap: triam 37.5 mg/*hydro* 25 mg
    Maxzide 1 tab once daily
      Tab: triam 75 mg/*hydro* 50 mg*
    Maxzide-25 1-2 tabs once daily
      Tab: triam 37.5 mg/*hydro* 25 mg*

NITRATE/PERIPHERAL VASODILATOR COMBINATION

▶ *isosorbide dinitrate/hydralazine* (C) initially 1 tab tid; may reduce to 1/2 tab tid if not tolerated; titrate as tolerated after 3-5 days; max 2 tabs tid
Pediatric: not recommended
    BiDil *Tab:* isosor 20 mg/hydral 37.5 mg
    Comment: BiDil is an adjunct to standard therapy in self-identified black persons to improve survival, to prolong time to hospitalization for heart failure, and to improve patient-reported functional status.

CARDIAC GLYCOSIDES

Comment: Therapeutic serum level of is 0.8-2 mcg/ml.
▶ *digoxin* (C)(G) 1-1.5 mg IM, IV, or PO in divided doses over 1-3 days as a loading dose; usual maintenance 0.125-0.5 mg/day
Pediatric: Total oral pediatric digitalizing dose (in 24 hours): <2 years: 40-50 mcg/kg; 2-10 years: 30-40 mcg/kg; >10 years: 0.75-1.5 mg; *Daily oral pediatric maintenance dose (single-dose):* <2 years: 10-12 mcg/kg; 2-10 years: 8-10 mcg/kg; >10 years: 0.125–0.5 mg
Comment: For more information on the use of digoxin in pediatric heart failure, see **Jain, S. & Vaidyanathan B.** Ann Pediatr Cardiol. 2009 Jul-Dec; 2(2): 149–152.
    Lanoxicaps
        Pediatric: <10 years: use elixir or parenteral form
        Cap: 0.05, 0.1, 0.2 mg soln-filled (alcohol)
    Lanoxin
        Pediatric: <10 years: use elixir or parenteral form
        Tab: 0.0625, 0.125*, 0.1875, 0.25*mg; *Elix:* 0.05 mg/ml (2 oz w. dropper) (lime) (alcohol 10%)
    Lanoxin Injection *Amp:* 0.25 mg/ml (2 ml)
    Lanoxin Injection Pediatric *Amp:* 0.1 mg/ml (1 ml)

OTHER

▶ *ivabradine* (D) initially 5 mg bid with food; assess after 2 weeks and adjust dose to achieve a resting heart rate 50-60 bpm; thereafter, adjust dose as needed based on resting heart rate and tolerability; max 7.5 mg bid; in patients with a history of conduction defects, or for whom bradycardia could lead to hemodynamic compromise, initiate at 2.5 mg bid before increasing the dose based on heart rate
Pediatric: <18 years: not established
    Corlanor *Tab:* 5, 7.5 mg
    Comment: **Corlanor** is indicated to reduce the risk of hospitalization for worsening heart failure inpatients with stable, symptomatic, chronic heart failure with left ventricular ejection fraction (LVEF) ≤35%, who are in sinus rhythm with resting heart rate ≤70 bpm and either are on maximally tolerated doses of beta-blockers or have a contraindication to beta-blocker use. **Corlanor** is contraindicated with acute decompensated heart failure, BP <90/50, sick sinus syndrome (SSS), sinoatrial block, and 3rd degree AV block (unless patient has a functioning demand pacemaker). **Corlanor** may cause fetal toxicity when administered pregnant women based on embryo-fetal toxicity and cardiac teratogenic to effects observed in animal studies. Therefore, females should be advised to use effective contraception when taking this drug.

◯ *HELICOBACTER PYLORI (H. PYLORI)* INFECTION

ERADICATION REGIMENS

Comment: There are many H2 receptor blocker-based and PPI-based treatment regimens suggested in the professional literature for the eradication of the *H. pylori* organism and subsequent ulcer healing. Generally, regimens range from 10-14 days for eradication and 2-6 more weeks of continued gastric acid suppression. A three- or four-antibiotic combination may increase treatment effectiveness and decrease the likelihood of resistant strain emergence. Empirical treatment is not recommended. Diagnosis should be confirmed before treatment is started. Antibiotic choices include *doxycycline*, *tetracycline*, *amoxicillin*, *amoxicillin/clavulanate*, *clarithromycin*, *clindamycin*, and *metronidazole*. Follow-up visits are recommended at 2 and 6 weeks to evaluate treatment outcomes.

▷ **Regimen 1: Helidac Therapy (D)** *bismuth subsalicylate* 525 mg qid + *tetracycline* 500 mg qid + *metronidazole* 250 mg qid x 14 days
  Pediatric: not recommended
  Pack: bismuth subsalicylate chew tab: 262.4 mg (112/pck); *tetracycline cap:* 500 mg (56/pck); *metronidazole Tab:* 250 mg (56/pck)

▷ **Regimen 2: PrevPac (D)(G)** *amoxicillin* 500 mg 2 caps bid + *lansoprazole* 30 mg bid + *clarithromycin* 500 mg bid x 14 days (one card per day)
  Pediatric: not recommended
  Kit: lansoprazole cap: 30 mg (2/card); *amoxicillin cap:* 500 mg (4/card); *clarithromycin tab:* 500 mg (2/card) (14 daily cards/carton)

▷ **Regimen 3: Pylera (D)** take 3 caps qid after meals and at bedtime x 10 days; take with 8 oz water (plus, take *omeprazole* 20 mg bid with breakfast and dinner for 10 days)
  Pediatric: not recommended
  Cap: bismuth subsalicylate 140 mg/*tetracycline* 125 mg/*metronidazole* 125 mg (120 caps)
  Comment: *omeprazole* not included with **Pylera**.

▷ **Regimen 4: Omeclamox-Pak (C)** *omeprazole* 20 mg bid + *amoxicillin* 1000 bid + *clarithromycin* 500 mg bid x 10 days
  Kit: omeprazole cap: 20 mg (2/pck); *amoxicillin cap:* 500 mg (4/pck); *clarithromycin tab:* 500 mg (2/pck) (10 pcks/carton)

▷ **Regimen 5: (C)** *omeprazole* 40 mg daily + *clarithromycin* 500 mg tid x 2 weeks; then continue *omeprazole* 10-40 mg daily x 6 more weeks

▷ **Regimen 6: (B)** *lansoprazole* 30 mg tid + *amoxicillin* 1 g tid x 10 days; then continue *lansoprazole* 15-30 mg daily x 6 more weeks

▷ **Regimen 7: (C)** *omeprazole* 40 mg daily + *amoxicillin* 1 g bid + *clarithromycin* 500 mg bid x 10 days; then continue *omeprazole* 10-40 mg daily x 6 more weeks

▷ **Regimen 8: (D)** *bismuth subsalicylate* 525 mg qid + *metronidazole* 250 mg qid + *tetracycline* 500 mg qid + H2 receptor agonist x 2 weeks; then continue H2 receptor agonist x 6 more weeks

▷ **Regimen 9: (not for use in 1st; B in 2nd, 3rd)** *bismuth subsalicylate* 525 mg qid + *metronidazole* 250 mg qid + *amoxicillin 500 mg qid + H2 receptor agonist x 2 weeks; then continue H2 receptor agonist x 6 more weeks* receptor agonist x 2 weeks; then continue H2 receptor agonist x 6 more weeks

▷ **Regimen 10: (C)** *ranitidine bismuth citrate* 400 mg bid + *clarithromycin* 500 mg bid x 2 weeks; then continue *ranitidine bismuth citrate* 400 mg bid x 2 more weeks

▷ **Regimen 11: (D)** *omeprazole* 20 mg or *lansoprazole* 30 mg q AM + *bismuth subsalicylate* 524 mg qid + *metronidazole* 500 mg tid + *tetracycline* 500 mg qid x 2 weeks; then continue *omeprazole* 20 mg or *lansoprazole* 30 mg q AM for 6 more weeks

HEMORRHOIDS

▷ *dibucaine* (C)(OTC)(G) 1 applicatorful or suppository bid and after each stool; max 6/day
Pediatric: not recommended
> **Nupercainal (OTC)** *Rectal oint:* 1% (30, 60 g); *Rectal supp:* 1% (12, 14/pck)

▷ *hydrocortisone* (C)(OTC)(G)
Pediatric: not recommended
> **Anusol-HC** 1 suppository rectally bid-tid or 2 suppositories bid x 2 weeks
> *Rectal supp:* 25 mg (12, 24/pck)
> **Anusol-HC Cream** 2.5% apply bid-qid prn
> *Rectal crm:* 2.5% (30 g)
> **Anusol HC-1** apply tid-qid prn; max 7 days
> *Rectal crm:* 1% (0.7 oz)
> **Hydrocortisone Rectal Cream**
> *Rectal crm:* 1, 2.5% (30 g)
> **Nupercainal** apply tid-qid prn
> *Rectal crm:* 1% (30 g)
> **Proctocort** 1 suppository rectally bid-tid prn or 2 suppositories bid
> x 2 weeks
> *Rectal supp:* 30 mg (12/pck)
> **Proctocream HC** 2.5% apply rectally bid-qid prn
> *Rectal crm:* 2.5% (30 g)
> **Proctofoam HC** 1% apply rectally tid-qid prn
> *Rectal foam:* 1% (14 applications/10 g)

▷ *hydrocortisone/pramoxine* (C) 1 applicatorful tid-qid and after each stool; max 2 weeks
Pediatric: not recommended
> **Procort** *Rectal crm:* hydro 1.85%/pramox 1.15% (30 g)

▷ *hydrocortisone/lidocaine* (B) apply bid-tid prn
Pediatric: not recommended
> **AnaMantle HC, LidaMantle HC** *Crm/Lotn:* hydrocort 5%/lido 3% (1 oz)

▷ *petrolatum/mineral oil/shark liver oil/phenylephrine* (C)(OTC)(G)
> **Preparation H Ointment** apply up to qid prn
> *Rectal oint:* 1, 2 oz

▷ *petrolatum/glycerin/shark liver oil/phenylephrine* (C)(OTC)(G)
> **Preparation H Cream** apply up to qid prn
> *Rectal crm:* 0.9, 1.8 oz

▷ *phenylephrine/cocoa butter/shark liver oil* (C)(OTC)(G)
> **Preparation H Suppositories** 1 suppository or 1 application of rectal ointment
> or cream, up to qid
> *Rectal supp:* phenyle 0.25%/cocoa 85.5%/shark 3% (12, 24, 45/pck); *Rectal
> oint:* phenyle 0.25%/petro 1.9%/mineral oil 14%/shark liv 3% (1, 2 oz); *Rectal
> crm:* phenyle 0.25%/petro 18%/gly 12%/shark liv 3% (0.9, 1.8 oz)

▷ *witch hazel* topical solution/gel (NR)(OTC)
> **Tucks** apply up to 6 x/day; leave on x 5-15 minutes
> *Pad:* 12, 40, 100/pck; *Gel:* 19.8 g

▷ *lidocaine* 3% cream (B) apply bid-tid prn
Pediatric: reduce dosage commensurate with age, body weight, and physical condition
> **LidaMantle** *Crm:* 3% (1 oz)

Bulk-forming Agents, Stool Softeners, and Stimulant Laxatives *see Constipation*
page 97

◯ HEPATITIS A (HAV)

Comment: Administer a 2-dose series. Schedule first immunization at least 2 weeks before expected exposure. Booster dose recommended 6-12 months later. Under 1 year-of-age administer in the vastus lateralis; over 1 year-of-age administer in deltoid.

PROPHYLAXIS (HEPATITIS A)

▷ *hepatitis A vaccine, inactivated* (C)
    Havrix 1,440 El.U IM; repeat in 6-12 months
      Pediatric: <2 years: not recommended; 2-18 years: 720 El.U IM; repeat in 6-12 months or 360 El.U IM; repeat in 1 month
    Vaqta 25 U (1 ml) IM; repeat in 6 months
      Pediatric: <2 years: not recommended; 2-18 years: 0.5 ml IM; repeat in 6-18 months
      Vial: 25 U/ml single-dose (preservative-free); *Prefilled syringe:* 25 U/ml, (0.5, 1 ml single-dose)

PROPHYLAXIS (HEPATITIS A AND B COMBINATION)

▷ *hepatitis A inactivated/hepatitis B surface antigen (recombinant vaccine)* (C)
    Pediatric: <18 years: not recommended
    Twinrix 1 ml IM in deltoid; repeat in 1 month and 6 months
      Vial (soln): hepatitis A inactivated 720 IU/*hepatitis B* surface antigen (recombinant) 20 mcg/ml (1, 10 ml); *Prefilled syringe: hepatitis A* inactivated 720 IU/ *hepatitis B* surface antigen (recombinant) 20 mcg/ml

◯ HEPATITIS B (HBV)

PROPHYLAXIS (HEPATITIS B)

Comment: Administer IM; under 1 year-of-age, administer in vastus lateralis. Over 1 year-of-age, administer in the deltoid. Administer a 3-dose series; *First dose:* newborn (or now); *Second dose:* 1-2 months after first dose; *Third dose:* 6 months after first dose.
▷ *hepatitis B recombinant vaccine* (C)
    Engerix-B Adult 20 mcg (1 ml) IM; repeat in 1 and 6 months
      Pediatric: infant-19 years: 10 mcg (1/2 ml) IM; repeat in 1 and 6 months
      Vial: 20 mcg/ml single-dose (preservative-free, thimerosal); *Prefilled syringe:* 20 mcg/ml
    Engerix-B Pediatric/Adolescent
      Pediatric: infant-19 years: 10 mcg IM; repeat in 1 and 6 months; *Vial:* 10 mcg/0.5 ml single-dose (preservative-free, thimerosal)
      Prefilled syringe: 10 mcg/0.5 ml
    Recombivax HB Adult 10 mcg (1 ml) IM in deltoid; repeat in 1 and 6 months
      Vial: 10 mcg/ml single-dose; *Vial:* 10 mcg/3 ml multi-dose
    Recombivax HB Pediatric/Adolescent 5 mcg (0.5 ml) IM; repeat in 1 and 6 months
      Pediatric: birth-19 years: 5 mcg (0.5 ml) IM; repeat in 1 and 6 months; >19 years: use adult formulation or 10 mcg (1 ml) pediatric/adolescent formulation
      Vial: 5 mcg/0.5 ml single-dose

PROPHYLAXIS (HEPATITIS A AND B COMBINATION)

Comment: Administer IM; under 1 year-of-age, administer in vastus lateralis. Over 1 year-of-age, administer in the deltoid. Administer a 3-dose series; *First dose:* newborn (or now); *Second dose:* 1-2 months after first dose; *Third dose:* 6 months after first dose.
➤ *hepatitis A inactivated/hepatitis B surface antigen (recombinant) vaccine* (C)
   Pediatric: <18 years: not recommended
      Twinrix 1 ml IM in deltoid; repeat in 1 months and 6 months
         Vial (soln): hepatitis A inactivated 720 IU/*hepatitis B* surface antigen (recombinant) 20 mcg/ml (1, 10 ml); *Prefilled syringe: hepatitis A* inactivated 720 IU/ *hepatitis B* surface antigen (recombinant) 20 mcg/ml

CHRONIC HBV INFECTION TREATMENT

Nucleoside Analogs (Reverse Transcriptase Inhibitors and HBV Polymerase Inhibitors)

Comment: Nucleoside analogs are indicated for chronic hepatitis infection with viral replication and either elevated ALT/AST or histologically active disease.
➤ *adefovir dipivoxil* (C) 10 mg daily; *CrCl 20-49 mL/min:* 10 mg q 48 hours; *CrCl 10-19 mL/min:* 10 mg q 72 hours
   Pediatric: not recommended
      Hepsera *Tab:* 10 mg
➤ *entecavir* (C)(G) take on an empty stomach
      Nucleoside naïve: 0.5 mg daily; *Nucleoside naïve, CrCl 30-49 mL/min:* 0.25 mg daily; *Nucleoside naïve, CrCl 10-29 mL/min:* 0.15 mg daily; *Nucleoside naïve, CrCl <10 mL/min:* 0.05 mg daily; *lamivudine-refractory:* 1 mg daily; *lamivudine-refractory, renal impairment:* see mfr literature
      Pediatric: <16 years: not recommended
      Baraclude *Tab:* 0.5, 1 mg; *Oral Soln:* 0.05 mg/ml (orange; parabens)
➤ *lamivudine* (C)(G) 100 mg daily; *CrCl <5 mL/min:* 35 mg for 1st dose, then 10 mg once daily; *CrCl 5-14 mL/min:* 35 mg for 1st dose, then 15 mg once daily; *CrCl 15-29 mL/min:* 100 mg for 1st dose, then 25 mg once daily; *CrCl 30-49 mL/min:* 100 mg for 1st dose, then 50 mg once daily
   Pediatric: <2 years: not recommended; 2-17 years: 3 mg/kg (max 100 mg) once daily
      Epivir-HBV *Tab:* 100 mg
      Epivir-HBV Oral Solution *Oral Soln:* 5 mg/ml (240 ml) (strawberry-banana)
➤ *telbivudine* (C) 600 mg daily; *CrCl <40 mL/min:* 600 mg q 72 hours; *CrCl 30-49 mL/ min:* 600 mg q 48 hours
   Pediatric: <16 years: not recommended
      Tyzeka *Tab:* 600 mg

Interferon Alpha

➤ *interferon alfa-2b* (C) 5 million IU SC or IM daily or 10 million IU SC or IM 3 times/ week x 16 weeks; reduce dose by half or interrupt dose if WBCs, granulocyte count, or platelet count decreases
   Pediatric: <1 year: not recommended; >1 year: 3 million IU/m^2 3 times/week x 1 week; then increase to 6 million IU/m^2 3 times/week to 16-24 weeks; max 10 million IU/dose; reduce dose by half or interrupt dose if WBCs, granulocyte count, or platelet count decreases

Intron A *Vial (pwdr):* 5, 10, 18, 25, 50 million IU/vial (pwdr + diluent; single-dose) (benzoyl alcohol); *Vial (soln):* 3, 5, 10 million IU/vial (single-dose); *Multi-dose vials (soln):* 18, 25 million IU/vial soln; *Multi-dose pens (soln):* 3, 5, 10 million IU/0.2 ml (6 doses/pen)

 HEPATITIS C (HCV)

CHRONIC HCV INFECTION TREATMENT

Nucleoside Analogs (Reverse Transcriptase Inhibitors)

Comment: Nucleoside analogs are indicated for patients with compensated liver disease previously untreated with *alpha interferon* or who have relapsed after *alpha interferon* therapy. Primary toxicity is hemolytic anemia. Contraindicated in male partners of pregnant women; use 2 forms of contraception during therapy and for 6 months after discontinuation.

▷ *ribavirin* (X) *Interferon-naïve:* treat for 24-48 weeks; *Relapse:* treat for 24 weeks; >18 years (>75 kg): 400 mg in AM and 600 mg in PM; >18 years (>75 kg): 600 mg in AM and 600 mg in PM
Pediatric: <4 years: not recommended; >3 years: 15 mg/kg per day in 2 divided doses; <25 kg: use solution; 25-36 kg: 200 mg twice daily; 37-49 kg: 200 mg in AM and 400 mg in PM; 50-61 kg: 400 mg twice daily; >61 kg: same as adult
    Copegus *Tab:* 200 mg
    Rebetol *Cap:* 200mg
    Rebetol Oral Solution *Oral soln:* 40 mg/ml (120 ml) (bubble gum)
    Ribashere RibaPak 600 mg *Tab:* 600 mg (14/pck)

Interferon Alpha

▷ *interferon alfacon-1* (C)
Pediatric: <18 years: not recommended
    Infergen 9 mcg SC 3 times/week x 24 weeks, then 15 mcg SC 3 times/week x 6 months; allow at least 48 hours between doses
    Vial (soln): 9, 15 mcg/vial soln (6-single dose/pck; preservative-free)
▷ *interferon alfa-2b* (C)
    Intron A *Vial (pwdr):* 5, 10, 18, 25, 50 million IU/vial (pwdr w. diluent; single-dose) (benzoyl alcohol); *Vial (soln):* 3, 5, 10 million IU/vial (single-dose); *Multi-dose vials (soln):* 18, 25 million IU/vial; *Multi-dose pens (soln):* 3, 5, 10 million IU/0.2 ml (6 doses/pen)
▷ *peginterferon alfa-2a* (C) administer 180 mcg SC once weekly (on the same day of the week); treat for 48 weeks; consider discontinuing if adequate response after 12-24 weeks
Pediatric: <18 years: not recommended
    PEGasys *Vial:* 180 mcg/ml (single-dose); *Monthly pck (vials):* 180 mcg/ml (1 ml, 4/pck)
▷ *peginterferon alfa-2b* (C) administer SC once weekly (on the same day of the week); treat for 1 year; consider discontinuing if inadequate response after 24 weeks; 37-45 kg: 40 mcg (100 mg/ml, 0.4 ml); 46-56 kg: 50 mcg (100 mg/ml, 0.5 ml); 57-72 kg: 64 mcg (160 mg/ml, 0.4 ml); 73-88 kg: 80 mcg (160 mg/ml, 0.5 ml); 89-106 kg: 96 mcg (240 mg/ml, 0.4 ml); 107-136 kg: 120 mcg (240 mg/ml, 0.5 ml); 137-160 kg: 150 mcg (300 mg/ml, 0.5 ml)

Pediatric: <18 years: not recommended
> **PEG-Intron** *Vial:* 50, 80, 120, 150 mcg/ml (single-dose)
> **PEG-Intron Redipen** *Pen:* 50, 80, 120, 150 mcg/ml (disposable pens)

HCV NS5A Inhibitor

▷ *daclatasvir* (X) 60 mg once daily for 12 weeks (with *sofosbuvir*); if *sofosbuvir* is discontinued, daclatasvir should also be discontinued; with concomitant CY3P inhibitors, reduce dose to 30 mg once daily; with concomitant CY3P inducers, increase dose to 90 mg once daily
> **Daklinza** *Tab:* 30, 60 mg
> Comment: **Daklinza** is indicated in combination with *sofosbuvir* with or without *ribavirin*, for the treatment of HCV genotypes 1 and 3, and in patients with co-morbid HIV-1 infection, advanced cirrhosis, or post-liver transplant recurrence of HCV.

HCV NS5A Inhibitor/HCV NS3/4A Protease Inhibitor Combinations

▷ *elbasvir/grazoprevir* (NR) 1 tab as a single dose once daily; see mfr literature for length of treatment
Pediatric: <18 years: not recommended
> **Zepatier** *Tab: elba* 50 mg/*grazo* 100/mg
> Comment: **Zepatier** is contraindicated with moderate or severe hepatic impairment, concomitant atazanavir, carbamazepine, cyclosporing, darunavir, efavirenz, lopinavir, phenatoin, rifampin, saquinavir, St. John's wort, tipranavir. When co-administered with ribavirin, pregnancy category (X)

HCV NS5A Inhibitor/HCV NS3/4A Protease Inhibitor/ CYP3A Inhibitor Combinations

▷ *ombitasvir/paritaprevir/ritonavir* (B) take 2 tabs once daily in the AM x 12 weeks
Pediatric: <18 years: not established
> **Technivie** *Tab: omvi* 25 mg/*pari* 75 mg/*rito* 50 mg (4 x 7 daily dose pcks/carton)
> Comment: **Technivie** is indicated for use in chronic HCV genotype 4 without cirrhosis. **Technivie** is not for use with moderate hepatic impairment.

HCV NS3/4A Protease Inhibitor Combinations

▷ *boceprevir* (C) 800 mg 3 times/day; take with food (not low-fat); not for monotherapy; start after 4 weeks therapy with *peginterferon* and discontinue if HCV-RNA levels indicate futility *ribavirin*; *Without cirrhosis:* continue as indicated by HCV-RNA levels at weeks 8, 12, and 24; *With cirrhosis:* continue for 44 weeks; do not reduce dose
Pediatric: <18 years: not recommended
> **Victrelis** *Cap:* 200 mg
▷ *simeprevir* (C) 150 mg once daily; swallow whole; take with food, not for monotherapy; do not reduce dose or interrupt therapy; if discontinued, do not reinitiate; discontinue if HCV-RNA levels indicate futility; discontinue if *peginterferon*, *ribavirin*, or *sofobuvir* is permanently discontinued; *Treatment naïve, treatment relapses, with or without cirrhosis:* treat x 12 weeks (*simeprevir* + *peginterferon* + *ribavirin*) followed by additional 12 weeks *peginterferon* + *ribavirin* (total = 24 weeks). *Partial and non-responders, with or without cirrhosis:* treat x 12 weeks (*simeprevir* + *peginterferon* + *ribavirin*) followed by additional

36 weeks *peginterferon* + *ribavirin* (total = 48 weeks); *Treatment naïve or treatment experienced without cirrhosis*: treat x 12 weeks (*simeprevir* + *sofosbuvir*); *Treatment naïve or treatment experienced with cirrhosis*: treat x 24 weeks (*simeprevir* + *sofosbuvir*)

Olysio *Cap*: 150 mg

HCV NS5A Inhibitor/HCV NS5B PALM Polymerase Inhibitor

▷ *ledipasvir/sofosbuvir* (NR) *Treatment naïve, without cirrhosis, with pretreatment HCV RNA <6 million IU/ml*: 1 tab daily x 8 weeks; *Treatment naïve with or without cirrhosis or treatment-experienced without cirrhosis*: 1 tab daily x 12 weeks; *Treatment-experienced with cirrhosis*: 1 tab daily x 24 weeks; *In combination with ribavirin*: 1 tab daily x 12 weeks;

Pediatric: <18 years: not established

Harvoni *Tab*: *ledi* 90 mg/*sofo* 400 mg

Comment: **Harvoni** is indicated for patients with advanced liver disease, genotytpe 1, 4, 5, or 6 infection: chronic HCV genotype 1- or 4-infected liver transplant recipients with or without cirrhosis or with compensated cirrhosis (Child-Pugh A), and for HCV genotype 1-infected patients with decompensated cirrhosis (Child-Pugh B/C), including those who have undergone liver transplantation. No adequate human data are available to establish whether or not **Harvoni** poses a risk to pregnancy outcomes; the background risk of major birth defects and miscarriage for the indicated population is unknown. If **Harvoni** is administered with *ribavirin*, the combination regimen is contraindicated (**X**) in pregnant women and in men whose female partners are pregnant. It is not known whether **Harvoni** and its metabolites are present in human breast milk, affect human milk production or have effects on the breastfed infant. If **Harvoni** is administered with *ribavirin*, the nursing mother's information for *ribavirin* also applies to this combination regimen.

HCV NS5A Inhibitor/HCV NS3/4A Protease Inhibitor/CYP3A Inhibitor PLUS HCV NS5B PALM Polymerase Inhibitor Combination

▷ *ombitasvir/paritaprevir/ritonavir* plus *dasabuvir* (B)
Pediatric: not established

Viekira Pak *ombitasvir/paritaprevir/ritonavir* fixed-dose combination tablet: 2 tablets orally once a day (in the morning); *dasabuvir*: 250 mg orally twice a day (morning and evening)

Tab: *omvi* 12.5 mg/*pari* 75 mg/*rito* 50 mg plus *Tab*: dasa 250 mg (28 day supply/ pck)

Comment: **Viekira Pak** is indicated for mild liver dysfunction (Child-Pugh A). **Viekira Pak** is contraindicated for moderate (Child-Pugh B) to severe (Child-Pugh C) liver dysfunction. No adjustment is recommended with mild, moderate, or severe renal dysfunction.

 HERPANGINA

ANALGESICS

▷ *acetaminophen* (B) *see Fever page* 143

➤ *tramadol* (C)(IV)(G)

    Rybix ODT initially 100 mg once daily; may increase by 100 mg every 5 days; max 300 mg/day; *CrCl <30 mL/min* or *severe hepatic impairment*: not recommended; *Cirrhosis*: max 50 mg q 12 hours

      Pediatric: <17 years: not recommended

      ODT: 50 mg (mint) (phenylalanine)

    Ryzolt initially 100 mg once daily; may increase by 100 mg every 5 days; max 300 mg/day; *CrCl <40 mL/min* or *severe hepatic impairment*: not recommended

      Pediatric: <16 years: not recommended; ≥16 years: same as adult

      Tab: 100, 200, 300 mg ext-rel

    Ultram 50-100 mg q 4-6 hours prn; max 400 mg/day; *CrCl <40 mL/min:* max 100 mg q 12 hours; *Cirrhosis:* max 50 mg q 12 hours

      Pediatric: <16 years: not recommended; ≥16 years: same as adult

      Tab: 50*mg

    Ultram ER initially 100 mg once daily; may increase by 100 mg every 5 days; max 300 mg/day; *CrCl <40 mL/min* or *severe hepatic impairment*: not recommended

      Pediatric: <18 years: not recommended

      Tab: 100, 200, 300 mg ext-rel

➤ *tramadol/acetaminophen* (C)(IV)(G) 2 tabs q 4-6 hours; max 8 tabs/day; 5 days; *CrCl <40 mL/min:* max 2 tabs q 12 hours; max 4 tabs/day x 5 days

    Pediatric: <16 years: not recommended; ≥16 years: same as adult

    Ultracet *Tab:* tram 37.5/acet 325 mg

Other Oral Analgesics see *Pain page 298*

TOPICAL ANESTHETICS

➤ *lidocaine* viscous soln (B) 15 ml gargle or mouthwash; repeat after 3 hours; max 8 doses/day

    Pediatric: <4 years: apply 1.25 ml to affected area with cotton-tipped applicator; may repeat after 3 hours; max 8 doses/day

    Xylocaine 2% Viscous Solution *Viscous soln:* 2% (20, 100, 450 ml)

    Antipyretics see *Fever page 143*

◯ HERPES GENITALIS (HSV TYPE II)

Comment: The following treatment regimens are published in the **2015 CDC Sexually Transmitted Diseases Treatment Guidelines**. Treatment regimens are for adults only; consult a specialist for treatment of patients less than 18 years-of-age. Treatment regimens are presented in alphabetical order by generic drug name, followed by brands and dose forms.

RECOMMENDED REGIMENS: FIRST CLINICAL EPISODE

Regimen 1

➤ *acyclovir* 400 mg tid x 7-10 days or 200 mg 5 times/day x 10 days or until clinically resolved

Regimen 2

➤ *acyclovir* cream apply q 3 hours 6 x/day x 7 days

Regimen 3

▷ *famciclovir* 250 mg tid x 7-10 days <u>or</u> until clinically resolved

Regimen 4

▷ *valacyclovir* 1 g bid x 10 days <u>or</u> until clinically resolved

RECOMMENDED RECURRENT/EPISODIC REGIMENS

Comment: Initiate treatment of recurrent episodes within 1 day of onset of lesions.

Regimen 1

▷ *acyclovir* 200 mg 5 times/day x 5 days

Regimen 2

▷ *famciclovir* 125 mg bid x 5 days

Regimen 3

▷ *valacyclovir* 500 mg bid x 3-5 days <u>or</u> until clinically resolved

SUPPRESSION THERAPY REGIMENS

Regimen 1

▷ *acyclovir* 400 mg bid x 1 year

Regimen 2

▷ *famciclovir* 250 mg bid x 1 year

Regimen 3

▷ *valacyclovir* 500 mg daily x 1 year (for ≤9 recurrences/year) <u>or</u> 1 g daily x 1 year (for ≥10 recurrences/year)

DAILY SUPPRESSIVE REGIMENS FOR PERSONS WITH HIV

Regimen 1

▷ *acyclovir* 400-800 mg bid-tid

Regimen 2

▷ *famciclovir* 500 mg bid

Regimen 3

▷ *valacyclovir* 500 mg bid

RECURRENT/EPISODIC REGIMENS FOR PERSONS WITH HIV

Regimen 1

▷ *acyclovir* 400 mg tid x 5-10 days

Regimen 2

▷ *famciclovir* 500 mg bid x 5-10 days

Regimen 3

▷ *valacyclovir* 1 g bid x 5-10 days

DRUG BRANDS AND DOSE FORMS

▷ *acyclovir* (B)(G)
> Zovirax *Cap:* 200 mg; *Tab:* 400, 800 mg
> Zovirax Oral Suspension *Oral susp:* 200 ml/5 ml (banana)
> Zovirax Cream *Crm:* 5% (3, 15 g); *Oint:* 5% (3, 15 g)
▷ *famciclovir* (B)
> Famvir *Tab:* 125, 250, 500 mg
▷ *valacyclovir* (B)
> Valtrex *Cplt:* 500, 1,000 mg

HERPES LABIALIS/HERPES FACIALIS (HERPES SIMPLEX VIRUS TYPE I, COLD SORE, FEVER BLISTER)

PRIMARY INFECTION

▷ *acyclovir* (B)(G) do not chew, crush, <u>or</u> swallow the buccal tab; apply within 1 hour of symptom onset and before appearance of lesion; apply a single buccal tab to the upper gum region on the affected side and hold in place for 30 seconds
> *Pediatric:* not established
> Sitavig *Buccal tab:* 50 mg
>> *Pediatric: see page 541 for dose by weight*
> **Comment:** **Sitavig** is contraindicated with allergy to milk protein concentrate.
▷ *valacyclovir* (B) 2 g q 12 hours x 1 day
> Valtrex *Cplt:* 500, 1,000 mg

SUPPRESSION THERAPY (FOR 6 <u>OR</u> MORE OUTBREAKS/YEAR)

▷ *acyclovir* (B)(G) 200 mg 2-5 x/day x 1 year
> *Pediatric:* <2 years: not recommended; >2 years, <40 kg: 20 mg/kg 2-5 times/day x 1 year; >2 years, >40 kg: 200 mg 2-5 times/day x 1 year; *see page 541 for dose by weight*
> Zovirax *Cap:* 200 mg; *Tab:* 400, 800 mg
> Zovirax Oral Suspension *Oral susp:* 200 mg/5 ml (banana)

TOPICAL ANTIVIRAL THERAPY

▷ *acyclovir* (B)(G) apply q 3 hours 6 times/day x 7 days
> *Pediatric:* <2 years: not recommended; ≥2 years: same as adult
> Zovirax Cream *Crm:* 5% (3, 15 g); *Oint:* 5% (3, 15 g)
▷ *docosanol* (B) apply and gently rub in 5 times daily until healed
> *Pediatric:* not recommended
> Abreva (OTC) *Crm:* 10% (2 g)

▷ *penciclovir* (B) apply q 2 hours while awake x 4 days
   Pediatric: not recommended
      Denavir *Crm:* 1% (2 g)

TOPICAL ANTIVIRAL/CORTICOSTEROID THERAPY

▷ *acyclovir/hydrocortisone* (B)(G) cream apply to affected area 5 x/day x 5 days
   Pediatric: <12 years: not recommended; ≥12 years: same as adult
      Crm: 1% (2, 5 g)

 # HERPES ZOSTER (SHINGLES)

ORAL ANTIVIRALS

▷ *famciclovir* (B) 500 mg tid x 7 days
   Pediatric: <18 years: not recommended
      Famvir *Tab:* 125, 250, 500 mg
▷ *valacyclovir* (B) 1 g tid x 7 days
   Pediatric: not recommended
      Valtrex *Cplt:* 500, 1,000 mg
▷ *acyclovir* (B)(G) 800 mg 5 x/day x 7-10 days
   Pediatric: <2 years: not recommended; ≥2 years, <40 kg: 20 mg/kg 5 x/day x 7-10
   days; >2 years, >40 kg: 800 mg 5 x/day x 7-10 days; *see page 541 for dose by weight*
      Zovirax *Cap:* 200 mg; *Tab:* 400, 800 mg
      Zovirax Oral Suspension *Oral susp:* 200 mg/5 ml (banana)

PROPHYLAXIS AGAINST SECONDARY INFECTION

▷ *silver sulfadiazine* (B) apply qid
   Pediatric: not recommended
      Silvadene *Crm:* 1% (20, 50, 85, 400, 1,000 g jar; 20 g tube)

ANALGESICS

▷ *acetaminophen* (B) *see Fever page 143*
▷ *aspirin* (D) *see Fever page 144*
   Comment: *aspirin*-containing medications are contraindicated with history of allergic-type reaction to *aspirin*, children and adolescents with *varicella* <u>or</u> other viral
illness, and 3rd trimester pregnancy.
▷ *tramadol* (C)(IV)(G)
   Rybix ODT initially 100 mg once daily; may increase by 100 mg every 5 days;
   max 300 mg/day; *CrCl <30 mL/min* <u>or</u> *severe hepatic impairment:* not recommended; *Cirrhosis:* max 50 mg q 12 hours
     Pediatric: <17 years: not recommended
     ODT: 50 mg (mint) (phenylalanine)
   Ryzolt initially 100 mg once daily; may increase by 100 mg every 5 days; max 300
   mg/day; *CrCl <30 mL/min* <u>or</u> *severe hepatic impairment,* not recommended
     Pediatric: <16 years: not recommended; ≥16 years: same as adult
     Tab: 100, 200, 300 mg ext-rel
   Ultram 50-100 mg q 4-6 hours prn; max 400 mg/day; *CrCl <40 mL/min:* max
   100 mg q 12 hours; *Cirrhosis:* max 50 mg q 12 hours
     Pediatric: <16 years: not recommended: ≥16 years: same as adult

Tab: 50*mg

Ultram ER initially 100 mg once daily; may increase by 100 mg every 5 days; max 300 mg/day; *CrCl <30 mL/min* or *severe hepatic impairment:* not recommended
Pediatric: <18 years: not recommended
Tab: 100, 200, 300 mg ext-rel
▷ *tramadol/acetaminophen* (C)(IV)(G) 2 tabs q 4-6 hours; max 8 tabs/day x 5 days; CrCl <40 mL/min: max 2 tabs q 12 hours; max 4 tabs/day x 5 days
Pediatric: <16 years: not recommended; ≥16 years: same as adult
Ultracet *Tab:* tram 37.5/acet 325 mg
Other Oral Analgesics *see Pain page* 298
Postherpetic Neuralgia *see page* 342

SECONDARY INFECTION PROPHYLAXIS

▷ *silver sulfadiazine* (B) apply qid
Pediatric: not recommended
Silvadene *Crm:* 1% (20, 50, 85, 400, 1,000 g/jar; 20 g tube)

◯ HICCUPS: INTRACTABLE

▷ *chlorpromazine* (C) 25-50 mg tid-qid
Pediatric: <6 months: not recommended; ≥6 months: 0.25 mg/lb orally q 4-6 hours prn or 0.5 mg/lb rectally q 6-8 hours prn
Thorazine *Tab:* 10, 25, 50, 100, 200 mg; *Spansule:* 30, 75, 150 mg sust-rel; *Syr:* 10 mg/5 ml (4 oz; orange custard); *Oral conc:* 30 mg/ml (4 oz); 100 mg/ml (2, 8 oz); *Supp:* 25, 100 mg

◯ HIDRADENITIS SUPPURATIVA

ORAL ANTI-INFECTIVES

▷ *doxycycline* (D)(G) 100 mg bid x 7-14 days
Pediatric: <8 years: not recommended; ≥8 years, <100 lb: 2 mg/lb on first day in 2 divided doses, followed by 1 mg/lb/day in 1-2 divided doses; ≥8 years, ≥100 lb: same as adult; *see page 561 for dose by weight*
Actilate *Tab:* 75, 150** mg
Adoxa *Tab:* 50, 75, 100, 150 mg ent-coat
Doryx *Tab:* 75, 100, 150 mg del-rel
Monodox *Cap:* 50, 75, 100 mg
Oracea *Cap:* 40 mg del-rel
Vibramycin *Cap:* 50, 100 mg; *Syr:* 50 mg/5 ml (raspberry; sulfites); *Oral susp:* 25 mg/5 ml (raspberry-apple)
Vibra-Tab *Tab:* 100 mg film-coat
Comment: *doxycycline* is contraindicated <8 years-of-age, in pregnancy, and lactation (discolors developing tooth enamel). A side effect may be photo-sensitivity (photophobia). Do not give with antacids, calcium supplements, milk or other dairy, or within two hours of taking another drug.
▷ *erythromycin base* (B)(G) 1-1.5 g divided qid x 7-14 days
Pediatric: <45 kg: 30-50 mg in 2-4 divided doses x 7-14 days; ≥45 kg: same as adult
Ery-Tab *Tab:* 250, 333, 500 mg ent-coat

PCE *Tab:* 333, 500 mg

Comment: *erythromycin* may increase INR with concomitant *warfarin*, as well as increase serum level of *digoxin*, benzodiazepines and statins.

▷ *erythromycin ethylsuccinate* (B)(G) 1200-1600 mg divided qid x 7-14 days
Pediatric: 30-50 mg/kg/day in 4 divided doses x 7 days; may double dose with severe infection; max 100 mg/kg/day; see page 563 for dose by weight

EryPed *Oral susp:* 200 mg/5 ml (100, 200 ml) (fruit); 400 mg/5 ml (60, 100, 200 ml) (banana); *Oral drops:* 200, 400 mg/5 ml (50 ml) (fruit); *Chew tab:* 200 mg wafer (fruit)

E.E.S. *Oral susp:* 200, 400 mg/5 ml (100 ml) (fruit)

E.E.S. Granules *Oral susp:* 200 mg/5 ml (100, 200 ml) (cherry)

E.E.S. 400 Tablets *Tab:* 400 mg

Comment: *erythromycin* may increase INR with concomitant *warfarin*, as well as increase serum level of *digoxin*, benzodiazepines and statins.

▷ *minocycline* (D)(G) 100 mg bid x 7-14 days
Pediatric: <8 years: not recommended, ≥8 years: same as adult

Dynacin *Cap:* 50, 100 mg

Minocin *Cap:* 50, 75, 100 mg; *Oral susp:* 50 mg/5 ml (60 ml) (custard) (sulfites, alcohol 5%)

Comment: *minocycline* is contraindicated <8 years-of-age, in pregnancy, and lactation (discolors developing tooth enamel). A side effect may be photo-sensitivity (photophobia). Do not give with antacids, calcium supplements, milk or other dairy, or within two hours of taking another drug.

▷ *tetracycline* (D)(G) 250 mg qid or 500 mg tid x 7-14 days
Pediatric: <8 years: not recommended; ≥8 years, <100 lb: 25-50 mg/kg/day in 2-4 divided doses x 7-14 days; ≥8 years, ≥100 lb: same as adult; *see page 574 for dose by weight*

Achromycin V *Cap:* 250, 500 mg

Sumycin *Tab:* 250, 500 mg; *Cap:* 250, 500 mg; *Oral susp:* 125 mg/5 ml (100, 200 ml) (fruit, sulfites)

Comment: *tetracycline* is contraindicated <8 years-of-age, in pregnancy, and lactation (discolors developing tooth enamel). A side effect may be photo-sensitivity (photophobia). Do not give with antacids, calcium supplements, milk or other dairy, or within two hours of taking another drug.

TOPICAL ANTI-INFECTIVES

▷ *clindamycin* (B) topical apply bid x 7-14 days
Cleocin T *Pad:* 1% (60/pck; alcohol 50%); *Lotn:* 1% (60 ml); *Gel:* 1% (30, 60 g); *Soln w. applicator:* 1% (30, 60 ml; alcohol 50%)

 HOOKWORM (UNCINARIASIS, CUTANEOUS LARVAE MIGRANS)

ANTIHELMINTICS

▷ *albendazole* (C) 400 mg as a single dose; may repeat in 3 weeks
Pediatric: <2 years: 200 mg daily x 3 days; may repeat in 3 weeks; ≥2-12 years: 400 mg daily x 3 days; may repeat in 3 weeks

Albenza *Tab:* 200 mg

➤ *mebendazole* **(C)(G)** 100 mg AM and PM x 3 consecutive days <u>or</u> 500 mg as a single dose; may repeat in 2-3 weeks if needed

Pediatric: same as adult (chew <u>or</u> crush and mix with food)

Vermox *Chew tab:* 100 mg

➤ *pyrantel pamoate* **(C)** 11 mg/kg x 1 dose; max 1 g/dose

Pediatric: 25-37 lb: 1/2 tsp x 1 dose; 38-62 lb: 1 tsp x 1 dose; 63-87 lb: 1 tsp x 1 dose; 88-112 lb: 2 tsp x 1 dose; 113-137 lb: 2 tsp x 1 dose; 138-162 lb: 3 tsp x 1 dose; 163-187 lb: 3 tsp x 1 dose; >187 lb: 4 tsp x 1 dose

Pin-X (OTC) *Cap:* 180 mg; *Liq:* 50 mg/ml (30 ml); 144 mg/ml (30 ml); *Oral susp:* 50 mg/ ml (30 ml)

➤ *thiabendazole* **(C)**

Pediatric: <40 lb: consult mfr literature; >30 lb: 2 divided doses/day with meals; 30-50 lbs: 250 mg bid with meals; >50 lb: 10 mg/lb/dose bid with meals; max 3g/day; Treat all bid x 7 days

Mintezol *Chew tab:* 500*mg (orange); *Oral susp:* 500 mg/5 ml (120 ml) (orange)

Comment: *thiabendazole* is not for prophylaxis. May impair mental alertness.

HUMAN IMMUNODEFICIENCY VIRUS (HIV) EXPOSURE, ANTIRETROVIRAL PEP/nPEP

Antiretroviral drug brand names and dose forms (*see Anti-HIV Drugs page 510*)

Comment: Antiretroviral prophylactic treatment regimens for occupational HIV exposure (PEP) and nonoccupational exposure (nPEP) are referenced from the **2015 CDC Sexually Transmitted Diseases Treatment Guidelines, MMWR, and NIH** available at: www.cdc.gov/mmwr/preview/mmwrhtml/rr5402a1.htm and www .aidsinfo.nih.gov/guidelines/default_db2.asp?id=50. Highly active antiretroviral treatment (HAART) regimens in this section are for adults only; consult a specialist for adult dosing and recommendations and for selection of age-appropriate dosing regimens for patients less than 18 years-of-age. For pediatric dosing information, see *Guidelines for Use of Antiretroviral Agents in Pediatric HIV Infection* available at https://www.aidsinfo.nih.gov/contentfiles/lvguidelines/pediatricguidelines. pdf. The 2015 CDC-recommended antiretroviral treatment (ART) regimens are followed by brand names with dose forms and recommended dosing. Initiation of PEP/nPEP with ART as soon as possible increases the likelihood of prophylactic benefit. Treatment regimens must be initiated ≥72 hours following exposure. A 28-day course of ART is recommended for persons with *substantial risk for HIV exposure* (i.e., exposure of vagina, rectum, eye, mouth, <u>or</u> other mucous membrane, non-intact skin, <u>or</u> percutaneous contact with blood, semen, vaginal secretions, breast milk, <u>or</u> any body fluid that is visibly contaminated with blood, when the source is known to be infected with HIV). ART is not recommended for persons with *negligible risk for HIV exposure* (i.e., exposure of vagina, rectum, eye, mouth, <u>or</u> other mucus membrane, intact <u>or</u> non-intact skin, <u>or</u> percutaneous contact with urine, nasal secretions, saliva, sweat, <u>or</u> tears, if not visibly contaminated with blood, regardless of the known <u>or</u> suspected HIV status of the source). There is no evidence indicating any specific antiretroviral medication, <u>or</u> combination of medications is optimal for suppressing local viral replication. There is no evidence to indicate that a 3-drug ART regimen is any more beneficial than a

2-drug regimen. When the source person is available for interview and testing, his or her history of retroviral medication use and most recent/current viral load measurement should be considered when selecting an ART treatment regimen (e.g., to help avoid prescribing an antiretroviral medication to which the source virus is likely to be resistant).

PREFERRED REGIMENS

Nonnucleoside Reverse Transcriptase Inhibitor (NNRTI)-Based Regimen

▷ *efavirenz* plus (*lamivudine* or *emtricitabine*) plus (*zidovudine* or *tenofovir*)

Protease Inhibitor (PI)-Based Regimen

▷ *lopinavir/ritonavir* (co-formulated as **Kaletra**) plus (*lamivudine* or *emtricitabine*) plus *zidovudine*

ALTERNATIVE REGIMENS

NNRTI-Based Regimen

▷ *efavirenz* plus (*lamivudine* or *emtricitabine*) plus (*abacavir* or *didanosine* or *stavudine*)
   Comment: *efavirenz* should be avoided in pregnant women and women of child-bearing potential.

PI-Based Regimens

Regimen 1

▷ *atazanavir* plus (*lamivudine* or *emtricitabine*) plus (*zidovudine* or *stavudine* or *abacavir* or *didanosine*) or (*tenofovir* plus *ritonavir* (100 mg/day)

Regimen 2

▷ *fosamprenavir* plus (*lamivudine* or *emtricitabine*) plus (*zidovudine* or *stavudine*) or (*abacavir* or *tenofovir* or *didanosine*)

Regimen 3

▷ *fosamprenavir/ritonavir* plus (*lamivudine* or *emtricitabine*) plus (*zidovudine* or *stavudine* or *abacavir* or *tenofovir* or *didanosine*)

Regimen 4

▷ *indinavir/ritonavir* plus (*lamivudine* or *emtricitabine*) plus (*zidovudine* or *stavudine* or *abacavir* or *tenofovir* or *didanosine*)
   Comment: Using *ritonavir* with *indinavir* may increase risk for renal adverse events.

Regimen 5

▷ *lopinavir/ritonavir* (co-formulated as **Kaletra**) plus (*lamivudine* or *emtricitabine*) plus (*stavudine* or *abacavir* or *tenofovir* or *didanosine*)

Regimen 6

▷ nelfinavir plus (lamivudine or emtricitabine) plus (zidovudine or stavudine or abacavir or tenofovir or didanosine)

Regimen 7

▷ saquinavir (hgc or sgc)/ritonavir plus (lamivudine or emtricitabine) plus (zidovudine or stavudine or abacavir or tenofovir or didanosine)
   Comment: hgc=hard gel capsule (**Invirase**); sgc=soft-gel capsule (**Fortovase**)

Triple Nucleoside Reverse Transcriptase Inhibitor (NRTI)-Based Regimen

abacavir plus lamivudine plus zidovudine
Comment: Triple NRTI therapy should be used only when an NNRTI- or PI-based regimen cannot or should not be used.

BRAND NAMES, DOSING, AND DOSE FORMS: SINGLE AGENTS

Nucleoside and Nonnucleoside Reverse Transcriptase Inhibitors (NRTIs/NNRTIs)

▷ abacavir sulfate (C)
   Ziagen Tab: 300*mg; Oral soln: 20 mg/ml (240 ml) (strawberry-banana; parabens, propylene glycol)
▷ didanosine (C)
   Videx EC Cap: 125, 200, 250, 400 mg ent-coat del-rel; Chew tab: 25, 50, 100, 150, 200 mg (mandarin orange; buffered with calcium carbonate and magnesium hydroxide, phenylalanine); Pwdr for oral soln: 2, 4 g (120, 240 ml)
▷ emtricitabine (B)
   Emtriva Cap: 200 mg; Oral soln: 10 mg/ml (170 ml) (cotton candy)
▷ lamivudine (C) (G)
   Epivir Tab: 150*, 300*mg; Oral soln: 10 mg/ml (240 ml) (strawberry-banana; sucrose 3 g/15 ml)
▷ stavudine (C)
   Zerit Cap: 15, 20, 30, 40 mg; Oral soln: 1 mg/ml pwdr for reconstitution (200 ml) (fruit; dye-free)
▷ tenofovir disoproxil fumarate (C)
   Viread Tab: 150, 200, 250, 300 mg; Oral pwdr: 40 mg/L
▷ zidovudine (C)
   Retrovir Tab: 300 mg; Cap: 100 mg; Syr: 50 mg/5 ml (240 ml) (strawberry); Vial: 10 mg/ml (20 ml vial for IV infusion) (peservative-free)

Nonnucleoside Reverse Transcriptase Inhibitors (NNRTIs)

▷ efavirenz (D) 600 mg once daily at bedtime
   Sustiva Tab: 600 mg; Cap: 50, 200 mg
   Comment: Do not use efavirenz with known or possible pregnancy.

Nucleoside and Nonnucleoside Reverse Transcriptase Inhibitors (NRTI/NNRTI) Combinations

▷ emtricitabine/tenofovir disoproxil fumarate/rilpivirine (B) take with a meal; 1 tab once daily; CrCl <50 mL/min: not recommended; if concomitant rifabutin needed, take additional rilpivirine 25 mg once daily

Pediatric: not established
>> **Complera** *Tab:* emtri 200 mg/tenof 300 mg/*rilpiv 25 mg*
Comment: Complera is indicated for treatment of HIV-1 in adults naïve to HIV-1 medications (where the virus has not developed resistance to these anti-HIV-1 medications) and who have no more than 100,000 copies/ml of HIV-1 RNA in their blood. **Rilpivirine** is an NNRTI. **Rilpivirine** is contraindicated with anticonvulsants (*carbamazepine, oxcarbazepine, phenytoin, phenobarbital*), antimycobacterials (*rifampin, rifapentine*), proton pump inhibitors (*esomeprazole, lansoprazole, omeprazole, pantoprazole, rabeprazole*), systemic dexamethasone (more than a single dose), or *St John's wort*. **Rifabutin** is used to prevent *mycobacterium avium complex* (MAC) in people with HIV-1 infection. **Rifabutin** is also used with other medicines to treat tuberculosis in people with HIV-1. **Rifabutin** has not been studied in patients under 18 years-of-age.

Protease Inhibitors (PIs)

▷ *atazanavir* (B) 400 mg once daily; if administered with *tenofovir* plus *ritonavir* 300 mg once daily
  Reyataz *Cap:* 100, 150, 200, 300 mg
▷ *fosamprenavir* (C) 1,400 mg twice daily
  Lexiva *Tab:* 700 mg; *Oral soln:* 50 mg/ml (grape, bubble gum) (peppermint)
▷ *indinavir sulfate* (C) 800 mg every 8 hours or 800 mg plus ritonavir 100 mg every 12 hours or 800 mg plus ritonavir 200 mg every 12 hours
  Crixivan *Cap:* 100, 200, 333, 400 mg
▷ *nelfinavir mesylate* (B) 750 mg 3 x/day or 1,250 mg 2 x/day
  Viracept *Tab:* 250, 625 mg; *Pwdr for oral soln:* 50 mg/g (144 g) (phenylalanine)
▷ *ritonavir* (B) see doses used in combination with other specific PIs
  Norvir *sgc:* 100 mg (alcohol); *Oral soln:* 80 mg/ml (8 oz) (peppermint-caramel) (alcohol)
▷ *saquinavir mesylate* (hgc or sgc) (B) 400 mg plus *ritonavir* 400 mg twice daily or 1,000 mg plus *ritonavir* 100 mg twice daily
  Invirase *hsc:* 200 mg
  Fortovase *sgc:* 200 mg

BRAND NAMES, DOSING, AND DOSE FORMS: COMBINATION AGENTS

▷ *abacavir sulfate/lamivudine* (B)
  Epzicom *Tab:* aba 600 mg/lami 300 mg
▷ *abacavir sulfate/lamivudine/zidovudine* (C) (G)
  Trizivir *Tab:* aba 300 mg/lami 150 mg/zido 300 mg
▷ *emtricitabine/tenofovir disoproxil fumarate* (B)
  Truvada *HIV-1 infection, ≥12 years-of-age and ≥35 kg:* 1 tab once daily; *CrCl 30-49 mL/min:* 1 tab every other day; *CrCl <30 mL/min, hemodialysis:* not recommended; *PrEP:* 1 tab once daily; *CrCl 60 mL/min:* do not use; confirm HIV-negative status immediately prior to initiating treatment and repeat every 3 months
    Pediatric: <12 years or <35 kg: not established
    Tab: **Truvada 100/150** *emt 100 mg/teno 150 mg*
      Truvada 133/200 *emt 133 mg/teno 200 mg*
      Truvada 167/250 *emt 167 mg/teno 250 mg*
      Truvada 200/300 *emt 200 mg/teno 300 mg*

Comment: **Truvada** is indicated for treatment of HIV-1 infection and pre-exposure prophylaxis (PrEP) to reduce the risk of sexually acquired HIV-1 in high risk adults in combination with safe sex practices.
➤ *lamivudine/zidovudine* (C)
  Combivir *Tab: lami* 150 mg/*zido* 300 mg
➤ *lopinavir/ritonavir* (C)
    Tab: **Kaletra 100/25** *lopin* 100 mg/*riton* 25 mg
        Kaletra 200/50 *lopin* 200 mg/*riton* 50 mg

HUMAN PAPILLOMAVIRUS (HPV)

PROPHYLAXIS

Comment: Administer IM in deltoid. Administer a 3-dose series; First dose females (10-25 years of age) and males (9-15 years of age); Second dose: 1-2 months after first dose; Third dose: 6 months after first dose. HPV vaccination is indicated for the prevention of cervical, vulvar, vaginal, and anal cancers. Register pregnant patients exposed to **Gardasil** by calling 800-986-8999.
➤ *bivalent human papillomavirus types 16 and 18 vaccine, aluminum adsorbed* (B)
  Pediatric: <10 years: not recommended
    Cervarix administer in the deltoid; 1st dose 0.5 ml IM on elected date; then, 2nd dose 0.5 ml IM 1 month later; then, 3rd dose 0.5 ml IM 6 months after the first dose
      Vial: susp for IM inj (single-dose; prefilled syringe) (preservative-free)
➤ *quadrivalent human papillomavirus types 6, 11, 16, and 18 vaccine, recombinant, aluminum adsorbed* (B)
  Pediatric: >9 years: not recommended
    Gardasil administer in the deltoid or upper thigh; 1st dose 0.5 ml IM on elected date; then, 2nd dose 0.5 ml IM 2 months later; then, 3rd dose 0.5 ml IM 6 months after the first dose
      Vial: susp for IM inj (single-dose; prefilled syringe w. needles or tip caps) (preservative-free)
➤ *quadrivalent human papillomavirus types 6, 11, 16, 18, 31, 33, 45, 52, and 58 vaccine, recombinant, aluminum adsorbed* (B)
    Gardasil 9 *Adults and Children: 9-26 Years-of-Age:* administer IM in the deltoid or thigh; administer the 1st dose; administer the 2nd dose 2 months after the 1st dose; administer the 3rd dose 6 months after the 1st dose (4 months after the 2nd dose).
      Vial: susp for IM inj (0.5 ml single-dose; prefilled syringe w. needles or tip caps) (preservative-free)

TREATMENT

see **Wart: Venereal** page 448

HYPERHIDROSIS (PERSPIRATION, EXCESSIVE)

➤ *aluminum chloride* (NR) 20% solution apply q HS; wash treated area the following morning; after 1-2 treatments, may reduce frequency to 1-2 times/week
  Drysol *Soln:* 35, 60 ml (alcohol 93%) cont-rel
Comment: Apply to clean dry skin (e.g., underarms). Do not apply to broken, irritated, or recently shaved skin.

⬤ HYPERHOMOCYSTEINEMIA

Comment: Elevated homocysteine is associated with cognitive impairment, vascular dementia, and dementia of the Alzheimer's type.

HOMOCYSTEINE-LOWERING NUTRITIONAL SUPPLEMENTS

▷ *L-methylfolate calcium (as metafolin)/pyridoxyl 5-phosphate/methyl-cobalamin* (NR) take 1 cap daily
Pediatric: not recommended
  Metanx *Cap: metafo* 3 mg/*pyrid* 35 mg/*methyl* 2 mg (gluten-free, yeast-free, lactose-free)
  Comment: **Metanx** is indicated as adjunct treatment of endothelial dysfunction and/or hyperhomocysteinemia in patients who have lower extremity ulceration.

▷ *L-methylfolate calcium (as metafolin)/methylcobalamin/N-acetylcysteine* (NR) take 1 cap daily
Pediatric: not recommended
  Cerefolin *Cap: metafo* 5.6 mg/*methyl* 2 mg/*N-ace* 600 mg (gluten-free, yeast-free, lactose-free)
  Comment: **Cerefolin** is indicated in the dietary management of patients treated for early memory loss, with emphasis on those at risk for neurovascular oxidative stress, hyperhomocysteinemia, mild to moderate cognitive impairment with or without vitamin B-12 deficiency, vascular dementia, or Alzheimer's disease.

⬤ HYPERKALEMIA (POTASSIUM EXCESS)

HYPERKALEMIA CATION EXCHANGE RESIN

▷ *Sodium polystyrene sulfonate* pwdr (sodium content 4.1 mg mEq/g **(C)**
Pediatrics: Use 1 g/1 mEq of K as basis of calculation; see mfr likterature
  Kayexalate *Susp:* 15 g 1-4 times daily; *Rectal Enema:* 30-50 g in 100 ml every 6 hours
Comment: Contraindicated in neonates and with obstructive bowel disease. Reduces absorption of *thyroxine* and *lithium*. **Digoxin** is potentiated by hypokalemia. May cause GI irritability, ulceration, necrosis, sodium retention, hypocalcemia, hypomagnesemia, fecal impaction, ischemic colitis. Avoid non-absorbable cation-donating antacids and laxatives (e.g., *magnesium hydroxide*, *aluminum hydroxide*. Concomitant sorbitol should be avoided because it may cause intestinal necrosis.

▷ *patiromer* **(B)** take once daily; mix pkt in 1 oz water, stir; add 2 more ounces of water; make sure all of the pwdr is dissolved and swallow immediately; do not add to heated water or heated food
  Veltassa
  Pwdr: 8.4, 16.8, 25.2 g/pkt (4, 30/carton)
  Comment: Take **Veltassa** at least 6 hours before or at least 6 hours after any other medicine taken by mouth.

HYPERPARATHYROIDISM

➤ *paricalcitol* (C)(G) administer 0.04-1 mcg/kg (2.8-7 mcg) IV bolus, during dialysis, no more than every other day; may be increased by 2-4 mcg every 2-4 weeks; monitor serum calcium and phosphorus during dose adjustment periods; if Ca x P >75, immediately reduce dose or discontinue until these levels normalize; discard unused portion of single-use vials immediately
Pediatric: <18 years: not established

Zemplar *Vial:* 2, 5 mcg/ml soln for inj

Comment: Zemplar is indicated for the prevention and treatment of secondary hyperparathyroidism associated with chronic kidney disease, stage 5.

HYPERPHOSPHATEMIA

PHOSPHATE BINDERS

Comment: Monitor for development of hypercalcemia. Normal serum PO_4^- is 2.5-4.5 mg/dL and normal serum calcium is 8.5-10.5 mg/dL.
➤ *calcium acetate* (C)(G) initially 2 tabs or caps with each meal; then titrate gradually to keep serum phosphate at <6 mg/dL; usual maintenance is 3-4 tabs or caps with each meal
Pediatric: not recommended

PhosLo *Tab:* 667 mg; *Cap:* 667 mg
➤ *lanthanum carbonate* (C) initially 750 mg to 1.5 g per day in divided doses; take with meals; titrate at 2-3-week intervals in increments of 750 mg/day based on serum phosphate; usual range 1.5-3 g/day; usual max 3,750 mg/day
Pediatric: not recommended

Fosrenol *Chew tab:* 250, 500, 750 mg; 1 g
➤ *sevelamer* (C) for patients not taking a phosphate binder, take tid with meals; swallow whole; titrate by 1 tab per meal at 1-week intervals to keep serum phosphorus 3.5-5.5 mg/dL; switching from calcium acetate to *sevelamer,* see mfr literature.
Serum phosphorus >5.5 to >7.5 mg/dL: 800 mg tid; *Serum phosphorus 7.5-9:* 1.2-1.6 g tid
Pediatric: not recommended

Renagel *Tab:* 400, 800 mg
Renvela *Tab:* 800 mg

HYPERPIGMENTATION

Comment: Depigmenting agents may be used for hyperpigmented skin conditions including chloasma, melasma, freckles, senile lentigenes. Limit treatments to small areas at one time. Sunscreen ≥30 SPF recommended.
➤ *hydroquinone* (C)(G) apply sparingly to affected area and rub in bid

Lustra *Crm:* 4% (1, 2 oz) (sulfites)
Lustra AF *Crm:* 4% (1, 2 oz) (sunscreen, sulfites)
➤ *monobenzone* (C) apply sparingly to affected area and rub in bid-tid; depigmentation occurs in 1-4 months

Benoquin *Crm:* 20% (1.25 oz)

▷ *tazarotene* (X)(G) apply daily at HS
   Pediatric: not recommended
        Avage Cream *Crm:* 0.1% (30 g)
        Tazorac Cream *Crm:* 0.05, 0.1% (15, 30, 60 g)
        Tazorac Gel *Gel:* 0.05, 0.1% (30, 100 g)
▷ *tretinoin* (C) apply daily at HS
   Pediatric: <12 years: not recommended; ≥12 years: same as adult
        Avita *Crm/Gel:* 0.025% (20, 45 g)
        Renova *Crm:* 0.02% (40 g); 0.05% (40, 60 g)
        Retin-A Cream *Crm:* 0.025, 0.05, 0.1% (20, 45 g)
        Retin-A Gel *Gel:* 0.01, 0.025% (15, 45 g) (alcohol 90%)
        Retin-A Liquid *Liq:* 0.05% (28 ml) (alcohol 55%)
        Retin-A Micro *Microspheres:* 0.04, 0.1% (20, 45 g)

COMBINATION AGENTS

▷ *hydroquinone/fluocinolone/tretinoin* (C) apply sparingly to affected area and rub in daily at HS
   Pediatric: not recommended
        Tri-Luma *Crm:* hydro 4%/fluo 0.01%/tretin 0.05% (30 g) (parabens, sulfites)
▷ *hydroquinone/padimate O/oxybenzone/octyl methoxcinnamate* (C) apply sparingly to affected area and rub in bid
   Pediatric: <12 years: not recommended; ≥16 years: same as adult
        Glyquin *Crm:* 4% (1 oz jar)
▷ *hydroquinone/ethyl dihydroxypropyl PABA/dioxybenzone/oxybenzone* (C) apply sparingly to affected area and rub in bid; max 2 months
        Pediatric: not recommended
        Solaquin *Crm:* hydro 2%/PABA 5%/dioxy 3%/oxy 2% (1 oz) (sulfites)
▷ *hydroquinone/padimate/dioxybenzone/oxybenzone* (C) apply sparingly to affected area and rub in bid; max 2 months
   Pediatric: not recommended
        Solaquin Forte *Crm:* hydro 4%/pad 0.5%/dioxy 3%/oxy 2% (1oz) (sunscreen, sulfites)
▷ *hydroquinone/padimate/dioxybenzone* (C) apply sparingly to affected area and rub in bid; max 2 months
   Pediatric: not recommended
        Solaquin Forte Gel: hydro 4%/pad 0.5%/dioxy 3% (1 oz) (alcohol, sulfites)

⬤ HYPERPROLACTINEMIA

DOPAMINE RECEPTOR AGONIST

▷ *dostinex* (B)(G) initial therapy is 0.25 mg twice a week; may increase by 0.25 mg twice weekly up to 1 mg twice a week according to the patient's serum prolactin level; dose increases should not occur more than every 4 weeks; after a normal serum prolactin level has been maintained for 6 months, may be discontinued, with periodic monitoring of serum prolactin level to determine if/when treatment should be reinstituted
   Pediatric: not established
        Cabergoline *Tab:* 0.5 mg
   Comment: Cabergoline is indicated to treat hyperprolactinemia disorders due to idiopathic <u>or</u> pituitary adenoma.

⬤ HYPERTENSION: PRIMARY

see JNC-8 Recommendations page 460

BETA-BLOCKERS: CARDIOSELECTIVE

Comment: Cardioselective beta-blockers are less likely to cause bronchospasm, peripheral vasoconstriction, or hypoglycemia than noncardioselective beta-blockers.
▷ *acebutolol* (B)(G) initially 400 mg in 1-2 divided doses; usual range 200-800 mg/day; max 1.2 g/day in 2 divided doses
    Pediatric: not recommended
        Sectral *Cap:* 200, 400 mg
▷ *atenolol* (D)(G) initially 50 mg daily; may increase after 1-2 weeks to 100 mg daily; max 100 mg/day
    Pediatric: not recommended
        Tenormin *Tab:* 25, 50, 100 mg
▷ *betaxolol* (C) initially 10 mg daily; may increase to 20 mg/day after 7-14 days; usual max 20 mg/day
    Pediatric: not recommended
        Kerlone *Tab:* 10*, 20 mg
▷ *bisoprolol* (C) 5 mg daily; max 20 mg daily
    Pediatric: not recommended
        Zebeta *Tab:* 5*, 10 mg
▷ *metoprolol succinate* (C)
    Pediatric: not recommended
        Toprol-XL initially 25-100 mg in a single dose once daily; increase weekly if needed; max 400 mg/day; as monotherapy or with a diuretic
          Tab: 25*, 50*, 100*, 200*mg ext-rel
▷ *metoprolol tartrate* (C)
    Pediatric: not recommended
        Lopressor (G) initially 25-50 mg bid; increase weekly if needed; max 400 mg/day; as monotherapy or with a diuretic
          Tab: 25, 37.5, 50, 75, 100 mg
▷ *nebivolol* (C)(G)
    Pediatric: not recommended
        Bystolic initially 5 mg daily; may increase at 2 week intervals; max 40 mg/day
          Tab: 2.5, 5, 10, 20 mg

BETA-BLOCKERS: NONCARDIOSELECTIVE

Comment: Noncardioselective beta-blockers are more likely to cause bronchospasm, peripheral vasoconstriction, and/or hypoglycemia than cardioselective beta-blockers.
▷ *nadolol* (C)(G) initially 40 mg daily; usual maintenance 40-80 mg daily; max 320 mg/day
    Pediatric: not recommended
        Corgard *Tab:* 20*, 40*, 80*, 120*, 160*mg
▷ *penbutolol* (C) 20 mg daily
    Pediatric: not recommended
        Levatol *Tab:* 20*mg

▷ *pindolol* (B)(G) initially 5 mg bid; may increase after 3-4 weeks in 10 mg increments; max 60 mg/day
Pediatric: not recommended
    Pindolol *Tab:* 5, 10 mg
    Visken *Tab:* 5, 10 mg
▷ *propranolol* (C)(G)
    Inderal initially 40 mg bid; usual maintenance 120-240 mg/day; max 640 mg/day
      Pediatric: initially 1 mg/kg/day; usual range 2-4 mg/kg/day in 2 divided doses; max 16 mg/kg/day
      Tab: 10*, 20*, 40*, 60*, 80*mg
    Inderal LA initially 80 mg daily in a single dose; increase q 3-7 days; usual range 120-160 mg/day; max 320 mg/day in a single dose
      Pediatric: not recommended
      Cap: 60, 80, 120, 160 mg sust-rel
    InnoPran XL initially 80 mg q HS; max 120 mg/day
      Pediatric: not recommended
      Cap: 80, 120 mg ext-rel
▷ *timolol* (C)(G) initially 10 mg bid, increase weekly if needed; usual maintenance 20-40 mg/day; max 60 mg/day in 2 divided doses
Pediatric: not recommended
    Blocadren *Tab:* 5, 10*, 20*mg

BETA-BLOCKER: (NONCARDIOSELECTIVE)/ALPHA-1 BLOCKER COMBINATIONS

▷ *carvedilol* (C)
Pediatric: <18 years: not recommended
    Coreg initially 6.25 mg bid; may increase at 1-2-week intervals to 12.5 mg bid; max 25 mg bid
      Tab: 3.125, 6.25, 12.5, 25 mg
    Coreg CR initially 20 mg once daily for 2 weeks; may increase at 1-2-week intervals; max 80 mg once daily
      Tab: 10, 20, 40, 80 mg cont-rel
▷ *carteolol* (C)
Pediatric: not recommended
    Cartrol initially 2.5 mg daily, gradually increase to 5 or 10 mg daily; usual maintenance 2.5-5 mg daily
      Tab: 2.5, 5 mg
▷ *labetalol* (C)(G) initially 100 mg bid; increase after 2-3 days if needed; usual maintenance 200-400 mg bid; max 2.4 g/day
Pediatric: not recommended
    Normodyne *Tab:* 100*, 200*, 300 mg
    Trandate *Tab:* 100*, 200*, 300*mg

DIURETICS

Thiazide Diuretics

▷ *chlorthalidone* (B)(G) initially 15 mg daily; may increase to 30 mg once daily based on clinical response; max 45-60 mg/day

    Pediatric: not established
>   **Chlorthalidone** *Tab:* 25, 50 mg
>   **Thalitone** *Tab:* 15 mg

▷ *chlorothiazide* (B)(G) 0.5-1 g/day in a single <u>or</u> divided doses; max 2 g/day
    Pediatric: <6 months: up to 15 mg/lb/day in 2 divided doses; ≥6 months: 10 mg/lb/
    day in 2 divided doses
>   **Diuril** *Tab:* 250*, 500*mg; *Oral susp:* 250 mg/5 ml (237 ml)

▷ *hydrochlorothiazide* (B)(G)
    Pediatric: not recommended
>   **Esidrix** 25-100 mg once daily
>   *Tab:* 25, 50, 100 mg
>   **Hydrochlorothiazide** *Tab:* 25*, 50*mg
>   **Microzide** 12.5 mg once daily; usual max 50 mg/day
>   *Cap:* 12.5 mg

▷ *methyclothiazide* (B) initially 2.5 mg daily; max 10 mg daily
    Pediatric: not recommended
>   **Enduronyl** *Tab: methy* 5 mg/*deser* 0.25 mg*
>   **Enduronyl Forte** *Tab: methy* 5 mg/*deser* 0.5 mg*

▷ *polythiazide* (C) 2-4 mg once daily
    Pediatric: not recommended
>   **Renese** *Tab:* 1, 2, 4 mg

Potassium-Sparing Diuretics

▷ *amiloride* (B)(C) initially 5 mg; may increase to 10 mg; max 20 mg
    Pediatric: not recommended
>   **Midamor** *Tab:* 5 mg

▷ *spironolactone* (D)(G) initially 50-100 mg in a single <u>or</u> divided doses; titrate at
    2-week intervals
    Pediatric: not established
>   **Aldactone** *Tab:* 25, 50*, 100*mg

▷ *triamterene* (B) 100 mg bid; max 300 mg
    Pediatric: not recommended
>   **Dyrenium**
>   *Cap:* 50, 100 mg

Loop Diuretics

▷ *bumetanide* (C)(G) 0.5-2 mg daily; may repeat at 4-5-hour intervals; max
    10 mg/day
    Pediatric: <18 years: not recommended
    Tab: 1* mg
    Comment: *bumetanide* is contraindicated with sulfa drug allergy.

▷ *ethacrynic acid* (B) initially 50-200 mg/day
    Pediatric: infant: not recommended; ≥1 month: initially 25 mg/day; then adjust
    dose in 25-mg increments
>   **Edecrin** *Tab:* 25, 50 mg

▷ *furosemide* (C)(G) initially 40 mg bid
    Pediatric: not recommended
>   **Lasix** *Tab:* 20, 40*, 80 mg; *Oral Soln:* 10 mg/ml (2, 4 oz w. dropper)
    Comment: *furosemide* is contraindicated with sulfa drug allergy.

▷ *torsemide* (B) 5 mg once daily; may increase to 10 mg once daily
    Pediatric: not recommended
        Demadex *Tab:* 5*, 10*, 20*, 100*mg

Other Diuretics

▷ *indapamide* (B) initially 1.25 mg daily; may titrate dosage upward q 4 weeks if needed; max 5 mg/day
    Pediatric: not recommended
        Lozol *Tab:* 1.25, 2.5 mg
    Comment: *indapamide* is contraindicated with sulfa drug allergy.
▷ *metolazone* (B)
    Pediatric: not recommended
        Zaroxolyn 2.5- 5 mg daily
         Tab: 2.5, 5, 10 mg
    Comment: *metolazone* is contraindicated with sulfa drug allergy.

DIURETIC COMBINATIONS

▷ *amiloride/hydrochlorothiazide* (B)(G) initially 1 tab daily; may increase to 2 tabs/day in a single <u>or</u> divided doses
    Pediatric: not recommended
        Moduretic *Tab:* amil 5 mg/*hydro* 50 mg*
▷ *deserpidine/methylchlothiazide* (C) titrate *methylchlothiazide* 2.5-10 mg daily
    Pediatric: not recommended
        Enduronyl
            Tab: **Enduronyl 0.25/5** *deser* 0.25 mg/*methylclo* 5 mg*
                Enduronyl 0.5/5 *deser* 0.5 mg/*methylclo* 5 mg*
▷ *spironolactone/hydrochlorothiazide* (D)(G)
    Pediatric: not recommended
        Aldactazide 25 usual maintenance 50-100 mg in a single <u>or</u> divided doses
            Tab: *spiro* 25 mg/*hctz* 25 mg
        Aldactazide 50 usual maintenance 50-100 mg in a single <u>or</u> divided doses
            Tab: *spiro* 50 mg/*hydro* 50 mg
▷ *triamterene/hydrochlorothiazide* (C)(G)
    Pediatric: not recommended
        Dyazide 1-2 caps once daily
            Cap: *triam* 37.5 mg/*hctz* 25 mg
        Maxzide 1 tab once daily
            Tab: *triam* 75 mg/*hctz* 50 mg*
        Maxzide-25 1-2 tabs once daily
            Tab: *triam* 37.5 mg/*hctz* 25 mg*

ANGIOTENSIN CONVERTING ENZYME INHIBITORS (ACEIs)

Comment: Black patients receiving ACEI monotherapy have been reported to have a higher incidence of angioedema compared to non-Blacks. Non-Blacks have a greater decrease in BP when ACEIs are used compared to Black patients.
▷ *benazepril* (D)(G) initially 10 mg daily; usual maintenance 20-40 mg/day in 1-2 divided doses; usual max 80 mg/day
    Pediatric: not recommended

     Lotensin *Tab:* 5, 10, 20, 40 mg
▷ *captopril* (D)(G) initially 25 mg bid-tid; after 1-2 weeks increase to 50 mg bid-tid
Pediatric: not recommended
     Capoten *Tab:* 12.5*, 25*, 50*, 100*mg
▷ *enalapril* (D)(G) initially 5 mg/day; max 40 mg/day; usual range 10-40 mg in 1-2
divided doses; *CrCl <40 mL/min:* initially 2.5 mg daily
Pediatric: <1 month: not recommended; ≥1 month: initially 0.08 mg/kg up to 5 mg
once daily; max 0.58 mg/kg (or 40 mg) daily; *CrCl <40 mL/min* or *on dialysis* (administer on dialysis days)
     Epaned *Oral soln:* 150 mg/150 ml pwdr for reconstitution (Kit: pwdr w. diluent)
     Vasotec *Tab:* 2.5*, 5*, 10*, 20* mg
▷ *fosinopril* (D) initially 10 mg daily; usual maintenance 20-40 mg/day in a single or
divided doses; max 80 mg/day
Pediatric: <6 years, <50 kg: not recommended; ≥6-12 years, >50 kg: 5-10 mg once daily
     Monopril *Tab:* 10*, 20, 40 mg
▷ *lisinopril* (D) initially 10 mg daily; usual range 20-40 mg/day
Pediatric: not recommended
     Prinivil *Tab:* 5*, 10*, 20*, 40 mg
     Zestril *Tab:* 2.5, 5*, 10, 20, 30, 40 mg
▷ *moexipril* (D) initially 7.5 mg daily; usual range 15-30 mg/day in 1-2 divided doses;
max 30 mg/day
Pediatric: not recommended
     Univasc *Tab:* 7.5*, 15*mg
▷ *perindopril* (D) 2-8 mg daily-bid; max 16 mg/day
Pediatric: not recommended
     Aceon *Tab:* 2*, 4*, 8*mg
▷ *quinapril* (D) initially 10 mg once daily; usual maintenance 20-80 mg daily in 1-2
divided doses
Pediatric: not recommended
     Accupril *Tab:* 5*, 10, 20, 40 mg
▷ *ramipril* (D)(G) initially 2.5 mg bid; usual maintenance 2.5-20 mg in 1-2 divided
doses
Pediatric: not established
     Altace *Tab/Cap:* 1.25, 2.5, 5, 10 mg
▷ *trandolapril* (C; D in 2nd, 3rd) initially 1-2 mg once daily; adjust at 1-week intervals;
usual range 2-4 mg in 1-2 divided doses; max 8 mg/day
Pediatric: not recommended
     Mavik *Tab:* 1*, 2, 4 mg

ANGIOTENSIN II RECEPTOR BLOCKERS (ARBs)

▷ *azilsartan medoxomil* (D) *Monotherapy, not volume depleted:* 80 mg once daily; *Vol-
ume-depleted (concomitant high-dose diuretic):* initially 40 mg once daily
Pediatric: not recommended
     Edarbi *Tab:* 40, 80 mg
▷ *candesartan* (D) initially 16 mg daily; range 8-32 mg in 1-2 divided doses
Pediatric: not recommended
     Atacand *Tab:* 4, 8, 16, 32 mg
▷ *eprosartan* (D)(G) initially 400 mg bid or 600 mg once daily; max 800 mg/day
Pediatric: not established
     Teveten *Tab:* 400, 600 mg

▷ *irbesartan* (D)(G) initially 150 mg daily; titrate up to 300 mg
  Pediatric: not recommended
      Avapro *Tab:* 75, 150, 300 mg
▷ *losartan* (D)(G) initially 50 mg daily; max 100 mg/day
  Pediatric: not recommended
      Cozaar *Tab:* 25, 50, 100 mg
▷ *olmesartan medoxomil* (D) initially 20 mg once daily; after 2 weeks, may increase
  to 40 mg daily
  Pediatric: <6 years: not recommended; ≥6-16 years: 20-35 kg: initially 10 mg once
  daily; after 2 weeks, may increase to max 20 mg once daily; ≥6-16 years: >35 kg:
  initially 20 mg once daily; after 2 weeks, may increase to max 40 mg once daily
      Benicar *Tab:* 5, 20, 40 mg
▷ *telmisartan* (D)(G) initially 40 mg once daily; usual dose 20-80 mg
  Pediatric: not recommended
      Micardis *Tab:* 20, 40, 80 mg
▷ *valsartan* (D)(G) initially 80 mg once daily; may increase to 160 or 320 mg once daily
  after 2-4 weeks; usual range 80-320 mg/day
  Pediatric: not recommended
      Diovan *Tab:* 40*, 80, 160, 320 mg

CALCIUM CHANNEL BLOCKERS (CCBs)

Benzothiazepines

▷ *diltiazem* (C)(G)
  Pediatric: not established
      Cardizem initially 30 mg qid; may increase gradually every 1-2 days; max 360
      mg/day in divided doses
        Tab: 30, 60, 90, 120 mg
      Cardizem CD initially 120-180 mg daily; adjust at 1-2-week intervals; max 480
      mg/day
        Cap: 120, 180, 240, 300, 360 mg ext-rel
      Cardizem LA initially 180-240 mg daily; titrate at 2-week intervals; max 540
      mg/day
        Tab: 120, 180, 240, 300, 360, 420 mg ext-rel
      Cardizem SR initially 60-120 mg bid; adjust at 2-week intervals; max 360 mg/
      day
        Cap: 60, 90, 120 mg sust-rel
      Cartia XT initially 180 or 240 mg once daily; max 540 mg once daily
        Cap: 120, 180, 240, 300 mg ext-rel
      Dilacor XR initially 180 or 240 mg in AM; usual range 180-480 mg/day; max
      540 mg/day
        Cap: 120, 180, 240 mg ext-rel
      Tiazac (G) initially 120-240 mg daily; adjust at 2-week intervals; usual max 540
      mg/day
        Cap: 120, 180, 240, 300, 360, 420 mg ext-rel
▷ *diltiazem maleate* (C) initially 120-180 mg daily; adjust at 2-week intervals; usual
  range 120-480 mg daily
  Pediatric: not recommended
      Tiamate *Cap:* 120, 180, 240 mg ext-rel

Dihydropyridines

▷ *amlodipine* (C) initially 5 mg once daily; max 10 mg/day
  Pediatric: not recommended
    Norvasc *Tab:* 2.5, 5, 10 mg
▷ *clevidipine butyrate* (C) administer by IV infusion; initially 1-2 mg/hour; double
  dose at 90-second intervals until BP approaches goal; then titrate slower; adjust at
  5-10-minute intervals; maintenance 4-6 mg/hour; usual max, 16-32 mg/hour; do
  not exceed 1,000 ml (21 mg/hour for 24 hours) due to lipid load
  Pediatric: <18 years: not recommended
    Cleviprex *Vial:* 0.5 mg/ml soln for IV infusion (single use, 50, 100 ml) (lipids)
      Comment: **Cleviprex** is indicated to reduce blood pressure when oral therapy is
      not feasible or desirable. **Cleviprex** is contraindicated with egg or soy allergy.
▷ *felodipine* (C)(G) initially 5 mg daily; usual range 2.5-10 mg daily; adjust at 2-week
  intervals; max 10 mg/day
  Pediatric: not recommended
    Plendil *Tab:* 2.5, 5, 10 mg ext-rel
▷ *isradipine* (C)
  Pediatric: not recommended
    DynaCirc initially 2.5 mg bid; adjust in increments of 5 mg/day at 2-4-week
    intervals; max 20 mg/day
      Cap: 2.5, 5 mg
    DynaCirc CR initially 5 mg daily; adjust in increments of 5 mg/day at 2-4-week
    intervals; max 20 mg/day
      Tab: 5, 10 mg cont-rel
▷ *nicardipine* (C)(G)
  Pediatric: <18 years: not recommended
    Cardene initially 20 mg tid; adjust at intervals of at least 3 days; max 120 mg/day
      Cap: 20, 30 mg
    Cardene SR 30-60 mg bid
      Cap: 30, 45, 60 mg sust-rel
▷ *nifedipine* (C)(G)
  Pediatric: not recommended
    Adalat initially 10 mg tid; usual range 10-20 mg tid; max 180 mg /day
      Cap: 10, 20 mg
    Adalat CC initially 10 mg tid; usual range 10-20 mg tid; max 180 mg/day
      Cap: 30, 60, 90 mg ext-rel
    Afeditab CR initially 30 mg once daily; titrate over 7-14 days; max 90 mg/day
      Cap: 30, 60 mg ext-rel
    Procardia initially 10 mg tid; titrate over 7-14 days: max 30 mg/dose and 180
    mg/day in divided doses
      Cap: 10, 20 mg
    Procardia XL initially 30-60 mg daily; titrate over 7-14 days; max dose 90 mg/day
      Tab: 30, 60, 90 mg ext-rel
▷ *nisoldipine* (C)
  Pediatric: not recommended
    Sular initially 20 mg daily; may increase by 10 mg weekly; usual maintenance
    20-40 mg/day; max 60 mg/day
      Tab: 10, 20, 30, 40 mg ext-rel

Diphenylalkylamines

▷ **verapamil** (C)(G)
> *Pediatric:* not recommended
>> **Calan** 80-120 mg tid; may titrate up; usual max 360 mg in divided doses
>>> *Tab:* 40, 80*, 120*mg
>> **Calan SR** initially 120 mg in the AM; may titrate up; max 480 mg/day in divided doses
>>> *Cplt:* 120, 180*, 240*mg sust-rel
>> **Covera HS** initially 180 mg q HS; titrate to 240 mg; then to 360 mg; then to 480 mg if needed
>>> *Tab:* 180, 240 mg ext-rel
>> **Isoptin** initially 80-120 mg tid
>>> *Tab:* 40, 80, 120 mg
>> **Isoptin SR** initially 120-180 mg in the AM; may increase to 240 mg in the AM; then 180 mg q 12 hours or 240 mg in the AM and 120 mg in the PM; then 240 mg q 12 hours
>>> *Tab:* 120, 180*, 240*mg sust-rel
>> **Verelan** initially 240 mg once daily; adjust in 120 mg increments; max 480 mg/day
>>> *Cap:* 120, 180, 240, 360 mg sust-rel
>> **Verelan PM** initially 200 mg q HS; may titrate upward to 300 mg; then 400 mg if needed
>>> *Cap:* 100, 200, 300 mg ext-rel

ALPHA-1 ANTAGONISTS

Comment: Educate the patient regarding potential side effects of hypotension when taking an alpha-1 antagonist, especially with first dose ("first dose effect"). Start at lowest dose and titrate upward.
▷ **doxazosin** (C)(G) initially 1 mg once daily at HS; increase dose slowly every 2 weeks if needed; max 16 mg/day
> *Pediatric:* not recommended
>> **Cardura** *Tab:* 1*, 2*, 4*, 8*mg
>> **Cardura XL** *Tab:* 4, 8 mg
▷ **prazosin** (C)(G) first dose at HS, 1 mg bid-tid; increase dose slowly; usual range 6-15 mg/day in divided doses; max 20-40 mg/day
> *Pediatric:* not recommended
>> **Minipress** *Cap:* 1, 2, 5 mg
▷ **terazosin** (C) 1 mg q HS, then increase dose slowly; usual range 1-5 mg q HS; max 20 mg/day
> *Pediatric:* not recommended
>> **Hytrin** *Cap:* 1, 2, 5, 10 mg

CENTRAL ALPHA-AGONISTS

▷ **clonidine** (C)
> *Pediatric:* <12 years: not recommended
>> **Catapres** initially 0.1 mg bid; usual range 0.2-0.6 mg/day in divided doses; max 2.4 mg/day; *Tab:* 0.1*, 0.2*, 0.3*mg
>> **Catapres-TTS** initially 0.1 mg patch weekly; increase after 1-2 weeks if needed; max 0.6 mg/day

    Patch: 0.1, 0.2 mg/day (12/carton); 0.3 mg/day (4/carton)
    Kapvay (G) initially 0.1 mg bid; usual range 0.2-0.6 mg/day in divided doses; max 2.4 mg/day; *Tab:* 0.1, 0.2 mg
    Nexiclon XR initially 0.18 mg (2 ml) suspension <u>or</u> 0.17 mg tab once daily; usual max 0.52 mg (6 ml suspension) once daily
    Tab: 0.17, 0.26 mg ext-rel; *Oral susp:* 0.09 mg/ml ext-rel (4 oz)

▷ *guanabenz* **(C)(G)** initially 4 mg bid; may increase by 4-8 mg/day every 1-2 weeks; max 32 mg/day
    Pediatric: not recommended
    Tab: 4, 8 mg

▷ *guanfacine* **(B)(G)** initially 1 mg/day q HS; may increase to 2 mg/day q HS; usual max 3 mg/day
    Pediatric: not recommended
    Tenex *Tab:* 1, 2 mg

▷ *methyldopa* **(B)(G)** initially 250 mg bid-tid; titrate at 2-day intervals; usual maintenance 500 mg/day to 2 g/day; max 3 g/day
    Pediatric: initially 10 mg/kg/day in 2-4 divided doses; max 65 mg/kg/day <u>or</u> 3 g/day, whichever is less
    Aldomet *Tab:* 125, 250, 500 mg; *Oral susp:* 250 mg/5 ml (473 ml)

ALDOSTERONE RECEPTOR BLOCKER

▷ *eplerenone* **(B)** initially 25-50 mg daily; may increase to 50 mg bid; max 100 mg/day
    Pediatric: not recommended
    Inspra *Tab:* 25, 50 mg
Comment: Contraindicated with concomitant potent CYP3A4 inhibitors. Risk of hyperkalemia with concomitant ACE-I <u>or</u> ARB. Monitor serum potassium at baseline, 1 week, and 1 month. Caution with serum Cr >2 mg/dL (male) <u>or</u> >1.8 mg/dL (female) <u>and/or</u> CrCl <50 mL/min, and DM with proteinuria.

PERIPHERAL ADRENERGIC BLOCKER

▷ *guanethidine* **(C)** initially 10 mg daily; may adjust dose at 5-7 day intervals; usual range 25-50 mg/day
    Pediatric: not recommended
    Ismelin *Tab:* 10, 25 mg

DIRECT RENIN INHIBITOR

▷ *aliskiren* **(D)** initially 150 mg once daily; max 300 mg/day
    Pediatric: <18 years: not recommended
    Tekturna *Tab:* 150, 300 mg

PERIPHERAL VASODILATORS

▷ *hydralazine* **(C)(G)** initially 10 mg qid x 2-4 days; then increase to 25 mg qid for remainder of 1st week; then increase to 50 mg qid; max 300 mg/day
    Pediatric: initially 0.75 mg/kg/day in 4 divided doses; increase gradually over 3-4 weeks; max 7.5 mg/kg/day <u>or</u> 2,000 mg /day
    Tab: 10, 25, 50, 100 mg

▷ *minoxidil* (C) initially 5 mg daily; may increase at 3-day intervals to 10 mg/day, then 20 mg/day, then 40 mg/day; usual range 10-40 mg/day; max 100 mg/day
Pediatric: initially 0.2 mg/kg daily; may increase in 50%-100% increments every 3 days; usual range 0.25-1 g/kg/day; max 50 mg/day
Loniten *Tab:* 2.5*, 10*mg

ACEI/DIURETIC COMBINATIONS

▷ *benazepril*/hydrochlorothiazide (D)
Lotensin HCT 1 tab once daily; titrate individual components
Pediatric: not recommended
Tab: **Lotensin HCT 5/6.25** *benaz* 5 mg/*hctz* 6.25 mg*
Lotensin HCT 10/12.5 *benaz* 10 mg/*hctz* 12.5 mg*
Lotensin HCT 20/12.5 *benaz* 20 mg/*hctz* 12.5 mg*
Lotensin HCT 20/25 *benaz* 20 mg/*hctz* 25 mg*
▷ *captopril*/hydrochlorothiazide (D)(G)
Pediatric: not recommended
Capozide 1 tab once daily; titrate individual components
Tab: **Capozide 25/15** *capt* 25 mg/*hctz* 15 mg*
Capozide 25/25 *capt* 25 mg/*hctz* 25 mg*
Capozide 50/15 *capt* 50 mg/*hctz* 15 mg*
Capozide 50/25 *capt* 50 mg/*hctz* 25 mg*
▷ *enalapril*/hydrochlorothiazide (D)
Pediatric: not recommended
Vaseretic 1 tab once daily; titrate individual components
Tab: **Vaseretic 5/12.5** *enal* 5 mg/*hctz* 12.5 mg
Vaseretic 10/25 *enal* 10 mg/*hctz* 25 mg
▷ *lisinopril*/hydrochlorothiazide (D)
Pediatric: not recommended
Prinzide 1 tab once daily; titrate individual components
Tab: **Prinzide 10/12.5** *lis* 10 mg/*hctz* 12.5 mg
Prinzide 20/12.5 *lis* 20 mg/*hctz* 12.5 mg
Prinzide 20/25 *lis* 20 mg/*hctz* 25 mg
Zestoretic 1 tab once daily; titrate individual components; *CrCl <40 mL/min:* not recommended
Tab: **Zestoretic 10/12.5** *lis* 10 mg/*hctz* 12.5 mg
Zestoretic 20/12.5 *lis* 20 mg/*hctz* 12.5 mg*
Zestoretic 20/25 *lis* 20 mg/*hctz* 25 mg
▷ *moexipril*/hydrochlorothiazide (D)
Pediatric: not recommended
Uniretic 1 tab once daily; titrate individual components
Tab: **Uniretic 7.5/12.5** *moex* 7.5 mg/*hctz* 12.5 mg*
Uniretic 15/12.5 *moex* 15 mg/*hctz* 12.5 mg*
Uniretic 15/25 *moex* 15 mg/*hctz* 25 mg*
▷ *quinapril*/hydrochlorothiazide (D)
Pediatric: not recommended
Accuretic 1 tab once daily; titrate individual components
Tab: **Accuretic 10/12.5** *quin* 10 mg/*hctz* 12.5 mg*
Accuretic 20/12.5 *quin* 20 mg/*hctz* 12.5 mg*
Accuretic 20/25 *quin* 20 mg/*hctz* 25 mg*

ARB/DIURETIC COMBINATIONS

▷ *azilsartan/chlorthalidone* (D)
  Pediatric: <18 years: not recommended
      Edarbyclor 1 tab once daily; titrate individual components
        Tab: **Edarbyclor 40/12.5** *azil* 40 mg/*chlor* 12.5 mg
          Edarbyclor 40/25 *azil* 40 mg/*chlor* 25 mg
▷ *candesartan/hydrochlorothiazide* (D) 1 tab once daily; titrate individual components
  Pediatric: not recommended
      Atacand HCT
        Tab: **Atacand HCT 16/12.5** *cande* 16 mg/*hctz* 12.5 mg
          Atacand HCT 32/12.5 *cande* 32 mg/*hctz* 12.5 mg
▷ *eprosartan/hydrochlorothiazide* (D)
  Pediatric: not recommended
      Teveten HCT 1 tab once daily; titrate individual components
        Tab: **Teveten HCT 600/12.5** *epro* 600 mg/*hctz* 12.5 mg
          Teveten HCT 600/25 *epro* 600 mg/*hctz* 25 mg
▷ *irbesartan/hydrochlorothiazide* (D)
  Pediatric: not recommended
      Avalide 1 tab once daily; titrate individual components
        Tab: **Avalide 150/12.5** *irbes* 150 mg/*hctz* 12.5 mg
          Avalide 300/12.5 *irbes* 300 mg/*hctz* 12.5 mg
▷ *losartan/hydrochlorothiazide* (D)(G)
  Pediatric: not recommended
      Hyzaar 1 tab once daily; titrate individual components
        Tab: **Hyzaar 50/12.5** *losar* 50 mg/*hctz* 12.5 mg
          Hyzaar 100/12.5 *losar* 100 mg/*hctz* 12.5 mg
          Hyzaar 100/25 *losar* 100 mg/*hctz* 25 mg
▷ *olmesartan medoxomil/hydrochlorothiazide* (D)
  Pediatric: not recommended
      Benicar HCT 1 tab once daily; titrate individual components
        Tab: **Benicar HCT 20/12.5** *olmi* 20 mg/*hctz* 12.5 mg
          Benicar HCT 40/12.5 *olmi* 40 mg/*hctz* 12.5 mg
          Benicar HCT 40/25 *olmi* 40 mg/*hctz* 25 mg
▷ *telmisartan/hydrochlorothiazide* (D)
  Pediatric: not recommended
      Micardis HCT 1 tab once daily; titrate individual components
        Tab: **Micardis HCT 40/12.5** *telmi* 40 mg/*hctz* 12.5 mg
          Micardis HCT 80/12.5 *telmi* 80 mg/*hctz* 12.5 mg
          Micardis HCT 80/25 *telmi* 80 mg/*hctz* 25 mg
▷ *valsartan/hydrochlorothiazide* (D)
  Pediatric: not recommended
      Diovan HCT 1 tab once daily; titrate individual components
        Tab: **Diovan HCT 80/12.5** *vals* 80 mg/*hctz* 12.5 mg
          Diovan HCT 160/12.5 *vals* 160 mg/*hctz* 12.5 mg
          Diovan HCT 160/25 *vals* 160 mg/*hctz* 25 mg
          Diovan HCT 320/12.5 *vals* 320 mg/*hctz* 12.5 mg
          Diovan HCT 320/25 *vals* 320 mg/*hctz* 25 mg

CENTRAL ALPHA-AGONIST/DIURETIC COMBINATIONS

▷ *clonidine/chlorthalidone* (C)
  Pediatric: not recommended
    Combipres 1 tab daily-bid
      Tab: **Combipres 0.1** *clon* 0.1 mg/*chlorthal* 15 mg*
        Combipres 0.2 *clon* 0.2 mg/*chlorthal* 15 mg*
        Combipres 0.3 *clon* 0.3 mg/*chlorthal* 15 mg*
▷ *methyldopa/hydrochlorothiazide* (C)(G)
  Pediatric: not recommended
    Aldoril initially **Aldoril 15** bid-tid <u>or</u> **Aldoril 25** bid; titrate individual components
      Tab: **Aldoril 15** *meth* 250 mg/*hctz* 15 mg
        Aldoril 25 *meth* 250 mg/*hctz* 25 mg
        Aldoril D30 *meth* 500 mg/*hctz* 30 mg
        Aldoril D50 *meth* 500 mg/*hctz* 50 mg

BETA-BLOCKER (CARDIOSELECTIVE)/DIURETIC COMBINATIONS

▷ *atenolol/chlorthalidone* (D)(G)
  Pediatric: not recommended
    Tenoretic initially *tenoretic* 50 mg once daily; may increase to *tenoretic* 100 mg
    once daily
      Tab: **Tenoretic 50/25** *aten* 50 mg/*chlor* 25 mg*
        Tenoretic 100/25 *aten* 100 mg/*chlor* 25 mg
▷ *bisoprolol/hydrochlorothiazide* (C)
  Pediatric: not recommended
    Ziac initially one 2.5/6.25 mg tab daily; adjust at 2 week intervals; max two
    10/6.25 mg tabs daily
      Tab: **Ziac 2.5** *biso* 2.5 mg/*hctz* 6.25 mg
        Ziac 5 *biso* 5 mg/*hctz* 6.25 mg
        Ziac 10 *biso* 10 mg/*hctz* 6.25 mg
▷ *metoprolol succinate/hydrochlorothiazide* (C)
  Pediatric: not recommendxed
    Lopressor HCT titrate individual components
      Tab: **Lopressor HCT 50/25** *meto succ* 50 mg/*hctz* 25mg*
        Lopressor HCT 100/25 *meto succ* 100 mg/*hctz* 25mg*
        Lopressor HCT 100/50 *meto succ* 100 mg/*hctz* 50mg*
▷ *metoprolol succinate/ext-rel hydrochlorothiazide* (C)
  Pediatric: not established
    Dutoprol titrate individual components; may titrate to max 200/25 mg once
    daily
      Tab: **Dutoprol 25/12.5** *meto succ* 25 mg/*ext-rel hctz* 12.5 mg
        Dutoprol 50/12.5 *meto succ* 50 mg/*ext-rel hctz* 12.5 mg
        Dutoprol 100/12.5 *meto succ* 100 mg/*ext-rel hctz* 12.5 mg

BETA-BLOCKER (NONCARDIOSELECTIVE)/DIURETIC COMBINATIONS

▷ *nadolol/bendroflumethiazide* (C)
  Pediatric: not recommended
    Corzide titrate individual components

Tab: **Corzide 40/5** *nado* 40 mg/*bend* 5 mg*
Corzide 80/5 *nado* 80 mg/*bend* 5 mg*

▷ *propranolol/hydrochlorothiazide* (C)(G)
Pediatric: not recommended
Inderide titrate individual components
Tab: **Inderide 40/25** *prop* 40 mg/*hctz* 25 mg*
Inderide 80/25 prop 80 mg/*hctz* 25 mg*
Inderide LA titrate individual components
Cap: **Inderide LA 80/50** *prop* 80 mg/*hctz* 50 mg sust-rel
Inderide LA 120/50 *prop* 120 mg/*hctz* 50 mg sust-rel
Inderide LA 160/50 *prop* 160 mg/*hctz* 50 mg sust-rel

▷ *timolol/hydrochlorothiazide* (C)
Pediatric: not recommended
Timolide usual maintenance 2 tabs/day in a single or 2 divided doses
Tab: *timo* 10 mg/*hctz* 25 mg

ALPHA-1 ANTAGONIST/DIURETIC COMBINATIONS

▷ *prazosin/polythiazide* (C)
Pediatric: not recommended
Minizide titrate individual components
Cap: **Minizide 1** *praz* 1 mg/*poly* 0.5 mg
Minizide 2 *praz* 2 mg/*poly* 0.5 mg
Minizide 5 *praz* 5 mg/*poly* 0.5 mg

PERIPHERAL ADRENERGIC BLOCKER/HCTZ COMBINATIONS

▷ *guanethidine/hydrochlorothiazide* (C)
Pediatric: not recommended
Esmil titrate individual components
Tab: **Esmil 10/25** *guan* 1 mg/*hctz* 25 mg

ACEI/CCB COMBINATIONS

▷ *amlodipine/benazepril* (D)
Pediatric: not recommended
Lotrel titrate individual components
Cap: **Lotrel 2.5/10** *amlo* 2.5 mg/*benaz* 10 mg
Lotrel 5/10 *amlo* 5 mg/*benaz* 10 mg
Lotrel 5/20 *amlo* 5 mg/*benaz* 20 mg
Lotrel 10/20 *amlo* 10 mg/*benaz* 20 mg
Lotrel 5/40 *amlo* 5 mg/*benaz* 40 mg
Lotrel 10/40 *amlo* 10 mg/*benaz* 40 mg

▷ *amlodipine/perindopril* (D)
Pediatric: not recommended
Prolastin titrate individual components
Cap: **Prolastin 2.5/3.5** *amlo* 2.5 mg/*peri* 3.5 mg
Prolastin 5/7 *amlo* 5 mg/*peri* 7 mg
Prolastin 5/14 *amlo* 5 mg/*peri* 14 mg

▷ *enalapril/diltiazem* (D)
    Pediatric: not recommended
        Teczem titrate individual components
        Tab: enal 5 mg/*dil* 180 mg ext-rel
▷ *enalapril/felodipine* (D)
    Pediatric: <18 years: not recommended
        Lexxel initially 1 tab daily; after 1-2 weeks may increase to 2 tabs/day; titrate
        individual components
            Tab: **Lexxel 5/2.5** *enal* 5 mg/*felo* 2.5 mg ext-rel
            Lexxel 5/5 *enal* 5 mg/*felo* 5 mg ext-rel
▷ *perindopril/amlodipine* (D)
    Pediatric: not established
        Prestalia titrate individual components; max 14/10 once daily
        Tab: **Prestalia 3.5/2.5** *peri* 3.5 mg/*amlo* 2.5 mg
            Prestalia 7/5 *peri* 7 mg/*amlo* 5 mg
            Prestalia 14/10 *peri* 14 mg/*amlo* 10 mg
▷ *trandolapril/verapamil* (D)
    Pediatric: not established
        Tarka titrate individual components
        Tab: **Tarka 1/240** *tran* 1 mg/*ver* 240 mg ext-rel
            Tarka 2/180 *tran* 2 mg/*ver* 180 mg ext-rel
            Tarka 2/240 *tran* 2 mg/*ver* 240 mg ext-rel
            Tarka 4/240 *tran* 4 mg/*ver* 240 mg ext-rel

DRI/HCTZ COMBINATIONS

▷ *aliskiren/hydrochlorothiazide* (D) initially *aliskiren* 150 mg once daily; max *aliskiren*
300 mg/day
    Pediatric: <18 years: not recommended
        Tekturna HCT
        Tab: **Tekturna HCT 150/12.5** *alisk* 150 mg/*hctz* 12.5 mg
            Tekturna HCT 150/25 *alisk* 150 mg/*hctz* 25 mg
            Tekturna HCT 300/12.5 *alisk* 300 mg/*hctz* 12.5 mg
            Tekturna HCT 300/25 *alisk* 300 mg/*hctz* 25 mg

DRI/ARB COMBINATIONS

▷ *aliskiren/valsartan* (D)
    Pediatric: not recommended
        Valturna initially 150/160 once daily; may increase to max 300/320 once daily
        Tab: **Valturna 150/160** *alisk* 150 mg/*vals* 160 mg
            Valturna 300/320 *alisk* 300 mg/*vals* 320 mg

DRI/CCB COMBINATIONS

▷ *aliskiren/amlodipine* (D)
    Pediatric: not recommended
        Tekamlo initially 150/5 once daily; may increase to max 300/10 once daily
        Tab: **Tekamlo 150/5** *alisk* 150 mg/*amlo* 5 mg
            Tekamlo 150/10 *alisk* 150 mg/*amlo* 10 mg
            Tekamlo 300/5 *alisk* 300 mg/*amlo* 5 mg
            Tekamlo 300/10 *alisk* 300 mg/*amlo* 10 mg

DRI/CCB/HCTZ COMBINATIONS

▷ *aliskiren/amlodipine/hydrochlorothiazide* (D)
  Pediatric: not established
    Amturnide initially 150/5/12.5 once daily; may increase to max 300/10/25 once daily
      Tab: **Amturnide 150/5/12.5** *alisk* 150 mg/*amlo* 5 mg/*hctz* 12.5 mg
        Amturnide 300/5/12.5 *alisk* 300 mg/*amlo* 5 mg/*hctz* 12.5 mg
        Amturnide 300/5/25 *alisk* 300 mg/*amlo* 5 mg/*hctz* 25 mg
        Amturnide 300/10/25 *alisk* 300 mg/*amlo* 10 mg/*hctz* 25 mg

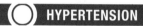

HYPERTENSION

ARB/CCB COMBINATIONS

▷ *amlodipine/valsartan medoxomil* (D)(G)
  Pediatric: not recommended
    Exforge 1 tab daily; titrate individual components at 1-week intervals; max 10/320 daily
      Tab: **Exforge 5/160** *amlo* 5 mg/*vals* 160 mg
        Exforge 5/320 *amlo* 5 mg/*vals* 320 mg
        Exforge 10/160 *amlo* 10 mg/*vals* 160 mg
        Exforge 10/320 *amlo* 10 mg/*vals* 320 mg
▷ *amlodipine/olmesartan* (D)
  Pediatric: not established
    Azor titrate individual components
      Tab: **Azor 5/20** *amlo* 5 mg/*olme* 20 mg
        Azor 10/20 *amlo* 10 mg/*olme* 20 mg
        Azor 5/40 *amlo* 5 mg/*olme* 40 mg
        Azor 10/40 *amlo* 10 mg/*olme* 40 mg
▷ *telmisartan/amlodipine* (D)
  Pediatric: not established
    Twynsta initially 40/5 once daily; titrate at 1 week intervals; max 80/10 once daily
      Tab: **Twynsta 40/5** *telmi* 40 mg/*amlo* 5 mg
        Twynsta 40/10 *telmi* 40 mg/*amlo* 10 mg
        Twynsta 80/5 *telmi* 80 mg/*amlo* 5 mg
        Twynsta 80/10 *telmi* 80 mg/*amlo* 10 mg

ARB/CCB/HCTZ COMBINATIONS

▷ *amlodipine/valsartan medoxomil/hydrochlorothiazide* (D)
  Pediatric: not recommended
    Exforge HCT: initially 5/160/12.5 once daily; may titrate at 1-week intervals to max 10/320/25 once daily
      Tab: **Exforge HCT 5/160/12.5** *amlo* 5 mg/*vals* 160 mg/*hctz* 12.5 mg
        Exforge HCT 5/160/25 *amlo* 5 mg/*vals* 160 mg/*hctz* 25 mg
        Exforge HCT 10/160/12.5 *amlo* 10 mg/*vals* 160 mg/*hctz* 12.5 mg
        Exforge HCT 10/160/25 *amlo* 10 mg/*vals* 160 mg/*hctz* 25 mg
        Exforge HCT 10/320/25 *amlo* 10 mg/*vals* 320 mg/*hctz* 25 mg

▷ *olmesartan medoxomil/amlodipine/hydrochlorothiazide* (D)
  Pediatric: not recommended
      Tribenzor: initially 40/5/12.5 once daily; may titrate at 1-week intervals to max
      40/10/25 daily
         Tab: **Tribenzor 40/5/12.5** *olme* 40 mg/*amlo* 5 mg/*hctz* 12.5 mg
               Tribenzor 40/5/25 *olme* 40 mg/*amlo* 5 mg/*hctz* 25 mg
               Tribenzor 40/10/12.5 *olme* 40 mg/*amlo* 10 mg/*hctz* 12.5 mg
               Tribenzor 40/10/25 *olme* 40 mg/*amlo* 10 mg/*hctz* 25 mg

OTHER COMBINATION AGENTS

▷ *clonidine/chlorthalidone* (C)
  Pediatric: not recommended
      Clorpres initially 0.1/15 once daily; may titrate to max 0.3/15 bid
         Tab: **Clorpres 0.1/15** *clon* 0.1 mg/*chlor* 15 mg
              Clorpres 0.2/15 *clon* 0.2 mg/*chlor* 15 mg
              Clorpres 0.3/15 *clon* 0.3 mg/*chlor* 15 mg
▷ *reserpine/hydroflumethiazide* (C)
  Pediatric: not recommended
      Salutensin initially 1.25/25 once daily; may titrate to 1.25/25 bid <u>or</u> 1.25/50
      once daily
         Tab: **Salutensin 1.25/25** *enal* 1.25 mg/*hydro* 25 mg
               Salutensin 1.25/50: *enal* 1.25 mg/*hydro* 50 mg

ANTIHYPERTENSION/ANTILIPID COMBINATIONS

CCB/Statin Combinations

▷ *amlodipine/atorvastatin* (X)
  Pediatric: <10 years: not established; ≥10 years (female postmenarche): same as adult
      Caduet select according to blood pressure and lipid values; titrate *amlodipine* over
      7-14 days; titrate ***atorvastatin*** according to monitored lipid values; max ***amlodip-***
      ine 10 mg/day and max ***atorvastatin*** 80 mg/day; refer to contraindications and
      precautions for CCB and statin therapy
         Tab: **Caduet 2.5/10** *amlo* 2.5 mg/*ator* 10 mg
               Caduet 2.5/20 *amlo* 2.5 mg/*ator* 20 mg
               Caduet 5/10 *amlo* 5 mg/*ator* 10 mg
               Caduet 5/20 *amlo* 5 mg/*ator* 20 mg
               Caduet 5/40 *amlo* 5 mg/*ator* 40 mg
               Caduet 5/80 *amlo* 5 mg/*ator* 80 mg
               Caduet 10/10 *amlo* 10 mg/*ator* 10 mg
               Caduet 10/20 *amlo* 10 mg/*ator* 20 mg
               Caduet 10/40 *amlo* 10 mg/*ator* 40 mg
               Caduet 10/80 *amlo* 10 mg/*ator* 80 mg

⊙ HYPERTHYROIDISM

▷ *methimazole* (D) initially 15-60 mg/day in 3 divided doses; maintenance 5-15 mg/day
  Pediatric: initially 0.4 mg/kg/day in 3 divided doses; maintenance 0.2 mg/kg/day <u>or</u>
  1/2 initial dose

Tapazole *Tab:* 5*, 10*mg
Comment: *methimazole* potentiates anticoagulants. Contraindicated in nursing mothers.
▷ *propylthiouracil (ptu)* (D)(G)
  Propyl-Thyracil initially 100-900 mg/day in 3 divided doses; maintenance usually 50-600 mg/day in 2 divided doses
    Pediatric: <6 years: not recommended; ≥6-10 years: initially 50-150 mg/day or 5-7 mg/kg/day in 3 divided doses; >10 years: initially 150-300 mg/day or 5-7 mg/kg/day in 3 divided doses; *maintenance:* 0.2 mg/kg/day or 1/2-2/3 of initial dose
    Tab: 50* mg

Comment: Preferred agent in pregnancy. Side effects include dermatitis, nausea, agranulocytosis, and hypothyroidism. Should be taken regularly for 2 years. Do not discontinue abruptly.

BETA-ADRENERGIC BLOCKER

▷ *propranolol* (C)(G) 40-240 mg daily
  Pediatric: not recommended
    Inderal *Tab:* 10*, 20*, 40*, 60*, 80*mg
    Inderal LA initially 80 mg daily in a single dose; increase q 3-7 days; usual range 120-160 mg/day; max 320 mg/day in a single dose
      Cap: 60, 80, 120, 160 mg sust-rel
    InnoPran XL initially 80 mg q HS; max 120 mg/day
      Cap: 80, 120 mg ext-rel

◯ HYPERTRIGLYCERIDEMIA

OMEGA 3-FATTY ACID ETHYL ESTERS

Comment: *Vascepa, Lovaza,* and **Epanova** are indicated for the treatment of TG ≥500 mg/dL.
▷ *icosapent ethyl (omega 3-fatty acid ethyl ester of EPA)* (C) 2 caps bid with food; max 4 g/day; swallow whole, do not crush or chew
  Pediatric: <18 years: not recommended
    Vascepa *sgc:* 1 g (α-tocopherol 4 mg/cap)
▷ *omega 3-fatty acid ethyl esters* (C) 2 g bid or 4 g daily; swallow whole, do not crush or chew
  Pediatric: <18 years: not recommended
▷ **Lovaza** *Gelcap:* 1 g (α-tocopherol 4 mg/cap) *omega 3-carcartonyl acids* (C) take 2-4 gel aps (2-4 g) daily without regard to meals
    Epanova *Gelcap:* 1 g

ISOBUTYRIC ACID DERIVATIVE

▷ *gemfibrozil* (C)(G)
  Pediatric: not recommended
    Lopid 600 mg bid 30 minutes before AM and PM meals
      Tab: 600*mg

FIBRATES (FIBRIC ACID DERIVATIVES)

▷ *fenofibrate* (C) take with meals; adjust at 4-8-week intervals; discontinue if inadequate response after 2 months; lowest dose or contraindicated with renal impairment and the elderly
Pediatric: not recommended
   Antara 43-130 mg once daily; max 130 mg/day
      Cap: 43, 87, 130 mg
   FibriCor 30-105 mg once daily; max 105 mg/day
      Tab: 30, 105 mg
   TriCor (G) 48-145 mg once daily; max 145 mg/day
      Tab: 48, 145 mg
   TriLipix (G) 45-135 mg once daily; max 135 mg/day
      Cap: 45, 135 mg del-rel
   Lipofen (G) 50-150 mg once daily; max 150 mg/day
      Cap: 50, 150 mg
   Lofibra 67-200 mg daily; max 200 mg/day
      Tab: 67, 134, 200 mg

NICOTINIC ACID DERIVATIVES

Comment: Contraindicated in liver disease. Decrease total cholesterol, LDL-C, and TG; increase HDL-C. Before initiating and at 4-6 weeks, 3 months, and 6 months of therapy, check fasting lipid profile or as indicated by manufacturer, LFT, glucose, and uric acid. Significant side effect of transient skin flushing. Take with food and take *aspirin* 325 mg 30 minutes before dose to decrease flushing.
▷ *niacin* (C)
   Niaspan 375 mg daily for 1st week, then 500 mg daily for 2nd week, then 750 mg daily for 3rd week, then 1 g daily for weeks 4-7; may increase by 500 mg q 4 weeks; usual range 1-3 g/day
      Tab: 500, 750, 1,000 mg ext-rel
   Slo-Niacin 250 mg or 500 mg or 750 mg q AM or HS
      Tab: 250, 500, 750 mg cont-rel

HMG-COA REDUCTASE INHIBITORS

▷ *atorvastatin* (X)(G) initially 10 mg daily; usual range 10-80 mg daily
Pediatric: <10 years: not recommended; ≥10 years (female postmenarche): same as adult
   Lipitor *Tab:* 10, 20, 40, 80 mg
▷ *fluvastatin* (X)(G) initially 20-40 mg q HS; usual range 20-80 mg/day
Pediatric: <18 years: not recommended
   Lescol *Cap:* 20, 40 mg
   Lescol XL *Tab:* 80 mg ext-rel
▷ *lovastatin* (X) initially 20 mg daily at evening meal; may increase at 4 week intervals; max 80 mg/day in a single or divided doses; *Concomitant fibrates,* **niacin,** *or CrCl <40 mL/min:* usual max 20 mg/day
Pediatric: <10 years: not recommended; 10-17 years: initially 10-20 mg daily at evening meal; may increase at 4 week intervals; max 40 mg daily; *Concomitant fibrates, niacin,* or *CrCl <40 mL/min:* usual max 20 mg/day
   Mevacor *Tab:* 10, 20, 40 mg

▷ **pravastatin (X)(G)** initially 10-20 mg q HS; usual range 10-80 mg/day; may start at
40 mg/day
Pediatric: <8 years: not recommended; 8-13 years: 20 mg q HS; 14-17 years: 40 mg q HS
Pravachol *Tab:* 10, 20, 40, 80 mg
▷ **rosuvastatin (X)** initially 20 mg q HS; usual range 5-40 mg/day; adjust at 4 week intervals
Pediatric: <10 years: not recommended; 10-17 years: 5-20 mg q HS; max 20 mg q HS
Crestor *Tab:* 5, 10, 20, 40 mg
▷ **simvastatin (X)(G)** initially 20 mg q HS; usual range 5-80 mg/day; adjust at 4 week intervals
Pediatric: <10 years: not recommended; 10-17 years: initially 10 mg q HS; may
increase at 4 week intervals; max 40 mg q HS
Zocor *Tab:* 5, 10, 20, 40, 80 mg

NICOTINIC ACID DERIVATIVE/HMG-COA REDUCTASE INHIBITOR

▷ **niacin/lovastatin (X)**
Advicor
Pediatric: <18 years: not recommended
Tab: **Advicor 500 mg/20 mg** *niac* 500 mg ext-rel/*lova* 20 mg
Advicor 750 mg/20 mg *niac* 750 mg ext-rel/*lova* 20 mg
Advicor 1,000 mg/20 mg *niac* 1,000 mg ext-rel/*lova* 20 mg

 HYPOCALCEMIA

Comment: Hypocalcemia resulting in metabolic bone disease may be secondary
to hyperparathyroidism, pseudoparathyroidism, and chronic renal disease.
Normal serum Ca^{++} range is approximately 8.5-12 mg/dL. Signs and symptoms of
hypocalcemia include confusion, increased neuromuscular excitability, muscle spasms,
paresthesias, hyperphosphatemia, positive Chvostek's sign, and positive Trousseau's
sign. Signs and symptoms of hypercalcemia include fatigue, lethargy, decreased
concentration and attention span, frank psychosis, anorexia, nausea, vomiting,
constipation, bradycardia, heart block, shortened QT interval. Foods high in calcium
include almonds, broccoli, baked beans, salmon, sardines, buttermilk, turnip greens,
collard greens, spinach, pumpkin, rhubarb, and bran. Recommended daily calcium
intake: 1-3 years: 700 mg; 4-8 years: 1,000 mg; 9-18 years: 1,300 mg; 19-50 years:
1,000 mg: 51-70 years (males): 1,000 mg; ≥51 years (females): 1,200 mg; pregnancy or
nursing: 1,000-1,300 mg. Recommended daily vitamin D intake: >1 year: 600 IU; 50+
years: 800-1,000 IU. The American Academy of Rheumatology (AAR) recommends
the following daily doses for anyone on a chronic oral corticosteroid regimen: Calcium
1,200-1,500 mg/day and vitamin D 800-1,000 IU/day.

CALCIUM SUPPLEMENTS

Comment: Take *calcium* supplements after meals to avoid gastric upset. Dosages
of *calcium* over 2,000 mg/day have not been shown to have any additional benefit.
Calcium decreases *tetracycline* absorption. *Calcium* absorption is decreased by
corticosteroids.
▷ **calcitonin-salmon (C)**
Miacalcin 200 units (1 spray intranasally) once daily; alternate nostrils each day
Nasal spray: 14 dose (2 ml)
Miacalcin injection 100 units/day SC or IM
Vial: 2 ml

▷ *calcium carbonate* (C)(OTC)(G)
    Rolaids chew 2 tabs bid; max 14 tabs/day
      Tab: calcium carbonate: 550 mg
    Rolaids Extra Strength chew 2 tabs bid; max 8 tabs/day
      Tab: 1,000 mg
    Tums chew 2 tabs bid; max 16 tabs/day
      Tab: 500 mg
    Tums Extra Strength chew 2 tabs bid; max 10 tabs/day
      Tab: 750 mg
    Tums Ultra chew 2 tabs bid; max 8 tabs/day
      Tab: 1,000 mg
    Os-Cal 500 (OTC) 1-2 tab bid-tid
      Tab: elemental calcium carbonate 500 mg
▷ *calcium carbonate/vitamin D* (C)(G)
    Os-Cal 250+D (OTC) 1-2 tabs tid
      Tab: elemental calcium carbonate 250 mg/*vit d* 125 IU
    Os-Cal 500+D (OTC) 1-2 tabs bid-tid
      Tab: elemental calcium carbonate 500 mg/*vit d* 125 IU
    Viactiv (OTC) 1 tab tid
      Chew tab: elemental calcium 500 mg/*vit d and vit a*100 IU/*Vit k* 40 mEq
▷ *calcium citrate*
    Citracal (OTC) 1-2 tabs bid
      Tab: elemental calcium citrate 200 mg
▷ *calcium citrate/vitamin D* (C)(G)
    Citracal+D (OTC) 1-2 cplts bid
      Cplt: elemental calcium citrate 315 mg/*vit d* 200 IU
    Citracal 250+D (OTC) 1-2 tabs bid
      Tab: elemental calcium citrate 250 mg/*vit d* 62.3 IU

VITAMIN D ANALOGS

Comment: Concurrent vitamin D supplementation is contraindicated for patients taking *calcitrol* **or** *doxecalciferol* due to the risk of vitamin D toxicity.
▷ *calcitriol* (C) *Predialysis:* initially 0.25 mcg daily; may increase to 0.5 mcg daily; *Dialysis:* initially 0.25 mcg daily; may increase by 0.25 mcg/day at 4-8-week intervals; usual maintenance 0.5-1 mcg/day; *Hypoparathyroidism:* initially 0.25 mcg q AM; may increase by 0.25 mcg/day at 4-8 week intervals; usual maintenance 0.5-2 mcg/day
Pediatric: Predialysis: <4 years: 10-15 ng/kg/day; >3 years: initially 0.25 mcg daily; may increase to 0.5 mcg/day; *Dialysis:* not recommended; *Hypoparathyroidism:* initially 0.25 mcg daily; may increase by 0.25 mcg/day at 2-4-week intervals; usual maintenance (1-5 years) 0.25-0.75 mcg/day, (>6 years) 0.5-2 mcg/day
    Rocaltrol *Cap:* 0.25, 0.5 mcg
    Rocaltrol Solution *Soln:* 1 mcg/ml (15 ml, single-use dispensers)
▷ *doxecalciferol* (C) initially 0.25 mcg q AM; may increase by 0.25 mcg/day at 4-8-week intervals; usual maintenance 0.5-2 mcg/day
Pediatric: initially 0.25 mcg daily; may increase by 0.25 mcg/day at 2-4 week intervals; usual maintenance (1-5 years) 0.25-0.75 mcg/day, (>6 years) 0.5-2 mcg/day
    Hectorol *Cap:* 0.25, 0.5 mcg

HUMAN PARATHYROID HORMONE

▶ *bioengineered replica of human parathyroid hormone* (C) initially inject mg IM into the thigh once daily; when initiating, decrease dose of active vitamin D by 50%, if serum calcium is above 7.5 mg/dL; monitor serum calcium levels every 3 to 7 days after starting or adjusting dose and when adjusting either active vitamin D or calcium supplements dose.

Natpara *Soln for inj:* 25, 50, 75, 100 mcg (2/pkg) multiple dose, dual-chamber glass cartridge containing a sterile powder and diluent

Comment: **Natpara** is indicated as an adjunct to calcium and vitamin D in patients with hypoparathyroidism.

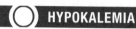

HYPOKALEMIA

Comment: Normal serum K⁺ range is approximately 3.5-5.5 mEq/L. Signs and symptoms of hypokalemia include neuromuscular weakness, muscle twitching and cramping, hyporeflexia, postural hypotension, anorexia, nausea and vomiting, depressed ST segments, flattened T waves, and cardiac tachyarrhythmias. Signs and symptoms of hyperkalemia include peaked T waves, elevated ST segment, and widened QRS complexes.

PROPHYLAXIS

Comment: Usual dose range is 8-10 mEq/day.

TREATMENT OF HYPOKALEMIA: NONEMERGENCY (K⁺ <2.5 mEq/l)

Comment: Usual dose range 40-120 mEq/day in divided doses. Solutions are preferred; potentially serious GI side effects may occur with tablet formulations or when taken on an empty stomach.

POTASSIUM SUPPLEMENTS

Comment: Potassium supplements should be taken with food. Solutions are the preferred form. Extended-release and sustained-release forms should be swallowed whole; do not crush or chew. Potassium supplementation is indicated for hypokalemia including that caused by diuretic use, and digitalis intoxication without atrioventricular (AV) block.

▶ *potassium* (C)(G)

Pediatric: not established

KCL Solution Oral soln: 10% (30 ml unit dose, 50/case)

K-Dur (as chloride) *Tab:* 10, 20* mEq sust-rel

K-Lor for Oral Solution (as chloride) *Pkts* for reconstitution: 20 mEq/pkt (fruit)

Klor-Con/25 (as chloride) *Pkts* for reconstitution: 25 mEq/pkt

Klor-Con/EF 25 (as bicarbonate) *Pkts* for reconstitution: 25 mEq/pkt (effervescent) (fruit)

Klor-Con Extended-Release (as chloride) *Tab:* 8, 10 mEq ext-rel

Klor-Con M (as chloride) *Tab:* 10, 15*, 20* mEq ext-rel

Klor-Con Powder (as chloride) 20, 25 mEq *Pkts* for reconstitution: (30/carton) (fruit)

Klorvess (as bicarbonate and citrate) *Tab:* 20 mEq effervescent for solution; *Granules:* 20 mEq/pkt effervescent for solution; *Oral liq:* 20 mEq/15 ml (16 oz)

Klotrix (as chloride) *Tab:* 10 mEq sust-rel

K-Lyte (as bicarbonate and citrate) *Tab:* 25 mEq effervescent for solution (lime, orange)
K-Lyte/CL (as chloride) *Tab:* 25 mEq effervescent for solution (citrus, fruit)
K-Lyte/CL 50 (as chloride) *Tab:* 50 mEq effervescent for solution (citrus, fruit)
K-Lyte/DS (as bicarbonate and citrate) *Tab:* 50 mEq effervescent for solution (lime, orange)
K-Tab (as chloride) *Tab:* 10 mEq sust-rel
Micro-K (as chloride) *Cap:* 8, 10 mEq sust-rel
Potassium Chloride Extended Release Caps *Cap:* 8, 10 mEq ext-rel
Potassium Chloride Sust-Rel Tabs *Tab/Cap:* 10 mEq sust-rel
Potassium Chloride ER *Tab:* 8mEq (600 mg), 10 mEq (750 mg)

 HYPOMAGNESEMIA

Comment: Normal serum Mg^{++} range is approximately 1.2-2.6 mEq/L. Signs and symptoms of hypomagnesemia include confusion, disorientation, hallucinations, hyperreflexia, tetany, convulsions, tachyarrhythmia, positive Chvostek's sign, and positive Trousseau's sign. Signs and symptoms of hypermagnesemia include drowsiness, lethargy, muscle weakness, hypoactive reflexes, slurred speech, bradycardia, hypotension, convulsions, and cardiac arrhythmias.

MAGNESIUM SUPPLEMENTS

▷ *magnesium* (B)
   Slow-Mag 2 tabs daily
      Tab: 64 mg (as chloride)/110 mg (as carbonate)
▷ *magnesium oxide* (B)
   Mag-Ox 400 1-2 tabs daily
      Tab: 400 mg

 HYPOPARATHYROIDISM

VITAMIN D ANALOGS

Comment: Concurrent vitamin D supplementation is contraindicated for patients taking *calcitrol* **or** *doxecalciferol* owing to the risk of vitamin D toxicity.
▷ *calcitrol* (C) initially 0.25 mcg q AM; may increase by 0.25 mcg/day at 4-8-week intervals; usual maintenance 0.5-2 mcg/day
Pediatric: initially 0.25 mcg daily; may increase by 0.25 mcg/day at 2-4-week intervals; usual maintenance (1-5 years) 0.25-0.75 mcg/day, (>6 years) 0.5-2 mcg/day
   Rocaltrol *Cap:* 0.25, 0.5 mcg
   Rocaltrol Solution *Soln:* 1 mcg/ml (15 ml, single-use dispensers)
▷ *doxecalciferol* (C) initially 0.25 mcg q AM; may increase by 0.25 mcg/day at 4-8-week intervals; usual maintenance 0.5-2 mcg/day
Pediatric: initially 0.25 mcg daily; may increase by 0.25 mcg/day at 2-4-week intervals; usual maintenance (1-5 years) 0.25-0.75 mcg/day, (>6 years) 0.5-2 mcg/day
   Hectorol *Cap:* 0.25, 0.5 mcg

HUMAN PARATHYROID HORMONE

▶ *teriparatide* (C) 20 mcg SC daily in the thigh <u>or</u> abdomen; may treat for up to 2 years
Pediatric: not recommended
    Forteo Multidose Pen *Multi-dose pen:* 250 mcg/ml (3 ml)
    Comment: **Forteo** is indicated for the treatment of postmenopausal osteoporosis in women who are at high risk for fracture and to increase bone mass in men with primary <u>or</u> hypogonadal osteoporosis who are at high risk for fracture.

BIOENGINEERED REPLICA OF HUMAN PARATHYROID HORMONE

▶ *bioengineered replica of human parathyroid hormone* (C) initially inject mg IM into the thigh once daily; when initiating, decrease dose of active vitamin D by 50% if serum calcium is above 7.5 mg/dL; monitor serum calcium levels every 3-7 days after starting <u>or</u> adjusting dose and when adjusting either active vitamin D <u>or</u> calcium supplements dose
    Natpara *Soln for inj:* 25, 50, 75, 100 mcg (2/pkg) multiple dose, dual-chamber glass cartridge containing a sterile powder and diluent
    Comment: **Natpara** is indicated as an adjunct to calcium and vitamin D in patients with parathyroidism.

HYPOPHOSPHATASIA (OSTEOMALACIA, RICKETS)

Comment: Hypophosphatasia (HPP) is an inborn error of metabolism marked by abnormally low serum alkaline phosphatase activity and phosphoethanolamine in the urine. It is manifested by osteomalacia in adults and rickets in infants and children. It is most severe in infants under 6 months-of-age. With congenital absence of alkaline phosphatase, an enzyme essential to the calcification of bone tissue, complications include vomiting, growth retardation, and often death in infancy. Surviving children have numerous skeletal abnormalities and dwarfism.

▶ *asfotase alfa* (NR)
Pediatric and Adult: 6 mg/kg/week SC, administered as 2 mg/kg <u>or</u> 1 mg/kg 6 x/week; max 9 mg/kg/week SC administered as 3 mg/kg 3 x/week
    Strensiq *Vial:* 18 mg/0.45 ml, 28 mg/0.7 ml, 40 mg/ml, 80 mg/0.8 ml for SC inj, single-use (1, 12/carton) (preservative-free)
    Comment: **Strensiq** is the first FDA-approved (2015) treatment for perinatal, infantile, and juvenile onset HPP. Prior to the availability of **Strensiq**, there was no effective treatment and patient prognosis was very poor.

HYPOTENSION: NEUROGENIC, ORTHOSTATIC

ALPHA-1 AGONIST

▶ *midodrine* (C)(G) 10 mg tid at 3-4-hour intervals; take while upright; take last dose at least 4 hours before bedtime
Pediatric: not recommended
    ProAmatine *Tab:* 2.5*, 5*, 10*mg

SYNTHETIC AMINO ACID PRECURSOR OF NOREPINEPHRINE

▷ **droxidopa** (C) initially 100 mg, taken 3 times/day (upon arising in the morning, at midday, and in the late afternoon at least 3 hours prior to bedtime (to reduce the potential for supine hypertension during sleep); administer with or without; swallow whole; titrate to symptomatic response, in increments of 100 mg tid every 24-48 hours; max 600 mg tid (max total 1,800 mg/day)
Pediatric: not recommended
  Northera *Cap:* 100, 200, 300 mg
  Comment: **Northera** is indicated for the treatment of orthostatic dizziness, lightheadedness, or feeling about to black out in adult patients with symptomatic neurogenic orthostatic hypotension (NOH) caused by primary autonomic failure [Parkinson's disease (PD), multiple system atrophy (MSA) and pure autonomic failure], dopamine beta-hydroxylase deficiency, and nondiabetic autonomic neuropathy. Effectiveness beyond 2 weeks of treatment has not been established. The continued effectiveness of **Northera** should be assessed. Administering **Northera** in combination with other agents that increase blood pressure (e.g., norepinephrine, ephedrine, midodrine, triptans) would be expected to increase the risk for supine hypertension.

 HYPOTHYROIDISM

Comment: Take thyroid replacement hormone in the morning on an empty stomach. For the elderly, start thyroid hormone replacement at 25 mcg/day. Target TSH is 0.4-5.5 mIU/L; target T4 is 4.5-12.5 ng/L. Signs and symptoms of thyroid toxicity include tachycardia, palpitations, nervousness, chest pain, heat intolerance, and weight loss.

ORAL THYROID HORMONE SUPPLEMENTS

T3

▷ **liothyronine** (A) initially 25 mcg daily; may increase by 25 mcg every 1-2 weeks as needed; usual maintenance 25-75 mcg/day
Pediatric: initially 5 mcg/day; may increase by 5 mcg/day every 3-4 days; *Cretinism:* maintenance dose: <1 year: 20 mcg/day; 1-3 years: 50 mcg/day; >3 years: same as adult
  Cytomel *Tab:* 5, 25, 50 mcg

T4

▷ **levothyroxine** (A)
  Levoxyl initially 25-100 mcg/day; increase by 25 mcg/day q 2-3 weeks as needed; maintenance 100-200 mcg/day
    Pediatric: <6 months: 8-10 mcg/kg/day; 6-12 months: 6-8 mcg/kg/day; >1-5 years: 5-6 mcg/kg/day; 6-12 years: 4-5 mcg/kg/day; >12 years: same as adult
    Tab: 25*, 50* (dye-free), 75*, 88*, 100*, 112*, 125*, 137*, 150*, 175*, 200*, 300*mcg
  Synthroid initially 50 mcg/day; increase by 25 mcg/day q 2-3 weeks as needed; max 300 mcg/day
    Pediatric: <6 months: 8-10 mcg/kg/day; 6-12 months: 6-8 mcg/kg/day; >1-5 years: 5-6 mcg/kg/day; 6-12 years: 4-5 mcg/kg/day; >12 years: same as adult
    Tab: 25*, 50* (dye-free), 75*, 88*, 100*, 112*, 125*, 137*, 150*, 175*, 200*, 300*mcg
  Unithroid initially 50 mcg/day; increase by 25 mcg/day q 2-3 weeks as needed; max 300 mcg/day

Pediatric: 0-3 months: 10-15 mcg/kg/day; 3-6 months: 8-10 mcg/kg/day; 6-12 months: 6-8 mcg/kg/day; 1-5 years: 5-6 mcg/kg/day; 6-12 years: 4-5 mcg/kg/day; >12 years: 2-3 mcg/kg/day; Growth and puberty complete: same as adult
Tab: 25*, 50* (dye-free), 75*, 88*, 100*, 112*, 125*, 150*, 175*, 200*, 300*mcg

T3/T4 Combination

▷ liothyronine/levothyroxine (A) initially 15-30 mg/day; increase by 15 mg/day q 2-3 weeks to target goal; usual maintenance 60-120 mg/day
Pediatric: <6 months: 4.6-6 mcg/kg/day; 6-12 months: 3.6-4.8 mcg/kg/day; >1-5 years: 3-3.6 mcg/kg/day; 6-12 years: 2.4-3 mcg/kg/day; >12 years: 1.2-1.8 mcg/kg/day; Growth and puberty complete: same as adult
  Armour Thyroid Tab Tab: per grain: T3 9 mcg/T4 38 mcg: 1/4, 1/2, 1, 1, 2, 3*, 4*, 5* gr; 15, 30, 60, 90, 120, 180*, 240*, 300*mg
  Thyrolar Tab: per grain: T3 12.5 mcg/ T4 50 mcg: 1/4, 1/5, 1, 2, 3 gr

PARENTERAL THYROID HORMONE SUPPLEMENT

▷ levothyroxine sodium (A) 1/2 oral dose by IV or IM and titrate; Myxedema Coma: 200-500 mcg IV x 1 dose; may administer 100-300 mcg (or more) IV on second day if needed; then 50-100 mcg IV daily; switch to oral form as soon as possible
Pediatric: not recommended
  T4 Inj: 200, 500 mcg (pwdr for IM or IV administration after reconstitution)

◯ IDIOPATHIC PULMONARY FIBROSIS (IPF)

▷ nintedanib (D) take with food at the same time each day; take 150 mg bid, 12 hours apart; max 300 mg/day
Pediatric: not established
  Ofev Cap: 100, 150 mg
Comment: Monitor liver enzymes. If elevated LFTs (3 < AST/ALT <5 XULN) without severe liver damage, interrupt therapy or reduce dose to 100 mg bid. When liver enzymes return to baseline, restart at 100 mg bid and titrate up.
▷ pirfenidone (C) take with food at the same time each day; Days 1-7: 1 cap tid; Days 8-14: 2 caps tid; Days 15 and ongoing: 3 caps tid; max 9 caps/day
Pediatric: not established
  Esbriet Gelcap: 267 mg

◯ IMPETIGO CONTAGIOSA (INDIAN FIRE)

Comment: The most common infectious organisms are Staphylococcus aureus and Streptococcus pyogenes.

TOPICAL ANTI-INFECTIVES

▷ mupirocin (B)(G) apply to lesions bid; apply to walls of nares bid
Pediatric: same as adult
  Bactroban Oint: 2% (22 g); Crm: 2% (15, 30 g)
  Centany Oint: 2% (15, 30 g)

ORAL ANTI-INFECTIVES

▷ *amoxicillin* (B)(G) 500-875 mg bid <u>or</u> 250-500 mg tid x 10 days
  Pediatric: <40 kg (88 lb): 20-40 mg/kg/day in 3 divided doses x 10 days <u>or</u> 25-45 mg/kg/day in 2 divided doses x 10 days; >40 kg: same as adult; *see page 543 for dose by weight*
    Amoxil *Cap:* 250, 500 mg; *Tab:* 875*mg; *Chew tab:* 125, 200, 250, 400 mg (cherry-banana-peppermint) (phenylalanine); *Oral susp:* 125, 250 mg/5 ml (80, 100, 150 ml) (strawberry); 200, 400 mg/5 ml (50, 75, 100 ml) (bubble gum); Oral drops: 50 mg/ml (30 ml) (bubble gum)
    Moxatag *Tab:* 775 mg ext-rel
    Trimox *Tab:* 125, 250 mg; *Cap:* 250, 500 mg; *Oral susp:* 125, 250 mg/5 ml (80, 100, 150 ml) (raspberry-strawberry)
▷ *amoxicillin/clavulanate* (B)(G) 500 mg tid <u>or</u> 875 mg bid x 10 days
    Augmentin *Tab:* 250, 500, 875 mg; *Chew tab:* 125, 250 mg (lemon-lime); 200, 400 mg (cherry-banana) (phenylalanine); *Oral susp:* 125 mg/5 ml (banana), 250 mg/5 ml (75, 100, 150 ml) (orange); 200, 400 mg/5 ml (50, 75, 100 ml) (orange) (phenylalanine)
      Pediatric: 40-45 mg/kg/day divided tid x 10 days <u>or</u> 90 mg/kg/day divided bid x 10 days *see page 545 for dose by weight*
    Augmentin ES-600 *Oral susp:* 600 mg/5 ml (50, 75, 100, 125, 150, 200 ml) (strawberry cream) (phenylalanine) every 12 hours
      Pediatric: <3 months: not recommended; ≥3 months, <40 kg: 90 mg/kg/day in 2 divided doses; ≥40 kg: not recommended
    Augmentin XR 2 tabs q 12 hours x 7-10 days
      Pediatric: <16 years: use other forms; ≥16 years: same as adult
      Tab: 1000*mg ext-rel
▷ *azithromycin* (B) 500 mg <u>x</u> 1 dose on day 1, then 250 mg daily on days 2-5 <u>or</u> 500 mg daily <u>x</u> 3 days <u>or</u> 2 g in a single dose
    Zithromax *Tab:* 250, 500, 600 mg; *Oral susp:* 100 mg/5 ml (15 ml); 200 mg/5 ml (15, 22.5, 30 ml) (cherry); *Pkt:* 1 g for reconstitution (cherry-banana)
    Zithromax Tri-pak *Tab:* 3 x 500 mg tabs/pck
    Zithromax Z-pak *Tab:* 6 x 250 mg tabs/pck
    Zmax *Oral susp:* 2 g ext-rel for reconstitution (cherry-banana) (148 mg Na⁺)
▷ *cefaclor* (B)(G) 250-500 mg q 8 hours <u>x</u> 10 days; max 2 g/day
  Pediatric: <1 month: not recommended; 20-40 mg/kg bid <u>or</u> q 12 hours x 10 days; max 1 g/day; *see page 549 for dose by weight*
  Tab: 500 mg; *Cap:* 250, 500 mg; *Susp:* 125 mg/5 ml (75, 150 ml) (strawberry); 187 mg/5 ml (50, 100 ml) (strawberry); 250 mg/5 ml (75, 150 ml) (strawberry); 375 mg/5 ml (50, 100 ml) (strawberry)
  Pediatric: <16 years: ext-rel not recommended; ≥16 years: same as adult
    Cefaclor Extended Release *Tab:* 375, 500 mg ext-rel
▷ *cefadroxil* (B) 1-2 g in 1-2 divided doses x 10 days
  Pediatric: 30 mg/kg/day in 2 divided doses x 10 days; *see page 550 for dose by weight*
    Duricef *Cap:* 500 mg; *Tab:* 1 g; *Oral susp:* 250 mg/5 ml (100 ml); 500 mg/5 ml (75, 100 ml) (orange-pineapple)
▷ *cefpodoxime proxetil* (B) 200 mg bid x 10 days
  Pediatric: <2 months: not recommended; 2 months-12 years: 10 mg/kg/day (max 400 mg/dose) <u>or</u> 5 mg/kg/day bid (max 200 mg/dose) x 10 days; *see page 553 for dose by weight*

Vantin *Tab*: 100, 200 mg; *Oral susp*: 50, 100 mg/5 ml (50, 75, 100 mg) (lemon creme)

▷ *cefprozil* (B) 500 mg bid x 10 days
Pediatric: ≤6 months: not recommended; 6 months-12 years: *see page 554 for dose by weight*
Cefzil *Tab*: 250, 500 mg; *Oral susp*: 125, 250 mg/5 ml (50, 75, 100 ml) (bubble gum) (phenylalanine)

▷ *ceftaroline fosamil* (B) administer by IV infusion after reconstitution every 12 hours x 5-14 days; *CrCl >50 mL/min:* 600 mg; *CrCl >30-<50 mL/min:* 400 mg; *CrCl >1 5-<30 mL/min:* 300 mg; ESRD: 200 mg
Teflaro *Vial:* 400, 600 mg

▷ *cefuroxime axetil* (B) (G) 250-500 mg bid x 10 days
Pediatric: 15 mg/kg bid x 10 days; *see page 556 for dose by weight*
Ceftin *Tab:* 250, 500 mg; *Oral susp:* 12, 250 mg/5 ml (50, 100 ml) (tutti-frutti)

▷ *cephalexin* (B) (G) 250-500 mg qid or 500 mg bid x 10 days
Pediatric: 25-50 mg/kg/day in 4 divided doses x 10 days; *see page 557 for dose by weight*
Keflex *Cap:* 250, 333, 500, 750 mg; *Oral susp:* 125, 250 mg/5 ml (100, 200 ml) (strawberry)

▷ *clarithromycin* (C)(G) 500 mg or 500 mg ext-rel daily x 7 days
Pediatric: <6 months: not recommended; ≥6 months: 7.5 mg/kg bid x 7 days; *see page 558 for dose by weight*
Biaxin *Tab:* 250, 500 mg
Biaxin Oral Suspension *Oral susp:* 125, 250 mg/5 ml (50, 100 ml) (fruit punch)
Biaxin XL *Tab:* 500 mg ext-rel

▷ *dicloxacillin* (B) (G) 500 mg q 6 hours x 10 days
Pediatric: 12.5-25 mg/kg/day in 4 divided doses x 10 days; *see page 560 for dose by weight*
Dynapen *Cap:* 125, 250, 500 mg; *Oral susp:* 62.5 mg/5 ml (80, 100, 200 ml)

▷ *erythromycin base* (B)(G) 250 mg qid, or 333 mg tid, or 500 mg bid x 7-10 days
Pediatric: ≤45 kg: 30-50 mg in 2-4 divided doses x 7-10 days; ≥45 kg: same as adult
Ery-Tab *Tab:* 250, 333, 500 mg ent-coat
PCE *Tab:* 333, 500 mg
Comment: *erythromycin* may increase INR with concomitant ***warfarin***, as well as increase serum level of ***digoxin***, benzodiazepines and statins.

▷ *erythromycin ethylsuccinate* (B)(G) 400 mg tid x 7-10 days
Pediatric: 30-50 mg/kg/day in 4 divided doses x 7-10 days; may double dose with severe infection; max 100 mg/kg/day; see page 563 for dose by weight
EryPed *Oral susp:* 200 mg/5 ml (100, 200 ml) (fruit); 400 mg/5 ml (60, 100, 200 ml) (banana); *Oral drops:* 200, 400 mg/5 ml (50 ml) (fruit); *Chew tab:* 200 mg wafer (fruit)
E.E.S. *Oral susp:* 200, 400 mg/5 ml (100 ml) (fruit)
E.E.S. Granules *Oral susp:* 200 mg/5 ml (100, 200 ml) (cherry)
E.E.S. 400 Tablets *Tab:* 400 mg
Comment: *erythromycin* may increase INR with concomitant ***warfarin***, as well as increase serum level of ***digoxin***, benzodiazepines and statins.

▷ *loracarbef* (B) 200 mg bid x 10 days
Pediatric: 15 mg/kg/day in 2 divided doses x 10 days; *see page 570 for dose by weight*

Pediatric: 30 mg/kg/day in 2 divided doses x 7 days

> **Lorabid** *Pulvule:* 200, 400 mg; *Oral susp:* 100 mg/5 ml (50, 100 ml); 200 mg/5 ml (50, 75, 100 ml) (strawberry bubble gum)

▶ *penicillin G (benzathine)* **(B)** 1.2 million units IM x 1 dose

Pediatric: <60 lb: 300,000-600,000 units IM x 1 dose; ≥60 lb: 900,000 units x 1 dose

> **Bicillin L-A** *Cartridge-needle unit:* 600,000 units (1 ml); 1.2 million units (2 ml)

▶ *penicillin G (benzathine/procaine)* **(B) (G)** 2.4 million units IM x 1 dose

Pediatric: <30 lb: 600,000 units IM x 1 dose; 30-60 lb: 900,000-1.2 million units IM x 1 dose

> **Bicillin C-R** *Cartridge-needle unit:* 600,000 units (1 ml); 1.2 million units (2 ml); 2.4 million units (4 ml)

▶ *penicillin V potassium* **(B)** 250-500 mg q 6 hours x 10 days

Pediatric: 50 mg/kg/day in 4 divided doses x 3 days; ≥12 years: same as adult; *see page 572 for dose by weight*

> **Pen-Vee K** *Tab:* 250, 500 mg; *Oral soln:* 125 mg/5 ml (100, 200 ml); 250 mg/5 ml (100, 150, 200 ml)

INCONTINENCE: FECAL

Comment: Treatment of fecal incontinence in patients who have failed conservative therapy (e.g., diet, fiber therapy, antimotility agents).

▶ *dextranomer microspheres/sodium hyaluronate* **(NR)**

Pediatric: ≤18 years: not recommended

> Pretreatment: bowel preparation using enema (required) and prophylactic antibiotics (recommended) prior to injection
>
> Treatment: inject slowly into the deep submucosal layer in the proximal part of the high pressure zone of the anal canal about 5 mm above the dentate line; four 1-ml injections in the following order: posterior, left lateral, anterior, right lateral; keep needle in place 15-30 seconds to minimize leakage; use a new needle for each syringe and injection site
>
> Posttreatment: avoid hot baths and physical activity during first 24 hours; avoid antidiarrheal drugs, sexual intercourse, and strenuous activity for 1 week; avoid anal manipulation for 1 month
>
> Retreatment: may repeat if needed with max 4 ml, no sooner than 4 weeks after the first injection; point of injection should be made in between initial injection sites (i.e., shifted 1/8 of a turn)
>
> **Solesta** *dex micro* 50 mg/*sod hyal* 15 mg per ml
>
> > *Syringe:* 1 ml (4 w. needles)

INCONTINENCE: URINARY (STRESS INCONTINENCE/ OVERACTIVE BLADDER/STRESS INCONTINENCE)

See **Enuresis** *page* 138

▶ *estrogen* replacement **(X)** *see* **Menopause** *page* 257

▶ *pseudoephedrine* **(C)(G)** 30-60 mg tid

> **Sudafed** (OTC) *Tab:* 30 mg; *Liq:* 15 mg/5 ml (1, 4 oz)

VASOPRESSIN

▷ *desmopressin acetate (DDAVP)* (B)(G)
   DDAVP usual dosage 0.1-1.2 mg/day in 2-3 divided doses; 0.2 mg q HS prn for nocturnal enuresis
   Pediatric: <6 years: not recommended; ≥6 years: 0.5 mg daily or q HS prn
   Tab: 0.1*, 0.2*mg
   DDAVP Rhinal Tube
   Pediatric: <6 years: not recommended; ≥6 years: 10 mcg or 0.1 ml of soln each nostril (20 mcg total dose) q HS prn; max 40 mcg total dose
   Rhinal tube: 0.1 mg/ml (2.5 ml)

BETA-3 ADRENERGIC AGONIST

▷ *mirabegron* (C) initially 25 mg once daily; max 50 mg once daily; severe renal impairment, 25 mg once daily
   Myrbetriq *Tab:* 25, 50 mg ext-rel

MUSCARINIC RECEPTOR ANTAGONISTS

▷ *fesoterodine* (C)(G) 4 mg daily; max 8 mg/day
   Pediatric: not recommended
   Toviaz *Tab:* 4, 8 mg ext-rel
▷ *tolterodine tartrate* (C)(G)
   Pediatric: not recommended
      Detrol 2 mg bid; may decrease to 1 mg bid
         Tab: 1, 2 mg
      Detrol LA 2-4 mg once daily
         Cap: 2, 4 mg ext-rel

ANTISPASMODIC/ANTICHOLINERGICS

▷ *darifenacin* (C) 7.5-15 mg daily with liquid; max 15 mg/day
   Pediatric: not recommended
      Enablex 7.5-15 mg daily with liquid; max 15 mg/day
         Tab: 7.5, 15 mg ext-rel
▷ *dicyclomine* (B)(G) 10-20 mg qid
   Pediatric: not recommended
      Bentyl *Tab:* 20 mg; *Cap:* 10 mg; *Syr:* 10 mg/5 ml (16 oz)
▷ *flavoxate* (B) 100-200 mg tid-qid
   Pediatric: not recommended
      Urispas *Tab:* 100 mg
▷ *hyoscyamine* (C)(G)
      Anaspaz 1-2 tabs q 4 hours prn; max 12 tabs/day
         Pediatric: <2 years: not recommended; 2-12 years: 0.0625-0.125 mg q 4 hours prn; max 0.75 mg/day
         Tab: 0.125*mg
      Levbid 1-2 tabs q 12 hours prn; max 4 tabs/day
         Pediatric: <12 years: not recommended; ≥12 years: same as adult

Tab: 0.375*mg ext-rel

Levsin 1-2 tabs q 4 hours prn; max 12 tabs/day
>   *Pediatric:* <6 years: not recommended; 6-12 years: 1 tab q 4 hours prn
>   *Tab:* 0.125*mg

Levsin Drops 1-2 ml q 4 hours prn; max 60 ml/day
>   *Pediatric:* 3.4 kg: 4 drops q 4 hours prn; max 24 drops/day; 5 kg: 5 drops q 4
>   hours prn; max 30 drops/day; 7 kg: 6 drops q 4 hours prn; max 36 drops/day;
>   10 kg: 8 drops q 4 hours prn; max 40 drops/day
>   *Oral drops:* 0.125 mg/ml (15 ml) (orange) (alcohol 5%)

Levsin Elixir 5-10 ml q 4 hours prn
>   *Pediatric:* <10 kg: use drops; 10-19 kg: 1.25 ml q 4 hours prn; 20-39 kg: 2.5
>   ml q 4 hours prn; 40-49 kg: 3.75 ml q 4 hours prn; ≥50 kg: 5 ml q 4 hours prn
>   *Elix:* 0.125 mg/5 ml (16 oz) (orange) (alcohol 20%)

Levsinex SL 1-2 tabs q 4 hours SL <u>or</u> PO; max 12 tabs/day
>   *Pediatric:* 2-12 years: 1 tab q 4 hours; max 6 tabs/day; >12 years: same as adult
>   *Tab:* 0.125 mg sublingual

Levsinex Timecaps 1-2 caps q 12 hours; may adjust to 1 cap q 8 hours
>   *Pediatric:* 2-12 years: 1 cap q 12 hours; max 2 caps/day; >12 years: same as
>   adult
>   *Cap:* 0.375 mg time-rel

NuLev dissolve 1-2 tabs on tongue, with <u>or</u> without water, q 4 hours prn; max
12 tabs/day
>   *Pediatric:* <2 years: not recommended; 2-12 years: dissolve 1 tab on tongue,
>   with <u>or</u> without water, q 4 hours prn; max 6 tabs/day; ≥12 years: same as adult
>   *ODT:* 0.125 mg (mint; phenylalanine)

➤ *oxybutynin chloride* (B)

Ditropan 5 mg bid-tid; max 20 mg/day
>   *Pediatric:* <5 years: not recommended; 5-12 years: 5 mg bid; max 15 mg/day;
>   ≥16 years: same as adult
>   *Tab:* 5*mg; *Syr:* 5 mg/5 ml

Ditropan XL initially 5 mg daily; may increase weekly in 5-mg increments as
needed; max 30 mg/day
>   *Pediatric:* <6 years: not recommended; ≥6 years: initially 5 mg once daily; may
>   increase weekly in 5-mg increments as needed; max 20 mg/day
>   *Tab:* 5, 10, 15 mg ext-rel

GelniQUE 3 mg Pump: apply 3 pumps (84 mg) once daily to clean dry intact
skin on the abdomen, upper arm, shoulders, <u>or</u> thighs; rotate sites; wash hands;
avoid washing application site for 1 hour after application
>   *Pediatric:* not recommended
>   *Gel:* 3% (92 g, metered pump dispenser) (alcohol)

GelniQUE 1 g Sachet: apply 1 g gel (1 sachet) once daily to dry intact skin on
abdomen, upper arms/shoulders, <u>or</u> thighs; rotate sites; wash hands; avoid
washing application site for 1 hour after application
>   *Pediatric:* not recommended
>   *Gel:* 10%, 1 g/sachet (30/carton) (alcohol)

Oxytrol Transdermal Patch (OTC): apply patch to clean dry area of the abdomen,
hip, <u>or</u> buttock; one patch twice weekly; rotate sites
>   *Pediatric:* not recommended
>   *Transdermal patch:* 3.9 mg/day

▷ *propantheline* (C) 15-30 mg tid
    Pediatric: not recommended
        Pro-Banthine *Tab:* 7.5, 15 mg
▷ *solifenacin* (C) 5-10 mg daily
    Pediatric: not recommended
        VESIcare *Tab:* 5, 10 mg
▷ *trospium chloride* (C)(G)
    Pediatric: not recommended
        Sanctura 20 mg twice daily; ≥75 years <u>or</u> CrCl ≤30 mL/min, 20 mg once daily
            Tab: 20 mg
        Sanctura XR 60 mg daily in the morning
            Cap: 60 mg ext-rel
    Comment: Take *trospium chloride* on an empty stomach.

OVERFLOW INCONTINENCE/ATONIC BLADDER

▷ *bethanechol* (C) 10-30 mg tid
        Urecholine *Tab:* 5, 10, 25, 50 mg

OVERFLOW INCONTINENCE/PROSTATIC ENLARGEMENT

Alpha-1 Blockers

Comment: Educate the patient regarding the potential side effect of hypotension when taking an alpha-1 blocker, especially with first dose. Start at lowest dose and titrate upward.
▷ *terazosin* (C) initially 1 mg q HS; titrate to 10 mg q HS; max 20 mg/day
        Hytrin *Cap:* 1, 2, 5, 10 mg
▷ *doxazosin* (C) initially 1 mg q HS; may double dose every 1-2 weeks; max 8 mg/day
        Cardura *Tab:* 1*, 2*, 4*, 8*mg
        Cardura XL *Tab:* 4, 8 mg
▷ *prazosin* (C)(G) 1-15 mg q HS; max 15 mg/day
        Minipress *Tab:* 1, 2, 5 mg
▷ *tamsulosin* (C) initially 0.4 mg daily; may increase to 0.8 mg daily after 2-4 weeks if needed
        Flomax *Cap:* 0.4 mg

5-ALPHA REDUCTASE INHIBITOR

▷ *finasteride* (X) 5 mg daily
        Proscar *Tab:* 5 mg

ALPHA 1A-BLOCKER

▷ *silodosin* (B) take 8 mg with food once daily; *CrCl 30-50 mL/min:* take 4 mg
        Rapaflo *Cap:* 4, 8 mg

 INFLUENZA (FLU)

Comment: With the exception of **Flucelvax**, flu vaccine is contraindicated with allergy to egg <u>or</u> chicken proteins, <u>or</u> egg products. All flu vaccines are contraindicated with allergy to latex, active infection, acute respiratory disease, active neurological disorder; history of Guillain-Barre syndrome. Have epinephrine 1:1,000 on hand. Flu vaccine is contraindicated for children under 18 years of age who are taking aspirin <u>and/or</u> an aspirin-containing product due to the risk of developing Reye's syndrome. Under 1 year of age, administer flu vaccine in the vastus lateralis. Over 1 year of age, administer flu vaccine in the deltoid. Flu vaccine formulations change annually. Administer flu vaccine 1 month before flu season. Spray may be administered earlier. The influenza vaccine reduces hospitalization by about 70% and mortality by about 80% in the elderly.

PROPHYLAXIS (NASAL SPRAY)

▷ *trivalent, live attenuated influenza* vaccine, types A and B (C) 1 spray each nostril; ≥50 years not recommended
  Pediatric: ≤5 years: not recommended; ≥5 years: same as adult
    Never vaccinated with **FluMist:** 5-8 years: 2 divided doses 46-74 days apart.
    Previously vaccinated with **FluMist:** 5-8 years: same as adult
    FluMist Nasal Spray 0.5 ml spray annually
      Nasal spray: 0.5 ml (0.25 ml/spray) (10/carton) (preservative-free)

PROPHYLAXIS (INJECTABLE)

▷ *quadrivalent inactivated influenza subvirion vaccine, types A and B* (C)
    Fluad 0.5 ml IM annually
    Comment: **Fluad** is the first seasonal influenza vaccine with adjuvant, indicated for persona ≥65 years-of-age. Adjuvants are incorporated into some vaccine formulations to enhance <u>or</u> direct the immune response.
    Fluarix Quadrivalent 0.5 ml IM annually
      Pediatric: <3 years: not recommended; ≥3 years: same as adult
      Prefilled syringes: 0.5 ml (10/carton; preservative-free, latex-free)
▷ *trivalent inactivated influenza subvirion vaccine, types A and B*
    Fluarix (B) 0.5 ml IM annually
      Pediatric: <3 years: not recommended; 3-9 years (previously unvaccinated <u>or</u> vaccinated for the first time last season with one dose of flu vaccine): 2 doses per season at least 1 month apart; 3-9 years (previously vaccinated with two doses of flu vaccine); and >9 years: 1 dose per season
      Prefilled syringe: 0.5 ml single-dose (5/carton) (may contain trace amounts of hydrocortisone, gentamicin; preservative-free)
    Flublok 0.5 ml IM annually; ≥49 years, not recommended
      Pediatric: <18 years: not recommended
      Vial: 0.5 ml single-dose (10/carton) (preservative-free, egg protein-free, antibiotic-free, latex-free)
    Comment: **Flublok** is a cell culture-derived vaccine and, therefore, is an alternative to the traditional egg-based vaccines. Contains 3 times the amount of active ingredient in traditional flu vaccines **Flucelvax** 0.5 ml IM annually
      Pediatric: <18 years: not recommended
      Prefilled syringes: 0.5 ml (10/carton; preservative-free, latex-free)
    Comment: **Flucelvax** is a cell culture-derived vaccine and, therefore, is an alternative to the traditional egg-based vaccines.
    FluLaval (C) 0.5 ml IM annually
      Pediatric: <18 years: not recommended
      Vial: (5 ml)

FluShield 0.5 ml IM annually
Pediatric: <6 months: not recommended; *Never vaccinated:* <9 years: 2 doses at least 4 weeks apart; 9-12 years: same as adult; *Previously vaccinated:* 6-35 months: 0.25 ml IM x 1 dose; 3-8 years: same as adult
Fluzone 0.5 ml IM annually
Vial: 5 ml (thimerosal)
Fluzone Preservative-Free: Adult Dose 0.5 ml IM annually
Pediatric: <6 months: not recommended; *Not previously vaccinated:* 6 months-8 years: 0.25 ml IM; repeat in 1 month; *Previously vaccinated:* 6-35 months: 0.25 ml IM x 1 dose; >3 years: same as adult
Prefilled syringe: 0.5 ml (10/carton) (preservative-free, trace thimerosal)
Fluzone Preservative-Free: Pediatric Dose
Pediatric: <6 months: not recommended; *Not previously vaccinated:* 6 months-8 years: 0.25 ml IM; repeat in 1 month; *Previously vaccinated:* 6-35 months: 0.25 ml IM x 1 dose; ≥3 years: 0.5 ml IM (use **Fluzone for Adult**)
Prefilled syringe: 0.5 ml (10/carton; preservative-free; trace thimerosal)

PROPHYLAXIS AND TREATMENT

Neuraminidase Inhibitors

Comment: Effective for influenza type A and B. Indicated for treatment of uncomplicated acute illness in patients who have been symptomatic for no more than 2 days; therefore, start within 2 days of symptom onset <u>or</u> exposure. Indicated for influenza prophylaxis in patients ≥3 months of age.
▷ *oseltamivir* (C)
Treatment: 75 mg bid x 5 days; initiate treatment only if symptomatic <2 days
Pediatric: <1 year: not recommended; 1-12 years: <15 kg: 30 mg bid x 5 days; 16-23 kg: 45 mg bid x 5 days; 24-40 kg: 60 mg bid x 5 days; >40 kg: same as adult
Prophylaxis: 75 mg daily for at least 7 days and up to 6 weeks for community outbreak
Pediatric: <1 year: not recommended; 1-12 years: <15 kg: 30 mg once daily x 10 days; 16-23 kg: 45 mg once daily x 10 days; 24-40 kg: 60 mg once daily x 10 days; >40 kg: same as adult
Tamiflu *Cap:* 30, 45, 75 mg; *Oral susp:* 6 mg/ml pwdr for reconstitution (60 ml w. oral dispenser) (tutti-frutti)
Comment: **Tamiflu** is effective for influenza type A and B.
▷ *zanamivir* (C) 2 inhalations (10 mg) bid x 5 days
Pediatric: <7 years: not recommended; ≥7 years: same as adult
Relenza Inhaler *Inhaler:* 5 mg/inh blister; 4 blisters/Rotadisk (5 Rotadisks/carton w. 1 inhaler)
Comment: **Relenza Inhaler** is effective for influenza type A and B. Use caution with asthma and COPD.
Antipyretics *see Fever page 143*

 INSECT BITE/STING

TOPICAL ANESTHETIC

▷ *lidocaine* 3% cream (B) apply bid-tid prn
Pediatric: reduce dosage commensurate with age, body weight, and physical condition

LidaMantle *Crm:* 3% (1 oz)
Oral Drugs for Allergy, Cough, and Cold *see page* 524
Topical Corticosteroids *see page* 494
Parenteral Corticosteroids *see page* 499
Oral Corticosteroids *see page* 497

OTHER AGENTS

▷ *epinephrine* (C)(G) 1:1,000 0.3-0.5 ml SC
  Pediatric: 0.01 ml/kg SC

TETANUS PROPHYLAXIS

▷ *tetanus toxoid* vaccine (C)(G) 0.5 ml IM x 1 dose if previously immunized
  Vial: 5 Lf units/0.5 ml (0.5, 5 ml); *Prefilled syringe:* 5 Lf units/0.5 ml (0.5 ml) (For
  patients not previously immunized *see Tetanus page* 398)

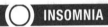 **INSOMNIA**

MELATONIN RECEPTOR AGONIST

▷ *ramelteon* (C)(IV) 8 mg within 30 minutes of bedtime; delayed effect if taken with
  a meal
  Pediatric: not recommended
    Rozerem *Tab:* 8 mg

NONBENZODIAZEPINES

▷ *zaleplon* (C)(IV) (imidazopyridine) 5-10 mg at HS <u>or</u> after going to bed if unable to
  sleep; do not take if unable to sleep for at least 4 hours before required to be active
  again; max 20 mg/day x 1 month; delayed effect if taken with a meal
  Pediatric: not recommended
    Sonata *Cap:* 5, 10 mg (tartrazine)
    Comment: **Sonata** is indicated for the treatment of insomnia when a middle-of-
    the-night awakening is followed by difficulty returning to sleep.
▷ *zolpidem* oral solution spray (C)(IV) (imidazopyridine hypnotic) 2 actuations (10
  mg) immediately before bedtime; elderly, debilitated, <u>or</u> hepatic impairment, 2 actuations (5 mg); max 2 actuations (10 mg)
  Pediatric: not recommended
    ZolpiMist *Oral soln spray:* 5 mg/actuation (60 metered actuations) (cherry)
    Comment: The lowest dose of *zolpidem* in all forms is recommended for women as
    drug elimination is slower than in men.
▷ *zolpidem* tabs (B)(IV)(G) (pyrazolopyrimidine hypnotic) 5-10 mg <u>or</u> 6.25-12.5 ext-
  rel q HS prn; max 12.5 mg/day x 1 month; do not take if unable to sleep for at least
  8 hours before required to be active again; delayed effect if taken with a meal
  Pediatric: ≤18 years: not recommended
    Ambien *Tab:* 5, 10 mg
    Ambien CR *Tab:* 6.25, 12.5 mg ext-rel
    Comment: The lowest dose of *zolpidem* in all forms is recommended for women as
    drug elimination is slower than in men.

➤ *zolpidem* sublingual tabs (C)(IV)(G) (imidazopyridine hypnotic) dissolve 1 tab under the tongue; allow to disintegrate completely before swallowing; take only once per night and only if at least 4 hours of bedtime remain before planned time for awakening

    Intermezzo *SL Tab:* 1.75, 3.5 mg

    Comment: **Intermezzo** is indicated for the treatment of insomnia when a middle-of-the-night awakening is followed by difficulty returning to sleep. The lowest dose of *zolpidem* in all forms is recommended for women as drug elimination is slower than in men.

➤ *eszopiclone* (C)(IV)(G) (pyrrolopyrazine) 1-3 mg; max 3 mg/day x 1 month; do not take if unable to sleep for at least 8 hours before required to be active again; delayed effect if taken with a meal

    Pediatric: <18 years: not recommended

    Lunesta *Tab:* 1, 2, 3 mg

OREXIN RECEPTOR ANTAGONIST

➤ *suvorexant* (C)(IV) use lowest effective dose; take 30 minutes before bedtime; do not take if unable to sleep for ≥7 hours, max 20 mg

    Pediatric: not recommended

    Belsomra *Tab:* 5, 10, 15, 20 mg (30/blister pck)

BENZODIAZEPINES

➤ *estazolam* (X)(IV)(G) initially 1 mg q HS prn; may increase to 2 mg q HS

    Pediatric: ≤18 years: not recommended

    ProSom *Tab:* 1*, 2*mg

➤ *flurazepam* (X)(IV)(G) 30 mg q HS prn; elderly <u>or</u> debilitated, 15 mg

    Pediatric: <15 years: not recommended; ≥15 years: same as adult

    Dalmane *Cap:* 15, 30 mg

➤ *temazepam* (X)(IV)(G) 7.5-30 mg q HS prn; short term, 7-10 days; max 30 mg; max 1 month

    Pediatric: <18 years: not recommended

    Restoril *Cap:* 7.5, 15, 22.5, 30 mg

➤ *triazolam* (X)(IV) 0.125-0.25 mg q HS prn; short term, 7-10 days; max 0.5 mg; max 1 month

    Pediatric: <18 years: not recommended

    Halcion *Tab:* 0.125, 0.25*mg

    Barbiturates

➤ *pentobarbital* (D)(II)(G)

    Nembutal 100 mg q HS prn

        Cap: 50, 100 mg

    Nembutal Suppository 120 <u>or</u> 200 mg suppository rectally q HS prn

        Pediatric: 2-12 months (10-20 lb): 30 mg supp; 1-4 years (21-40 lb): 30 <u>or</u> 60 mg supp; 5-12 years (41-80 lb): 60 mg supp; 12-14 years (81-110 lb): 60 <u>or</u> 120 mg sup

        Rectal supp: 30, 60, 120, 200 mg

ORAL H₁ RECEPTOR AGONIST (1ST GENERATION ANTIHISTAMINE)

➤ *doxepin* (C)

    Silenor 3-6 mg q HS prn; elderly, hepatic impairment, tendency to urinary retention, initially 3 mg

    Tab: 3, 6 mg

Other Oral 1st Generation Antihistamines *see page* 524

ANALGESIC/1ST GENERATION ANTIHISTAMINE COMBINATIONS

▷ *acetaminophen/diphenhydramine* (B)
    Excedrin PM (OTC) 2 tabs q HS prn
      Pediatric: <12 years: not recommended; ≥12 years: same as adult
      Tab/Geltab: acet 500 mg/*diphen* 38 mg
    Tylenol PM (OTC) 2 caps q HS prn
      Pediatric: <12 years: not recommended; ≥12 years: same as adult
      Tab/Cap/Gel cap: acet 500 mg/*diphen* 25 mg
    Tricyclic Antidepressants *see Depression page* 108

⊙ INTERSTITIAL CYSTITIS

Comment: Avoid peppers and spicy food, citrus, vinegar, caffeine (e.g., coffee, tea, colas), alcohol, carbonated beverages, and other GU tract irritants.

MANAGEMENT OF PAIN AND URINARY URGENCY

Acetaminophen for IV Infusion *see Pain page* 296
Oral Prescription NSAIDs *see page* 489
▷ *phenazopyridine* (B)(G) 95-200 mg q 6 hours prn; max 2 days
  Pediatric: not recommended
    AZO Standard, Prodium, Uristat (OTC) *Tab:* 95 mg
    AZO Standard Maximum Strength (OTC) *Tab:* 97.5 mg
    Pyridium, Urogesic *Tab:* 100, 200 mg *phenazopyridine* (B)(G) 190-200 mg tid;
    max 2 days
  Pediatric: not recommended
    Azo Standard (OTC) *Tab:* 95 mg
    Azo Standard Maximum Strength (OTC) *Tab:* 97.5 mg
    Pyridium *Tab:* 100, 200 mg ent-coat
    Uristat (OTC) *Tab:* 95 mg
    Urogesic *Tab:* 100, 200 mg
▷ *hyoscyamine* (C)(G)
    Anaspaz 1-2 tabs q 4 hours prn; max 12 tabs/day
      Pediatric: <2 years: not recommended; 2-12 years: 0.0625-0.125 mg q 4 hours
      prn; max 0.75 mg/day; ≥12 years: same as adult
      Tab: 0.125*mg
    Levbid 1-2 tabs q 12 hours prn; max 4 tabs/day
      Pediatric: <12 years: not recommended; ≥12 years: same as adult
      Tab: 0.375*mg ext-rel
    Levsin 1-2 tabs q 4 hours prn; max 12 tabs/day
      Pediatric: <6 years: not recommended; 6-12 years: 1 tab q 4 hours prn; ≥12
      years: same as adult
      Tab: 0.125*mg
    Levsin Drops 1-2 ml q 4 hours prn; max 60 ml/day
      Pediatric: 3.4 kg: 4 drops q 4 hours prn; max 24 drops/day; 5 kg: 5 drops q 4
      hours prn; max 30 drops/day; 7 kg: 6 drops q 4 hours prn; max 36 drops/day;
      10 kg: 8 drops q 4 hours prn; max 40 drops/day

Oral drops: 0.125 mg/ml (15 ml) (orange) (alcohol 5%)

Levsin Elixir 5-10 ml q 4 hours prn
   Pediatric: <10 kg: use drops; 10-19 kg: 1.25 ml q 4 hours prn; 20-39 kg: 2.5 ml q 4 hours prn; 40-49 kg: 3.75 ml q 4 hours prn; ≥50 kg: 5 ml q 4 hours prn; *Elix:* 0.125 mg/5 ml (16 oz) (orange) (alcohol 20%)

Levsin SL 1-2 tabs q 4 hours SL <u>or</u> po; max 12 tabs/day
   Pediatric: <2 years: not recommended; 2-12 years: 1 tab q 4 hours; max 6 tabs/day; ≥12 years: same as adult
   SL tab: 0.125 mg

Levsinex Timecaps 1-2 caps q 12 hours; may adjust to 1 cap q 8 hours
   Pediatric: <2 years: not recommended; 2-12 years: 1 cap q 12 hours; max 2 caps/day; ≥12 years: same as adult
   Cap: 0.375 mg time-rel

NuLev dissolve 1-2 tabs on tongue, with <u>or</u> without water, q 4 hours prn; max 12 tabs/day
   Pediatric: <2 years: not recommended; 2-12 years: dissolve 1 tab on tongue, with <u>or</u> without water, q 4 hours prn; max 6 tabs/day; ≥12 years: same as adult
   ODT: 0.125 mg (mint; phenylalanine)

➤ *methenamine/na phosphate monobasic/phenyl salicylate/methylene blue/hyoscyamine sulfate* (C) 1 cap qid
   Pediatric: <6 years: not recommended; ≥6 years: individualize dose
      Uribel *Cap:* meth 118 mg/*na phos* 40.8 mg/*phenyl sal* 36 mg/*meth blue* 10 mg/*hyoscy* 0.12 mg

➤ *methenamine/phenyl salicylate/methylene blue/benzoic acid/atropine sulfate/hyoscyamine sulfate* (C)(G) 2 tabs qid
   Pediatric: <6 years: not recommended; ≥6 years: same as adult
      Urised *Tab:* meth 40.8 mg/*phenyl sal* 18.1 mg/*meth blue* 5.4 mg/*benz acid* 4.5 mg/*atro sul* 0.03 mg/*hyoscy* 0.03 mg

   Comment: Urised imparts a blue-green color to urine which may stain fabrics.

➤ *oxybutynin chloride* (B)
   Ditropan 5 mg bid-tid; max 20 mg/day
      Pediatric: <5 years: not recommended; 5-12 years: 5 mg bid; max 15 mg/day; ≥12 years: same as adult
      Tab: 5*mg; *Syr:* 5 mg/5 ml

   Ditropan XL initially 5 mg daily; may increase weekly in 5-mg increments as needed; max 30 mg/day
      Tab: 5, 10, 15 mg ext-rel

➤ *pentosan* (B) 100 mg tid; reevaluate at 3 and 6 months
   Pediatric: <16 years: not recommended; ≥16 years: same as adult
      Elmiron *Cap:* 100 mg

URINARY TRACT ANALGESIA

➤ *phenazopyridine* (B)(G) 95-200 mg q 6 hours prn; max 2 days
   Pediatric: not recommended
      AZO Standard, Prodium, Uristat (OTC) *Tab:* 95 mg
      AZO Standard Maximum Strength (OTC) *Tab:* 97.5 mg
      Pyridium, Urogesic *Tab:* 100, 200 mg

Pediatric: not recommended
Azo Standard (OTC) *Tab:* 95 mg
Azo Standard Maximum Strength (OTC) *Tab:* 97.5 mg
Pyridium *Tab:* 100, 200 mg ent-coat
Uristat (OTC) *Tab:* 95 mg
Urogesic *Tab:* 100, 200 mg
Comment: *Phenazopyridine* imparts an orange-red color to urine which may stain fabrics.
▷ *propantheline* (C) 15-30 mg tid
Pro-Banthine *Tab:* 7.5, 15 mg
▷ *tolterodine tartrate* (C) 2 mg bid; may decrease to 1 mg bid
Detrol 2 mg bid; may decrease to 1 mg bid
Tab: 1, 2 mg
Detrol XL 2-4 mg daily
Cap: 2, 4 mg ext-rel

ANTICHOLINERGIC/SEDATIVE COMBINATION

▷ *chlordiazepoxide/clidinium* (D)(IV) 1-2 caps ac and HS; max 8 caps/day
Pediatric: not recommended
Librax *Cap:* chlor 5 mg/clid 2.5 mg

TRICYCLIC ANTIDEPRESSANTS (TCAs)

▷ *amitriptyline* (C)(G) 25-50 mg q HS
Pediatric: not recommended
Tab: 10, 25, 50, 75, 100, 150 mg
▷ *imipramine* (C)(G)
Pediatric: not recommended
Tofranil initially 75 mg daily (max 200 mg); adolescents initially 30-40 mg daily (max 100 mg/day); if maintenance dose exceeds 75 mg daily, may switch to **Tofranil PM** for divided or bedtime dose
Tab: 10, 25, 50 mg
Tofranil PM initially 75 mg daily 1 hour before HS; max 200 mg
Cap: 75, 100, 125, 150

INTERTRIGO

Comment: Intertrigo is an irritation and rash secondary to adjacent skin surfaces rubbing together. Treatment is dependent on symptoms and presence of infection.
Topical Corticosteroids *see page* 494
Topical Antifungals *see Tinea Corporis page* 400
Topical Anti-infectives *see Skin Infection: Bacterial page* 387

IRITIS: ACUTE

▷ *loteprednol etabonate* (C) 1-2 drops qid; may increase to 1 drop hourly as needed
Pediatric: not recommended

Lotemax Ophthalmic Solution *Ophth soln:* 0.3% (2.5, 5, 10, 15 ml)
▶ *prednisone acetate* (C) 1 drop q 1 hour x 24-48 hours, then 1 drop q 2 hours while
awake x 24-48 hours, then 1 drop bid-qid until resolved
Pediatric: not recommended
Pred Forte *Ophth soln:* 1% (1, 5, 10, 15 ml)

IRON OVERLOAD

IRON CHELATING AGENTS

▶ *deferasirox (tridentate ligand)* (C) initially 20 mg/kg/day; titrate; may increase 5-10
mg/kg q 3-6 months based on serum ferritin trends; max 30 mg/kg/day
Pediatric: <2 years: not recommended; ≥2 years: same as adult
Exjade *Tab for oral soln:* 125, 250, 500 mg
Jadenu *Tab:* 90, 180, 360 mg film-coat
Comment: *deferasirox* is an orally active chelator selective for iron. It is indicated
for the treatment of chronic iron overload due to blood transfusions (transfusional
hemosiderosis). Monitor serum ferritin monthly. Consider interrupting therapy
if serum ferritin falls below 500 mcg/L. Take *deferasirox* (**Jadenu, Exjade**) on an
empty stomach. Completely disperse tablet(s) for oral solution in 3.5 oz liquid if
dose is ≤1 g or 7 oz liquid if dose is ≥1 g.
▶ *Succimer* (C) initially 10 mg/kg q 8 hours x 5 days; then, reduce frequency to every 12
hours x 14 more days; allow at least 14 days between courses unless blood lead levels
indicate need for prompt treatment
Pediatric: <12 months: not recommended; ≥12 monhs: same as adult
Chemet Cap: 100 mg
Comment: *Chemet is* indicated for the treatment of lead poisoning when blood
lead level 45 mcg/dL. Treatment for more than 3 consecutive weeks is not
recommended. Monitor hydration, renal, and hepatic function.

IRRITABLE BOWEL SYNDROME WITH CONSTIPATION (IBS-C)

Bulk-Producing Agents, Laxatives, Stool Softeners *see Constipation page 95*

GUANYLATE CYCLASE-C AGONIST

▶ *linaclotide* (C) 290 mcg once daily; take on an empty stomach at least 30 minutes
before the first meal of the day; swallow whole
Pediatric: <6 years: not recommended; 6-17 years: avoid
Linzess Cap: 145, 290 mcg
Comment: May open **Linzess** cap and sprinkle on applesauce or in water for
administration
▶ *lubiprostone* (C) 8 mcg bid; take with food and water; *Severe hepatic impairment
(Child-Pugh Class C):* 8 mcg once daily
Pediatric: <18 years: not recommended
Amitiza Cap: 8, 24 mcg

IRRITABLE BOWEL SYNDROME WITH DIARRHEA (IBS-D)

Bulk-Producing Agents *see Constipation* page 95

CONSTIPATING AGENTS

▷ *difenoxin/atropine* (C) 2 tabs, then 1 tab after each loose stool <u>or</u> 1 tab q 3-4 hours as needed; max 8 tab/day x 2 days
Pediatric: <12 years: not recommended; ≥12 years: same as adult
 Motofen *Tab:* difen 1 mg/*atro* 0.025 mg

▷ *diphenoxylate/atropine* (C)(G) 2 tabs <u>or</u> 10 ml qid
Pediatric: <2 years: not recommended; 2-12 years: initially 0.3-0.4 mg/kg/day in 4 divided doses; ≥12 years: same as adult
 Lomotil *Tab:* difen 2.5 mg/*atro* 0.025 mg; *Liq:* difen 2.5 mg/*atro* 0.025 mg per 5 ml (2 oz)

▷ *eluxadoline* (NA)(IV) 100 mg bid; 75 mg bid if unable to tolerate 100 mg, <u>or</u> without a gall bladder, <u>or</u> mild-to-moderate hepatic impairment, <u>or</u> receiving concomitant OATP1B1 inhibitors
Pediatric: not established
 Viberzi 4 mg initially, then 2 mg after each loose stool; max 16 mg/day
 Tab: 75, 100 mg film-coat
Comment: *Eluxadoline* is a mu-opioid receptor agonist. It is contraindicated with biliary obstruction, Sphincter of Oddi disease <u>or</u> dysfunction, alcohol abuse <u>or</u> addiction, pancreatitis, pancreatic duct obstruction, severe hepatic impairment, and mechanical GI obstruction.

▷ *loperamide* (B)(G)
 Imodium (OTC) 4 mg initially, then 2 mg after each loose stool; max 16 mg/day
  Pediatric: <5 years: not recommended; ≥5 years: same as adult
  Cap: 2 mg
 Imodium A-D (OTC) 4 mg initially, then 2 mg after each loose stool; usual max 8 mg/day x 2 days
  Pediatric: <2 years: not recommended; 2-5 years (24-47 lb): 1 mg up to tid x 2 days; 6-8 years (48-59 lb): 2 mg initially, then 1 mg after each loose stool; max 4 mg/day x 2 days; 9-11 years (60-95 lb): 2 mg initially, then 1 mg after each loose stool; max 6 mg/day x 2 days; ≥12 years: same as adult
  Cplt: 2 mg; *Liq:* 1 mg/5 ml (2, 4 oz)

▷ *loperamide/simethicone* (B)(G)
 Imodium Advanced (OTC) 2 tabs chewed after loose stool, then 1 after the next loose stool; max 4 tabs/day
  Pediatric: <6 years: not recommended; 6-8 years: 1 tab chewed after loose stool, then 1/2 after next loose stool; max 2 tabs/day; 9-11 years: 1 tab chewed after loose stool, then 1/2 after next loose stool; max 3 tabs/day; ≥12 years: same as adult
  Chew tab: lop 2 mg/*sim* 125 mg

5-HT3 RECEPTOR ANTAGONIST

▷ *alosetron* (B)(G) initially 0.5 mg bid; may increase to 1 mg bid after 4 weeks if starting dose is tolerated but inadequate
Pediatric: not recommended
 Lotronex *Tab:* 0.5, 1 mg

ANTISPASMODIC/ANTICHOLINERGIC COMBINATIONS

▶ *dicyclomine* (B)(G) initially 20 mg bid-qid; may increase to 40 mg qid PO; usual IM dose 80 mg/day divided qid; do not use IM route for more than 1-2 days
Pediatric: not recommended
> **Bentyl** *Tab:* 20 mg; *Cap:* 10 mg; *Syr:* 10 mg/5 ml (16 oz); *Vial:* 10 mg/ml (10 ml); *Amp:* 10 mg/ml (2 ml)

▶ *methscop olamine bromide* (B) 1 tab q 6 hours prn
Pediatric: not recommended
> **Pamine** *Tab:* 2.5 mg
> **Pamine Forte** *Tab:* 5 mg

ANTICHOLINERGICS

▶ *hyoscyamine* (C)(G)
> **Anaspaz** 1-2 tabs q 4 hours prn; max 12 tabs/day
> *Pediatric:* <2 years: not recommended; 2-12 years: 0.0625-0.125 mg q 4 hours prn; max 0.75 mg/day; ≥12 years: same as adult
> *Tab:* 0.125*mg

> **Levbid** 1-2 tabs q 12 hours prn; max 4 tabs/day
> *Pediatric:* <12 years: not recommended; ≥12 years: same as adult
> *Tab:* 0.375*mg ext-rel

> **Levsin** 1-2 tabs q 4 hours prn; max 12 tabs/day
> *Pediatric:* <6 years: not recommended; 6-12 years: 1 tab q 4 hours prn; >12 years: same as adult
> *Tab:* 0.125*mg

> **Levsinex SL** 1-2 tabs q 4 hours SL <u>or</u> po; max 12 tabs/day
> *Pediatric:* <2 years: not recommended; 2-12 years: 1 tab q 4 hours; max 6 tabs/day; >12 years: same as adult
> *Tab:* 0.125 mg sublingual

> **Levsinex Timecaps** 1-2 caps q 12 hours; may adjust to 1 cap q 8 hours
> *Pediatric:* <2 years: not recommended; 2-12 years: 1 cap q 12 hours; max 2 caps/day; >12 years: same as adult
> *Cap:* 0.375 mg time-rel

> **NuLev** dissolve 1-2 tabs on tongue, with <u>or</u> without water, q 4 hours prn; max 12 tabs/day
> *Pediatric:* <2 years: not recommended; 2-12 years: dissolve 1 tab on tongue, with <u>or</u> without water, q 4 hours prn; max 6 tabs/day; >12 years: same as adult
> *ODT:* 0.125 mg (mint; phenylalanine)

▶ *simethicone* (C)(G) 0.3 ml qid pc and HS
> **Mylicon Drops** (OTC) *Oral drops:* 40 mg/0.6 ml (30 ml)

▶ *phenobarbital/hyoscyamine/atropine/scopolamine* (C)(IV)(G)
> **Donnatal** 1-2 tabs ac and HS
> *Pediatric:* not recommended
> *Tab:* pheno 16.2 mg/*hyo* 0.1037 mg/*atro* 0.0194 mg/*scop* 0.0065 mg

> **Donnatal Elixir** 1-2 tsp ac and HS
> *Pediatric:* 20 lb: 1 ml q 4 hours <u>or</u> 1.5 ml q 6 hours; 30 lb: 1.5 ml q 4 hours <u>or</u> 2 ml q 6 hours; 50 lb: 1/2 tsp q 4 hours <u>or</u> 3/4 tsp q 6 hours; 75 lb: 3/4 tsp q 4 hours <u>or</u> 1 tsp q 6 hours; 100 lb: 1 tsp q 4 hours <u>or</u> 1 tsp q 6 hours
> *Elix:* pheno 16.2 mg/*hyo* 0.1037 mg/*atro* 0.0194 mg/*scop* 0.0065 mg per 5 ml (4, 16 oz)

> **Donnatal Extentabs** 1 tab q 12 hours

Pediatric: not recommended
Tab: pheno 48.6 mg/*hyo* 0.3111 mg/*atro* 0.0582 mg/*scop* 0.0195 mg ext-rel

ANTICHOLINERGIC/SEDATIVE COMBINATION

▷ *chlordiazepoxide/clidinium* (D)(IV) 1-2 caps ac and HS: max 8 caps/day
Pediatric: not recommended
　　Librax *Cap: chlor* 5 mg/*clid* 2.5 mg

TRICYCLIC ANTIDEPRESSANTS (TCAs)

▷ *amitriptyline* (C)(G) 25-50 mg q HS
Pediatric: not recommended
　　Tab: 10, 25, 50, 75, 100, 150 mg
▷ *imipramine* (C)(G) 25-50 mg tid
Pediatric: not recommended
　　Tofranil initially 75 mg daily (max 200 mg); adolescents initially 30-40 mg daily
　　(max 100 mg/day); if maintenance dose exceeds 75 mg daily, may switch to
　　Tofranil PM for divided <u>or</u> bedtime dose
　　　　Tab: 10, 25, 50 mg
　　Tofranil PM initially 75 mg daily 1 hour before HS; max 200 mg
　　　　Cap: 75, 100, 125, 150
　　Tofranil Injection 50 mg IM; lower dose for adolescents; switch to oral form as
　　soon as possible
　　　　Amp: 25 mg/2 ml (2 ml)

⬤ JUVENILE RHEUMATOID ARTHRITIS (JRA)

Acetaminophen for IV Infusion *see Pain page* 296
Oral Prescription NSAIDs *see Pain page* 489
Other Oral Analgesics *see Pain page* 298
Topical/Transdermal NSAIDs *see Pain page* 297
Parenteral Corticosteroids *see page* 499
Oral Corticosteroids *see page* 497
Topical Analgesic and Anesthetic Agents *see page* 499

TOPICAL ANALGESICS

▷ *capsaicin* (B)(G) apply tid-qid prn to intact skin
Pediatric: <2 years: not recommended; ≥2 years: same as adult
　　Axsain *Crm:* 0.075% (1, 2 oz)
　　Capsin *Lotn:* 0.025, 0.075% (59 ml)
　　Capzasin-P (OTC) *Crm:* 0.025% (1.5 oz); *Lotn:* 0.025% (2 oz)
　　Dolorac *Crm:* 0.025% (28 g)
　　Double Cap (OTC) *Crm:* 0.05% (2 oz)
　　R-Gel *Gel:* 0.025% (15, 30 g)
　　Zostrix (OTC) *Crm:* 0.025% (0.7, 1.5, 3 oz)
　　Zostrix HP (OTC) *Emol crm:* 0.075% (1, 2 oz)
Comment: Provides some relief by 1-2 weeks; optimal benefit may take 4-6 weeks.

ORAL SALICYLATE

▷ *indomethacin* (C) initially 25 mg bid-tid, increase as needed at weekly intervals by 25-50 mg/day; max 200 mg/day
Pediatric: <14 years: usually not recommended; ≥2 years, if risk warranted: 1-2 mg/kg/day in divided doses; max 3-4 mg/kg/day (or total 150-200 mg/day, whichever is less); ≤14 years, ER cap not recommended
Cap: 25, 50 mg; Susp: 25 mg/5 ml (pineapple-coconut, mint; alcohol 1%); Supp: 50 mg; ER Cap: 75 mg ext-rel
Comment: *Indomethacin* is indicated only for acute painful flares. Administer with food and/or antacids. Use lowest effective dose for shortest duration.

▷ *methotrexate* (X) 7.5 mg x 1 dose per week or 2.5 mg x 3 at 12-hour intervals once a week; max 20 mg/week; therapeutic response begins in 3-6 weeks; administer methotrexate injection SC only into the abdomen or thigh
Pediatric: <2 years: not recommended; ≥2 years: 10 mg/m² once weekly; max 20 mg/m²
   Rasuvo *Autoinjector:* 7.5 mg/0.15 ml, 10 mg/0.20 ml, 12.5 mg/ 0.25 ml, 15 mg/0.30 ml, 17.5 mg/0.35 ml, 20 mg/0.40 ml, 22.5 mg/0.45 ml, 25 mg/0.50 ml, 27.5 mg/0.55 ml, 30 mg/0.60 ml (solution concentration for SC injection is 50 mg/ml)
   Rheumatrex *Tab:* 2.5*mg (5, 7.5, 10, 12.5, 15 mg/week, 4/card unit-of-use dose pack)
   Trexall *Tab:* 5*, 7.5*, 10*, 15*mg (5, 7.5, 10, 12.5, 15 mg/week, 4/card unit-of-use dose pack)
Comment: *methotrexate* (MTX) is contraindicated with immunodeficiency, blood dyscrasias, alcoholism, and chronic liver disease.

○ KERATITIS/KERATOCONJUNCTIVITIS: HERPES SIMPLEX

▷ *ganciclovir* (C) instill 1 drop 5 times per day (every 3 hours) while awake until corneal ulcer heals; then 1 drop tid x 7 days
Pediatric: <2 years: not recommended; ≥2 years: same as adult
   Zirgan *Ophth gel:* 0.15% (5 gm)(benzalkonium chloride)

▷ *idoxuridine* (C) instill 1 drop q 1 hour during day and every other hour at night or 1 drop every minute for 5 minutes and repeat q 4 hours during day and night
   Herplex *Ophth soln:* 0.1% (15 ml)

▷ *trifluridine* (C) instill 1 drop q 2 hours while awake (max 9 drops/day until reepithelialization; then 1 drop q 4 hours x 7 more days (at least 5 drops/day); max 21 days
Pediatric: <6 years: not recommended; ≥6 years: same as adult
   Viroptic *Ophth soln:* 1% (7.5 ml) (thimerosal)

▷ *vidarabine* (C) apply 1/2 inch in lower conjunctival sac 5 times/day q 3 hours until reepithelialization occurs, then bid x 7 more days
Pediatric: <2 years: not recommended; ≥2 years: same as adult
   Vira-A *Ophth oint:* 3% (3.5 g)

○ KERATITIS/KERATOCONJUNCTIVITIS: VERNAL

OPHTHALMIC MAST CELL STABILIZERS

Comment: Contact lens wear is contraindicated

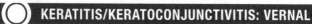

▷ *cromolyn sodium* (B) 1-2 drops 4-6 times/day
  Pediatric: <4 years: not recommended; ≥4 years: same as adult
    Crolom, Opticrom *Ophth soln:* 4% (10 ml) (benzalkonium chloride)
▷ *lodoxamide tromethamine* (B) 1-2 drops qid; max 3 months
  Pediatric: <2 years: not recommended; ≥2 years: same as adult
    Alomide *Ophth susp:* 0.1% (10 ml)

LABYRINTHITIS

▷ *meclizine* (B) 25 mg tid
  Pediatric: not recommended
    Antivert *Tab:* 12.5, 25, 50*mg
    Bonine (OTC) *Cap:* 15, 25, 30 mg; *Tab:* 12.5, 25, 50 mg; *Chew tab/Film-coated tab:* 25 mg
    Dramamine II (OTC) *Tab:* 25*mg
    Zentrip *Strip:* 25 mg orally disintegrating
▷ *promethazine* (C)(G) 25 mg tid
  Pediatric: <2 years: not recommended; ≥2 years: 0.5 mg/lb or 6.25-25 mg tid
    Phenergan *Tab:* 12.5*, 25*, 50 mg; *Plain syr:* 6.25 mg/5 ml; *Fortis syr:* 25 mg/5 ml; *Rectal supp:* 12.5, 25, 50 mg
▷ *scopolamine* (C)
    Transderm Scop 1 patch behind ear at least 4 hours before travel; each patch is effective for 3 days
      Transdermal patch: 1.5 mg (4/carton)

LACTOSE INTOLERANCE

▷ *lactase* enzyme (NR) 9,000 FCC units taken with dairy food; adjust based on abatement of symptoms; usual max 18,000 units/dose
  Pediatric: same as adult
    Lactaid Drops (OTC) 5-7 drops to each quart of milk and shake gently; may increase to 10-15 drops if needed; hydrolyzes 70%-99% of lactose at refrigerator temperature in 24 hours
      Oral drops: 1,250 units/5 gtts (7 ml w. dropper)
    Lactaid Extra (OTC) *Cplt:* 4,500 FCC units
    Lactaid Fast ACT (OTC) *Cplt:* 9,000 FCC units; *Chew tab:* 9,000 FCC units (vanilla twist)
    Lactaid Original (OTC) *Cplt:* 3,000 FCC units
    Lactaid Ultra (OTC) *Cplt:* 9,000 FCC units; *Chew tab:* 9,000 FCC units (vanilla twist)

LARVA MIGRANS: CUTANEOUS/VISCERAL

▷ *thiabendazole* (C) Adult and pediatric dosing schedules are the same; dosing is bid, is based on weight in pounds, and must be taken with meals.
    Cutaneous Larva Migrans: treat bid x 2 days
    Visceral Larva Migrans: treat bid x 7 days
      <30 lbs: consult mfr literature; 30 lbs: 250 mg bid; 50 lbs: 500 mg bid; 75 lbs: 750 mg bid; 100 lbs: 1000 mg bid; 125 lbs: 1250 mg bid; ≥150 lbs: 1500 mg bid; max 3000 mg/day.

Mintezol *Chew tab:* 500*mg (orange); *Oral susp:* 500 mg/5 ml (120 ml) (orange)
Comment: *thiabendazole* is not for prophylaxis.

⬤ LEAD POISONING

Comment: Chelation therapy for lead poisoning requires maintenance of adequate hydration, close monitoring of renal and hepatic function, and monitoring for neutropenia; discontinue therapy at first sign of toxicity. Contraindicated with severe renal disease or anuria.

CHELATING AGENTS

➢ *deferoxamine mesylate* (C) initially 1 g IM, followed by 500 mg IM every 4 hours x 2 doses; then repeat every 4-12 hours if needed; max 6 g/day
Pediatric: <3 months: not recommended; ≥3 months: same as adult
   Desferal *Vial:* 250 mg/ml after reconstitution (500 mg)
➢ *edetate calcium disodium (EDTA)* (B) administer IM or IV; use IM route of administration for children and overt lead encephalopathy
Pediatric: same as adult; *Serum lead level:* 20-70 mcg/dL: 1 g/m² per day; *IV:* infuse over 8-12 hours; *IM:* divided doses q 8-12 hours; Treat for 5 days; then stop for 2-4 days; may repeat if serum lead level is >70 mcg/dL
   Calcium Disodium Versenate *Amp:* 200 mg/ml (5 ml)
➢ *succimer* (C) may swallow caps whole or put contents onto a small amount of soft food or a spoon and swallow, followed by a fruit drink
Pediatric: <12 months: not recommended; ≥12 months: same as adult; *Serum lead level:* >45 mcg/dL: initially 10 mg/kg (or 350 mg/m²) every 8 hours for 5 days; then reduce frequency to every 12 hours for 14 more days; allow at least 14 days between courses unless serum lead levels indicate a need for more prompt treatment; for more than 3 consecutive weeks not recommended
   Chemet *Cap:* 100 mg

⬤ LEG CRAMPS: NOCTURNAL, RECUMBENCY

➢ *quinine sulfate* (C)(G) 1 tab or cap q HS
Pediatric: <16 years: not recommended; ≥16 years: same as adult
Tab: 260 mg; *Cap:* 260, 300, 325 mg
   Qualaquin *Cap:* 324 mg
Comment: If hypokalemia is the cause of leg cramps, treat with potassium supplementation (see page 220).

⬤ LENTIGINES: BENIGN, SENILE

Comment: Wash affected area with a soap-free cleanser; pat dry and wait 20-30 minutes; then apply agent sparingly to affected area; use only once daily in PM. Avoid eyes, ears, nostrils, mouth, and healthy skin. Avoid sun exposure. Cautious use of concomitant astringents, alcohol-based products, sulfur-containing products, salicylic acid-containing products, soap, and other topical agents.

TOPICAL RETINOIDS

▶ *tazarotene* (X) apply daily at HS
  Pediatric: not recommended
      Avage Cream *Crm:* 0.1% (30 g)
      Tazorac Cream *Crm:* 0.05, 0.1% (15, 30, 60 g)
      Tazorac Gel *Gel:* 0.05, 0.1% (30, 100 g)
▶ *tretinoin* (C) apply daily at HS
  Pediatric: <12 years: not recommended; ≥12 years: same as adult
      Avita *Crm:* 0.025% (20, 45 g); *Gel:* 0.025% (20, 45 g)
      Renova *Crm:* 0.02% (40 g); 0.05% (40, 60 g)
      Retin-A Cream *Crm:* 0.025, 0.05, 0.1% (20, 45 g)
      Retin-A Gel *Gel:* 0.01, 0.025% (15, 45 g; alcohol 90%)
      Retin-A Liquid *Liq:* 0.05% (28 ml; alcohol 55%)
      Retin-A Micro *Microspheres:* 0.04, 0.1% (20, 45 g)

LISTERIOSIS

▶ *erythromycin base* (B)(G) 500 mg qid x 10 days
  Pediatric: <45 kg: 30-40 mg/kg/day in 4 divided doses x 10 days; ≥45 kg: same as adult
      Ery-Tab *Tab:* 250, 333, 500 mg ent-coat
      PCE *Tab:* 333, 500 mg

  Comment: *erythromycin* may increase INR with concomitant *warfarin*, as well as increase serum level of *digoxin*, benzodiazepines and statins.
▶ *erythromycin ethylsuccinate* (B)(G) 400 mg po qid x 10 days
  Pediatric: 30-50 mg/kg/day in 4 divided doses x 10 days; may double dose with severe infection; max 100 mg/kg/day; *see page 563 for dose by weight*
      EryPed *Oral susp:* 200 mg/5 ml (100, 200 ml) (fruit); 400 mg/5 ml (60, 100, 200 ml; banana); *Oral drops:* 200, 400 mg/5 ml (50 ml) (fruit); *Chew tab:* 200 mg wafer (fruit)
      E.E.S. *Oral susp:* 200, 400 mg/5 ml (100 ml) (fruit)
      E.E.S. Granules *Oral susp:* 200 mg/5 ml (7.5 ml) (thimerosal)
      E.E.S. 400 Tablets *Tab:* 400 mg

  Comment: *erythromycin* may increase INR with concomitant *warfarin*, as well as increase serum level of *digoxin*, benzodiazepines and statins.

LOW BACK STRAIN

Acetaminophen for IV Infusion *see Pain page 296*
Oral Prescription NSAIDs *see page 489*
Other Oral Analgesics *see Pain page 298*
Topical/Transdermal NSAIDs *see Pain page 297*
Parenteral Corticosteroids *see page 499*
Oral Corticosteroids *see page 497*
Topical Analgesic and Anesthetic Agents *see page 487*

LOW LIBIDO, HYPOACTIVE SEXUAL DESIRE DISORDER (HSDD)

5-HT1A AGONIST/5-HT2A

▷ *flibanserin* (NR) 1 tab once daily at bedtime; discontinue if no improvement in 8 weeks
  Pediatric: <18 years: not recommended
    Tab: < 100 mg
    Comment: **Addyi** is for use in premenopausal women. **Addyi** is not for use in men, postmenopausal women, and is not recommended in pregnancy, or lactation. Potential ASEs include dry mouth, nausea, hypotension, dizziness, syncope, fatigue, somnolence, and insomnia.

LYME DISEASE (ERYTHEMA CHRONICUM MIGRANS)

Comment: The bite of the deer tick (*Ioxodes scapularis*) carries the *Borrelia burgdorferi* organism causing Lyme disease. Proper removal of the tick, and early diagnosis and treatment are essential to effective management of this disease.

STAGE 1

▷ *amoxicillin* (B)(G) 500-875 mg bid or 250-500 mg tid x 10 days
  Pediatric: <40 kg (88 lb): 20-40 mg/kg/day in 3 divided doses x 10 days or 25-45 mg/kg/day in 2 divided doses x 10 days; ≥40 kg: same as adult; *see page 543 for dose by weight*
    Amoxil *Cap:* 250, 500 mg; *Tab:* 875*mg; *Chew tab:* 125, 200, 250, 400 mg (cherry-banana-peppermint) (phenylalanine); *Oral susp:* 125, 250 mg/5 ml (80, 100, 150 ml) (strawberry); 200, 400 mg/5 ml (50, 75, 100 ml) (bubble gum); *Oral drops:* 50 mg/ml (30 ml) (bubble gum)
    Moxatag *Tab:* 775 mg ext-rel
    Trimox *Tab:* 125, 250 mg; *Cap:* 250, 500 mg; *Oral susp:* 125, 250 mg/5 ml (80, 100, 150 ml) (raspberry-strawberry)
▷ *cefuroxime axetil* (B)(G) 500 mg bid x 20 days
  Pediatric: <3 months: not recommended; ≥3 months: 15 mg/kg bid x 20 days
    Ceftin *Tab:* 250, 500 mg; *Oral susp:* 125, 250 mg/5 ml (50, 100 ml) (tutti-frutti)
▷ *clarithromycin* (C)(G) 500 mg bid or 500 mg ext-rel daily x 14-21 days
  Pediatric: <6 months: not recommended; ≥6 months: 7.5 mg/kg bid x 7 days; *see page 558 for dose by weight*
    Biaxin *Tab:* 250, 500 mg
    Biaxin Oral Suspension *Oral susp:* 125, 250 mg/5 ml (50, 100 ml)
    Biaxin XL *Tab:* 500 mg ext-rel
▷ *doxycycline* (D)(G) 100 mg bid x 14-21 days
  Pediatric: <8 years: not recommended; ≥8 years, ≤100 lb: 2 mg/lb on first day in 2 divided doses, followed by 1 mg/lb/day in 1-2 divided doses; ≥8 years, >100 lb: same as adult; *see page 561 for dose by weight*
    Actilate *Tab:* 75, 150** mg
    Adoxa *Tab:* 50, 75, 100, 150 mg ent-coat
    Doryx *Tab:* 75, 100, 150 mg del-rel

Monodox *Cap:* 50, 75, 100 mg
Oracea *Cap:* 40 mg del-rel
Vibramycin *Cap:* 50, 100 mg; *Syr:* 50 mg/5 ml (raspberry; sulfites); *Oral susp:* 25 mg/5 ml (raspberry-apple)
Vibra-Tab *Tab:* 100 mg film-coat

Comment: *doxycycline* is contraindicated <8 years-of-age, in pregnancy, and lactation (discolors developing tooth enamel). A side effect may be photo-sensitivity (photophobia). Do not give with antacids, calcium supplements, milk or other dairy, or within two hours of taking another drug.

▶ *minocycline* (D)(G) 200 mg on first day; then 100 mg q 12 hours x 9 more days
Pediatric: ≤8 years: not recommended; ≥8 years, <100 lb: 2 mg/lb on first day in 2 divided doses, followed by 1 mg/lb q 12 hours x 9 more days; ≥8 years, >100 lb: same as adult

Dynacin *Cap:* 50, 100 mg
Minocin *Cap:* 50, 75, 100 mg; *Oral susp:* 50 mg/5 ml (60 ml) (custard) (sulfites, alcohol 5%)

Comment: *minocycline* is contraindicated <8 years-of-age, in pregnancy, and lactation (discolors developing tooth enamel). A side effect may be photo-sensitivity (photophobia). Do not give with antacids, calcium supplements, milk or other dairy, or within two hours of taking another drug.

▶ *tetracycline* (D)(G) 250-500 mg qid ac x 21 days
Pediatric: <8 years: not recommended; ≥8 years, ≤100 lb: 25-50 mg/kg/day in 2-4 divided doses x 7 days; ≥8 years, >100 lb: same as adult; *see page 574 for dose by weight*

Achromycin V *Cap:* 250, 500 mg
Sumycin *Tab:* 250, 500 mg; *Cap:* 250, 500 mg; *Oral susp:* 125 mg/5 ml (100, 200 ml) (fruit) (sulfites)

Comment: *tetracycline* is contraindicated <8 years-of-age, in pregnancy, and lactation (discolors developing tooth enamel). A side effect may be photo-sensitivity (photophobia). Do not give with antacids, calcium supplements, milk or other dairy, or within two hours of taking another drug.

◯ LYMPHADENITIS

Comment: Therapy should continue for no less than 5 days after resolution of symptoms.

▶ *amoxicillin/clavulanate* (B)(G) 500 mg tid or 875 mg bid x 10 days
Augmentin *Tab:* 250, 500, 875 mg; *Chew tab:* 125, 250 mg (lemon-lime); 200, 400 mg (cherry-banana) (phenylalanine); *Oral susp:* 125 mg/5 ml (banana), 250 mg/5 ml (75, 100, 150 ml) (orange); 200, 400 mg/5 ml (50, 75, 100 ml) (orange) (phenylalanine)
Pediatric: 40-45 mg/kg/day divided tid x 10 days or 90 mg/kg/day divided bid x 10 days *see pages 545-546 for dose by weight*
Augmentin ES-600 *Oral susp:* 600 mg/5 ml (50, 75, 100, 125, 150, 200 ml) (strawberry cream) (phenylalanine) every 12 hours
Pediatric: <3 months: not recommended; ≥3 months, <40 kg: 90 mg/kg/day in 2 divided doses; ≥40 kg: not recommended
Augmentin XR 2 tabs q 12 hours x 7-10 days
Pediatric: <16 years: use other forms; ≥16 years: same as adult
Tab: 1000*mg ext-rel

▷ *cephalexin* (B)(G) 500 mg bid x 10 days
   Pediatric: 25-50 mg/kg/day in 4 divided doses x 10 days; *see page 557 for dose by weight*
      Keflex *Cap:* 250, 333, 500, 750 mg; *Oral susp:* 125, 250 mg/5 ml (100, 200 ml)
      (strawberry)
▷ *dicloxacillin* (B) 500 mg qid x 10 days
   Pediatric: 12.5-25 mg/kg/day in 4 divided doses x 10 days; *see page 560 for dose by
   weight*
      Dynapen *Cap:* 125, 250, 500 mg; *Oral susp:* 62.5 mg/5 ml (80, 100, 200 ml)

◯ LYMPHOGRANULOMA VENEREUM

Comment: The following treatment regimens are published in the **2015 CDC Sexually
Transmitted Diseases Treatment Guidelines**. This section contains treatment regimens
for adults only; consult a specialist for treatment of patients less than 18 years of age.
Treatment regimens are presented in alphabetical order by generic drug name, followed
by brands and dose forms. Treat all sexual contacts. Persons with both LGV and HIV
infection should receive the same treatment regimens as those who are HIV-negative;
however, prolonged treatment may be required and delay in resolution of symptoms may
occur.

RECOMMENDED REGIMEN

Regimen 1

▷ *doxycycline* 100 mg bid x 21 days

ALTERNATIVE REGIMEN

Regimen 1

▷ *erythromycin base* 500 mg qid x 21 days <u>or</u> *erythromycin ethylsuccinate* 400 mg qid
   x 21 days

RECOMMENDED REGIMENS FOR THE MANAGEMENT OF SEXUAL CONTACTS

Comment: LGV is caused by *C. trachomatis* serovars L1, L2, <u>or</u> L3. Persons who have
had sexual contact with a patient who has LGV within 60 days before onset of the
patient's symptoms should be examined, tested for urethral <u>or</u> cervical chlamydial
infection, and treated with a chlamydia regimen.

Regimen 1

▷ *azithromycin* 1 g in a single dose

Regimen 2

▷ *doxycycline* 100 mg bid x 7 days

DRUG BRANDS AND DOSE FORMS

▷ *azithromycin* (B)
      Zithromax *Tab:* 250, 500, 600 mg; *Oral susp:* 100 mg/5 ml (15 ml);
      200 mg/5 ml (15, 22.5, 30 ml) (cherry); *Pkt:* 1 g for reconstitution (cherry-banana)

Zithromax Tri-pak *Tab:* 3 x 500 mg tabs/pck
Zithromax Z-pak *Tab:* 6 x 250 mg tabs/pck
Zmax *Oral susp:* 2 g ext-rel for reconstitution (cherry-banana) (148 mg Na$^+$)

▷ *doxycycline* (D)(G)
Actilate *Tab:* 75, 150** mg
Adoxa *Tab:* 50, 75, 100, 150 mg ent-coat
Doryx *Tab:* 75, 100, 150 mg del-rel
Monodox *Cap:* 50, 75, 100 mg
Vibramycin *Cap:* 50, 100 mg; *Syr:* 50 mg/5 ml (raspberry; sulfites); *Oral susp:*
25 mg/5 ml (raspberry-apple)
Vibra-Tab *Tab:* 100 mg film-coat

Comment: *doxycycline* is contraindicated <8 years-of-age, in pregnancy, and
lactation (discolors developing tooth enamel). A side effect may be photo-
sensitivity (photophobia). Do not give with antacids, calcium supplements, milk or
other dairy, or within two hours of taking another drug.

▷ *erythromycin base* (B)(G)
Ery-Tab *Tab:* 250, 333, 500 mg ent-coat
PCE *Tab:* 333, 500 mg

Comment: *erythromycin* may increase INR with concomitant *warfarin*, as well as
increase serum level of *digoxin*, benzodiazepines and statins.

▷ *erythromycin ethylsuccinate* (B)(G)
EryPed *Oral susp:* 200 mg/5 ml (100, 200 ml) (fruit); 400 mg/5 ml (60, 100,
200 ml) (banana); *Oral drops:* 200, 400 mg/5 ml (50 ml) (fruit); *Chew tab:*
200 mg wafer (fruit)
E.E.S. *Oral susp:* 200, 400 mg/5 ml (100 ml) (fruit)
E.E.S. Granules *Oral susp:* 200 mg/5 ml (100, 200 ml) (cherry)
E.E.S. 400 Tablets *Tab:* 400 mg

Comment: *erythromycin* may increase INR with concomitant *warfarin*, as well as
increase serum level of *digoxin*, benzodiazepines and statins.

MALARIA (*PLASMODIUM FALCIPARUM*, *PLASMODIUM VIVAX* MALARIA)

▷ *doxycycline* (D)(G) 100 mg daily; initiate 1-2 days prior to travel; take during travel;
continue for 4 weeks after leaving the endemic area
Pediatric: ≤8 years: not recommended; ≥8 years, ≤100 lb: 1 mg/lb/day prior to travel;
take during travel; continue for 4 weeks after leaving the endemic area; ≥8 years,
≥100 lb: same as adult; *see page 561 for dose by weight*
Actilate *Tab:* 75, 150** mg
Adoxa *Tab:* 50, 75, 100, 150 mg ent-coat
Doryx *Tab:* 75, 100, 150 mg del-rel
Monodox *Cap:* 50, 75, 100 mg
Vibramycin *Cap:* 50, 100 mg; *Syr:* 50 mg/5 ml (raspberry; sulfites); *Oral susp:*
25 mg/5 ml (raspberry-apple)
Vibra-Tab *Tab:* 100 mg film-coat

Comment: *doxycycline* is contraindicated <8 years-of-age, in pregnancy, and
lactation (discolors developing tooth enamel). A side effect may be photo-
sensitivity (photophobia). Do not give with antacids, calcium supplements, milk or
other dairy, or within two hours of taking another drug.

▷ *minocycline* (D)(G) 100 mg daily; initiate 1-2 days prior to travel; take during travel; continue for 4 weeks after leaving the endemic area
Pediatric: <8 years: not recommended; ≥8 years, ≤100 lb: 2 mg/lb on first day in 2 divided doses, followed by 1 mg/lb q 12 hours x 9 more days; ≥8 years, >100 lb: same as adult
    Dynacin *Cap:* 50, 100 mg
    Minocin *Cap:* 50, 75, 100 mg; *Oral susp:* 50 mg/5 ml (60 ml) (custard) (sulfites, alcohol 5%)
Comment: *minocycline* is contraindicated <8 years-of-age, in pregnancy, and lactation (discolors developing tooth enamel). A side effect may be photo-sensitivity (photophobia). Do not give with antacids, calcium supplements, milk or other dairy, or within 2 hours of taking another drug.

▷ *tetracycline* (D) 250 mg daily; initiate 1-2 days prior to travel; take during travel; continue for 4 weeks after leaving the endemic area
Pediatric: <8 years: not recommended; ≥8 years, ≤100 lb: 25-50 mg/kg/day in 4 divided doses x 10 days; ≥8 years, >100 lb: same as adult; *see page 574 for dose by weight*
    Achromycin V *Cap:* 250, 500 mg
    Sumycin *Tab:* 250, 500 mg; *Cap:* 250, 500 mg; *Oral susp:* 125 mg/5 ml (100, 200 ml) (fruit) (sulfites)
Comment: *tetracycline* is contraindicated <8 years-of-age, in pregnancy, and lactation (discolors developing tooth enamel). A side effect may be photo-sensitivity (photophobia). Do not give with antacids, calcium supplements, milk or other dairy, or within 2 hours of taking another drug.

ANTIMALARIALS

▷ *quinine sulfate* (C)(G) 1 tab <u>or</u> cap every 8 hours x 7 days
Pediatric: <16 years: not recommended; ≥16 years: same as adult
    Tab: 260 mg; *Cap:* 260, 300, 325 mg
    Qualaquin *Cap:* 324 mg
    Comment: **Qualaquin** is indicated in the treatment of uncomplicated *P. falciparum* malaria (including chloroquine-resistant strains).

▷ *atovaquone* (C)(G) take as a single dose with food <u>or</u> a milky drink at the same time each day; repeat dose if vomited within 1 hour; *Prophylaxis:* 1,500 mg once daily; *Treatment:* 750 mg bid x 21 days
    Mepron *Susp:* 750 mg/5 ml

▷ *atovaquone/proguanil* (C)(G) take as a single dose with food <u>or</u> a milky drink at the same time each day; repeat dose if vomited within 1 hour; *Prophylaxis:* 1 tab daily starting 1-2 days before entering endemic area, during stay, and for 7 days after return; *Treatment (acute, uncomplicated):* 4 tabs daily x 3 days
Pediatric: <5 kg: not recommended; 5-40 kg
Prophylaxis: daily dose starting 1-2 days before entering endemic area, during stay, and for 7 days after return; 5-20 kg: 1 ped tab; 21-30 kg: 2 ped tabs; 31-40 kg: 3 ped tabs; ≥40 kg: same as adult; *Treatment (acute, uncomplicated):* daily dose x 3 days; 5-8 kg: 2 ped tabs; 9-10 kg: 3 ped tabs; 11-20 kg: 1 adult tab; 21-30 kg: 2 adult tabs; 31-40 kg: 3 adult tabs; >40 kg: same as adult
    Malarone *Tab:* atov 250 mg/prog 100 mg
    Malarone Pediatric *Tab:* atov 62.5 mg/prog 25 mg
Comment: *atovaquone* is antagonized by *tetracycline* and *metoclopramide*. Concomitant *rifampin* is not recommended (may elevate LFTs).

▷ *chloroquine* (C)(G) *Prophylaxis:* 500 mg once weekly (on the same day of each week); start 2 weeks prior to exposure, continue while in the endemic area, and continue 4 weeks after departure; *Treatment:* initially 1 g; then 500 mg 6 hours, 24 hours, and 48 hours after initial dose or initially 200-250 mg IM; may repeat in 6 hours; max 1 g in first 24 hours; continue to 1.875 g in 3 days
Pediatric: Suppression: 8.35 mg/kg (max 500 mg) weekly (on the same day of each week); *Treatment:* initially 16.7 mg/kg (max 1 g); then 8.35 mg/kg (max 500 mg) 6 hours, 24 hours, and 48 hours after initial dose, or initially 6.25 mg/kg IM; may repeat in 6 hours; max 12.5 mg/kg/day
    Aralen *Tab:* 500 mg; *Amp:* 50 mg/ml (5 ml)

▷ *hydroxychloroquine* (C)(G) *Prophylaxis:* 400 mg once weekly (on the same day of each week); start 2 weeks prior to exposure, continue while in the endemic area, and continue 8 weeks after departure; *Treatment:* initially 800 mg; then 400 mg 6 hours, 24 hours, and 48 hours after initial dose
Pediatric: Suppression: 6.45 mg/kg (max 400 mg) weekly (on the same day of each week) beginning 2 weeks prior to arrival, continuing while in endemic area, and continuing 4 weeks after departure; *Treatment:* initially 12.9 mg/kg (max 800 mg); then 6.45 mg/kg (max 400 mg) 6 hours, 24 hours, and 48 hours after initial dose hours after initial dose
    Plaquenil *Tab:* 200 mg

▷ *mefloquine* (C) *Prophylaxis:* 250 mg once weekly (on the same day of each week); start 1 week prior to exposure, continue while in the endemic area, and continue for 4 weeks after departure; *Treatment:* 1,250 mg as a single dose
Pediatric: <6 months: not recommended; *Prophylaxis:* ≥6 months: 3-5 mg/kg (max 250 mg) weekly (on the same day of each week); start 1 week prior to exposure, continue while in the endemic area, and continue for 4 weeks after departure; *Treatment:* ≥6 months: 25-50 mg/kg as a single dose; max 250 mg
    Lariam *Tab:* 250*mg

Comment: *mefloquine* is contraindicated with active or recent history of depression, generalized anxiety disorder, psychosis, schizophrenia or any other psychiatric disorder or history of convulsions.

⃝ MASTITIS (BREAST ABSCESS)

ANTI-INFECTIVES

▷ *amoxicillin/clavulanate* (B)(G) 500 mg tid or 875 mg bid x 10 days
    Augmentin *Tab:* 250, 500, 875 mg; *Chew tab:* 125, 250 mg (lemon-lime); 200, 400 mg (cherry-banana) (phenylalanine); *Oral susp:* 125 mg/5 ml (banana), 250 mg/5 ml (75, 100, 150 ml) (orange); 200, 400 mg/5 ml (50, 75, 100 ml) (orange) (phenylalanine)
      Pediatric: 40-45 mg/kg/day divided tid x 10 days or 90 mg/kg/day divided bid x 10 days *see pages 545-546 for dose by weight*
    Augmentin ES-600 *Oral susp:* 600 mg/5 ml (50, 75, 100, 125, 150, 200 ml) (strawberry cream) (phenylalanine) every 12 hours
      Pediatric: <3 months: not recommended; ≥3 months, <40 kg: 90 mg/kg/day in 2 divided doses; ≥40 kg: not recommended
    Augmentin XR 2 tabs q 12 hours x 7-10 days
      Pediatric: <16 years: use other forms; ≥16 years: same as adult
      Tab: 1000*mg ext-rel

➤ *cefaclor* (B)(G) 250-500 mg q 8 hours x 10 days; max 2 g/day
  Pediatric: <1 month: not recommended; 20-40 mg/kg bid <u>or</u> q 12 hours x 10 days;
  max 1 g/day; *see page 549 for dose by weight*
  Tab: 500 mg; *Cap:* 250, 500 mg; *Susp:* 125 mg/5 ml (75, 150 ml) (strawberry);
  187 mg/5 ml (50, 100 ml) (strawberry); 250 mg/5 ml (75, 150 ml) (strawberry);
  375 mg/5 ml (50, 100 ml) (strawberry)
  Pediatric: <16 years: ext-rel not recommended; ≥12 years: same as adult
     Cefaclor Extended Release *Tab:* 375, 500 mg ext-rel
➤ *ceftriaxone* (B)(G) 1-2 grams IM daily continued 2 days after signs of infection have
  disappeared; max 4 g/day
  Pediatric: 50 mg/kg IM daily continued 2 days after signs of infection have disappeared
     Rocephin *Vial:* 250, 500 mg; 1, 2 g
➤ *cephalexin* (B)(G) 500 mg bid x 10 days
  Pediatric: 25-50 mg/kg/day in 4 divided doses x 10 days; *see page 557 for dose by weight*
     Keflex *Cap:* 250, 333, 500, 750 mg; *Oral susp:* 125, 250 mg/5 ml (100, 200 ml)
     (strawberry)
➤ *clindamycin* (B)(G) 300 mg tid x 10 days
  Pediatric: not recommended
     Cleocin *Cap:* 75 (tartrazine), 150 (tartrazine), 300 mg
     Cleocin Pediatric Granules *Oral susp:* 75 mg/5 ml (100 ml) (cherry)
➤ *erythromycin base* (B)(G) 250-500 mg qid x 10 days
  Pediatric: <45 kg: 30-40 mg/kg/day in 4 divided doses x 10 days; ≥45 kg: same as
  adult
     Ery-Tab *Tab:* 250, 333, 500 mg ent-coat
     PCE *Tab:* 333, 500 mg
  Comment: *erythromycin* may increase INR with concomitant *warfarin*, as well as
  increase serum level of *digoxin*, benzodiazepines and statins.

⃝ MELASMA

SKIN DEPIGMENTING AGENTS

➤ *hydroquinone* (C) apply a thin film to clean dry affected areas bid; discontinue if
  lightening does not occur after 2 months
  Pediatric: not recommended
     Lustra *Crm: hydro* 4% (1, 2 oz) (sulfites)
     Lustra AF *Crm: hydro* 4% (1, 2 oz) (sunscreens, sulfites)
➤ *hydroquinone/fluocinolone acetonide/tretinoin* (C) apply a thin film to clean dry affected areas once daily at least 30 minutes before bedtime
  Pediatric: not recommended
     Tri-Luma *Crm: hydro* 4%/*fluo acet* 0.01%/*tret* 0.05% (30 g) (sulfites, parabens)

⃝ MENIERE'S DISEASE

➤ *diazepam* (D)(IV)(G) initially 1-2.5 mg tid-qid; may increase gradually
  Pediatric: <6 months: not recommended; ≥6 months: same as adult
     Diastat *Rectal gel delivery system:* 2.5 mg
     Diastat AcuDial *Rectal gel delivery system:* 10, 20 mg

Valium *Tab:* 2*, 5*, 10*mg
Valium Intensol *Conc oral soln:* 5 mg/ml (30 ml w. dropper) (alcohol 19%)
Valium Oral Solution *Oral soln:* 5 mg/5 ml (500 ml) (wintergreen-spice)

▷ *dimenhydrinate* (B) 50 mg q 4-6 hours
Pediatric: <2 years: not recommended; 2-6 years: 12.5-25 mg q 6-8 hours; max 75 mg/day; >6-11 years: 25-50 mg q 6-8 hours; max 150 mg/day; >11 years: same as adult

Dramamine (OTC) *Tab:* 50*mg; *Chew tab:* 50 mg (phenylalanine, tartrazine); *Liq:* 12.5 mg/5 ml (4 oz)

▷ *diphenhydramine* (B)(OTC)(G) 25-50 mg q 6-8 hours; max 100 mg/day
Pediatric: <2 years: not recommended; 2-6 years: 6.25 mg q 4-6 hours; max 37.5 mg/day; >6-12 years: 12.5-25 mg q 4-6 hours; max 150 mg/day; >12 years: same as adult

Benadryl (OTC) *Chew tab:* 12.5 mg (grape; phenylalanine); *Liq:* 12.5 mg/5 ml (4, 8 oz); *Cap:* 25 mg; *Tab:* 25 mg; *dye-free softgel:* 25 mg; Dye-free liq: 12.5 mg/5 ml (4, 8 oz)

▷ *meclizine* (B)(G) 25-100/day in divided doses
Pediatric: not recommended

Antivert *Tab:* 12.5, 25, 50*mg; *Amp:* 50 mg/ml (1 ml); *Vial:* 50 mg/ml (1 ml single-use); 50 mg/ml (10 ml multi-dose)
Bonine (OTC) *Cap:* 15, 25, 30 mg; *Tab:* 12.5, 25, 50 mg; *Chew tab/Film-coat tab:* 25 mg
Dramamine II 25 mg bid; max 50 mg/day
Tab: 25*mg
Zentrip *Strip:* 25 mg orally disintegrating

▷ *promethazine* (C) 12.5-25 q 4-6 hours po or rectally
Pediatric: <2 years: not recommended; ≥2 years: 0.5 mg/lb or 6.25-25 mg q 4-6 hours PO or rectally

Phenergan *Tab:* 12.5*, 25*, 50 mg; *Plain syr:* 6.25 mg/5 ml; *Fortis syr:* 25 mg/5 ml; *Rectal supp:* 12.5, 25, 50 mg

▷ *scopolamine* transdermal patch (C) 1 patch behind ear; each patch is effective for 3 days; change patch every 4th day; alternate sites
Pediatric: not recommended

Transderm Scop *Patch:* 1.5 mg (4/carton)

 MENINGITIS (*NEISSERIA MENINGITIDIS*)

PROPHYLAXIS

Comment: Meningitis vaccine is a 3-dose series (0, 2, 6 month schedule) indicated for persons age ≥10-25 years. Have epinephrine 1:1,000 readily available and monitor for 15 minutes post-dose of meningitis vaccine.

▷ *Meningococcal group b vaccine [recombinant, absorbed]* administer first dose IM in the deltoid; administer second dose 2 months later; administer the third dose 6 months from the first dose;
Pediatric: <10 years: not established; ≥10 years: same as adult

Bexsero *Susp for IM inj:* 0.5 ml single-dose prefilled syringes (1, 10/carton)
Trumenba *Susp for IM inj:* 0.5 ml single-dose prefilled syringes (5, 10/carton)

▷ *Neisseria meningitides oligosaccharide conjugate* quadrivalent meningonococcal vaccine **(B)** contains *Corynebacterium diphtheria* CRM197 protein; 10 mcg of Group A + 5 mcg each of Group C, Y, and W-135 + 32.7-64.1 mcg of diphtheria CRM 197 protein per 0.5 m.
   Pediatric: <11 years: not recommended; ≥11-55 years: 0.5 ml IM x 1 dose in the deltoid
      Menveo *Vial multi-dose:* 5 doses/vial (MenA conjugate component pwdr for reconstitution + 1 vial liquid MenCWY conjugate component for reconstitution) (preservative-free)
▷ *Neisseria meningitidis polysaccharides* vaccine **(C)** 0.5 ml SC x 1 dose; if at high risk, may revaccinate after 3-5 years; age ≥55 years contact mfr
      Menactra (A/C/Y/W-135)
        Pediatric: <2 years: contact mfr; ≥2 years: same as adult; if at high risk, may revaccinate children first vaccinated ≤4 years-of-age after 2-3 years
        Vial (single-dose): 4 mcg each of group A, C, Y, and W-135 per 0.5 ml (pwdr for SC inj after reconstitution) (preservative-free diluent); *Vial (multi-dose):* 4 mcg each of group A, C, Y, and W-130 per 0.5 ml [pwdr for SC inj after reconstitution (5 doses/vial) (preservative-free)]
      Comment: Latex allergy is a contraindication to **Menactra.**
      Menomune-A/C/Y/W-135
        Pediatric: <2 years: not recommended (except ≥3 months of age as short-term protection against group A); ≥2 years: same as adult; if at high risk, may revaccinate children first vaccinated ≤4 years of age after 2-3 years (older children after 3-5 years)
        Vial (single-dose): 50 mcg each of group A, C, Y, and W-135 per 0.5 ml (pwdr for SC inj after reconstitution; preservative-free diluent); *Vial (multi-dose):* 50 mcg each of group A, C, Y, and W-130 per 0.5 ml [pwdr for SC inj after reconstitution (10 doses/vial) (thimerosal-preserved diluent)]
Comment: Use precaution with latex allergy.

 MENOPAUSE

Comment: *Estrogen* replacement lowers LDL and raises HDL. *Estrogen* replacement is indicated for osteoporosis prevention. Exogenous *estrogen* administration increases risk for endometrial cancer, MI, stroke, invasive breast cancer, pulmonary embolism, and DVT. *Estrogen* replacement is contraindicated in known or suspected pregnancy, known or suspected cancer of the breast, known or suspected *estrogen*-dependent neoplasia, undiagnosed genital bleeding, and active thrombophlebitis or thromboembolic disorders. Use HRT with caution in patients with cardiovascular or peripheral vascular disease.

VAGINAL RINGS

▷ *estradiol, acetate* **(X)**
      Femring Vaginal Ring insert high into vagina; replace every 90 days
▷ *estradiol, micronized* **(X)**
      Estring Vaginal Ring insert high into vagina; replace every 90 days
        Vag ring: 7.5 mcg/24 hours (1/pck)

REGIMENS FOR PATIENTS WITH INTACT UTERUS

Vaginal Preparations (With Uterus)

Comment: Vaginal preparations provide relief from vaginal and urinary symptoms only (i.e., atrophic vaginitis, dyspareunia, dysuria, and urinary frequency).

▷ *estradiol* (X)(G)
> **Vagifem Tabs** insert one 10 mcg or 25 mcg vaginal tablet once daily x 2 weeks; then twice weekly for 2 weeks (e.g., tues/fri); consider the addition of a progestin
> > *Vag tab:* 10, 25 mcg (8, 18/blister pck with applicator)

▷ *estradiol, micronized* (X) **Estrace Vaginal Cream** 2-4 g daily x 1-2 weeks, then gradually reduced to 1/2 initial dose x 1-2 weeks, then maintenance dose of 1 g 1-3 times/week
> *Vag crm:* 0.01% (12, 42.5 g w. calib applicator)

▷ *estrogen, conjugated equine* (X)
> **Premarin Vaginal Cream** 0.5-2 g/day intravaginally; cyclically (3 weeks on, 1 week off)
> > *Vag crm:* 1.5 oz w. applicator marked in 1/2 g increments to max of 2 g

Transdermal Systems (With Uterus)

Comment: Alternate sites. Do not apply patches on or near breasts.

▷ *estradiol* (X)
> **Climara** initially 0.025 mg/day patch once/week to trunk (3 weeks on and 1 week off)
> > *Transdermal patch:* 0.025, 0.0375, 0.05, 0.075, 0.1 mg/day (4/pck)
> **Esclim** apply twice weekly x 3 weeks, then 1 week off; use with an oral progestin to prevent endometrial hyperplasia
> > *Transdermal patch:* 0.025, 0.0375, 0.05, 0.075, 0.1 mg/day (8, 48/pck)
> **Vivelle** initially one 0.0375 mg/day patch twice weekly to trunk area; use with an oral progestin to prevent endometrial hyperplasia
> > *Transdermal patch:* 0.025, 0.0375, 0.05, 0.075, 0.1 mg/day (8, 48/pck)
> **Vivelle-Dot** initially one 0.05 mg/day patch twice weekly to lower abdomen, below the waist; use with an oral progestin to prevent endometrial hyperplasia
> > *Transdermal patch:* 0.025, 0.0375, 0.05, 0.075, 0.1 mg/day (8, 24/pck)

▷ *estradiol/levonorgestrel* (X) apply 1 patch weekly to lower abdomen; avoid waistline; alternate sites
> **Climara Pro** *Transdermal patch: estra* 0.045 mg/*levo* 0.015 mg per day (4/pck)

▷ *estradiol/norethindrone* (X)
> **CombiPatch** apply twice weekly or q 3-4 days
> > *Transdermal patch:* 9 cm^2: *estra* 0.05 mg/*noreth* 0.14 mg; 16 cm^2: *estra* 0.05 mg/*noreth* 0.25 mg

Comment: May cause irregular bleeding in first 6 months of therapy, but usually decreases over time (often to amenorrhea).

ORAL AGENTS (WITH UTERUS)

▷ *estradiol* (X)(G)
> **Estrace** 1-2 mg daily cyclically (3 weeks on and 1 week off)
> > *Tab:* 0.5, 1, 2*mg (tartrazine)

▷ *estradiol/drospirenone* (X)
> **Angeliq** 1 tab daily
> > *Tab:* **Angeliq 0.5/0.25**: *estra* 0.5 mg/*dros* 0.25 mg

      Angeliq 1/0.5: *estra* 1 mg/*dros* 0.5 mg
▷ *estradiol/norethindrone* (X) 1 tab daily
      Activella (G) *Tab:* estra 1 mg/*noreth* 0.5 mg
      FemHRT (G) 1/5 *Tab:* estra 5 mcg/*noreth* 1 mg
      Fyavolv (G) *Tab:* estra 0.25 mg/*noreth* 1 mg; *Tab:* estra 0.5 mg/*noreth* 1 mg
      Mimvey LO *Tab:* estra 0.5 mg/*noreth* 0.1 mg
▷ *estradiol/norgestimate* (X) 1 x *estradiol* 1 mg tab once daily x 3 days, then 1 x *estradiol* 1 mg/*norgestimate* 0.09 mg tab daily x 3 days; repeat this pattern continuously
      Ortho-Prefest *Tab:* estra 1 mg/*norgest* 0.09 mg (30/blister pck)
▷ *estrogen, conjugated/medroxyprogesterone* (X)
      Prempro 1 tab daily
         Tab: **Prempro 0.3/1.5:** *conj estra* 0.3 mg/*medroxy* 1.5 mg
            Prempro 0.45/1.5: *conj estra* 0.45 mg/*medroxy* 1.5 mg
            Prempro 0.625/2.5: *conj estra* 0.625 mg/*medroxy* 2.5 mg
            Prempro 0.625/5: *conj estra* 0.625 mg/*medroxy* 5 mg
            Premphase 0.625 *estrogen* on days 1-14, then 0.625 mg *estrogen*/5 mg *medroxyprogesterone* on days 15-28
         Tab (in dial dispenser): conj estra 0.625 mg (14 maroon tabs) + *medroxy* 5 mg (14 blue tabs)
▷ *estrogen, esterified (plant derived)* (X)
      Menest 0.3-2.5 mg daily cyclically, 3 weeks on and 1 week off (with progestins in the latter part of the cycle to prevent endometrial hyperplasia)
         Tab: 0.3, 0.625, 1.25, 2.5 mg
▷ *estrogen, esterified/methyltestosterone* (X)
      Estratest 1 tab daily cyclically, 3 weeks on and 1 week off
         Tab: ester estra 1.25 mg/*meth* 2.5 mg
      Estratest HS 1-2 tabs daily cyclically, 3 weeks on and 1 week off
         Tab: ester estra 0.625 mg/*meth* 1.25 mg
▷ *ethinyl estradiol* (X) 0.02-0.05 mg q 1-2 days cyclically, 3 weeks on and 1 week off (with progestins in the latter part of the cycle to prevent endometrial hyperplasia)
      Estinyl *Tab:* 0.02 (tartrazine), 0.05 mg
▷ *estropipate, piperazine estrone sulfate* (X)(G)
      Ogen 0.625-1.25 mg daily cyclically (3 weeks on and 1 week off)
         Tab: 0.625, 1.25, 2.5 mg
      Ortho-Est 0.75-6 mg daily cyclically (3 weeks on and 1 week off)
         Tab: 0.625, 1.25 mg
▷ *medroxyprogesterone* (X) 5-10 mg daily for 12 sequential days of each 28-day cycle to prevent endometrial hyperplasia in the postmenopausal women with an intact uterus receiving conjugated estrogens
      Provera *Tab:* 2.5, 5, 10 mg
▷ *norethindrone acetate* (X) 2.5-10 mg daily x 5-10 days during second half of menstrual cycle
      Aygestin *Tab:* 5*mg
▷ *progesterone, micronized* (X)(G)
      Prometrium 200 mg daily in the PM for 12 sequential days of each 28-day cycle to prevent endometrial hyperplasia in the postmenopausal woman with an intact uterus receiving conjugated estrogens
         Cap: 100, 200 mg (peanut oil)

ESTROGENS, CONJUGATED/ESTROGEN AGONIST-ANTAGONIST

▷ *estrogen, conjugated/bazedoxifene* (X)
    Duavee 1 tab daily
      Tab: conj estra 0.45 mg/*baze* 20 mg

REGIMENS FOR PATIENTS WITHOUT UTERUS

Oral Agents (Without Uterus)

▷ *estradiol* (X)(G)
    Estrace 1-2 mg daily
      Tab: 0.5*, 1*, 2*mg (tartrazine)
▷ *estrogen, conjugated (equine)* (X)
    Premarin 1 tab daily
      Tab: 0.3, 0.45, 0.625, 0.9, 1.25, 2.5 mg
▷ *estrogen, conjugated (synthetic)* (X) 1 tab daily; may titrate up to max 1.25 mg/day
    Cenestin *Tab:* 0.3, 0.625, 0.9, 1.25 mg
    Enjuvia *Tab:* 0.3, 0.45, 0.625 mg
▷ *estrogen, esterified (plant derived)* (X) 1 tab daily
    Estratab *Tab:* 0.3, 0.625, 2.5 mg
    Menest *Tab:* 0.3, 0.625, 1.25, 2.5 mg
▷ *ethinyl estradiol* (X) 0.02-0.05 mg q 1-2 days
    Estinyl *Tab:* 0.02 (tartrazine), 0.05 mg

Vaginal Preparations (Without Uterus)

Comment: Vaginal preparations provide relief from vaginal and urinary symptoms only (i.e., atrophic vaginitis, dyspareunia, dysuria, and urinary frequency).
▷ *estradiol* (X)(G)
    Vagifem Tabs insert one 10 mcg <u>or</u> 25 mcg vaginal tablet once daily x 2 weeks; then twice weekly for 2 weeks (e.g., tues/fri); consider the addition of a progestin
      Vag tab: 10, 25 mcg (8, 18/blister pck with applicator)

Topical Agents (Without Uterus)

▷ *estradiol* (X)
    Estrasorb apply 3.48 g (2 pouches) every morning; apply one pouch to each leg from the upper thigh to the calf; rub in for 3 minutes; rub excess on hands onto buttocks
      Emul: 0.025 mg/day/pouch (2.5 mg/g; 1.74 g/pouch)
    EstroGel apply 1.25 g (one compression) to one arm from wrist to shoulder once daily at the same time each day
      Gel: 0.06% per compression (93 g)

Transdermal Systems (Without Uterus)

Comment: Do not apply patches on <u>or</u> near breasts. Alternate sites.
▷ *estradiol* (X)
    Alora initially 0.05 mg/day apply patch twice weekly to lower abdomen, upper quadrant of buttocks <u>or</u> outer aspect of hip
      Transdermal patch: 0.025, 0.05, 0.075, 0.1 mg/day (8, 24/pck)

Climara initially 0.025 mg/day patch once/week to trunk
    Transdermal patch: 0.025, 0.0375, 0.05, 0.075, 0.1 mg/day (4, 8, 24/pck)
Esclim initially 0.025 mg/day apply patch twice weekly to buttocks, femoral triangle, <u>or</u> upper arm
    Transdermal patch: 0.025, 0.0375, 0.05, 0.075, 0.1 mg/day (8/pck)
Estraderm initially apply one 0.05 mg/day patch twice weekly to trunk
    Transdermal patch: 0.05, 0.1 mg/day (8, 24/pck)
Menostar apply one patch weekly to lower abdomen, below the waist; avoid the breasts; alternate sites
    Transdermal patch: 14 mcg/day (4/pck)
Minivelle initially one 0.0375 mg/day patch twice weekly to trunk area; adjust after one month of therapy
    Transdermal patch: 0.025, 0.0375, 0.05, 0.075, 0.1 mg/day (8/pck)
Vivelle initially one 0.0375 mg/day patch twice weekly to trunk area; adjust after one month of therapy
    Transdermal patch: 0.025, 0.0375, 0.05, 0.075, 0.1 mg/day (8, 48/pck)
Vivelle-Dot initially apply one 0.05 mg/day patch twice weekly to lower abdomen, below the waist; adjust after one month of therapy
    Transdermal patch: 0.025, 0.0375, 0.05, 0.075, 0.1 mg/day (8, 24/pck)
Comment: The *estrogens* in **Alora**, **Climara**, **Estraderm**, and **Vivelle-Dot** are plant derived.

MENOMETORRHAGIA: IRREGULAR HEAVY MENSTRUAL BLEEDING/MENORRHAGIA: HEAVY CYCLICAL MENSTRUAL BLEEDING

ANTIFIBROLYTIC AGENT

➤ *tranexamic acid* (B)(G) 1,300 mg tid; treat for up to 5 days during menses; *Normal renal function (SCr ≤1.4 mg/dL):* 1,300 mg tid; *SCr ≥1.4-2.8 mg/dL:* 1,300 mg bid; *SCr ≥2.8-5.7 mg/dL:* 1,300 mg once daily; *SCr ≥5.7 mg/dL:* 650 mg once daily
Pediatric: <18 years: not recommended
    Lysteda *Tab:* 650 mg

Injectible Progesterone Only Contraceptives

➤ *medroxyprogesterone* (X)(G)
    Depo-Provera 150 mg deep IM q 3 months
    Vial: 150 mg/ml (1 ml)
        Prefilled syringe: 150 mg/ml
    Depo-SubQ 104 mg SC q 3 months
        Prefilled syringe: 104 mg/ml (0.65 ml; parabens)
Comment: Administer first dose within 5 days of onset of normal menses, within 5 days postpartum if not breastfeeding, <u>or</u> at 6 weeks postpartum if breastfeeding exclusively. Do not use for >2 years unless other methods are inadequate.
Combined Oral Contraceptives *see page 474*
Intrauterine Devices *see page 486*

MITRAL VALVE PROLAPSE (MVP)

▷ *propranolol* (C)(G)
Inderal 10-30 mg tid-qid
Tab: 10*, 20*, 40*, 60*, 80*mg
Inderal LA initially 80 mg daily in a single dose; increase q 3-7 days; usual range
120-160 mg/day; max 320 mg/day in a single dose
Cap: 60, 80, 120, 160 mg sust-rel
InnoPran XL initially 80 mg q HS; max 120 mg/day
Cap: 80, 120 mg ext-rel

MONONUCLEOSIS (MONO)

ANALGESICS

▷ *acetaminophen* (B) see *Fever page* 143
Acetaminophen for IV Infusion *see page* 489
Other Oral Analgesics *see Pain page* 298
Parenteral Corticosteroids *see page* 499
Oral Corticosteroids *see page* 497
▷ *prednisone* (C) initially 40-80 mg/day, then taper off over 5-7 days
Comment: Corticosteroids recommended in patients with significant pharyngeal edema.

MOTION SICKNESS

▷ *dimenhydrinate* (B)(OTC) 50-100 mg q 4-6 hours; start 1 hour before travel; max
400 mg/day
Pediatric: <2 years: not recommended; 2-6 years: 12.5-25 mg; max 75 mg/day; start
1 hour before travel; may repeat q 6-8 hours; 6-11 years: 25-50 mg; max 150 mg/
day; start 1 hour before travel; may repeat q 6-8 hours; ≥12 years: same as adult
Dramamine
Tab: 50*mg; *Chew tab:* 50 mg (phenylalanine, tartrazine); *Liq:* 12.5 mg/5 ml
(4 oz)
▷ *meclizine* (B)(G) 25-50 mg 1 hour before travel; may repeat q 24 hours as needed;
max 50 mg/day
Pediatric: not recommended
Antivert *Tab:* 12.5, 25, 50*mg
Bonine (OTC) *Cap:* 15, 25, 50 mg; *Tab:* 12.5, 25, 50 mg;
Chew tab/Film-coat tab: 25 mg
Dramamine II (OTC) *Tab:* 25 mg
Zentrip *Strip:* 25 mg orally-disint
▷ *prochlorperazine* (C)(G)
Compazine 5-10 mg q 4 hours as needed
Pediatric: not recommended
Tab: 5 mg; *Syr:* 5 mg/5 ml (4 oz; fruit); *Rectal supp:* 2.5, 5, 25 mg
Compazine Spansule 15 mg q AM or 10 mg q 12 hours
Spansules: 10, 15 mg sust-rel

➤ *promethazine* (C)(G) 25 mg 30-60 minutes before travel; may repeat in 8-12 hours
  Pediatric: <2 years: not recommended; ≥2 years: 12.5-25 mg 30-60 minutes before travel; may repeat in 8-12 hours
    Phenergan *Tab:* 12.5*, 25*, 50 mg; *Plain syr:* 6.25 mg/5 ml; *Fortis syr:* 25 mg/5 ml; *Rectal supp:* 12.5, 25, 50 mg
➤ *scopolamine* (C)
    Scopace 0.4-0.8 mg 1 hour before travel; may repeat in 8 hours
      Pediatric: not recommended
      Tab: 0.4 mg
    Transderm Scop 1 patch behind ear at least 4 hours before travel; each patch is effective for 3 days
      Pediatric: not recommended
      Transdermal patch: 1.5 mg (4/carton)

◯ MULTIPLE SCLEROSIS (MS)

NICOTINIC ACID RECEPTOR AGONIST

➤ *dimethyl fumarate* (C) initially 120 mg bid x 7 days; then maintenance 240 mg bid
  Pediatric: <18 years: not recommended
    Tecfidera *Cap:* 120, 240 mg del-rel; *Starter Pack:* 14 x 120 mg, 46 x 240 mg
  Comment: The mechanism by which *dimethyl fumarate* (DMF) exerts its therapeutic effect in multiple sclerosis is unknown. DMF and the metabolite, *monomethyl fumarate* (MMF), have been shown to activate the nuclear factor (erythroid-derived 2)-like 2 (Nrf2) pathway in vitro and in vivo in animals and humans. The Nrf2 pathway is involved in the cellular response to oxidative stress. MMF has been identified as a nicotinic acid receptor agonist in vitro.

POTASSIUM CHANNEL BLOCKER

➤ *dalfampridine* (C) 10 mg q 12 hours
  Pediatric: <18 years: not recommended
    Ampyra *Tab:* 10 mg ext-rel
  Comment: *dalfampridine* is indicated to improve walking speed.

PYRIMIDINE SYNTHESIS INHIBITOR (DMARD)

➤ *teriflunomide* (X) 7 mg <u>or</u> 14 mg once daily
  Pediatric: not recommended
    Aubagio *Tab:* 7, 14 mg
  Comment: Contraindicated with severe hepatic impairment and women of childbearing potential not using reliable contraception. Co-administer *teriflunomide* with the DMARD *leflunomide* (**Arava**).

IMMUNOMODULATORS

Comment: The role of immunomodulators in the treatment of MS is to slow the progression of physical disability and to decrease frequency of clinical exacerbations.

➤ *alemtuzumab* (C) administer two treatment courses:

First treatment course: 12 mg/day x 5 days (total 60 mg); *Second treatment course:* 12 months later, administer 12 mg/day x 3 days (total 36 mg); complete all immunizations 6 weeks prior to the first treatment; premedicate with 1000 mg methylprednisolone or equivalent immediately prior to the first 3 treatment days in each treatment course
Pediatric: <18 years: not recommended

> **Lemtrada** *Vial:* 12 mg/1.2 ml soln for IV infusion, single-use vial

> Comment: **Lemtrada** is indicated for the treatment of patients with relapsing forms of MS. Because of its safety profile, the use of **Lemtrada** should generally be reserved for patients who have had an inadequate response to two or more drugs indicated for the treatment of MS. **Lemtrada REMS** is a restricted distribution program, which allows early detection and management of some of the serious risks associated with its use.

▷ *fingolimod* (C) 0.5 mg once daily
Pediatric: <18 years: not recommended

> **Gilenya** *Cap:* 0.5 mg

Comment: First-dose monitoring for bradycardia. In the first 2 weeks, first-dose monitoring is recommended after an interruption of 1 day or more. During weeks 3 and 4, first-dose monitoring is recommended after an interruption of more than 7 days.

▷ *glatiramer acetate* (B)(G) 20-40 mg SC daily
Pediatric: <18 years: not recommended

> **Copaxone** *Prefilled syringe:* 20, 40 mg/ml (mannitol, preservative-free)

▷ *interferon beta-1a* (C)
Pediatric: <18 years: not recommended

> **Avonex** 30 mcg IM weekly; rotate sites; may titrate to reduce flu-like symptoms; may use concurrent analgesics/antipyretics on treatment days; *Titration Schedule:* 7.5 mcg week 1; 15 mcg week 2; 22.5 mcg week 3; 30 mcg week 4 and ongoing

> > *Vial:* 30 mcg/vial pwdr for reconstitution (single-dose w. diluent, 4 vials/kit) (albumin [human], preservative-free); *Prefilled syringe:* 30 mcg single-dose (0.5 ml) (4/dose pck)

> **Rebif,** administer SC 3x/week (at least 48 hours apart and preferably in the late afternoon or evening); increase over 4 weeks to usual dose 22-44 mcg 3x/week; *Titration Schedule (22 mcg prescribed dose):* 4.4 mcg week 1 & 2; 11 mcg week 3 & 4; 22 mcg week 5 and ongoing; *Titration Schedule (44 mcg prescribed dose):* 8.8 mcg week 1 & 2; 22 mcg week 3 & 4; 44 mcg week 5 and ongoing

> > *Prefilled syringe:* 22, 44 mcg/0.5 ml w. needle (12/carton) (albumin [human], preservative-free); (titration pack, 6 doses of 8.8 mcg [0.2 ml] w. needle per carton) (albumin [human], preservative-free)

Comment: Only prefilled syringes (**Rebif**) can be used to titrate to the 22 mcg prescribed dose. Prefilled syringes or autoinjectors (**Rebif Rebidose**) can be used to titrate to the 44 mcg prescribed dose.

> **Rebif Rebidose** administer SC 3x/week (at least 48 hours apart and preferably in the late afternoon or evening) after titration to 22 mcg or 44 mcg

> > Titration Schedule: *see* **Rebif.**

> > *Prefilled autoinjector:* 22, 44 mcg/0.5 ml (0.5ml, 12/carton) (titration pack, 6 doses of 8.8 mcg [0.2 ml] per carton (albumin [human], preservative-free)

Comment: Only prefilled syringes (**Rebif**) can be used to titrate to the 22 mcg prescribed dose. Prefilled syringes or autoinjectors (**Rebif Rebidose**) can be used to titrate to the 44 mcg prescribed dose.

▷ *interferon beta-1b* (C)
  Pediatric: <18 years: not recommended
      Actimmune *BSA ≤0.5m²*: 1.5 mgc/kg SC in a single dose 3 times weekly; *BSA ≥0.5m²*: 50 mgc/m² SC in a single dose 3 times weekly *Vial:* 100 mcg/0.5 ml single-dose for SC injection
      Betaseron, Extavia 0.0625 mg (0.25 ml) SC every other day; increase over 6 weeks to 0.25 mg (1 ml) SC every other day
          Vial: 0.3 mg/vial pwdr for reconstitution (single-dose w. prefilled diluents syringes) (albumin [human], mannitol, preservative-free)
▷ *natalizumab* (C) administer 300 mg by IV infusion over 1 hour every 4 weeks; monitor during infusion and for 1 hour postinfusion
  Pediatric: <18 years: not recommended
      Tysabri *Vial:* 300 mg/15 ml (15 ml)

◯ MUMPS (INFECTIOUS PAROTITIS)

PROPHYLAXIS

▷ *measles, mumps, rubella, live, attenuated, neomycin vaccine* (C)
      MMR II 25 mcg SC (preservative-free)
  Comment: Contraindications: hypersensitivity to *neomycin* or eggs, primary or acquired immune deficiency, immunosuppressant therapy, bone marrow or lymphatic malignancy, and pregnancy (within 3 months after vaccination).
  see **Childhood Immunizations** *page* 462
  Parenteral Corticosteroids *see page* 499
  Oral Corticosteroids *see page* 497
  Antipyretics *see Fever page* 143

◯ MUSCLE STRAIN

Comment: Usual length of treatment for acute injury is approximately 5 days.
Acetaminophen for IV Infusion *see Pain page* 296
Narcotic Analgesics *see Pain page* 298
Parenteral Corticosteroids *see page* 499
Oral Corticosteroids *see page* 497

SKELETAL MUSCLE RELAXANTS

▷ *baclofen* (C)(G) 5 mg tid; titrate up by 5 mg every 3 days to 20 mg tid; max 80 mg/day
  Pediatric: not recommended
      Lioresal *Tab:* 10*, 20*mg
  Comment: *baclofen* is indicated for muscle spasm pain and chronic spasticity associated with multiple sclerosis and spinal cord injury or disease. Potential for seizures or hallucinations on abrupt withdrawal.
▷ *carisoprodol* (C)(G) 1 tab tid or qid
  Pediatric: not recommended
      Soma *Tab:* 350 mg

▷ *chlorzoxazone* (NR)(G) 1 caplet qid; max 750 mg qid
  Pediatric: not recommended
    Parafon Forte DSC *Cplt:* 500*mg
▷ *cyclobenzaprine* (B)(G) 10 mg tid; usual range 20-40 mg/day in divided doses; max 60 mg/day x 2-3 weeks or 15 mg ext-rel once daily; max 30 mg ext-rel/day x 2-3 weeks
  Pediatric: <15 years: not recommended
    Amrix *Cap:* 15, 30 mg ext-rel
    Fexmid *Tab:* 7.5 mg
    Flexeril *Tab:* 5, 10 mg
▷ *dantrolene* (C) 25md daily x 7 days; then 25 mg tid x 7 days; then 50 mg tid x 7 days; max 100 mg qid
  Pediatric: 0.5 mg/kg daily x 7 days; then 0.5 mg/kg tid x 7 days; then 1 mg/kg tid x 7 days; then 2 mg/kg tid; max 100 mg qid
    Dantrium *Tab:* 25, 50, 100 mg
  Comment: *dantrolene* is indicated for chronic spasticity associated with multiple sclerosis and spinal cord injury or disease.
▷ *diazepam* (C)(IV) 2-10 mg bid-qid; may increase gradually
  Pediatric: <6 months: not recommended; >6 months: initially 1-2.5 mg bid-qid; may increase gradually
    Diastat *Rectal gel delivery system:* 2.5 mg
    Diastat AcuDial *Rectal gel delivery system:* 10, 20 mg
    Valium *Tab:* 2, 5, 10 mg
    Valium Intensol *Conc oral soln:* 5 mg/ml (30 ml w. dropper)(alcohol 19%)
    Valium Oral Solution *Oral soln:* 5 mg/5 ml (500 ml) (wintergreen spice)
▷ *metaxalone* (B) 1 tab tid-qid
  Pediatric: not recommended
    Skelaxin *Tab:* 800*mg
▷ *methocarbamol* (C)(G) initially 1.5 g qid x 2-3 days; maintenance, 750 mg every 4 hours or 1.5 g 3 times daily; max 8 g/day
  Pediatric: <16 years: not recommended
    Robaxin *Tab:* 500 mg
    Robaxin 750 *Tab:* 750 mg
    Robaxin Injection 10 ml IM or IV; max 30 ml/day; max 3 days; max 5 ml/gluteal injection q 8 hours; max IV rate 3 ml/min
      Vial: 100 mg/ml (10 ml)
▷ *nabumetone* (C)
  Pediatric: not recommended
    Relafen *Tab:* 500, 750 mg
    Relafen 500 *Tab:* 500 mg
▷ *orphenadrine citrate* (C)(G) 1 tab bid
  Pediatric: not recommended
    Norflex *Tab:* 100 mg sust-rel
▷ *tizanidine* (C) 1-4 mg q 6-8 hours; max 36 mg/day
  Pediatric: not recommended
    Zanaflex *Tab:* 2*, 4**mg; *Cap:* 2, 4, 6 mg

SKELETAL MUSCLE RELAXANT/NSAID COMBINATIONS

Comment: *aspirin*-containing medications are contraindicated with history of allergic-type reaction to *aspirin*, children and adolescents with *Varicella* or other viral illness, and 3rd trimester pregnancy.

▷ *carisoprodol/aspirin* (C)(III)(G) 1-2 tabs qid
  Pediatric: not recommended
      Soma Compound *Tab: caris* 200 mg/*asa* 325 mg (sulfites)
▷ *meprobamate/aspirin* (D)(IV) 1-2 tabs tid or qid
  Pediatric: not recommended
      Equagesic *Tab: mepro* 200 mg/*asa* 325*mg

SKELETAL MUSCLE RELAXANT/NSAID/CAFFEINE COMBINATIONS

▷ *orphenadrine/aspirin/caffeine* (D)(G)
  Pediatric: not recommended
      Norgesic 1-2 tabs tid-qid
          Tab: orphen 25 mg/*asa* 385 mg/*caf* 30 mg
      Norgesic Forte 1 tab tid or qid; max 4 tabs/day
          Tab: orphen 50 mg/*asa* 770 mg/*caf* 60*mg

SKELETAL MUSCLE RELAXANT/NSAID/CODEINE COMBINATIONS

▷ *carisoprodol/aspirin/codeine* (D)(III)(G)
  Pediatric: not recommended
      Soma Compound w. Codeine 1-2 tabs qid
          Tab: caris 200 mg/*asa* 325 mg/*cod* 16 mg (sulfites)

TOPICAL/TRANSDERMAL NSAIDs

▷ *capsaicin* (B)(G) apply tid-qid prn to intact skin
  Pediatric: <2 years: not recommended; ≥2 years: apply sparingly tid-qid prn
      Axsain *Crm:* 0.075% (1, 2 oz)
      Capsin *Lotn:* 0.025, 0.075% (59 ml)
      Capzasin-P (OTC) *Crm:* 0.025% (1.5 oz); *Lotn:* 0.025% (2 oz)
      Dolorac *Crm:* 0.025% (28 g)
      Double Cap (OTC) *Crm:* 0.05% (2 oz)
      R-Gel *Gel:* 0.025% (15, 30 g)
      Zostrix (OTC) *Crm:* 0.025% (0.7, 1.5, 3 oz)
      Zostrix HP (OTC) *Emol crm:* 0.075% (1, 2 oz)
▷ *capsaicin* 8% patch (B) apply up to 4 patches for one 60-minute application to clean
  dry skin; may prep area with topical anesthetic; wear nonlatex gloves; patches may be
  cut to size/ shape; treatment may be repeated every 3 months; remove with cleansing
  gel after treatment
  Pediatric: <18 years: not recommended
      Qutenza *Patch:* 8% 1640 mcg/cm (179 mg; 1 or 2 patches, each w. 1-50 g tube
      cleansing gel/carton)
▷ *diclofenac epolamine transdermal patch* (C; D ≥30 wks) apply one patch to affected
  area bid; remove during bathing; avoid non-intact skin
  Pediatric: not recommended
      Flector Patch *Patch:* 180 mg/patch (30/carton)

ORAL NSAIDs

▷ *diclofenac* (C)
  Pediatric: <18 years: not recommended
      Zorvolex take on empty stomach; 35 mg tid; *Hepatic impairment:* use lowest dose
      Gelcap: 18, 35 mg

▷ *diclofenac sodium* (C)
 Pediatric: <18 years: not recommended
  Voltaren 50 mg bid-qid <u>or</u> 75 mg bid <u>or</u> 25 mg qid with an additional 25 mg at HS if necessary
   Tab: 25, 50, 75 mg ent-coat
  Voltaren XR 100 mg once daily; rarely, 100 mg bid may be used
   Tab: 100 mg ext-rel
For an expanded list of Oral Prescription NSAIDs *see page* 489

ORAL NSAIDS/PPI COMBINATIONS

▷ *esomeprazole/naproxen* (C) 1 tab bid; use lowest effective dose for the shortest duration swallow whole; take at least 30 minutes before a meal
 Pediatric: <18 years: not recommended
  Vimovo *Tab: nap* 375 mg/*eso* 20 mg ext-rel; *nap* 500 mg/*eso* 20 mg ext-rel
  Comment: Vimovo is indicated to improve signs/symptoms, and risk of gastric ulcer in patients at risk of developing NSAID-associated gastric ulcer.

COX-2 INHIBITORS

Comment: Cox-2 inhibitors are contraindicated with history of asthma, urticaria, and allergic-type reactions to **aspirin**, other NSAIDs, and sulfonamides, 3rd trimester of pregnancy, and coronary artery bypass graft (CABG) surgery.
▷ *celecoxib* (C)(G) 100-400 mg daily bid; max 800 mg/day
 Pediatric: <18 years: not recommended
  Celebrex *Cap:* 50, 100, 200, 400 mg
▷ *meloxicam* (C)(G) initially 7.5 mg once daily; max 15 mg once daily
 Pediatric: <2 years: not recommended; ≥2 years: 0.125 mg/kg; max 7.5 mg once daily
  Mobic *Tab:* 7.5, 15 mg; *Oral susp:* 7.5 mg/5 ml (100 ml) (raspberry)
  Vivlodex *Cap:* 5, 10 mg

TOPICAL/TRANSDERMAL NSAIDs

▷ *capsaicin* (B)(G) apply tid-qid prn to intact skin
 Pediatric: <2 years: not recommended; ≥2 years: apply sparingly tid-qid prn
  Axsain *Crm:* 0.075% (1, 2 oz)
  Capsin *Lotn:* 0.025, 0.075% (59 ml)
  Capzasin-P (OTC) *Crm:* 0.025% (1.5 oz); *Lotn:* 0.025% (2 oz)
  Dolorac *Crm:* 0.025% (28 g)
  Double Cap (OTC) *Crm:* 0.05% (2 oz)
  R-Gel *Gel:* 0.025% (15, 30 g)
  Zostrix (OTC) *Crm:* 0.025% (0.7, 1.5, 3 oz)
  Zostrix HP (OTC) *Emol crm:* 0.075% (1, 2 oz)
▷ *capsaicin* 8% patch (B) apply up to 4 patches for one 60-minute application to clean dry skin; may prep area with topical anesthetic; wear nonlatex gloves; patches may be cut to size/ shape; treatment may be repeated every 3 months; remove with cleansing gel after treatment
 Pediatric: <18 years: not recommended
  Qutenza *Patch:* 8% 1640 mcg/cm (179 mg; 1 <u>or</u> 2 patches, each w. 1-50 g tube cleansing gel/ carton)

▸ *diclofenac epolamine transdermal patch* (C; D ≥30 wks) apply one patch to affected area bid; remove during bathing; avoid nonintact skin
Pediatric: not recommended
    Flector Patch *Patch:*180 mg/patch (30/carton)
▸ *diclofenac sodium* (C; D ≥30 wks) (G) apply gel qid prn; avoid non-intact skin
Pediatric: not recommended
    Voltaren Gel *Gel:* 1% (100 g)

TOPICAL/TRANSDERMAL LIDOCAINE

▸ *lidocaine* transdermal patch (C)(G) apply one patch to affected area for 12 hours (then off for 12 hours); remove during bathing; avoid non-intact skin
Pediatric: not recommended
    Lidoderm *Patch:* 5% (10 cm x14 cm; 30/carton)

 NARCOLEPSY

STIMULANTS

▸ *amphetamine sulfate* (C)(II) administer first dose on awakening, and additional doses at 4- to 6-hour intervals; usual range 5-60 mg/day
Pediatric: <6 years: not recommended; 6-12 years: 5 mg daily in the AM; may increase by 5 mg/day at weekly intervals; >12-18 years: initially 10 mg in the AM; may increase by 10 mg daily at weekly intervals
    Evekeo initially 10 mg once <u>or</u> twice daily at the same time(s) each day; may increase by 10 mg/day at weekly intervals; max 40 mg/day
        Pediatric: <6 years: not recommended; 6-12 years: initially 5 mg once <u>or</u> twice daily at the same time(s) each day; may increase by 5 mg/day at weekly intervals; max 40 mg/day; >12 years: same as adult
        Tab: 5, 10 mg
▸ *armodafinil* (C)(IV) *OSAHS:* 150-250 mg once daily in the AM; *SWSD:* 150 mg 1 hour before starting shift; reduce dose with severe hepatic impairment hepatic impairment
Pediatric: <17 years: not recommended
    Nuvigil *Tab:* 50, 150, 200, 250 mg
▸ *modafinil* (C)(IV)(G) 100-200 mg q AM; max 400 mg/day
Pediatric: <17 years: not recommended
    Provigil *Tab:* 100, 200*mg
    Comment: **Provigil** also promotes wakefulness in patients with shift work sleep disorder and excessive sleepiness due to obstructive sleep apnea/hypopnea syndrome.
▸ *sodium oxybate* (B) take dose at bedtime while in bed and repeat 2.5-4 hours later; titrate to effect; initially 4.5 grams/night in 2 divided doses; may increase by 1.5 g/night in 2 divided doses; max 9 g/night
Pediatric: <16 years: not recommended; ≥16 years: same as adult
    Xyrem *Oral soln:* 100, 200*mg
    Comment: **Xyrem** is used to reduce the number of cataplexy attacks (sudden loss of muscle strength) and reduce daytime sleepiness in patients with narcolepsy. Contraindicated with *alcohol* <u>or</u> CNS depressant (may impair consciousness; may lead to respiratory depression, coma, <u>or</u> death). Prepare both doses

prior to bedtime and do not attempt to get out of bed after taking the first dose. Place both doses within reach at the bedside. Set the bedside clock to awaken for the second dose. Dilute each dose in 60 ml (1/4 cup, 4 tblsp) water in child resistant dosing containers. Food significantly reduces the bioavailability of *sodium oxybate*; take at least 2 hours after ingesting food.

STIMULANTS

▷ *dextroamphetamine sulfate* (C)(II)(G) initially start with 10 mg daily; increase by 10 mg at weekly intervals if needed; may switch to daily dose with sust-rel spansules when titrated

Pediatric: <3 years: not recommended; 3-5 years: 2.5 mg daily; may increase by 2.5 mg daily at weekly intervals if needed; 6-12 years: initially 5 mg daily-bid; may increase by 5 mg/day at weekly intervals; usual max 40 mg/day; >12 years: initially 10 mg daily; may increase by mg/day at weekly intervals; max 40 mg/day 10

Dexedrine *Tab:* 5*mg (tartrazine)
Dexedrine Spansule *Cap:* 5, 10, 15 mg sust-rel
Dextrostat *Tab:* 5, 10 mg (tartrazine)

▷ *dextroamphetamine saccharate/dextroamphetamine sulfate/amphetamine aspartate/ amphetamine sulfate* (C)(II)(G)

Adderall initially 10 mg daily; may increase weekly by 10 mg/day; usual max 60 mg/day in 2-3 divided doses; first dose on awakening and then q 4-6 hours prn

Pediatric: <6 years: not indicated; 6-12 years: initially 5 mg daily; may increase weekly by 5 mg/day; usual max 40 mg/day in 2-3 divided doses; >12 years: same as adult

Tab: 5**, 7.5**, 10**, 12.5**, 15**, 20**, 30**mg

Adderall XR

Pediatric: <6 years: not recommended; 6-12 years: initially 10 mg daily in the AM; may increase by 10 mg weekly; max 30 mg/day; 13-17 years: initially 10 mg daily; may increase to 20 mg/day after 1 week; max 30 mg/day; Do not chew; may sprinkle on apple sauce

Cap: 5, 10, 15, 20, 25, 30 mg ext-rel

Comment: Adderall is also indicated to improve wakefulness in patients with shift-work sleep disorder and excessive sleepiness due to obstructive sleep apnea/hypopnea syndrome.

▷ *dexmethylphenidate* (C)(II) take once daily in the AM

Pediatric: <6 years: not recommended; ≥6 years: same as adult

Focalin initially 2.5 mg bid; allow at least 4 hours between doses; may increase at 1 week intervals; max 40 mg/day

Tab: 2.5, 5, 10*mg (dye-free)

Focalin XR 20-40 mg q AM; max 40 mg/day

Tab: 5, 10, 15, 20, 30, 40 mg ext-rel (dye-free)

▷ *methamphetamine* (C)(II)(G)

Desoxyn Granumets

Pediatric: <6 years: not recommended; ≥6 years: initially 5 mg daily bid; may increase by 5 mg/day at weekly intervals; usual effective dose; 20-25 mg/day

Tab: 5, 10, 15 mg sust-rel

▷ *methylphenidate (regular-acting)* (C)(II)(G)

Methylin, Methylin Chewable, Methylin Oral Solution usual dose 20-30 mg/day in 2-3 divided doses 30-45 minutes before a meal; may increase to 60 mg/day

Pediatric: <6 years: not recommended; ≥6 years: initially 5 mg twice daily before breakfast and lunch; may increase 5-10 mg/week; max 60 mg/day

Tab: 5, 10*, 20*mg; *Chew tab:* 2.5, 5, 10 mg (grape) (phenylalanine); *Oral soln:* 5, 10 mg/5 ml) (grape)

Ritalin 10-60 mg/day in 2-3 divided doses 30-45 minutes ac; max 60 mg/day

Pediatric: <6 years: not recommended; ≥6 years: initially 5 mg bid ac (before breakfast and lunch); may gradually increase by 5-10 mg at weekly intervals as needed; max 60 mg/day

Tab: 5, 10*, 20*mg

▷ *methylphenidate (long-acting)* (C)(II)

Concerta initially 18 mg q AM; may increase in 18 mg increments as needed; max 54 mg/ day; do not crush <u>or</u> chew

Tab: 18, 27, 36, 54 mg sust-rel

Metadate CD (G) 1 cap daily in the AM; may sprinkle on food; do not crush <u>or</u> chew

Pediatric: <6 years: not recommended; ≥6 years: initially 20 mg daily; may gradually increase by 20 mg/day at weekly intervals as needed; max 60 mg/day

Cap: 10, 20, 30, 40, 50, 60 mg immed- and ext-rel beads

Metadate ER 1 tab daily in the AM; do not crush <u>or</u> chew

Pediatric: <6 years: not recommended; ≥6 years: use in place of regular-acting **methylphenidate** when the 8-hour dose of **Metadate-ER** corresponds to the titrated 8-hour dose of regular-acting **methylphenidate**

Tab: 10, 20 mg ext-rel (dye-free)

Ritalin LA 1 cap daily in the AM

Pediatric: <6 years: not recommended; ≥6 years: use in place of regular-acting **methylphenidate** when the 8-hour dose of **Ritalin LA** corresponds to the titrated 8-hour dose of regular-acting **methylphenidate**; max 60 mg/day

Cap: 10, 20, 30, 40 mg ext-rel (immed- and ext-rel beads)

Ritalin SR 1 cap daily in the AM

Pediatric: <6 years: not recommended; ≥6 years: use in place of regular-acting **methylphenidate** when the 8-hour dose of **Ritalin SR** corresponds to the titrated 8-hour dose of regular-acting **methylphenidate**; max 60 mg/day

Tab: 20 mg sust-rel (dye-free)

▷ *methylphenidate (transdermal patch)* (C)(II)(G) 1 patch daily in the AM

Pediatric: <6 years: not recommended; ≥6 years: initially 10 mg patch daily in the AM; may increase by 5-10 mg/week; max 60 mg/day

Transdermal patch: 10, 15, 20, 30 mg

▷ *pemoline* (B)(IV) 18.75-112.5 mg/day; usually start with 37.5 mg in AM; increase weekly by 18.75 mg/day if needed; max 112.5 g/day

Pediatric: <6 years: not recommended; ≥6 years: same as adult

Cylert *Tab:* 18.75*, 37.5*, 75*mg

Cylert Chewable *Chew tab:* 37.5*mg

Comment: Monitor baseline serum ALT and repeat every 2 weeks thereafter.

NAUSEA/VOMITING

PROPHYLAXIS (FOR PREVENTION OF MOTION SICKNESS AND POST-OP NAUSEA AND VOMITING)

Anticholinergic Agents

▷ *scopolamine* (C)
> **Scopace** 0.4-0.8 mg 1 hour before travel; may repeat in 8 hours
> > *Pediatric:* not recommended
> > *Tab:* 0.4 mg
> **Transderm Scop** 1 patch behind ear at least 4 hours before travel; each patch is effective for 3 days
> > *Pediatric:* not recommended
> > *Transdermal patch:* 1.5 mg (4/carton)

MILD NAUSEA

▷ *phosphorylated carbohydrate* solution (C)(G) 1-2 tblsp q 15 minutes until nausea subsides; max 5 doses/day
Pediatric: 1-2 tsp q 15 minutes until nausea subsides; max 5 doses/day
> **Emetrol** (OTC) *Soln:* dextrose 1.87 g/fructose 1.87 g/phosphoric acid 21.5 mg per 5 ml (4, 8, 16 oz)

Cannabinoid

▷ *dronabinol* (C)(III) initially 5 mg/m² 1-3 hours before chemotherapy; then q 2-4 hours prn; max 4-6 doses/day, 15 mg/m²
> **Marinol** *Cap:* 2.5, 5, 10 mg (sesame seed oil)
▷ *nabilone* (C)(II) 1-2 mg bid; max 6 mg/day in 3 divided doses; initially 1-3 hours before chemotherapy; may give 1-2 mg the night before chemo; may continue 48 hours after each chemo cycle
> **Cesamet** *Cap:* 1 mg (sesame seed oil)

Antihistamines

▷ *diphenhydramine* (C)(G) 10-50 mg IV <u>or</u> deep IM q 6-8 hours prn; max 400 mg/day
Pediatric: 5 mg/kg/day in 4 divided doses; max 300 mg/day
> **Benadryl** *Vial:* 50 mg/ml (1 ml single-use); 50 mg/ml (10 ml multi-dose); *Amp:* 50 mg/ml (1 ml); *Prefilled syringe:* 50 mg/ml (1 ml)
▷ *meclizine* (C)(G) *Travel:* 25-50 mg 1 hour prior to travel; repeat every 24 hours; *Vertigo of vestibular origin:* 25-100 mg/day in divided doses
Pediatric: 5 mg/kg/day in 4 divided doses; max 300 mg/day
> **Antivert** *Tab:* 12.5, 25, 50*mg; *Amp:* 50 mg/ml (1 ml)
> > *Vial:* 50 mg/ml (1 ml single-use); 50 mg/ml (10 ml multi-dose)
> **Bonine** (OTC) *Cap:* 15, 25, 50 mg; *Tab:* 12.5, 25, 50 mg;
> > *Chew tab/Film-coat tab:* 25 mg
> **Dramamine II** (OTC) *Tab:* 25 mg
> **Zentrip** *Strip:* 25 mg orally-disint

MODERATE TO SEVERE NAUSEA

Phenothiazines

▷ *chlorpromazine* (C)(G) 10-25 mg PO q 4 hours prn <u>or</u> 50-100 mg rectally q 6-8 hours prn

Pediatric: <6 months: not recommended; ≥6 months: 0.25 mg/lb orally q 4-6 hours prn <u>or</u> 0.5 mg/lb rectally q 6-8 hours prn

> **Thorazine** *Tab:* 10, 25, 50, 100, 200 mg; *Spansule:* 30, 75, 150 mg sust-rel; *Syr:* 10 mg/5 ml (4 oz; orange custard); *Conc:* 30 mg/ml (4 oz); 100 mg/ml (2, 8 oz); *Supp:* 25, 100 mg

▷ *perphenazine* (C) 5 mg IM (may repeat in 6 hours) <u>or</u> 8-16 mg/day PO in divided doses; max 15 mg/day IM; max 24 mg/day po

Pediatric: not recommended

> **Trilafon** *Tab:* 2, 4, 8, 16 mg; *Oral conc:* 16 mg/ 5 ml (118 ml); *Amp:* 5 mg/ml (1 ml)

▷ *prochlorperazine* (C)(G) 5-10 mg tid-qid prn; usual max 40 mg/day

> **Compazine**
> *Pediatric:* <2 years <u>or</u> <20 lb: not recommended; 20-29 lb: 2.5 mg daily bid prn; max 7.5 mg/day; 30-39 lb: 2.5 mg bid-tid prn; max 10 mg/day; 40-85 lb: 2.5 mg tid <u>or</u> 5 mg bid prn; max 15 mg/day
> *Tab:* 5, 10 mg; *Syr:* 5 mg/5 ml (4 oz) (fruit)
> **Compazine Suppository** 25 mg rectally bid prn; usual max 50 mg/day
> *Pediatric:* <2 years <u>or</u> <20 lb: not recommended; 20-29 lb: 2.5 mg daily-bid prn; max 7.5; mg/day; 30-39 lb: 2.5 mg bid-tid prn; max 10 mg/day; 40-85 lb: 2.5 mg tid <u>or</u> 5 mg bid prn; max 15 mg/day
> *Rectal supp:* 2.5, 5, 25 mg
> **Compazine Injectable** 5-10 mg tid <u>or</u> qid prn
> *Pediatric:* <2 years <u>or</u> <20 lb: not recommended; ≥2 years <u>or</u> ≥20 lb: 0.06 mg/kg x 1 dose
> *Vial:* 5 mg/ml (2, 10 ml)
> **Compazine Spansule** 15 mg q AM prn <u>or</u> 10 mg q 12 hours prn usual max 40 mg/day
> *Pediatric:* not recommended
> *Spansule:* 10, 15 mg sust-rel

▷ *promethazine* (C)(G) 25 mg PO <u>or</u> rectally q 4-6 hours prn

Pediatric: <2 years: not recommended; ≥2 years: 0.5 mg/lb <u>or</u> 6.25-25 mg q 4-6 hours prn

> **Phenergan** *Tab:* 12.5*, 25*, 50 mg; *Plain syr:* 6.25 mg/5 ml; *Fortis syr:* 25 mg/5 ml; *Rectal supp:* 12.5, 25, 50 mg

Substance P/Neurokinin 1 Receptor Antagonist

▷ *aprepitant* (B) administer with corticosteroid and 5-HT-3 receptor antagonist; *Day 1 of chemotherapy cycle:* 125 mg 1 hour prior to chemotherapy *Day 2 & 3:* 80 mg in the morning

Pediatric: <6 months: years: not recommended; ≥6 months: use oral suspension (see mfr literature for dose by weight

> **Emend** *Cap:* 40, 80, 125 mg (2 x 80 mg bifold pck; 1 x 25 mg/2 x 80 mg tri-fold pck); *Oral susp:* 125 mg pwdr for oral suspension, single dose pouch w dispenser; *Vial:* 150 mg pwdr for reconstitution and IV infusion

5-HT-3 Receptor Antagonists

Comment: The selective 5-HT-3 receptor antagonists indicated for prevention of nausea and vomiting associated with moderately to highly emetogenic chemotherapy.

▷ **dolasetron** (B) administer 100 mg IV over 30 seconds, 30 min prior to administration of chemotherapy or 2 hours before surgery; max 100 mg /dose
  Pediatric: <2 years: not recommended; 2-16 years: 1.8 mg/kg; >16 years: same as adult
  Anzemet *Tab:* 50, 100 mg; *Amp:* 12.5 mg/0.625 ml; *Prefilled carpuject syringe:* 12.5 mg (0.625 ml); *Vial:* 100 mg/5 ml (single- use); *Vial:* 500 mg/25 ml (multi-dose)

▷ **granisetron** (B)
  Kytril administer IV over 30 seconds, 30 min prior to administration of chemo-therapy; max 1 dose/week
    Pediatric: <2 years: not recommended; ≥2 years: 10 mcg/kg
    Tab: 1 mg; *Oral soln:* 2 mg/10 ml (30 ml; orange); *Vial:* 1 mg/ml (1 ml single-dose; preservative-free); 1 mg/ml (4 ml multi-dose) (benzyl alcohol)
  Sancuso apply 1 patch 24-48 hours before chemo; remove 24 hours (minimum) to 7 days (maximum) after completion of treatment
    Transdermal patch: 3.1 mg/day

▷ **ondansetron** (C)(G)
  Oral Forms: *Highly emetogenic chemotherapy:* 24 mg x 1 dose 30 min prior to start of single-day chemotherapy; *Moderately emetogenic chemotherapy:* 8 mg q 8 hours x 2 doses beginning 30 minutes prior to start of chemotherapy; then 8 mg q 12 hours x 1-2 days following
    Pediatric: <4 years: not recommended; 4-11 years, moderately emetogenic chemotherapy: 4 mg q 4 hours x 3 doses beginning 30 min prior to start; then 4 mg q 8 hours x 1-2 days following
  Zofran *Tab:* 4, 8, 24 mg
  Zofran ODT *ODT:* 4, 8 mg (strawberry) (phenylalanine)
  Zofran Oral Solution *Oral soln:* 4 mg/5 ml (50 ml) (strawberry) (phenylala-nine); *Parenteral form:* see mfr literature
  Zofran Injection *Vial:* 2 mg/ml (2 ml single-dose); 2 mg/ml (20 ml multi-dose); 32 mg/50 ml (50 ml multi-dose); *Prefilled syringe:* 4 mg/2 ml, single-use (24/carton)
  Zuplenz Oral Soluble Film: 4, 8 mg oral-dis (10/carton) (peppermint)

▷ **palonosetron** (B)(G) *Chemotherapy:* administer 0.25 mg IV over 30 seconds, 30 min prior to administration of chemo; max 1 dose/week or 1 cap 1 hour before chemo; *Post-op:* administer 0.075 mg IV over 10 seconds immediately before induction of anesthesia
  Pediatric: <1 month: not recommended; 1 month to 17 years: 20 mcg/kg; max 1.5 mg single-dose; infuse over 15 minutes beginning 30 minutes prior to administration of chemo
  Aloxi *Vial (single-use):* 0.075 mg/1.5 ml; 0.25 mg/5 ml (mannitol)

ANTI-DOPAMINERGIC (PROMOTILITY) AGENTS

▷ **metoclopramide** (B) 10 mg 30 minutes before each meal and at HS for 2-8 weeks
  Metozolv ODT *ODT:* 5, 10 mg (mint)
  Reglan *Tab:* 5, 10*mg

Comment: *metoclopramide* is contraindicated when stimulation of GI motility may be dang6erous. Observe for tardive dyskinesia and Parkinsonism.
Avoid concomitant drugs which may cause an extrapyramidal reaction (e.g., phenothiazines, *haloperidol*).
Substance P/Neurokinin-1 (NK-1) Receptor Antagonist
➤ *rolapitant* (NR) take 180 mg in a single dose 1-2 hours before chemotherapy treatment; administer in combination with dexamethasone and 5-HT3 receptor antagonist
Pediatric: not established
  Varubi *Tab:* 90 mg film-coat
  Comment: Varubi is indicated in combination with other antiemetic agents in adults for the prevention of delayed nausea and vomiting associated with emetogenic cancer chemotherapy.

SUBSTANCE P/NEUROKININ-1 (NK-1) RECEPTOR ANTAGONIST/5-HT-3 RECEPTOR ANTAGONIST COMBINATION

➤ *netupitant/palonosetron* (C) take one cap approximately 1 hour prior to chemotherapy; administer in combination with dexamethasone
Pediatric: not established
  Akynzeo *Gelcap:* netu 300 mg/*palo* 0.5 mg
  Comment: Akynzeo is indicated in combination with other antiemetic agents in adults for the prevention of delayed nausea and vomiting associated with emetogenic cancer chemotherapy.

◯ NERVE AGENT POISONING

➤ *atropine sulfate* (NR)(G) 2 mg IM
Pediatric: <15 lb: not recommended; ≥15-40 lb: 0.5 mg IM; ≥40-90 lb: 1 mg IM; >90 lb: same as adult
  AtroPen *Pen (single-use):* 0.5, 1, 2 mg (0.5 ml)

◯ NON-24 SLEEP-WAKE DISORDER

Comment: For other drug options (stimulants, sedative hypnotics), *see* Insomnia *page* 233, Sleepiness: Excessive, Shift Work Sleep Disorder *page* 391

MELATONIN RECEPTOR AGONIST

➤ *tasimelteon* (C) take 1 gelcap before bedtime at the same time every night; do not take with food
Pediatric: not established
  Hetlioz *Gel cap:* 20 mg

OREXIN RECEPTOR ANTAGONIST

➤ *suvorexant* (C)(IV) use lowest effective dose; take 30 minutes before bedtime; do not take if unable to sleep for ≥7 hours; max 20 mg
Pediatric: not recommended
  Belsomra *Tab:* 5, 10, 15, 20 mg (30/blister pck)

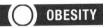 **OBESITY**

Comment: Target BMI is 25-30 (≤27 preferred).

STIMULANTS

▷ *amphetamine sulfate* (C)(II)
> **Evekeo** initially 5 mg 30-60 minutes before meals; usually up to 30 mg/day
> *Pediatric:* <12 years: not recommended; ≥12 years: same as adult
> *Tab:* 5, 10 mg

LIPASE INHIBITOR

▷ *orlistat* (X)(G) 1 cap tid 1 hour before or during each main meal containing fat
> *Pediatric:* <12 years: not recommended; ≥12 years: same as adult
> **Alli** (OTC) *Cap:* 60 mg
> **Xenical** *Cap:* 120 mg

Comment: For use when BMI >30 kg/m² or BMI >27 kg/m² in the presence of other risk factors (i.e., HTN, DM, dyslipidemia).

ANOREXIGENICS

Sympathomimetics

Comment: Side effects include hypertension, tachycardia, restlessness, insomnia, and dry mouth.

▷ *benzphetamine* (X)(III) initially 25-50 mg daily in the mid-morning or mid-afternoon; may increase to bid-tid as needed
> *Pediatric:* not recommended
> **Didrex** *Tab:* 50*mg

▷ *naltrexone/bupropion* (X) swallow whole; avoid high-fat meals; initially 10 mg bid; evaluate weight loss after 12 weeks; discontinue if less than 5% weight loss
> *Pediatric:* <18 years: not recommended
> **Contrave** *Tab:* nal 8 mg/bup 900 mg ext-rel

▷ *methamphetamine* (C)(II) 10-15 mg q AM
> *Pediatric:* <12 years: not recommended; ≥12 years: same as adult
> **Desoxyn** *Tab:* 5, 10, 15 mg sust-rel

▷ *phendimetrazine* (C)(III)
> *Pediatric:* <12 years: not recommended; ≥12 years: same as adult
> **Bontril PDM** 35 mg bid-tid 1 hour ac; may reduce to 17.5 mg (1/2 tab)/dose; max 210 mg/ day in 3 divided doses
> > *Tab:* 35*mg
> **Bontril Slow-Release** 105 mg in the AM 30-60 minutes before breakfast
> > *Cap:* 105 mg slow-rel

▷ *phentermine* (C)(IV)
> *Pediatric:* <16 years: not recommended; ≥16 years: same as adult
> **Adipex-P** (G) 1 cap or tab before breakfast or 1/2 tab bid ac
> > *Cap:* 37.5 mg; *Tab:* 37.5*mg
> **Fastin** (G) 1 cap before breakfast
> > *Cap:* 30 mg
> **Ionamin** (G) 1 cap before breakfast or 10-14 hours prior to HS
> > *Cap:* 15, 30 mg

Suprenza ODT (X)(IV) dissolve 1 tab on top of tongue once daily in the morning, with or without food; use lowest effective dose
Tab: 15, 30, 37.5 mg orally-disint
Comment: Contraindicated with history of cardiovascular disease (e.g., coronary artery disease, stroke, arrhythmias, congestive heart failure, uncontrolled hypertension, during or within 14 days following the administration of an MOAI, hyperthyroidism, glaucoma, agitated states, history of drug abuse, pregnancy, nursing).

Sympathomimetic/Antiepileptic Combination

▶ *phentermine/topiramate ext-rel* **(X)(IV)(G)** initially 3.75 mg/23 mg daily in the AM x 14 days; then increase to 7.5 mg/46 mg and evaluate weight loss on this dose after 12 weeks; if ≤3% weight loss from baseline, discontinue or increase dose to 11.25 mg/69 mg x 14 days; then increase to 15 mg/92 mg and evaluate weight loss on this dose after 12 weeks; if ≤5% weight loss from baseline, discontinue by taking a dose every other day for at least one week prior to stopping; max 7.5 mg/46 mg for moderate to severe renal impairment or moderate hepatic impairment.
Pediatric: <16 years: not established; ≥16 years: same as adult
Qsymia
Cap: **Qsymia 3.75/23:** *phen* 3.75 mg/*topir* 23 mg ext-rel
Qsymia 7.5/46: *phen* 7.5 mg/*topir* 46 mg ext-rel
Qsymia 11.25/69: *phen* 11.25 mg/*topir* 69 mg ext-rel
Qsymia 15/92: *phen* 15 mg/*topir* 92 mg ext-rel
Comment: Side effects include hypertension, tachycardia, restlessness, insomnia, and dry mouth. Contraindicated with glaucoma, hyperthyroidism, and within 14 days of taking an MAOI. **Qsymia 3.75/23** and **Qsymia 11.25/69** are for titration purposes only.

Serotonin 2C Receptor Agonist

▶ *lorcaserin* **(X)(G)** 10 mg bid; discontinue if 5% weight loss is not achieved by week 12
Pediatric: <18 years: not recommended
Belviq *Tab:* 10 mg film-coat
Comment: **Belviq** is indicated as an adjunct to a reduced-calorie diet and increased physical activity for chronic weight management in adults with an initial body mass index (BMI) of 30 kg/m² or greater (obese) or 27 kg/m² or greater (overweight) in the presence of at least one weight-related comorbid condition (e.g., hypertension, dyslipidemia, type 2 diabetes). Serotonin 2C receptor agonists interact with serotonergic drugs (selective serotonin reuptake inhibitors (SSRIs), serotonin-norepinephrine reuptake inhibitors (SNRIs), monoamine oxidase inhibitors (MAOIs), triptans, *bupropion, dextromethorphan, St. John's wort*); therefore, use with extreme caution due to the risk of serotonin syndrome.

GLUCAGON-LIKE PEPTIDE-1 (GLP-1) RECEPTOR AGONIST

▶ *liraglutide* **(C)** administer SC in the upper arm, abdomen, or thigh once daily; escalate dose gradually over 5 weeks to 3 mg SC daily; *Week 1:* 0.6 mg SC daily; *Week 2:* 1.2 mg SC daily; *Week 3:* 1.8 mg SC daily; *Week 4:* 2.4 mg SC daily; *Week 5:* 3 mg SC daily;
Pediatric: <18 years: not recommended
Saxenda Soln for SC inj: 6 mg/ml multi-dose prefilled pen (3 ml; 3, 5 pens/carton)

Comment: **Saxenda** is indicated as an adjunct to a reduced-calorie diet and increased physical activity for chronic weight management in adults with an initial body mass index (BMI) of 30 kg/m² or greater (obese) or 27 kg/m² or greater overweight) in the presence of at least one weight-related comorbid condition (e.g., hypertension, dyslipidemia, type 2 diabetes). Not indicated for treatment of T2DM. Do not use with Victoza, other GLP-1 receptor agonists, or insulin. Contraindicated with personal or family history of medullary thyroid carcinoma (MTC) and multiple endocrine neoplasia syndrome (MENS) type 2. Monitor for signs/ symptoms pancreatitis. Discontinue if gastroparesis, renal, or hepatic impairment.

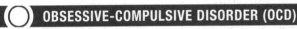

OBSESSIVE-COMPULSIVE DISORDER (OCD)

SELECTIVE SEROTONIN REUPTAKE INHIBITORS (SSRIs)

Comment: Co-administration of SSRIs with TCAs requires extreme caution. Concomitant use of MAOIs and SSRIs is absolutely contraindicated. Avoid other serotonergic drugs. A potentially fatal adverse event is *Serotonin Syndrome*, caused by serotonin excess. Milder symptoms require HCP intervention to avert severe symptoms which can be rapidly fatal without urgent/emergent medical care. Symptoms include restlessness, agitation, confusion, hallucinations, tachycardia, hypertension, dilated pupils, muscle twitching, muscle rigidity, loss of muscle coordination, diaphoresis, diarrhea, headache, shivering, piloerection, hyperpyrexia, cardiac arrhythmias, seizures, loss of consciousness, coma, death. Abrupt withdrawal or interruption of treatment with an antidepressant medication is sometimes associated with an *Antidepressant Discontinuation Syndrome* which may be mediated by gradually tapering the drug over a period of two weeks or longer, depending on the dose strength and length of treatment. Common symptoms of the *Serotonin Discontinuation Syndrome* include flu-like symptoms (nausea, vomiting, diarrhea, headaches, sweating), sleep disturbances (insomnia, nightmares, constant sleepiness), mood disturbances (dysphoria, anxiety, agitation), cognitive disturbances (mental confusion, hyperarousal), sensory and movement disturbances (imbalance, tremors, vertigo, dizziness, electric-shock-like sensations in the brain, often described by sufferers as "brain zaps."

➤ *fluoxetine* (C)(G)
  Prozac initially 20 mg daily; may increase after 1 week; doses >20 mg/day may be divided into AM and noon doses; max 80 mg/day
    Pediatric: <7 years: not recommended; 7-17 years: initially 10 mg/day; may increase after 2 weeks to 20 mg/day; range 20-60 mg/day; range for lower weight children 20-30 mg/day
    Cap: 10, 20, 40 mg; *Tab:* 30*, 60*mg; *Oral soln:* 20 mg/5 ml (4 oz) (mint)
  Prozac Weekly following daily *fluoxetine* therapy at 20 mg/day for 13 weeks, may initiate **Prozac Weekly** 7 days after the last 20 mg *fluoxetine* dose
    Pediatric: not recommended
    Cap: 90 mg ent-coat del-rel pellets

➤ *fluvoxamine* (C)
  Luvox initially 50 mg q HS; adjust in 50 mg increments at 4-7 day intervals; range 100-300 mg/day; over 100 mg/day, divide into 2 doses giving the larger dose at HS

Pediatric: <8 years: not recommended; 8-17 years: initially 25 mg q HS; adjust in 25 mg increments q 4-7 days; usual range 50-200 mg/day; over 50 mg/day, divide into 2 doses giving the larger dose at HS
> *Tab:* 25, 50*, 100*mg

Luvox CR initially 100 mg once daily at HS; may increase by 50 mg increments at 1 week intervals; max 300 mg/day; swallow whole
Pediatric: <18 years: not recommended
> *Cap:* 100, 150 mg ext-rel

▷ *paroxetine maleate* (D)(G)
Pediatric: not recommended

Paxil initially 20 mg daily in AM; may increase by 10 mg/day at weekly intervals as needed; max 60 mg/day
> *Tab:* 10*, 20*, 30, 40 mg

Paxil CR initially 25 mg daily in AM; may increase by 12.5 mg at weekly intervals as needed; max 62.5 mg/day
> *Tab:* 12.5, 25, 37.5 mg cont-rel ent-coat

Paxil Suspension initially 20 mg daily in AM; may increase by 10 mg/day at weekly intervals as needed; max 60 mg/day
> *Oral susp:* 10 mg/5 ml (250 ml) (orange)

▷ *sertraline* (C) initially 50 mg daily; increase at 1 week intervals if needed; max 200 mg daily
Pediatric: <6 years: not recommended; 6-12 years: initially 25 mg daily; max 200 mg/day; 13-17 years: initially 50 mg daily; max 200 mg/day

Zoloft *Tab:* 15*, 50*, 100*mg; *Oral conc:* 20 mg per ml (60 ml [dilute just before administering in 4 oz water, ginger ale, lemon-lime soda, lemonade, <u>or</u> orange juice]) (alcohol 12%)

TRICYCLIC ANTIDEPRESSANT (TCA) COMBINATIONS

▷ *clomipramine* (C)(G) initially 25 mg daily in divided doses; gradually increase to 100 mg during first 2 weeks; max 250 mg/day; total maintenance dose may be given at HS
Pediatric: <10 years: not recommended; ≥10 years: initially 25 mg daily in divided doses; gradually increase; max 3 mg/kg <u>or</u> 100 mg, whichever is smaller
Anafranil *Cap:* 25, 50, 75 mg

▷ *imipramine* (C)(G)
Tofranil initially 75 mg/day; max 200 mg/day
Pediatric: adolescents initially 30-40 mg/day; max 100 mg/day
> *Tab:* 10, 25, 50 mg

Tofranil PM initially 75 mg/day; max 200 mg/day
Pediatric: not recommended
> *Cap:* 75, 100, 125, 150 mg

 ONYCHOMYCOSIS (FUNGAL NAIL)

ORAL AGENTS

▷ *griseofulvin, microsize* (C)(G) 1 g daily for at least 4 months for fingernails and at least 6 months for toenails
Pediatric: 5 mg/lb/day; *see page 525 for dose by weight*
Grifulvin V *Tab:* 250, 500 mg; *Oral susp:* 125 mg/5 ml (120 ml; alcohol 0.02%)

➤ *griseofulvin, ultramicrosize* (C) 750 mg in a single <u>or</u> divided doses for at least 4 months for fingernails and at least 6 months for toenails
  Pediatric: <2 years: not recommended; ≥2 years: 3.3 mg/lb in a single <u>or</u> divided doses
    Gris-PEG *Tab:* 125, 250 mg
➤ *itraconazole* (C)(G) 200 mg daily x 12 consecutive weeks for toenails; 200 mg bid x 1 week, off 3 weeks, then 200 mg bid x 1 additional week for fingernails
  Pediatric: not recommended
      Sporanox *Cap:* 100 mg; *Soln:* 10 mg/ml (150 ml) (cherry-caramel)
      Pulse Pack: 100 mg caps (7/pck)
➤ *terbinafine* (B)(G) 250 mg daily x 6 weeks for fingernails; 250 mg daily x 12 weeks for toenails
  Pediatric: not recommended
      Lamisil *Tab:* 250 mg

TOPICAL AGENTS

Comment: File and trim nail while nail is free from drug. Remove unattached infected nail as frequently as monthly. For use with mild to moderate onychomycosis of the fingernails and toenails, without lunula involvement due to *Trichophyton rubrum* immunocompetent patients as part of a comprehensive treatment program. For use on nails and adjacent skin only. Apply evenly to entire onycholytic nail and surrounding 5 mm of skin daily, preferably at HS <u>or</u> 8 hours before washing; apply to nail bed, hyponychium, and under surface of nail plate when it is free of the nail bed; apply over previous coats, then remove with alcohol once per week; treat for up to 48 weeks.

➤ *ciclopirox* (B)
  Pediatric: not established
      Penlac Nail Lacquer *Topical soln (lacquer):* 8% (6.6 ml w. applicator)
➤ *efinaconazole* (C)
  Pediatric: not established
      Jublia *Topical soln:* 5% (10 ml w. brush applicator)
➤ *tavaborole* (C)
  Pediatric: not established
      Kerydin *Topical soln:* 10% (10 ml w. dropper)

 OPHTHALMIA NEONATORUM: CHLAMYDIAL

PROPHYLAXIS

➤ *erythromycin* ophthalmic ointment 0.5-1 cm ribbon into lower conjunctival sac of each eye x 1 application
      Ilotycin Ophthalmic Ointment *Ophth oint:* 5 mg/g (1/8 oz)
Comment: The following treatment regimens are published in the **2015 CDC Sexually Transmitted Diseases Treatment Guidelines**. Treatment regimens are presented by generic drug name first, followed by information about brands and dose forms.

RECOMMENDED REGIMENS

Regimen 1

➤ *erythromycin base* 50 mg/kg/day in 4 doses x 14 days

Regimen 2

▷ *erythromycin ethylsuccinate* 50 mg/kg/day in 4 doses x 14 days

DRUG BRANDS AND DOSE FORMS

▷ *erythromycin base* (B)(G)
  Pediatric: <45 kg: 30-50 mg in 2-4 divided doses x 7-10 days; ≥45 kg: same as adult
    Ery-Tab *Tab:* 250, 333, 500 mg ent-coat
    PCE *Tab:* 333, 500 mg
  Comment: *erythromycin* may increase INR with concomitant *warfarin*, as well as increase serum level of *digoxin*, benzodiazepines and statins.
▷ *erythromycin ethylsuccinate* (B)(G)
  Pediatric: 30-50 mg/kg/day in 4 divided doses x 7 days; may double dose with severe infection; max 100 mg/kg/day for at least 14 days; *see page 563 for dose by weight*
    EryPed *Oral susp:* 200 mg/5 ml (100, 200 ml) (fruit); 400 mg/5 ml (60, 100, 200 ml) (banana); *Oral drops:* 200, 400 mg/5 ml (50 ml) (fruit); *Chew tab:* 200 mg wafer (fruit)
    E.E.S. *Oral susp:* 200, 400 mg/5 ml (100 ml) (fruit)
    E.E.S. Granules *Oral susp:* 200 mg/5 ml (100, 200 ml) (cherry)
  Comment: *erythromycin* may increase INR with concomitant *warfarin*, as well as increase serum level of *digoxin*, benzodiazepines and statins.

OPHTHALMIA NEONATORUM: GONOCOCCAL

Comment: The following prophylaxis and treatment regimens for gonococcal conjunctivitis is published in the **2015 CDC Sexually Transmitted Diseases Treatment Guidelines.**

Regimen 1

▷ *erythromycin 0.5%* ophthalmic ointment 0.5-1 cm ribbon into lower conjunctival sac of each eye x 1 application
    Ilotycin Ophthalmic Ointment *Ophth oint:* 5 mg/g (1/8 oz)

Regimen 2

▷ *ceftriaxone* (B)(G) 25-50 mg/kg IV or IM in a single dose, not to exceed 125 mg
  Pediatric: 1 g IM in a single dose
    Rocephin *Vial:* 250, 500 mg; 1, 2 g

OPIOID DEPENDENCE OPIOID WITHDRAWAL SYNDROME

Safety labeling for all immediate-release (IR) opioids has been issued by the FDA. The boxed warning includes serious risks of misuse, abuse, addiction, overdose, and death. The dosing section offers clear steps regarding administration and patient monitoring including initial dose, dose changes, and the abrupt cessation of treatment in physical dependence. Chronic maternal use of opioids during pregnancy can lead to potentially life-threatening neonatal opioid withdrawal. The American Pain Society (APS) has released new evidence-based clinical practice guidelines that include 32 recommendations related to post-op pain management in adults and children.

NARCOTIC ANALGESIC

▷ *methadone* (C) *Narcotic Detoxification:* 15-40 mg daily in decreasing doses not to exceed 21 days; *Narcotic Maintenance:* >21 days; see mfr literature
  Pediatric: not established
    Dolphine *Tab:* 5, 10 mg; *Dispersible tab:* 40 mg (dissolve in 120 ml orange juice or other citrus drink); *Oral conc:* 5, 10 mg/5 ml; 10 mg/10 ml
  Comment: *methadone* maintenance is allowed only by approved providers with strict state and federal regulations.

OPIOID ANTAGONIST

▷ *naltrexone* (C)
  Pediatric: not established
    ReVia 50 mg daily
      Tab: 50 mg
    Vivitrol 380 mg IM once monthly; alternate buttocks
      Vial: 380 mg

OPIOID PARTIAL AGONIST-ANTAGONIST

Comment: **Butrans, Subutex, Sucartonone,** and **Zubsolv** maintenance are allowed only by approved providers with strict state and federal regulations.
▷ *buprenorphine* (C)(III)
    Belbuca *(buccal film)* (III)
      Pediatric: not established
      Buccal film: 75, 150, 300, 450, 600, 750, 900 mcg
    Butrans Transdermal System
      Pediatric: not established
      Transdermal patch: 5, 10, 20 mcg/hour (4/pck)
    Subutex (G) 8 mg in a single dose on day 1; then 16 mg in a single dose on day 2; target dose is 16 mg/day in a single dose; dissolve under tongue; do not chew or swallow whole
      Pediatric: not established
      SL tab (lemon-lime) or *SL film (lime):* 2, 8 mg (30/pck)

OPIOID PARTIAL AGONIST-ANTAGONIST/OPIOID ANTAGONIST

▷ *buprenorphine/naloxone* (C)(III) administer one buccal film once daily at the same time each day; target dose is 8.4/1.4 once daily; place the side of the **Bunavail** film with the text (BN2, BN4, or BN6) against the inside of the cheek; press and hold the film in place for 5 seconds; maintenance is usually 2.1/0.3 to 12.6/2.1
  Pediatric: <16 years: not recommended; ≥16 years: same as adult
    Bunavail
      SL film (lime):
    Bunavail 2.1/0.3 *bup* 2.1 mg/*nal* 0.3 mg (30/carton)
    Bunavail 4.2/0.7 *bup* 4.2 mg/*nal* 0.7 mg (30/carton)
    Bunavail 6.3/1 *bup* 6.3 mg/*nal* 1 mg (30/carton)

Comment: A **Bunavail** 4.2/0.7 mg buccal film provides equivalent buprenorphine exposure to a **Sucartonone** 8/2 mg sublingual tablet.

Sucartonone adjust in 2-4 mg of *buprenorphine*/day in a single dose; usual range is 4-24 mg/day in a single dose; target dose is 6 mg/day in a single dose; dissolve under tongue; do not chew or swallow whole

  Pediatric: <16 years: not recommended; ≥16 years: same as adult
  SL film (lime):
Sucartonone 2/0.5 *bup* 2 mg/*nal* 0.5 mg (30/pck)
Sucartonone 4/1 *bup* 4 mg/*nal* 1 mg (30/pck)
Sucartonone 8/2 *bup* 8 mg/*nal* 2 mg (30/pck)
Sucartonone 12/3 *bup* 12 mg/*nal* 3 mg (30/pck)
Zubsolv initial induction with buprenorphine sublingual tabs; administer as a single dose once daily; titrate dose in increments of 1.4/0.36 or 2.9/0.72 per day; recommended target dose is 11.4/2.9 per day; usual max 17.2/4.2 per day

  Pediatric: <16 years: not recommended; ≥16 years: same as adult
  SL tab:
Zubsolv 1.4/0.36 *bup* 1.4 mg/*nal* 0.36 mg
Zubsolv 2.9/0.72 *bup* 2.9 mg/*nal* 0.71 mg
Zubsolv 5.7/1.4 *bup* 5.7 mg/*nal* 1.4 mg
Zubsolv 8.6/2.1 *bup* 8.6 mg/*nal* 2.1 mg
Zubsolv 11.4/2.9 *bup* 11.4 mg/*nal* 2.9 mg
Comment: One **Subutex 5.7/1.4** S L tab is bioequivalent to one **Sucartonone** 8/2 SL film.

◯ OPIOID-INDUCED CONSTIPATION (OIC)

➤ *lubiprostone* (C) swallow whole; take with food and water; initially 24 mcg bid; *Moderate hepatic impairment (Child Pugh Class B):* 16 mg bid; *Severe hepatic impairment (Child Pugh Class C):* 8 mg bid
  Pediatric: not recommended
    Amitiza *Cap:* 8, 24 mg
➤ *methylnaltrexone bromide* (C) administer 12 mg SC once daily or once every other day, in the upper arm, abdomen, or thigh; max one dose/24 hrs; discontinue other laxatives; <38 kg-14 kg: 0.15 mg/kg; 38-<62 kg: 8 mg; 62-114 kg: 12 mg; *CrCl <30 mL/min:* reduce dose by half
  Pediatric: not established
    Relistor *Vial:* 8 mg/0.4 ml; 12 mg/0.6 ml single-use (7/carton); *Prefilled syringes* (7/carton)
➤ *naloxegol* (C) swallow whole; take on an empty stomach; initially 25 mg once daily in the AM; discontinue other laxatives; *CrCl <60 mL/min:* 12.5 mg
  Pediatric: not established
    Movantik *Tab:* 12.5, 25 mg

◯ OPIOID OVERDOSE

OPIOID ANTAGONISTS

➤ *nalmefene* (B) initially 0.25 mcg/kg IV, IM, or SC, then incremental doses of 0.25 mcg/kg at 2-5 minute intervals; cumulative max 1 mcg/kg; if opioid dependency suspected use 0.1 mg/70 kg initially and then proceed as usual if no response in 2 minutes

Pediatric: not recommended

    Revex *Amp:* 100 mcg/1 ml (1 ml); 1 mg/ml (2 ml)

▷ *naloxone* **(B)(G)** 0.4-2 mg; repeat in 2-3 minutes if no response

Pediatric: 0.01 mg/kg initially, repeat in 2-3 minutes at 0.1 mg/kg if response inadequate

    Evzio *Prefilled autoinjector:* 0.4 mg/0.4 ml IM/SC only

    Narcan *Vial/Amp:* 0.4 mg/ml (1 ml), 1 mg/ml (2 ml); *Prefilled syringe:* 0.4 mg ml (1 ml), 1 mg/ml (2 ml) IV, IM, <u>or</u> SC (parabens-free)

    Comment: If the electronic voice instruction system does not operate properly, **Evzio** will still deliver the intended dose of *naloxone* when used according to the printed instructions on the flat surface of the autoinjector label. **Evzio** cannot be administered IV. Due to the short duration of action of naloxone, as compared to opioids which are longer acting, monitoring of the patient is critical as the opioid reversal effects of naloxone may wear off before the effects of the opioid.

    Narcan Nasal Spray position supine with head tilted back; 1 spray in one nostril; if an additional dose is needed, spray into the opposite nostril

    Nasal spray: 4 mg/0.1 ml, single dose, single use (2 blister pcks, each w a single nasal spray/ carton)

OSGOOD-SCHLATTER DISEASE

Acetaminophen for IV Infusion *see Pain page* 296
Oral Prescription NSAIDs *see page* 489
Other Oral Analgesics *see Pain page* 298
Topical/Transdermal NSAIDs *see Pain page* 297
Parenteral Corticosteroids *see page* 499
Oral Corticosteroids *see page* 497
Topical Analgesic and Anesthetic Agents *see page* 487

OSTEOARTHRITIS

Acetaminophen for IV Infusion *see Pain page* 296
Oral Prescription NSAIDs *see page* 489
Other Oral Analgesics *see Pain page* 298
Topical/Transdermal NSAIDs *see Pain page* 297
Parenteral Corticosteroids *see page* 499
Oral Corticosteroids *see page* 497
Topical Analgesic and Anesthetic Agents *see page* 487

TOPICAL ANALGESICS

▷ *capsaicin* **(B)(G)** apply tid to qid prn to intact skin

Pediatric: <2 years: not recommended; ≥2 years: same as adult

    Axsain *Crm:* 0.075% (1, 2 oz)

    Capsin *Lotn:* 0.025, 0.075% (59 ml)

    Capzasin-P (OTC) *Crm:* 0.025% (1.5 oz); *Lotn:* 0.025% (2 oz)

    Dolorac *Crm:* 0.025% (28 g)

> **Double Cap (OTC)** *Crm:* 0.05% (2 oz)
> **R-Gel** *Gel:* 0.025% (15, 30 g)
> **Zostrix (OTC)** *Crm:* 0.025% (0.7, 1.5, 3 oz)
> **Zostrix HP (OTC)** *Emol crm:* 0.075% (1, 2 oz)

Comment: Provides some relief by 1-2 weeks; optimal benefit may take 4-6 weeks.

ORAL SALICYLATE

▷ *indomethacin* (C) initially 25 mg bid to tid, increase as needed at weekly intervals by 25-50 mg/day; max 200 mg/day
Pediatric: <14 years: usually not recommended; >2 years, if risk warranted: 1-2 mg/kg/day in divided doses; max 3-4 mg/kg/day (or 150-200 mg/day, whichever is less); <14 years, ER cap not recommended
> *Cap:* 25, 50 mg; *Susp:* 25 mg/5 ml (pineapple-coconut, mint) (alcohol 1%); *Supp:* 50 mg; *ER Cap:* 75 mg ext-rel

Comment: *indomethacin* is indicated only for acute painful flares. Administer with food and/or antacids. Use lowest effective dose for shortest duration.

ORAL NSAIDs

See more **Oral NSAIDs** *page 489*

▷ *diclofenac* (C)
Pediatric: <18 years: not recommended
> **Zorvolex** take on empty stomach; 35 mg tid; *Hepatic Impairment:* use lowest dose
> *Gelcap:* 18, 35 mg
▷ *diclofenac sodium* (C)
Pediatric: <18 years: not recommended
> **Voltaren** 50 mg bid to qid or 75 mg bid or 25 mg qid with an additional 25 mg at HS if necessary
> *Tab:* 25, 50, 75 mg ent-coat
> **Voltaren XR** 100 mg once daily; rarely, 100 mg bid may be used
> *Tab:* 100 mg ext-rel

ORAL NSAIDs PLUS PPI

▷ *esomeprazole/naproxen* (C) 1 tab bid; use lowest effective dose for the shortest duration swallow whole; take at least 30 minutes before a meal
Pediatric: <18 years: not recommended
> **Vimovo** *Tab:* nap 375 mg/*eso* 20 mg ext-rel; *nap* 500 mg/*eso* 20 mg ext-rel
> Comment: **Vimovo** is indicated to improve signs/symptoms, and risk of gastric ulcer in patients at risk of developing NSAID-associated gastric ulcer.

COX-2 INHIBITORS

Comment: Cox-2 inhibitors are contraindicated with history of asthma, urticaria, and allergic-type reactions to *aspirin*, other NSAIDs, and sulfonamides, 3rd trimester of pregnancy, and coronary artery bypass graft (CABG) surgery.
▷ *celecoxib* (C)(G) 100-400 mg daily bid; max 800 mg/day
Pediatric: <18 years: not recommended
> **Celebrex** *Cap:* 50, 100, 200, 400 mg

▷ *meloxicam* (C)(G) initially 7.5 mg once daily; max 15 mg once daily
  Pediatric: <2 years: not recommended; ≥2 years: 0.125 mg/kg; max 7.5 mg once daily
    Mobic *Tab:* 7.5, 15 mg; *Oral susp:* 7.5 mg/5 ml (100 ml) (raspberry)
    Vivlodex *Cap:* 5, 10 mg

INTRA-ARTICULAR INJECTION

▷ *sodium hyaluronate* (B) 20 mg by intra-articular injection weekly x 5 weeks; proceed
  with *lidocaine* or other anesthetic; remove joint effusion prior to injection
  Pediatric: not recommended
    Hyalgan *Vial:* 20 mg (2 ml); *Prefilled syringe:* 20 mg (2 ml)
    Hylan *Syringe:* 48 mg/ml soln for intra-articular injection, prefilled
    Synvisc One *Syringe:* 46 mg/6 ml soln for intraarticular injection, prefilled

OSTEOPOROSIS

Comment: Indications for bone density screening include: Postmenopausal women
not receiving HRT, maternal history of hip fracture, personal history of fragility
fracture, presence of high serum markers of bone resorption, smoker, height
>67 inches, weight <125 lb, taking a steroid, GnRH agonist, or antiseizure drug,
immobilization, hyperthyroidism, posttransplantation, malabsorption syndrome,
hyperparathyroidism, prolactinemia. The mnemonic ABONE [Age >65, Bulk (weight
<140 lbs at menopause), and Never Estrogens (for more than 6 months)], represent
other indications for bone density screening. Foods high in calcium include almonds,
broccoli, baked beans, salmon, sardines, buttermilk, turnip greens, collard greens,
spinach, pumpkin, rhubarb, and bran. Recommended Daily Calcium Intake: 1-3 years:
700 mg; 4-8 years: 1000 mg; 9-18 years: 1300 mg; 19-50 years: 1000 mg: 51-70 years
(males): 1000 mg; ≥51 years (females): 1200 mg; pregnancy or nursing: 1000-1300 mg
Recommended Daily Vitamin D Intake: >1 year: 600 IU; 50+ years: 800-1000 IU.

ESTROGEN REPLACEMENT THERAPY

Comment: *estrogen* plus progesterone is indicated for postmenopausal women with
an intact uterus. *estrogen* monotherapy is indicated in women without a uterus. The
following list is not inclusive; for more estrogen replacement therapies *see Menopause*
page 254)
▷ *estradiol* (X)
    Alora initially 0.05 mg/day apply patch twice weekly to lower abdomen, upper
    quadrant of buttocks or outer aspect of hip
      Transdermal patch: 0.025, 0.05, 0.075, 0.1 mg/day (8, 24/pck)
    Climara initially 0.025 mg/day patch once/week to trunk
      Transdermal patch: 0.025, 0.0375, 0.05, 0.075, 0.1 mg/day (4, 8, 24/pck)
    Estrace 1-2 mg daily cyclically (3 weeks on and 1 week off)
      Tab: 0.5, 1, 2*mg (tartrazine)
    Estraderm initially apply one 0.05 mg/day patch twice weekly to trunk
      Transdermal patch: 0.05, 0.1 mg/day (8, 24/pck)
    Menostar apply one patch weekly to lower abdomen, below the waist; avoid the
    breasts; alternate sites; *Transdermal patch:* 14 mcg/day (4/pck)

Minivelle initially one 0.0375 mg/day patch twice weekly to trunk area; adjust after one month of therapy
   Transdermal patch: 0.025, 0.0375, 0.05, 0.075, 0.1 mg/day (8/pck)
Vivelle initially one 0.0375 mg/day patch twice weekly to trunk area; use with an oral progestin to prevent endometrial hyperplasia
   Transdermal patch: 0.025, 0.0375, 0.05, 0.075, 0.1 mg/day (8, 48/pck)
Vivelle-Dot initially one 0.05 mg/day patch twice weekly to lower abdomen, below the waist; use with an oral progestin to prevent endometrial hyperplasia
   Transdermal patch: 0.025, 0.0375, 0.05, 0.075, 0.1 mg/day (8, 24/pck)

➤ *estradiol/levonorgestrel* (X) apply 1 patch weekly to lower abdomen; avoid waistline; alternate sites
Climara Pro *Transdermal patch: estra* 0.045 mg/*levo* 0.015 mg per day (4/pck)
➤ *estradiol/norethindrone* (X) 1 tab daily
Activella (G) *Tab: estra* 1 mg/*noreth* 0.5 mg
FemHRT 1/5 *Tab: estra* 5 mcg/*noreth* 1 mg
➤ *estradiol/norgestimate* (X) one-1mg estradiol tab daily x 3 days, then 1-*estradiol* 1 mg/*norgestimate* 0.09 mg tab once daily x 3 days; repeat this pattern continuously
Ortho-Prefest *Tab: estra* 1 mg/*norgest* 0.09 mg (30/blister pck)
➤ *estrogen, conjugated (equine)* (X)
Premarin 1 tab daily
   Tab: 0.3, 0.45, 0.625, 0.9, 1.25, 2.5 mg
➤ *estropipate, piperazine estrone sulfate* (X)(G)
Ogen 0.625-1.25 mg daily cyclically (3 weeks on and 1 week off)
   Tab: 0.625, 1.25, 2.5 mg
Ortho-Est 0.75-6 mg daily cyclically (3 weeks on and 1 week off)
   Tab: 0.625, 1.25 mg

ESTROGENS, CONJUGATED/ESTROGEN AGONIST-ANTAGONIST COMBINATION

➤ *estrogen, conjugated/bazedoxifene* (X)
Duavee 1 tab daily
   Tab: conj estra 0.45 mg/*baze* 20 mg

CALCIUM SUPPLEMENTS

Comment: Take *calcium* supplements after meals to avoid gastric upset. Dosages of calcium over 2000 mg/day have not been shown to have any additional benefit. *calcium* decreases *tetracycline* absorption. *calcium* absorption is decreased by corticosteroids.
➤ *calcitonin-salmon* (C)
Fortical 200 IU intranasally daily; alternate nostrils each day
   Nasal spray: 200 IU/actuation (30 doses, 3.7 ml)
Miacalcin Nasal spray 200 IU spray in one nostril once daily; alternate nostrils each day
   Nasal spray: 200 IU/actuation (30 doses, 3.7 ml)
Miacalcin Injection 100 units SC or IM every other day
   Vial: 200 units/ml (2 ml)
Comment: Supplement diet with calcium (1 g/day) and vitamin D (400 IU/day).
➤ *calcium carbonate* (C)(OTC)(G)
Rolaids chew 2 tabs bid; max 14 tabs/day

　　　　Chew tab: 550 mg
　　Rolaids Extra Strength chew 2 tabs bid; max 8 tabs/day
　　　　Chew tab: 1000 mg
　　Tums chew 2 tabs bid; max 16 tabs/day
　　　　Chew tab: 500 mg
　　Tums Extra Strength chew 2 tabs bid; max 10 tabs/day
　　　　Chew tab: 750 mg
　　Tum Sultra chew 2 tabs bid; max 8 tabs/day
　　　　Chew tab: 1000 mg
　　Os-Cal 500 (OTC) 1-2 tab bid to tid
　　　　Chew tab: elemental calcium carbonate 500 mg
▷ *calcium carbonate/vitamin d* (C)(G)
　　Os-Cal 250+D (OTC) 1-2 tab tid
　　　　Tab: elemental calcium carbonate 250 mg/*vit d* 125 IU
　　Os-Cal 500+D (OTC) 1-2 tab bid-tid
　　　　Tab: elemental calcium carbonate 500 mg/*vit d* 125 IU
　　Viactiv (OTC) 1 tab tid
　　　　Chew tab: elemental calcium 500 mg/*vit d* 100 IU/*vitamin k* 40 mcg
▷ *calcium citrate* (C)(G)
　　Citracal (OTC) 1-2 tabs bid
　　　　Tab: elemental calcium citrate 200 mg
▷ *calcium citrate/vitamin d* (C)(G)
　　Citracal +D (OTC) 1-2 cplts bid
　　　　Cplt: elemental calcium citrate 315 mg/*vit d* 200 IU
　　Citracal 250+D (OTC) 1-2 tabs bid
　　　　Tab: elemental calcium citrate 250 mg/*vit d* 62.3 IU

VITAMIN D ANALOGS

Comment: Concurrent *vitamin D* supplementation is contraindicated for patients taking *calcitrol* or *doxercalciferol* due to the risk of *vitamin D* toxicity.
▷ *calcitrol* (C) *Predialysis:* initially 0.25 mcg daily; may increase to 0.5 mcg daily; *Dialysis:* initially 0.25 mcg daily; may increase by 0.25 mcg/day at 4-8 week intervals; usual maintenance 0.5-1 mcg/day; *Hypoparathyroidism:* initially 0.25 mcg q AM; may increase by 0.25 mcg/day at 4- to 8-week intervals; usual maintenance 0.5-2 mcg/day *Pediatric: Predialysis:* <3 years: 10-15 ng/kg/day; ≥3 years: initially 0.25 mcg daily; may increase to 0.5 mcg/day; *Dialysis:* not recommended; *Hypoparathyroidism:* initially 0.25 mcg daily; may increase by 0.25 mcg/day at 2-4 week intervals; usual maintenance (1-5 years) 0.25-0.75 mcg/day, (>6 years) 0.5-2 mcg/day
　　Rocaltrol *Cap:* 0.25, 0.5 mcg
　　Rocaltrol Solution *Soln:* 1 mcg/ml (15 ml, single-use dispensers)
▷ *doxercalciferol* (C) initially 0.25 mcg q AM; may increase by 0.25 mcg/day at 4-8 week intervals; usual maintenance 0.5-2 mcg/day
Pediatric: initially 0.25 mcg daily; may increase by 0.25 mcg; 0.25 mcg/day at 2-4 week intervals; usual maintenance (1-5 years) 0.25-0.75 mcg/day, (≥6 years) 0.5-2 mcg/day
　　Hectorol *Cap:* 0.25, 0.5 mcg

BISPHOSPHONATES (CALCIUM MODIFIERS)

Comment: Biphosphonates should be swallowed whole in the AM with 6-8 oz of plain water 30 minutes before first meal, beverage, or other medications of the day.

Monitor serum alkaline phosphatase. Contraindications include abnormalities of the esophagus which delay esophageal emptying such as stricture or achalasia, inability to stand or sit upright for at least 30 minutes postdose, patients at risk of aspiration, and hypocalcemia. Co-administration of biphosphonates and *calcium*, antacids, or oral medications containing multivalent cations will interfere with absorption of the bophosphonate. Therefore, instruct patients to wait at least half hour after taking the biphosphonate before taking any other oral medications.

▶ *alendronate (as sodium)* (C) take once weekly, in the AM, 30 minutes before the first food, beverage, or medication of the day; do not lie down (remain upright) for at least 30 minutes and after the first food of the day; *CrCl <35 mL/min:* not recommended with
   Pediatric: not recommended

   Binosto dissolve the effervescent tab in 4 oz (120 ml) of plain, room temperature, water (not mineral or flavored); wait 5 minutes after the effervescence has subsided, then stir for 10 seconds, then drink
   Tab: 70 mg effervescent for buffered solution (4, 12/carton) (strawberry)
   Fosamax (G) swallow tab whole; dosing regimens are the same for men and postmenopausal women; *Prevention:* 5 mg once daily or 35 mg once weekly; *Treatment:* 10 mg once daily or 70 mg once weekly
   Tab: 5, 10, 35, 40, 70 mg

▶ *alendronate/cholecalciferol (vit d3)* (C)(G) take 1 tab once weekly, in the AM, with plain water (not mineral) 30 minutes before the first food, beverage, or medication of the day; do not lie down (remain upright) for at least 30 minutes and after the first food of the day
   Pediatric: not recommended

   Fosamax Plus D
   Tab: **Fosamax Plus D 70/2800:** *alen* 70 mg/*chole* 2800 IU
   Fosamax Plus D 70/5600: *alen* 70 mg/*chole* 5600 IU

▶ *ibandronate (as monosodium monohydrate)* (C)(G)
   Pediatric: not recommended

   Boniva take 2.5 mg once daily or 150 mg once monthly on the same day; take in the AM, with plain water (not mineral) 60 minutes before the first food, beverage, or medication of the day; do not lie down (remain upright) for at least 30 minutes and after the first food of the day
   Tab: 2.5, 150 mg
   Boniva Injection administer 3 mg every 3 months by IV bolus over 15-30 seconds; if dose is missed, administer as soon as possible; then every 3 months from the date of the last dose
   Prefilled syringe: 3 mg/3 ml (5 ml)
   Comment: Boniva Injection must be administered by a health care professional.

▶ *risedronate (as sodium)* (C)(G) take in the AM; swallow whole with a full glass of plain water (not mineral); do not lie down (remain upright) for 30 minutes afterward
   Pediatric: not recommended

   Actonel take at least 30 minutes before any food or drink; *Women:* 5 mg once daily or 35 mg once weekly or 75 mg on two consecutive days monthly or 150 mg once monthly; *Men:* 35 mg once weekly
   Tab: 5, 30, 35, 75, 150 mg
   Atelvia 35 mg once weekly immediately after breakfast
   Tab: 35 mg del-rel

▶ *risedronate/calcium* (C) 1 x 5 mg *risedronate* tab weekly plus 1 x 500 mg *calcium* tab on days 2-7 weekly

> **Actonel with Calcium** *Tab: risedronate* 5 mg and *Tab: calcium* 500 mg (4 *rise-dronate* tabs + 30 *calcium* tabs/pck)

▷ *zoledronic acid* (D)

Pediatric: not recommended

> **Reclast** administer 5 mg via IV infusion over at least 15 minutes mg once a year (for osteoporosis) or once every 2 years (for osteopenia or prophylaxis)
>
> *Bottle:* 5 mg/100 ml (single-dose)

Comment: **Reclast** is indicated for the treatment of postmenopausal osteoporosis in women who are at high risk for fracture and to increase bone mass in men with primary or hypogonadal osteoporosis who are at high risk for fracture. Administered by a health care professional. Contraindicated in hypocalcemia.

Zometa *Bottle:* 4 mg/5 ml administer 4 mg via IV infusion over at least 15 minutes every 3-4 weeks; optimal duration of treatment not known

Vial: 4 mg/5 ml (single-dose)

Comment: **Zometa** is indicated for the treatment of hypercalcemia of malignancy. The safety and efficacy of **Zometa** in the treatment of hypercalcemia associated with hyperparathyroidism or with other nontumor-related conditions has not been established.

SELECTIVE ESTROGEN RECEPTOR MODULATOR (SERMs)

▷ *raloxifene* (X)(G) 60 mg once daily

> **Evista** *Tab:* 60 mg

Comment: Contraindicated in women who have history of, or current, venous thrombotic event.

HUMAN PARATHYROID HORMONE

▷ *teriparatide* (C) 20 mcg SC daily in the thigh or abdomen; may treat for for up to 2 years

Pediatric: not recommended

> **Forteo Multidose Pen** *Multi-dose pen:* 250 mcg/ml (3 ml)

Comment: **Forteo** is indicated for the treatment of postmenopausal osteoporosis in women who are at high risk for fracture and to increase bone mass in men with primary or hypogonadal osteoporosis who are at high risk for fracture.

BIOENGINEERED REPLICA OF HUMAN PARATHYROID HORMONE

▷ *bioengineered replica of human parathyroid hormone* (C) initially inject mg IM into the thigh once daily; when initiating, decrease dose of active *vitamin D* by 50% if serum *calcium* is above 7.5 mg/dL; monitor serum *calcium* levels every 3 to 7 days after starting or adjusting dose and when adjusting either active *vitamin D* or *calcium* supplements dose

> **Natpara** *Soln for inj:* 25, 50, 75, 100 mcg (2/pkg) multi-dose, dual-chamber glass cartridge containing a sterile powder and diluent

Comment: **Natpara** is indicated as adjunct to *calcium* and *vitamin D* in patients with parathyroidism.

OSTEOCLAST INHIBITOR (RANKL INHIBITOR)

▷ *denosumab* (X) for SC injection 60 mcg SC once every 6 months in the upper arm, abdomen, or upper thigh

Pediatric: not established
> **Prolia** *Vial/Pen:* 60 mg/ml (1 ml) single-dose
> **Comment:** **Prolia** is indicated for the treatment of postmenopausal osteoporosis in women who are at high risk for fracture defined as a history of osteoporotic fracture, <u>or</u> multiple risk factors for fracture, <u>or</u> patients who have failed <u>or</u> are intolerant to other therapy. Administered by a health care professional. Contraindicated in hypocalcemia.

 OTITIS EXTERNA

OTIC ANALGESIC

▷ *antipyrine/benzocaine/zinc acetate dihydrate* (C) fill ear canal with solution; then insert a cotton pluge into meatus; may repeat every 1-2 hours prn
  Pediatric: same as adult
  > **Otozin** *Otic soln: antipyr* 5.4%/*benz* 1%/*zinc*1% per ml (10 ml w. dropper)

OTIC ANALGESIC/ANESTHETIC/ANTIBACTERIAL COMBINATION

▷ *acetic acid/antipyrine/benzocaine/u-policosanol 410* (C) fill ear canal with solution; then insert a cotton plug into meatus; may repeat every 1-2 hours prn
  Pediatric: same as adult
  > **AuralganOtic** *Otic soln: acet acid* 0.01%/*antipyr* 5.4%/*benz* 1.4% /*u-poly* 0.01% per ml (14 ml w. dropper)

OTIC ANTI-INFECTIVE

▷ *chloroxylenol/pramoxine* (C) 4-5 drops tid x 5-10 days
  Pediatric: <1 year: not recommended; 1-12 years: 5 drops bid x 10 days
  > **PramOtic** *Otic drops: chlorox/pramox* (5 ml w. dropper)
▷ *finafloxacin* (C) otic 4-5 drops tid x 5-10 days
  Pediatric: <1 year: not recommended; ≥1 year: same as adult
  > **Xtoro** *Otic soln:* 0.3% (5, 8 ml)
▷ *ofloxacin* (C)(G) 10 drops bid x 10 days
  Pediatric: <1 year: not recommended; 1-12 years: 5 drops bid x 10 days
  > **Floxin Otic** *Otic soln:* 0.3% (5, 10 ml w. dropper; 0.25 ml, 5 drop singles, 20/carton)
  > **Comment:** **Floxin Otic** is indicated for adult patients with perforated tympanic membranes and pediatric patients with PE tubes.

OTIC ANTI-INFECTIVE /CORTICOSTEROID COMBINATIONS

▷ *chloroxylenol/pramoxine/hydrocortisone* (C) drops 4 drops tid-qid x 5-10 days
  Pediatric: 3 drops tid-qid x 5-10 days
  > **Cortane B, Cortane B Aqueous** *Otic soln: chlo* 1 mg/*pram* 10 mg/*hydro* 10 mg per ml (10 ml w. dropper)
Comment: **Cortane B Aqueous** may be used to saturate a cotton wick.
▷ *ciprofloxacin/hydrocortisone* (C) susp 3 drops bid x 7 days
  Pediatric: <1 year: not recommended; ≥1 year: same as adult
  > **Cipro HC Otic** *Otic susp: cipro* 0.2%/*hydro* 1% (10 ml w. dropper)

▷ *ciprofloxacin/dexamethasone* (C) 4 drops bid x 7 days
    Pediatric: <6 months: not recommended; ≥6 months: same as adult
        Ciprodex *Otic susp:* cipro 0.3%/*dexa* 1% (7.5 ml)
        Comment: Ciprodex is indicated for the treatment of otitis media in pediatric
        patients with tympanostomy tubes.
▷ *colistin/neomycin/hydrocortisone/thonzonium* (C) 5 drops tid or qid x 5-10 days
    Pediatric: 4 drops tid-qid x 5-10 days
        Coly-Mycin S *Otic susp:* 5, 10 ml
        Cortisporin-TC Otic *Otic susp: colis* 3 mg/*neo* 3.3 mg/*hydro* 10 mg/*thon* 0.5 mg
        per ml (10 ml w. dropper) (thimerosal)
▷ *polymyxin B/neomycin/hydrocortisone* (C) 4 drops tid-qid; max 10 days
    Pediatric: 3 drops tid-qid; max 10 days
        Cortisporin Otic Suspension *Otic susp: poly b* 10,000 u/*neo* 3.5 mg/*hydro* 10 mg
        per 5 ml (10 ml w. dropper)
        Cortisporin Otic Solution *Otic soln: poly b* 10000 u/*neo* 3.5 mg/*hydro* 10 mg per
        5 ml (10 ml w. dropper)

OTIC ASTRINGENTS

▷ *acetic acid 2% in aluminum sulfate* (C) 4-6 drops q 2-3 hours
    Pediatric: same as adult
        Domeboro Otic *Otic soln:* 60 ml w. dropper
▷ *acetic acid/propylene glycol/benzethonium chloride/sodium acetate* (C) 3-5 drops q
    4-6 hours
    Pediatric: same as adult
        VoSol *Otic soln: acet* 2% (15, 30 ml)
▷ *acetic acid/propylene glycol/hydrocortisone/benzethonium chloride/sod-ium acetate*
    (C) 3-5 drops q 4-6 hours
    Pediatric: same as adult
        VoSol HC *Otic soln: acet* 2%/*hydro* 1% (10 ml)

OTIC ANESTHETIC/ANALGESIC COMBINATIONS

▷ *antipyrine/benzocaine/glycerine* (C) fill ear canal and insert cotton plug; may repeat
    q 1-2 hours as needed
    Pediatric: same as adult
        A/B Otic *Otic soln:* 15 ml w. dropper
▷ *benzocaine* (C) 4-5 drops q 1-2 hours
    Pediatric: <1 year: not recommended; ≥1 year: same as adult
        Americaine Otic *Otic soln:* 20% (15 ml w. dropper)
        Benzotic *Otic soln:* 20% (15 ml w. dropper)

SYSTEMIC ANTI-INFECTIVES

Comment: Used for severe disease or with culture.
▷ *amoxicillin/clavulanate* (B)(G) 500 mg tid or 875 mg bid x 10 days
        Augmentin *Tab:* 250, 500, 875 mg; *Chew tab:* 125, 250 mg (lemon-lime); 200,
        400 mg (cherry-banana) (phenylalanine); *Oral susp:* 125 mg/5 ml (banana), 250
        mg/5 ml (75, 100, 150 ml) (orange); 200, 400 mg/5 ml (50, 75, 100 ml) (orange)
        (phenylalanine)
            Pediatric: 40-45 mg/kg/day divided tid x 10 days or 90 mg/kg/day divided
            bid x 10 days *see pages 545-546 for dose by weight*

Augmentin ES-600 *Oral susp:* 600 mg/5 ml (50, 75, 100, 125, 150, 200 ml) (strawberry cream) (phenylalanine) every 12 hours
    Pediatric: <3 months: not recommended; ≥3 months, <40 kg: 90 mg/kg/day in 2 divided doses; ≥40 kg: not recommended

Augmentin XR 2 tabs q 12 hours x 7-10 days
    Pediatric: <16 years: use other forms; ≥16 years: same as adult
    Tab: 1000*mg ext-rel

▶ *cefaclor* **(B)(G)** 250-500 mg q 8 hours x 7-10 days
Pediatric: <1 month: not recommended; 20-40 mg/kg bid <u>or</u> q 12 hours x 10 days; max 1 g/day; *see page 549 for dose by weight*
Tab: 500 mg; *Cap:* 250, 500 mg; *Susp:* 125 mg/5 ml (75, 150 ml) (strawberry); 187 mg/5 ml (50, 100 ml) (strawberry); 250 mg/5 ml (75, 150 ml) (strawberry); 375 mg/5 ml (50, 100 ml) (strawberry)

    Cefaclor Extended Release
        Pediatric: <16 years: ext-rel not recommended; ≥16 years: same as adult
        Tab: 375, 500 mg ext-rel

▶ *dicloxacillin* **(B)** 500 mg qid x 7-10 days
Pediatric: 12.5-25 mg/kg/day in 4 divided doses x 7-10 days; *see page 560 for dose by weight*

    Dynapen *Cap:* 125, 250, 500 mg; *Oral susp:* 62.5 mg/5 ml (80, 100, 200 ml)

▶ *trimethoprim/sulfamethoxazole* **(C)(G)**
Pediatric: <2 months: not recommended; ≥2 months: 40 mg/kg/day of *sulfamethoxazole* in 2 doses bid x 10 days; *see page 576 for dose by weight*

    Bactrim, Septra 2 tabs bid x 10 days
        Tab: trim 80 mg/*sulfa* 400 mg*
    Bactrim DS, Septra DS 1 tab bid x 10 days
        Tab: trim 160 mg/*sulfa* 800 mg*
    Bactrim Pediatric Suspension, Septra Pediatric Suspension
        Oral susp: trim 40 mg/*sulfa* 200 mg per 5 ml (100 ml) (cherry) (alcohol 0.3%)

Comment: *trimethoprim/sulfamethoxazole* is not recommended in pregnancy <u>or</u> lactation. *CrCl 15-30 mL/min:* reduce dose by 1/2; *CrCl <15 mL/min:* not recommended.

OTITIS MEDIA: ACUTE

OTIC ANALGESIC

▶ *antipyrine/benzocaine/zinc acetate dihydrate* otic **(C)** fill ear canal with solution; then insert cotton plug into meatus; may repeat every 1-2 hours prn
Pediatric: same as adult
    Otozin *Otic soln: antipyr* 5.4%/*benz* 1%/*zinc*1% per ml (10 ml w. dropper)

OTIC ANALGESIC/ANESTHETIC/ANTIBACTERIAL COMBINATION

▶ *acetic acid/antipyrine/benzocaine/u-policosanol 410* otic **(C)** fill ear canal with solution; then moisten cotton plug with solution and insert into meatus; may repeat every 1-2 hours prn
Pediatric: same as adult
    Auralgan Otic *Otic soln: acet acid* 0.01%/*antipyr* 5.4%/*benz* 1.4%/*u-poly* 0.01% per ml (14 ml w. dropper)

SYSTEMIC ANTI-INFECTIVES

▷ *amoxicillin* (B)(G) 500-875 mg bid or 250-500 mg tid x 10 days
Pediatric: <40 kg (88 lb): 20-40 mg/kg/day in 3 divided doses x 10 days or 25-45 mg/kg/day in 2 divided doses x 10 days; *see page 543 for dose by weight*

> **Amoxil** *Cap:* 250, 500 mg; *Tab:* 875*mg; *Chew tab:* 125, 200, 250, 400 mg (cherry-banana-peppermint) (phenylalanine); *Oral susp:* 125, 250 mg/5 ml (80, 100, 150 ml) (strawberry); 200, 400 mg/5 ml (50, 75, 100 ml) (bubble gum); *Oral drops:* 50 mg/ml (30 ml) (bubble gum)
> **Moxatag** *Tab:* 775 mg ext-rel
> **Trimox** *Tab:* 125, 250 mg; *Cap:* 250, 500 mg; *Oral susp:* 125, 250 mg/5 ml (80, 100, 150 ml) (raspberry-strawberry)

Comment: Consider 80-90 mg/kg/day in 3 divided doses for resistant for cases

▷ *amoxicillin/clavulanate* (B)(G) 500 mg tid or 875 mg bid x 10 days
> **Augmentin** *Tab:* 250, 500, 875 mg; *Chew tab:* 125, 250 mg (lemon-lime); 200, 400 mg (cherry-banana) (phenylalanine); *Oral susp:* 125 mg/5 ml (banana), 250 mg/5 ml (75, 100, 150 ml) (orange); 200, 400 mg/5 ml (50, 75, 100 ml) (orange) (phenylalanine)
>> *Pediatric:* 40-45 mg/kg/day divided tid x 10 days or 90 mg/kg/day divided bid x 10 days *see pages 545-546 for dose by weight*
> **Augmentin ES-600** *Oral susp:* 600 mg/5 ml (50, 75, 100, 125, 150, 200 ml) (strawberry cream) (phenylalanine) every 12 hours
>> *Pediatric:* <3 months: not recommended; ≥3 months, <40 kg: 90 mg/kg/day in 2 divided doses; ≥40 kg: not recommended
> **Augmentin XR** 2 tabs q 12 hours x 7-10 days
>> *Pediatric:* <16 years: use other forms; ≥16 years: same as adult
>> *Tab:* 1000*mg ext-rel

▷ *ampicillin* (B) 250-500 mg qid x 10 days
Pediatric: 50-100 mg/kg/day in 4 divided doses x 10 days; *see page 547 for dose by weight*
> **Omnipen, Principen** *Cap:* 250, 500 mg; *Oral susp:* 125, 250 mg/5 ml (100, 150, 200 ml) (fruit)

▷ *azithromycin* (B)(G) 500 mg x 1 dose on day 1, then 250 mg daily on days 2-5 or 500 mg daily x 3 days or **Zmax** 2 g in a single dose
Pediatric: 12 mg/kg/day x 5 days; max 500 mg/day; *see page 548 for dose by weight*
> **Zithromax** *Tab:* 250, 500, 600 mg; *Oral susp:* 100 mg/5 ml (15 ml); 200 mg/5 ml (15, 22.5, 30 ml) (cherry); *Pkt:* 1 g for reconstitution (cherry-banana)
> **Zithromax Tri-pak** *Tab:* 3 x 500 mg tabs/pck
> **Zithromax Z-pak** *Tab:* 6 x 250 mg tabs/pck
> **Zmax** *Oral susp:* 2 g ext-rel for reconstitution (cherry-banana) (148 mg Na$^+$)

▷ *cefaclor* (B)(G) 250-500 mg q 8 hours x 7-10 days
Pediatric: <1 month: not recommended; 20-40 mg/kg bid or q 12 hours x 10 days; max 1 g/ day; *see page 549 for dose by weight*
Tab: 500 mg; *Cap:* 250, 500 mg; *Susp:* 125 mg/5 ml (75, 150 ml) (strawberry); 187 mg/5 ml (50, 100 ml) (strawberry); 250 mg/5 ml (75, 150 ml) (strawberry); 375 mg/5 ml (50, 100 ml) (strawberry)
> **Cefaclor Extended Release**
>> *Pediatric:* <16 years: ext-rel not recommended
>> *Tab:* 375, 500 mg ext-rel

▷ *cefdinir* (B) 300 mg bid <u>or</u> 600 mg daily x 5-10 days
  Pediatric: <6 months: not recommended; 6 months-12 years: 14 mg/kg/day in
  1-2 divided doses x 10 days; *>12 years: same as adult; see page 551 for dose by
  weight*
    Omnicef *Cap:* 300 mg; *Oral susp:* 125 mg/5 ml (60, 100 ml) (strawberry)
▷ *cefixime* (B)
  Pediatric: <6 months: not recommended; 6 months-12 years, <50 kg: 8 mg/kg/day in
  1-2 divided doses x 10 days; >12 years, ≥50 kg: same as adult; *see page 552 for dose by
  weight*
    Suprax *Tab:* 400 mg; *Cap:* 400 mg; *Oral susp:* 100, 200 mg/5 ml (50, 75, 100 ml)
    (strawberry)
▷ *cefpodoxime proxetil* (B) 100 mg bid x 5 days
  Pediatric: <2 months: not recommended; 2 months-12 years: 10 mg/kg/day (max
  400 mg/dose) <u>or</u> 5 mg/kg/day bid (max 200 mg/dose) x 5 days; >12 years: same as
  adult; *see page 553 for dose by weight*
    Vantin *Tab:* 100, 200 mg; *Oral susp:* 50, 100 mg/5 ml (50, 75, 100 ml) (lemon
    creme)
▷ *cefprozil* (B) 250-500 mg bid <u>or</u> 500 mg daily x 10 days
    Pediatric: <2 years: same as adult; 2-12 years: 7.5 mg/kg bid x 10 days; >12
    years: same as adult
    see page 554 for dose by weight
    Cefzil *Tab:* 250, 500 mg; *Oral susp:* 125, 250 mg/5 ml (50, 75, 100 ml) (bubble
    gum) (phenylalanine)
▷ *ceftibuten* (B) 400 mg daily x 10 days
  Pediatric: 9 mg/kg daily x 10 days; max 400 mg/day; *see page 555 for dose by
  weight*
    Cedax *Cap:* 400 mg; *Oral susp:* 90 mg/5 ml (30, 60, 90, 120 ml); 180 mg/5 ml
    (30, 60, 120 ml) (cherry)
▷ *ceftriaxone* (B)(G) 1-2 g IM x 1 dose; max 4 g
  Pediatric: 50 mg/kg IM x 1 dose
    Rocephin *Vial:* 250, 500 mg; 1, 2 g
▷ *cefuroxime axetil* (B)(G) 250-500 mg bid x 10 days
  Pediatric: 15 mg/kg bid x 10 days; *see page 556 for dose by weight*
    Ceftin *Tab:* 250, 500 mg; *Oral susp:* 125, 250 mg/5 ml (50, 100 ml) (tutti-
    frutti)
▷ *cephalexin* (B)(G) 250 mg qid x 10 days
  Pediatric: 25-50 mg/kg/day in 4 doses x 10 days; *see page 557 for dose by weight*
    Keflex *Cap:* 250, 333, 500, 750 mg; *Oral susp:* 125, 250 mg/5 ml (100, 200 ml)
    (strawberry)
▷ *clarithromycin* (C)(G) 500 mg bid <u>or</u> 500 mg ext-rel daily
  Pediatric: <6 months: not recommended; ≥6 months: 7.5 mg/kg divided bid x 7
  days; *see page 558 for dose by weight*
    Biaxin *Tab:* 250, 500 mg
    Biaxin Oral Suspension *Oral susp:* 125, 250 mg/5 ml (50, 100 ml) (fruit-punch)
    Biaxin XL *Tab:* 500 mg ext-rel
▷ *erythromycin/sulfisoxazole* (C)(G)
  Pediatric: <2 months: not recommended; ≥2 months: 50 mg/kg/day in 3 divided
  doses x 10 days
    Eryzole *Oral susp:* eryth 200 mg/sulf 600 mg per 5 ml (100, 150, 200, 250 ml)

Pediazole *Oral susp:* *eryth* 200 mg/*sulf* 600 mg per 5 ml (100, 150, 200 ml) (strawberry-banana)

Comment: *erythromycin* may increase INR with concomitant **warfarin**, as well as increase serum level of **digoxin**, benzodiazepines and statins. *sulfamethoxazole* is not recommended in pregnancy or lactation. *CrCl 15-30 mL/min:* reduce dose by 1/2; *CrCl <15 mL/min:* not recommended.

▷ *loracarbef* (B) 400 mg bid x 10 days
Pediatric: 30 mg/kg/day in divided bid x 7 days; *see page 570 for dose by weight*
Lorabid *Pulvule:* 200, 400 mg; *Oral susp:* 100 mg/5 ml (50, 100 ml); 200 mg/5 ml (50, 75, 100 ml) (strawberry bubble gum)

▷ *trimethoprim/sulfamethoxazole* (C)(G)
Pediatric: <2 months: not recommended; >2 months: 40 mg/kg/day of *sulfamethoxazole* in divided doses bid x 10 days; *see page 576 for dose by weight*
Bactrim, Septra 2 tabs bid x 10 days
Tab: trim 80 mg/*sulfa* 400 mg*
Bactrim DS, Septra DS 1 tab bid x 10 days
Tab: trim 160 mg/*sulfa* 800 mg*
Bactrim Pediatric Suspension, Septra Pediatric Suspension
Oral susp: trim 40 mg/*sulfa* 200 mg per 5 ml (100 ml) (cherry) (alcohol 0.3%)
Comment: *trimethoprim/sulfamethoxazole* is not recommended in pregnancy or lactation. *CrCl 15-30 mL/min:* reduce dose by 1/2; *CrCl <15 mL/min:* not recommended.

OTIC ANTI-INFECTIVE

▷ *ofloxacin* (C)(G) 10 drops bid x 14 days
Pediatric: <6 months: not recommended; 6 months-12 years: 5 drops bid x 14 days; >12 years: same as adult
Floxin Otic *Otic soln:* 0.3% (5, 10 ml w. dropper)
Comment: *ofloxacin* may be used with patients with perforated tympanic membrane or tympanostomy tubes.

Otic Anti-infective/Corticosteroid Combinations

Comment: *neomycin* may cause ototoxicity. Do not use with known or suspected tympanic membrane rupture.

▷ *chloroxylenol/pramoxine/hydrocortisone* (C) 4 drops tid-qid x 5-10 days
Pediatric: 3 drops tid-qid x 5-10 days
Cortane Ear Drops, *Otic drops:* 10 ml

▷ *ciprofloxacin/hydrocortisone* (C) otic susp 3 drops bid x 7 days
Pediatric: <1 year: not recommended; ≥1 year: same as adult
Cipro HC *Otic susp:* cipro 0.3%/*dexa* 0.1% (10 ml)

▷ *ciprofloxacin/dexamethasone* (C) otic susp 4 drops bid x 7 days
Pediatric: <6 months: not recommended; ≥6 months: same as adult
Ciprodex *Otic susp:* cipro 0.3%/*dexa* 1% (7.5 ml)
Comment: **Ciprodex** is indicated for the treatment of otitis media in pediatric patients with tympanostomy tubes (PE tubes).

▷ *colistin/neomycin/hydrocortisone/thonzonium* (C) 5 drops tid-qid x 5-10 days
Pediatric: 4 drops tid-qid x 5-10 days
Coly-Mycin S *Otic susp:* 5, 10 ml

➤ *polymyxin B/neomycin/hydrocortisone* (C) 4 drops tid-qid; max 10 days
  Pediatric: 3 drops tid-qid; max 10 days
      Cortisporin *Otic susp:* 10 ml w. dropper; *Otic soln:* 10 ml w. dropper
      PediOtic *Otic susp:* 7.5 ml w. dropper
➤ *polymyxin B/neomycin/hydrocortisone/surfactant* (C) 4 drops tid-qid
  Pediatric: 3 drops tid-qid; max 10 days
      Cortisporin-TC *Otic susp:* 10 ml w. dropper

OTIC ANESTHETIC/ANALGESIC COMBINATIONS

➤ *antipyrine/benzocaine/glycerine* (C) fill ear canal and insert cotton plug; may repeat
  q 1-2 hours as needed
  Pediatric: same as adult
      A/B Otic *Otic soln:* antipy 5.4%/benzo 1.4% 15 ml w. dropper
➤ *benzocaine* (C)(OTC) 4-5 drops q 1-2 hours
  Pediatric: <1 year: not recommended; ≥1 year: same as adult
      Otic drops: 20% (15 ml dropper-top bottle)
      Americaine Otic *Otic soln:* 15 ml w. dropper
      Benzotic *Otic soln:* 20% (15 ml w. dropper)

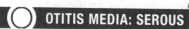

OTITIS MEDIA: SEROUS

Anti-infectives *see Otitis Media: Acute page* 290
Oral Drugs for Allergy, Cough, and Cold *see page* 524
Oral Corticosteroids *see page* 497

PAGET'S DISEASE: BONE

Comment: Calcium decreases *tetracycline* absorption. **calcium** absorption is decreased
by corticosteroids. **calcium** absorption is decreased by foods such as rhubarb, spinach,
and bran.

BISPHOSPHONATES (CALCIUM MODIFIERS)

Comment: Biphosphonates should be swallowed whole in the AM with 6-8 oz of
plain water 30 minutes before first meal, beverage, <u>or</u> other medications of the day.
Monitor serum alkaline phosphatase. Contraindications include abnormalities of the
esophagus which delay esophageal emptying such as stricture <u>or</u> achalasia, inability
to stand <u>or</u> sit upright for at least 30 minutes post-dose, patients at risk of aspiration,
and hypocalcemia. Coadministration of biphosphonates and calcium, antacids, <u>or</u>
oral medications containing multivalent cations will interfere with absorption of the
bophosphonate. Therefore, instruct patients to wait at least half hour after taking the
biphosphonate before taking any other oral medications.
➤ *alendronate (as sodium)* (C) take once weekly, in the AM, 30 minutes before the
  first food, beverage, <u>or</u> medication of the day; do not lie down (remain upright) for
  at least 30 minutes and after the first food of the day; not recommended with *CrCl
  <35 mL/min.*
  Pediatric: not recommended

Binosto dissolve the effervescent tab in 4 oz (120 ml) of plain, room temperature, water (not mineral or flavored); wait 5 minutes after the effervescence has subsided, then stir for 10 seconds, then drink

> *Tab:* 70 mg effervescent for buffered solution (4, 12/carton) (strawberry)

Fosamax (G) swallow tab whole; dosing regimens are the same for men and post-menopausal women; *Prevention:* 5 mg once daily or 35 mg once weekly; *Treatment:* 10 mg once daily or 70 mg once weekly

> *Tab:* 5, 10, 35, 40, 70 mg

➤ *alendronate/cholecalciferol (vit d3)* (C)(G) take 1 tab once weekly, in the AM, with plain water (not mineral) 30 minutes before the first food, beverage, or medication of the day; do not lie down (remain upright) for at least 30 minutes and after the first food of the day
Pediatric: not recommended

Fosamax Plus D

> *Tab:* **Fosamax Plus D 70/2800** *alen* 70 mg/*chole* 2800 IU
> **Fosamax Plus D 70/5600** *alen* 70 mg/*chole* 5600 IU

➤ *ibandronate (as monosodium monohydrate)* (C)(G)
Pediatric: not recommended

Boniva take 2.5 mg once daily or 150 mg once monthly on the same day; take in the AM, with plain water (not mineral) 60 minutes before the first food, beverage, or medication of the day; do not lie down (remain upright) for at least 30 minutes and after the first food of the day

> *Tab:* 2.5, 150 mg

Boniva Injection administer 3 mg every 3 months by IV bolus over 15-30 seconds; if dose is missed, administer as soon as possible, then every 3 months from the date of the last dose

> *Prefilled syringe:* 3 mg/3 ml (5 ml)

Comment: **Boniva Injection** must be administered by a qualified health care professional.

➤ *risedronate (as sodium)* (C)(G) take in the AM; swallow whole with a full glass of plain water (not mineral) do not lie down (remain upright) for 30 minutes afterward
Pediatric: not recommended

Actonel take at least 30 minutes before any food or drink; *Women:* 5 mg once daily or 35 mg once weekly or 75 mg on two consecutive days monthly or 150 mg once monthly; *Men:* 35 mg once weekly; *Tab:* 5, 30, 35, 75, 150 mg

Atelvia 35 mg once weekly immediately after breakfast

> *Tab:* 35 mg del-rel

➤ *risedronate/calcium* (C) 1 x 5 mg *risedronate* tab weekly and 1 x 500 mg *calcium* tab on days 2-7 weekly

Actonel with Calcium *Tab: risedronate* 5 mg and *Tab:* calcium 500 mg (4 *risedronate* tabs + 30 *calcium* tabs/pck)

➤ *zoledronic acid* (D)
Pediatric: not recommended

Reclast administer 5 mg via IV infusion over at least 15 minutes mg once a year (for osteoporosis) or once every 2 years (for osteopenia or prophylaxis)

> *Bottle:* 5 mg/100 ml (single-dose)

Comment: **Reclast** is indicated for the treatment of postmenopausal osteoporosis in women who are at high risk for fracture and to increase bone mass in men with primary or hypogonadal osteoporosis who are at high risk for fracture. Administered by a qualified health care professional. Contraindicated in hypocalcemia.

Zometa administer 4 mg via IV infusion over at least 15 minutes every 3-4 weeks; optimal duration of treatment not known

    Bottle: 4 mg/5 ml; *Vial:* 4 mg/5 ml (single-dose)

Comment: **Zometa** is indicated for the treatment of hypercalcemia of malignancy. The safety and efficacy of **Zometa** in the treatment of hypercalcemia associated with hyperparathyroidism <u>or</u> with other nontumor-related conditions has not been established.

 PAIN

Antidepressants *see Depression* page 105
Skeletal Muscle Relaxants *see Muscle Strain* page 262

ACETAMINOPHEN FOR IV INFUSION

▷ *acetaminophen* injectable **(B)** administer by IV infusion over 15 minutes; 1,000 mg q 6 hours prn <u>or</u> 650 mg q 4 hours prn; max 4,000 mg/day
Pediatric: <2 years: not recommended; 2-13 years <50 kg: 15 mg/kg q 6 hours prn <u>or</u> 2.5 mg/kg q 4 hours prn; max 750 mg single-dose; max 75 mg/kg per day; >13 years: same as adult

    Ofirmev *Vial:* 10 mg/ml (100 ml) (preservative-free)

    Comment: The **Ofirmev** vial is intended for single-use. If any portion is withdrawn from the vial, use within 6 hours. Discard the unused portion. For pediatric patients, withdraw the intended dose and administer via syringe pump. Do not admix **Ofirmev** with any other drugs. **Ofirmev** is physically incompatible with *diazepam* and *chlorpromazine hydrochloride*.

IBUPROFEN FOR IV INFUSION

▷ *ibuprofen* **(B)** dilute dose in 0.9% NS, D5W, <u>or</u> Lactated Ringers (LR) solution; administer by IV infusion over at least 10 minutes; do not administer via IV bolus <u>or</u> IM; 400-800 mg q 6 hours prn; maximum 3,200 mg/day
Pediatric: <6 months: not recommended; 6 months-<12 years: 10 mg/kg q 4-6 hours prn; max 400 mg/dose; max 40 mg/kg <u>or</u> 2,400 mg/24 hours, whichever is less; 12-17 years: 400 mg q 4-6 hours prn; max 2,400 mg/24 hours

    Caldolor *Vial:* 800 mg/8 ml single-dose

    Comment: Prepare Caldolor dolutiion for IV administration as follows: 100 mg dose: dilute 1 ml of **Caldolor** in at least 100 ml of diluent (IVF); 200 mg dose: dilute 2 ml of **Caldolor** in at least 100 ml of diluent; 400 mg dose: dilute 4 ml of **Caldolor** in at least 100 ml of diluent; 800 mg dose: dilute 8 ml of **Caldolor** in at least 200 ml of diluent. **Caldolor** is also indicated for management of fever. For adults with fever, 400 mg via IV infusion, followed by 400 mg q 4-6 hours <u>or</u> 100-200 mg q 4 hours prn.

OCULAR PAIN

▷ *difluprednate* **(C)** apply 1 drop to affected eye qid; for postop ocular pain, begin treatment 24 hours postop and continue x 2 weeks; then bid daily x 1 week; then taper
Pediatric: not recommended

    Durezol *Ophth emul:* 0.05% (5 ml)

Comment: **Durezol** is an ophthalmic steroid.
▶ *nepafenac* (C) apply 1 drop to affected eye tid; for postop ocular pain, begin
treatment 24 hours before surgery and continue day of surgery and for two weeks
post-op
Pediatric: <10 years: not recommended; ≥10 years: same as adult
  Nevanac *Ophth susp:* 0.1% (3 ml) (benzalkonium chloride)
  Comment: **Nevanac** is an ophthalmic NSAID.

TOPICAL/TRANSDERMAL NSAIDs

▶ *capsaicin* (B)(G) apply tid-qid prn to intact skin
Pediatric: <2 years: not recommended; ≥2 years: apply sparingly tid-qid prn
  Axsain *Crm:* 0.075% (1, 2 oz)
  Capsin *Lotn:* 0.025, 0.075% (59 ml)
  Capzasin-P (OTC) *Crm:* 0.025% (1.5 oz); *Lotn:* 0.025% (2 oz)
  Dolorac *Crm:* 0.025% (28 g)
  Double Cap (OTC) *Crm:* 0.05% (2 oz)
  R-Gel *Gel:* 0.025% (15, 30 g)
  Zostrix (OTC) *Crm:* 0.025% (0.7, 1.5, 3 oz)
  Zostrix HP (OTC) *Emol crm:* 0.075% (1, 2 oz)
▶ *capsaicin* 8% patch (B) apply up to 4 patches for one 60-minute application to clean
dry skin; may prep area with topical anesthetic; wear nonlatex gloves; patches may be
cut to size/shape; treatment may be repeated every 3 months; remove with cleansing
gel after treatment
Pediatric: <18 years: not recommended
  Qutenza *Patch:* 8% 1640 mcg/cm (179 mg) (1 or 2 patches, each w. 1-50 g tube
cleansing gel/carton)
▶ *diclofenac epolamine transdermal patch* (C; D ≥30 wks) apply one patch to affected
area bid; remove during bathing; avoid non-intact skin
Pediatric: not recommended
  Flector Patch *Patch:* 180 mg/patch (30/carton)
▶ *diclofenac sodium* (C; D ≥30 wks)
Pediatric: not established
  Pennsaid 1.5% in 10 drop increments, dispense and rub into front, side, and
back of knee: usually; 40 drops (40 mg) qid
    Topical soln: 1.5% (150 ml)
  Pennsaid 2% apply 2 pump actuations (40 mg) and rub into front, side, and
back of knee bid
    Topical soln: 2% (20 mg/pump actuation, 112 g)
  Comment: **Pennsaid** is indicated for the treatment of pain associated with
osteoarthritis of the knee.
    Pediatric: not recommended
  Voltaren Gel apply qid; avoid nonintact skin
    Gel: 1% (100 g)
  Comment: *diclofenac* is contraindicated with *aspirin* allergy. As with other
NSAIDs, **Voltaren Gel** should be avoided in late pregnancy (≥30 weeks) because
it may cause premature closure of the ductus arteriosus.
  Other Prescription NSAIDs *see page 489*

TOPICAL/TRANSDERMAL LIDOCAINE

▷ *lidocaine* transdermal patch (C)(G) apply one patch to affected area for 12 hours (then off for 12 hours); remove during bathing; avoid nonintact skin; do not re-use
Pediatric: not recommended
    Lidoderm *Patch:* 5% (10 cm x14 cm, 30/carton)

OPIOIDS AND OTHER ORAL ANALGESICS

▷ *butalbital/acetaminophen* (C)(G) 1 tab q 4 hours prn; max 6 tabs/day
    Pediatric: <12 years: not recommended; ≥12 years: same as adult
        Tab: but 50 mg/acet 325 mg
      Phrenilin 1-2 tabs q 4 hours prn; max 6 tabs/day
        Tab: but 50 mg/acet 325 mg
      Phrenilin Forte 1 tab or cap q 4 hours prn; max 6 caps/day
        Cap: but 50 mg/acet 325 mg; *Tab:* but 50 mg/acet 325 mg
▷ *butalbital/acetaminophen/caffeine* (C)(G)
    Pediatric: not recommended
      Fioricet 1-2 tabs q 4 hours prn; max 6/day
        Tab: but 50 mg/acet 325 mg/caf 40 mg
      Zebutal 1 cap q 4 hours prn; max 5/day
        Cap: but 50 mg/acet 325 mg/caf 40 mg
▷ *butalbital/aspirin/caffeine* (C)(III)(G)
    Pediatric: <12 years: not recommended; ≥12 year: same as adult
      Fiorinal 1-2 tabs or caps q 4 hours prn; max 6 caps/day
        Tab/Cap: but 50 mg/asa 325 mg/caf 40 mg
▷ *butalbital/aspirin/codeine/caffeine* (C)(III)(G)
    Pediatric: <12 years: not recommended; ≥12 year: same as adult
      Fiorinal with Codeine 1-2 caps q 4 hours prn; max 6 caps/day
        Cap: but 50 mg/asp 325 mg/cod 30 mg/caf 40 mg
▷ *codeine sulfate* (C)(III)(G) 15-60 q 4-6 hours prn; max 60 mg/day
    Tab: 15, 30, 60 mg
▷ *codeine/acetaminophen* (C)(III)(G) 15-60 mg of *codeine* q 4 hours prn; max 360 mg of *codeine*/day
    Pediatric: not recommended
      Tab: **Tylenol #1** cod 7.5 mg/acet 300 mg (sulfites)
        Tylenol #2 cod 15 mg/acet 300 mg (sulfites)
        Tylenol #3 cod 30 mg/acet 300 mg (sulfites)
        Tylenol #4 cod 60 mg/acet 300 mg (sulfites)
      Tylenol with Codeine Elixir (C)(III)
        Pediatric: 1 mg of *codeine*/kg/dose q 4-6 hours prn; max 60 mg of *codeine*/dose; <3 years: not recommended; 3-6 years: 5 ml tid-qid; 7-12 years: 10 ml tid-qid; >12 years: same as adult
        Elix: cod 12 mg/acet 120 mg per 5 ml (cherry) (alcohol)
▷ *dihydrocodeine/acetaminophen/caffeine* (C)(III)(G)
    Pediatric: not recommended
      Panlor DC 1-2 caps q 4-6 hours prn; max 10 caps/day
        Cap: dihydro 16 mg/acet 325 mg/caf 30 mg
      Panlor SS 1 tab q 4 hours prn; max 5 tabs/day
        Tab: dihydro 32 mg/acet 325 mg/caf 60*mg

▷ *dihydrocodeine/aspirin/caffeine* (D)(III)(G) 1-2 caps q 4 hours prn
  Pediatric: not recommended
    Synalgos-DC
      Cap: dihydro 16 mg/*asa* 356.4 mg/*caf* 30 mg
▷ *hydrocodone bitartrate* (C)(II)
  Pediatric: <18 years: not recommended
    Hysingla ER swallow whole; 1 tab once daily at the same time each day
      Tab: 20, 30, 40, 60, 80, 100, 120 mg ext-rel
    Zohydro ER swallow whole; *Opioid naïve:* 10 mg q 12 hours; may increase by 10 mg
    q 12 hours every 3-7 days; when discontinuing, titrate downward every 2-4 days
      Cap: 10, 15, 20, 30, 40, 50 mg ext-rel
▷ *hydrocodone bitartrate/acetaminophen* (C)(II)(G)
  Pediatric: not recommended
    Hycet 3 tsp (15 ml) q 4-6 hours prn; max 18 tsp/day
      Liq: hydro 7.5 mg/*acet* 325 mg per 15 ml
    Lorcet 1-2 caps q 4-6 hours prn; max 8 caps/day
      Cap: hydro 5 mg/*acet* 325 mg
    Lorcet 10/650 1 tab q 4-6 hours prn; max 6 tabs/day
      Tab: hydro 10 mg/*acet* 325 mg
    Lorcet-HD 1 cap q 4-6 hours prn; max 6 tabs/day
      Cap: hydro 5 mg/*acet* 325 mg
    Lorcet Plus 1 tab q 4-6 hours prn; max 6 tabs/day
      Tab: hydro 7.5 mg/*acet* 325 mg
    Lortab 2.5/500 1-2 tabs q 4-6 hours prn; max 8 tabs/day
      Tab: hydro 2.5 mg/*acet* 325*mg
    Lortab 5/500 1-2 tabs q 4-6 hours prn; max 8 tabs/day
      Tab: hydro 5 mg/*acet* 325*mg
    Lortab 7.5/500 1 tab q 4-6 hours prn; max 6 tabs/day
      Tab: hydro 7.5 mg/*acet* 325*mg
    Lortab 10/500 1 tab q 4-6 hours prn; max 6 tabs/day
      Tab: hydro 10 mg/*acet* 325*mg
    Lortab Elixir 3 tsp q 4-6 hours prn; max 18 tsp/day
      Liq: hydro 7.5 mg/*acet* 300 mg per 15 ml (tropical fruit punch) (alcohol)
    Maxidone 1 tab q 4-6 hours prn; max 5 tabs/day
      Tab: hydro 10 mg/*acet* 325*mg
    Norco 5/325 1 tab q 4-6 hours prn; max 8 tabs/day
      Tab: hydro 5 mg/*acet* 325*mg
    Norco 7.5/325 1 tab q 4-6 hours prn; max 6 tabs/day
      Tab: hydro 7.5 mg/*acet* 325*mg
    Norco 10/325 1 tab q 4-6 hours prn; max 6 tabs/day
      Tab: hydro 10 mg/*acet* 325*mg
    Vicodin 1-2 tabs q 4-6 hours prn; max 8 tabs/day
      Tab: hydro 5 mg/*acet* 300*mg
    Vicodin ES 1 tab q 4-6 hours prn; max 6 tabs/day
      Tab: hydro 7.5 mg/*acet* 300*mg
    Vicodin HP 1 tab q 4-6 hours prn; max 6 tabs/day
      Tab: hydro 10 mg/*acet* 300*mg
    Xodol 5/300 1-2 tabs q 4-6 hours prn; max 8 caps/day
      Tab: hydro 5 mg/*acet* 300*mg

        Xodol 7.5/300 1 tab q 4-6 hours prn; max 6 caps/day
           Tab: hydro 7.5 mg/*acet* 300*mg
        Xodol 10/300 1 tab q 4-6 hours prn; max 6 caps/day
           Tab: hydro 10 mg/*acet* 300*mg
        Zamicet 10/325 1-2 tabs q 4-6 hours prn; max 8 caps/day
           Liq: hydro 10 mg/*acet* 325 mg per 15 ml
        Zydone 5/400 1-2 tabs q 4-6 hours prn; max 8 caps/day
           Tab: hydro 5 mg/*acet* 400 mg
        Zydone 7.5/400 1 tab q 4-6 hours prn; max 6 caps/day
           Tab: hydro 7.5 mg/*acet* 400 mg
        Zydone 10/400 1 tab q 4-6 hours prn; max 6 caps/day
▶ *hydrocodone/ibuprofen* (C; not for use in 3rd)(II)(G)
   Pediatric: not recommended
        Ibudone 5/200 1 tab q 4-6 hours prn; max 5 tabs/day
           Tab: hydro 5 mg/*ibup* 200 mg
        Ibudone 10/200 1 tab q 4-6 hours prn; max 5 tabs/day
           Tab: hydro 10 mg/*ibup* 200 mg
        Reprexain 1 tab q 4-6 hours prn; max 5 tabs/day
           Tab: hydro 5 mg/*ibup* 200 mg
        Vicoprofen 1 tab q 4-6 hours prn; max 5 tabs/day
           Tab: hydro 7.5 mg/*ibup* 200 mg
▶ *hydromorphone* (C)(II)(G)
   Pediatric: not recommended
        Dilaudid initially 2-4 mg q 4-6 hours prn
           Tab: 2, 4, 8 mg (sulfites)
        Dilaudid Oral Liquid 2.5-10 mg q 3-6 hours prn
           Liq: 5 mg/5 ml (sulfites)
        Dilaudid Rectal Suppository 2.5-10 mg q 6-8 hours prn
           Rectal supp: 3 mg
        Dilaudid Injection initially 1-2 mg SC or IM q 4-6 hours prn
           Amp: 1, 2, 4 mg/ml (1 ml)
        Dilaudid-HP Injection initially 1-2 mg SC or IM q 4-6 hours prn
           Amp: 10 mg/ml (1 ml)
        Exalgo initially 8-64 mg once daily
           Tab: 8, 12, 16, 32 mg ext-rel (sulfites)
▶ *meperidine* (C; D in 2nd, 3rd)(II)(G) 50-150 mg q 3-4 hours prn
   Pediatric: 0.5-0.8 mg/lb q 3-4 hours prn; max adult dose
        Demerol *Tab:* 50, 100 mg; *Syr:* 50 mg/5 ml (banana) (alcohol-free)
▶ *meperidine/promethazine* (C; D in 2nd, 3rd)(II)(G)
   Pediatric: not recommended
        Mepergan 1-2 tsp q 3-4 hours prn
           Syr: mep 25 mg/*prom* 25 mg per ml
        Mepergan Fortis 1-2 tsp q 4-6 hours prn
           Tab: mep 50 mg/*prom* 25 mg
▶ *methadone* (C)(II) 2.5-10 mg PO, SC, or IM q 3-4 hours prn
   Pediatric: not recommended
        Dolophine *Tab:* 5, 10 mg; *Dispersible tab:* 40 mg (dissolve in 120 ml orange juice or other citrus drink); *Oral conc:* 5, 5 mg/5 ml; 10 mg/10 ml; *Inj:* 10 mg/ml

Comment: *methadone* maintenance is allowed only by approved treatment programs with strict state and federal regulations.
▶ *morphine sulfate* (C)(II)(G) tabs, usually 15-30 mg q 4 hours prn; solution, usually 10-20 mg q 4 hours prn
Pediatric: <18 years: not recommended
Tab: 15*, 30*mg; *Oral soln:* 10 mg/5 ml, 20 mg/5 ml (100, 500 ml), 100 mg/5 ml (30, 120 ml)
▶ *morphine sulfate (immed- and sust-rel)* (C)(II)
Comment: Dosage dependent upon previous opioid dosage; see product literature for conversion guidelines; not for prn use; swallow whole or sprinkle contents of caps on applesauce (do not crush, chew, or dissolve). Generic *morphine sulfate* is available in the following forms: *Tab:* 15*, 30*mg; *Oral soln:* 10, 20 mg/5 ml (100 ml); 100 mg/5 ml (30, 120 ml w. oral syringe).
Pediatric: <18 years: not recommended
    Duramorph administer per anesthesia
       IV/Intrathecal/Epidural: 0.5, 1 mg/ml
    Infumorph administer per anesthesia
       Intrathecal/Epidural: 10, 20 mg/ml
    Kadian (G) 1 cap every 12-24 hours
       Cap: 10, 20, 30, 50, 60, 80, 100, 200 mg sust-rel
    MS Contin (G) 1 tab every 24 hours
       Tab: 15, 30, 60, 100, 200 mg sust-rel
    MSIR 5-30 mg q 4 hours prn
       Tab: 15*, 30*mg; *Cap:* 15, 30 mg
    MSIR Oral Solution 5-30 mg q 4 hours prn
       Oral soln: 10, 20 mg/5 ml (120 ml)
    MSIR Oral Solution Concentrate 5-30 mg q 4 hours prn
       Oral conc: 20 mg/ml (30, 120 ml w. dropper)
    Oramorph SR 1 cap every 12-24 hours
       Tab: 15, 30, 60, 100 mg sust-rel
    Roxanol Oral Solution 10-30 mg q 4 hours prn
       Oral soln: 20 mg/ml (1, 4, 8 oz)
    Roxanol Rescudose
       Oral soln: 10 mg/2.5 ml (25 single-dose)
▶ *morphine sulfate/naltrexone* (C)(II)
Pediatric: <18 years: not recommended
    Embeda 1 cap q 12-24 hours
       Cap: **Embeda 20/0.8** *morph* 20 mg/*nal* 0.8 mg ext-rel
    Embeda 30/1.2 *morph* 30 mg/*nal* 1.2 mg ext-rel
    Embeda 50/2 *morph* 50 mg/*nal* 2 mg ext-rel
    Embeda 60/2.4 *morph* 60 mg/*nal* 2.4 mg ext-rel
    Embeda 80/3.2 *morph* 80 mg/*nal* 3.2 mg ext-rel
    Embeda 100/4 *morph* 100 mg/*nal* 4 mg ext-rel
    Comment: **Embeda** is not for prn use; for use in opioid-tolerant patients only; swallow whole or sprinkle contents of caps on applesauce (do not crush, chew, or dissolve); do not administer via NG or gastric tube (PEG tube).
▶ *nalbuphine* (B)(G) 10 mg/70 kg IM, SC, or IV q 3-6 hours prn
Pediatric: <18 years: not recommended
    Nubain *Amp:* 10, 20 mg/ml (1 ml) (sulfite-free, parabens-free)

▷ *oxycodone* (B)(II) 5-15 mg q 4-6 hours prn

Comment: Concomitant use os CYP3A4 inhibitors may increase opioid effects and CYP3A4 inducers may decrease effects <u>or</u> possibly cause development of an abstinence syndrome (withdrawal symtoms) in patients who are physically *oxycodone* dependent/addicted.

Pediatric: <18 years: not recommended

  Oxaydo *Tab:* 5, 7.5 mg

  Comment: Oxaydo is the first and only immediate-release oral *oxycodone* that discourages intranasal abuse. Oxaydo is formulated with sodium lauryl sulfate, an inactive ingredient that may cause nasal burning and throat irritation when snorted and, thus potentially reducing abuse liability. There is no generic equivalent.

  Oxecta *Tab:* 5, 7.5 mg

  Oxycodone Oral Solution (G) *Oral soln:* 5 mg/5 ml (15, 30 ml)

  OxyIR (G) *Cap:* 5 mg

  Roxycodone *Tab:* 5, 15*, 30*mg; *Oral soln:* 5 mg/ml

  Roxycodone Intensol *Oral soln:* 20 mg/ml

▷ *oxycodone cont-rel* (B)(II)(G) dosage dependent upon previous opioid dosages; see product literature for conversion guidelines

Pediatric: <11 years: not recommended; 11-16 years: must already tolerate minimum opium dose equal to *oxycodone* 20 mg/day x 5 days; >16 year: same as adult

  OxyContin dose q 12 hours

    Tab: 10, 15, 20, 30, 40, 60, 80 mg cont-rel

  OxyFast dose q 6 hours

    Oral conc: 20 mg/ml (30 ml w. dropper)

  Xtampza ER dose q 12 hours

    Pediatric: not recommended

    Cap: 10, 15, 20, 30, 40 mg ext-rel

  Comment: May open the Xtampza ER capsule and sprinkle in water <u>or</u> on soft food.

▷ *oxycodone/acetaminophen* (C)(II)(G)

  Comment: Maximum 4 grams acetaminophen per day.

  Pediatric: not recommended

    Magnacet 2.5/400 1 tab q 6 hours prn; max 10 tabs/day

      Tab: oxy 2.5 mg/*acet* 325 mg

    Magnacet 5/400 1 tab q 6 hours prn; max 10 tabs/day

      Tab: oxy 5 mg/*acet* 325 mg

    Magnacet 7.5/400 1 tab q 6 hours prn; max 8 tabs/day

      Tab: oxy 7.5 mg/*acet* 325 mg

    Magnacet 10/400 1 tab q 6 hours prn; max 6 tabs/day

      Tab: oxy 10 mg/*acet* 325 mg

    Percocet 2.5/325 1 tab q 6 hours prn; max 4 g acet/day

      Tab: oxy 2.5 mg/*acet* 325 mg

    Percocet 5/325 1 tab q 6 hours prn; max 4 g acet/day

      Tab: oxy 5 mg/*acet* 325*mg

    Percocet 7.5/325 1 tab q 6 hours prn; max 4 g acet/day

      Tab: oxy 7.5 mg/*acet* 325 mg

    Percocet 7.5/500 1 tabs q 6 hours prn; max 4 g acet/day

      Tab: oxy 7.5 mg/*acet* 325 mg

    Percocet 10/325 1 tabs q 6 hours prn; max 4 g acet/day

      Tab: oxy 10 mg/*acet* 325 mg

    Percocet 10/650 1 tab q 6 hours prn; max 4 g acet/day
      Tab: oxy 10 mg/*acet* 325 mg
    Roxicet 5/325 1 tab/tsp q 6 hours prn
      Tab: oxy 5 mg/*acet* 325 mg; *Oral soln: oxy* 5 mg/*acet* 325 mg per 5 ml
    Roxicet 5/500 1 caplet q 6 hours prn
      Cplt: oxy 5 mg/*acet* 325 mg
    Roxicet Oral Solution 1 tsp q 6 hours prn
      Oral soln: oxy 5 mg/*acet* 325 mg per 5 ml (alcohol 0.4%)
    Tylox 1 cap q 6 hours prn
      Cap: oxy 5 mg/*acet* 325 mg
    Xartemis XR 2 tabs q 12 hours prn
      Tab: oxy 7.5 mg/*acet* 325 mg
▷ *oxycodone/aspirin* (D)(II)(G)
    Percodan 1 tab q 6 hours prn
      Pediatric: not recommended
      Tab: oxy 4.8355 mg/*asa* 325*mg
    Percodan-Demi 1-2 tabs q 6 hours prn
      Pediatric: 6-12 years: 1/4 tab q 6 hours prn; >12-18 years: 1/2 tab q 6 hours prn
      Tab: oxy 2.25 mg/*oxy tere* 0.19 mg/*asa* 325 mg
▷ *oxycodone/ibuprofen* (C)(II)(G)
    Pediatric: <14 years: not recommended; ≥14 years: same as adult
    Combunox 1 tab q 6 hours prn
      Tab: oxy 5 mg/*ibu* 400*mg
▷ *oxycodone/naloxone* (C)(II) 1 tab q 3-4 hours prn
    Pediatric: not recommended
    Targiniq
      Tab: **Targiniq 10/5** oxy 10 mg/*nal* 5 mg
            Targiniq 20/10 oxy 20 mg/*nal* 10 mg
            Targiniq 40/20 oxy 40 mg/*nal* 20 mg
▷ *oxymorphone* (C)(II)(G)
    Pediatric: <18 years: not recommended
    Numorphan 1supp q 4-6 hours prn
      Rectal supp: 5 mg; *Vial:* 1 mg/ml (1 ml), *Amp:* 1.5 mg/ml (10 ml);
    Comment: Store in refrigerator in original package. 1 mg of
    Numorphan is approximately equivalent in analgesic activity to 10 mg of
    morphine sulfate.
    Opana 1-1 tab q 4-6 hours prn
      Tab: 5, 10 mg
    Opana ER 1 tab q 12 hours prn
      Tab: 5, 7.5, 10, 15, 20, 30, 40 mg ext-rel crush-resistant
    Opana Injection initially 0.5 mg IV <u>or</u> IM; 1 x 1 mg IM <u>or</u> IV q 4-6 hours prn
      Amp: 1 mg/ml (1 ml) (paraben/sodium dithionite-free)
▷ *pentazocine/aspirin* (D)(IV) 2 cplts tid <u>or</u> qid prn
    Pediatric: not recommended
    Talwin Compound *Cplt: pent* 12.5 mg/*asa* 325 mg
▷ *pentazocine/naloxone* (C)(IV) 1 tab q 3-4 hours prn
    Pediatric: not recommended
    Talwin NX *Tab: pent* 50 mg/*nal* 0.5*mg
▷ *pentazocine lactate* (C)(IV) 30 mg IM, SC, <u>or</u> IV q 3-4 hours; max 360 mg/day
    Pediatric: <1 year: not recommended; >1 year: 0.5 mg/kg IM

Talwin Injectable *Amp: pent* 30 mg/ml (1, 1.5, 2 ml)
▶ *propoxyphene napsylate/acetaminophen* (C)(IV)(G)
　　Comment: Max 4 g acetaminophen per day.
　　Pediatric: not recommended
　　　　Balacet 325 1 tab q 4 hours prn; max 6 tabs/day
　　　　　　Tab: prop 100 mg/*acet* 325 mg
▶ *tramadol* (C)(IV)(G)
　　　　Rybix ODT initially 100 mg once daily; may increase by 100 mg every 5 days; max 300 mg/day; *CrCl <30 mL/min or severe hepatic impairment:* not recommended; *Cirrhosis:* max 50 mg q 12 hours
　　　　　　Pediatric: <17 years: not recommended
　　　　　　ODT: 50 mg (mint) (phenylalanine)
　　　　Ryzolt initially 100 mg once daily; may increase by 100 mg every 5 days; max 300 mg/day; *CrCl <30 mL/min or severe hepatic mpairment:* not recommended
　　　　　　Pediatric: <16 years: not recommended; ≥16 years: same as adult
　　　　　　Tab: 100, 200, 300 mg ext-rel
　　　　Ultram 50-100 mg q 4-6 hours prn; max 400 mg/day; *CrCl <30 mL/min:* max 100 mg q 12 hours; *Cirrhosis:* max 50 mg q 12 hours
　　　　　　Pediatric: <16 years: not recommended; ≥16 year: same as adult
　　　　　　Tab: 50*mg
　　　　Ultram ER initially 100 mg once daily; may increase by 100 mg every 5 days; max 300 mg/day; *CrCl <30 mL/min or severe hepatic impairment:* not recommended
　　　　　　Pediatric: <18 years: not recommended
　　　　　　Tab: 100, 200, 300 mg ext-rel
▶ *tramadol/acetaminophen* (C)(IV)(G) 2 tabs q 4-6 hours; max 8 tabs/day; 5 days; *CrCl <30 mL/min:* max 2 tabs q 12 hours; max 4 tabs/day x 5 days
　　Pediatric: <16 years: not recommended; ≥16 year: same as adult
　　　　Ultracet *Tab: tram* 37.5/*acet* 325 mg
▶ *buprenorphine* (C)(III) change patch every 7 days; do not increase the dose until previous dose has been worn for at least 72 hours; after removal, do not re-use the site for at least 3 weeks; do not expose the patch to heat
　　Pediatric: <16 years: not recommended; ≥16 years: same as adult
　　　　Butrans Transdermal System
　　　　　　Transdermal patch: 5, 10, 20 mcg/hour (4/pck)
▶ *fentanyl* transdermal system (C)(II) apply to clean, dry, non-irritated, intact, skin; hold in place for 30 seconds; start at lowest dose and titrate upward; *Opioid-naïve:* change patch every 3 days (72 hours)
　　Pediatric: <18 years or <110 lb: not recommended
　　　　Duragesic *Transdermal patch:* 12, 25, 37.5, 50, 62.5, 75, 87.5, 100 mcg/hour (5/pck)
▶ *fentanyl iontophoretic transdermal system*
　　　　Ionsys is a transdermal patient-controlled device that sticks to the arm or chest; it is activated when the patient pushes the button
　　　　Comment: Ionsys is for in-hospital use only and should be discontinued prior to hospital discharge. It is indicated for postop pain relief.

TRANSMUCOSAL OPIOID

Comment: For chronic severe pain. For management of breakthrough pain in patients with cancer who are already receiving and who are tolerant to opioid therapy. Opioid-tolerant patients are those taking oral *morphine* ≥60 mg/day, transdermal *fentanyl* ≥25 mcg/hr, *oxycodone* ≥30 mg/day, oral *hydromorphone* ≥8 mg/day, or an equianalgesic dose of another opioid, for ≥1 week

OPIOID PARTIAL AGONIST-ANTAGONIST

▷ *buprenorphine* (C)
    Pediatric: <16 year: not recommended; ≥16 year: same as adult
        Subutex 8 mg in a single dose on day 1; then 16 mg in a single dose on day 2; target dose is 16 mg/day in a single dose; dissolve under tongue; do not chew or swallow whole
            SL tab (lemon-lime) or *SL film (lime):* 2, 8 mg (30/pck)
▷ *fentanyl* buccal soluble film (C)(II) dissolve 1 film on moistened area inside cheek; initially 200 mcg; no more than 4 doses/day at least 2 hours apart; max 1200 mcg/dose; do not cut film
    Pediatric: <18 years: not recommended
        Onsolis *Buccal film:* 200, 400, 600, 800, 1200 mcg (30 films/pck)
▷ *fentanyl citrate* transmucosal unit (C)(II)(G) initially one 200 mcg unit placed between cheek and lower gum; move from side to side; suck (not chew); use 6 units before titrating; titrate dose as needed; max 4 units/day
    Pediatric: <18 years: not recommended
        Actiq *Unit:* 200, 400, 600, 800, 1200, 1600 mcg (24 units/pck)
        Fentora *Unit:* 100, 200, 400, 600, 800 mcg (24 units/pck)
▷ *fentanyl* sublingual tab (C)(II) initially one 100 mcg dose; if inadequate after 30 minutes, may repeat; titrate in increments of 100 mcg; max 2 doses per episode, up to 4 episodes per day; wait at least 2 hours before treating another episode; *Maintenance:* use only one tablet of appropriate strength; do not chew, suck, or swallow tablets; do not convert from other *fentanyl* products on a mcg-per-mcg basis or interchange with other *fentanyl* products
    Pediatric: <18 years: not recommended
        Abstral *SL tab:* 100, 200, 300, 400, 600, 800 mcg (32 tabs/pck)
▷ *fentanyl sublingual spray* (C)(II)
    Pediatric: <18 years: not recommended
        Subsys 100, 200, 400, 600, 800 mcg/S L spray
        Comment: Subsys is not bioequivalent with other *fentanyl* products. Do not convert patients from other *fentanyl* products to **Subsys** on a mcg-per-mcg basis. There are no conversion directions available for patients on any other *fentanyl* products other than **Actiq.** (Note: This includes oral, transdermal, or parenteral formulations of *fentanyl.*)

PARENTERAL OPIOID (AGONIST/ANTAGONIST)

▷ *pentazocine/naloxone* (C)(IV) 1-2 tabs q 3-4 hours prn; max 12 tabs/day
    Pediatric: <12 years: not recommended; ≥12 year: same as adult
        Talwin-NX *Tab:* pent 50 mg/nal 0.5*mg

INTRANASAL TRANSMUCOSAL NARCOTIC ANALGESICS

▷ *butorphanol* nasal spray (C)(IV) initially 1 spray (1 mg) in one nostril and may repeat after 60-90 minutes (*Elderly* 90-120 minutes) in opposite nostril if needed or 1 spray in each nostril and may repeat in 3-4 hours
    Pediatric: <18 years: not recommended
        Butorphanol Nasal Spray, Stadol Nasal Spray *Nasal spray:* 10 mg/ml, 1 mg/actuation (2.5 ml)

➤ *fentanyl* nasal spray (C)(II) initially 1 spray (100 mcg) in one nostril and may repeat after 2 hours; when adequate analgesia is achieved, use that dose for subsequent breakthrough episodes

Titration steps: 100 mcg using 1 x 100 mcg spray; 200 mcg using 2 x 100 mcg spray (1 in each nostril); 400 mcg using 1 x 400 mcg spray; 800 mcg using 2 x 400 mcg (1 in each nostril); max 800 mcg; limit to ≤4 doses per day

Pediatric: <18 years: not recommended

> **Lazanda Nasal Spray** *Nasal spray:* 100, 400 mcg/100 mcl (8 sprays/bottle)
>
> **Comment:** **Lazanda Nasal Spray** is available by restricted distribution program. Call 855-841-4234 or visit www.LazandaREMS.com to enroll. **Lazanda Nasal Spray** is indicated for the management of breakthrough pain in cancer patients who are already receiving and who are tolerant to opioid therapy for their underlying persistent cancer pain. Patients considered opioid tolerant are those who are taking at least 60 mg of oral morphine/day, 25 mcg of transdermal *fentanyl*/hour, 30 mg oral *oxycodone*/day, 8 mg oral *hydromorphone*/day, 25 mg oral *oxymorphone*/day, or an equianalgesic dose of another opioid for a week or longer. Patients must remain on around-the-clock opioids when using **Lazanda Nasal Spray**. As such, it is contraindicated in the management of acute or post-op pain, including headache/migraine, or dental pain.

➤ *ziconotide* intrathecal (IT) infusion (C) initially no more than 2.4 mcg/day (0.1 mcg/hour) and titrate to upward by up to 2.4 mcg/day (0.1 mcg/day at intervals of no more than 2-3 times per week, up to a recommended maximum of 19.2 mcg/day (0.8 mcg/hr) by Day 21; dose increases in increments of less than 2.4 mcg/day (0.1 mcg/hr) and increases in dose less frequently than 2-3 times per week may be used.

Pediatric: not recommended

> **Prialt** *Vial:* 25 mcg/ml (20 ml), 100 mcg/ml (1, 2, 5 ml)
>
> **Comment:** Patients with a pre-existing history of psychosis should not be treated with *ziconotide*. Contraindications to the use of IT analgesia include conditions such as the presence of infection at the microinfusion injection site, uncontrolled bleeding diathesis, and spinal canal obstruction that impairs circulation of CSF.

⬤ PANCREATIC ENZYME DEFICIENCY

Comment: Seen in chronic pancreatitis, postpancreatectomy, cystic fibrosis, steatorrhea, post-GI tract bypass surgery, and ductal obstruction from neoplasia. May sprinkle cap; however, do not crush or chew cap or tab. May mix with applesauce or other acidic food; follow with water or juice. Do not let any drug remain in mouth. Take dose just prior to each meal or snack. Base dose on lipase units; adjust per diet and clinical response (i.e., steatorrhea). Pancrelipase products are interchangeable. Contraindicated with pork protein hypersensitivity.

PANCRELIPASE PRODUCTS

➤ *pancreatic enzymes* (C)

> **Creon** 500 units/kg per meal; max 2,500 units/kg per meal or <10,000 units/kg per day or <4,000 units/g fat ingested per day
>
> *Pediatric:* <12 months: 2,000-4,000 units per 120 ml formula or per breast-feeding (do not mix directly into formula or breast milk; 12 months to 4 years: 1,000 units/kg per meal; max 2,500 units/kg per meal <10,000 units/kg per day; >4 years: same as adult

Cap: **Creon 3000** *lip* 3,000 units/*pro* 9,500 units/*amyl* 15,000 units del-rel
Creon 6000 *lip* 6,000 units/*pro* 19,000 units/ *amyl* 30,000 units del-rel
Creon 12000 *lip* 12,000 units/*pro* 38,000 units/ amyl 60,000 units del-rel
Creon 24000 *lip* 24,000 units/*prot* 76,000 units/*amyl* 120,000 units del-rel
Creon 36000 *lip* 36,000 units/*pro*114,000 units/*amyl* 180,000 units del-rel

Cotazym 1-3 tabs just prior to each meal or snack
  Pediatric: not recommended
  Tab: **Cotazym** *lip* 1,000 units/*pro* 12,500 units/*amyl* 12,500 units del-rel
    Cotazym-S *lip* 5,000 units/*pro* 20,000 units/ *amyl* 20,000 units del-rel
Donnazyme 1-3 caps just prior to each meal or snack
  Pediatric: not recommended
  Cap: **Donnazyme** *lip* 5,000 units/*pro* 20,000 units/*amyl* 20,000 units del-rel
Ku-Zyme 1-2 caps just prior to each meal or snack
  Pediatric: not recommended
  Cap: **Ku-Zyme:** *lip* 12,000 units/*pro* 15,000 units/*amyl* 15,000 units del-rel
Kutrase 1-2 caps just prior to each meal or snack
  Pediatric: not recommended
  Cap: **Kutrase:** *lip* 12,000 units/*pro* 30,000 units/*amyl* 30,000 units del-rel
Pancreaze 2,500 lipase units/kg per meal or <10,000 lipase units/kg per day or
<4,000 lipase units/gram fat ingested per day
  Pediatric: <12 months: 2,000-4,000 lipase units per 120 ml formula or per
  breastfeeding; >12 months to <4 years 1,000 lipase units/kg per meal; >4
  years: 500 lipase units/kg per meal; max: adult dose
  Cap: **Pancreaze 4200** *lip* 4,200 units/*pro* 10,000 units/*amyl* 17,500 units
    ec-microtabs
    Pancreaze 10500 *lip* 10,500 units/*pro* 25,000 units/*amyl* 43,750 units
    ec microtabs
    Pancreaze 16800 *lip* 16,800 units/*pro* 40,000 units/*amyl* 70,000 units
    ec-microtabs
    Pancreaze 21000 *lip* 21,000 units/*pro* 37,000 units/*amyl* 61,000 units
    ec-microtabs
Pertyze *12 months to 4 years and ≥8 kg:* initially 1,000 lipase units/kg per meal; *≥4
years and ≥16 kg:* initially 500 lipase units/kg per meal; *Both:* 2,500 lipase units/kg
per meal or <10,000 units/kg per day or <4,000 lipase units/g fat ingested per day
  Cap: **Pertyze 8000** *lip* 8,000 units/*pro* 28,750 units *amyl* 30,250 units del-rel
Pertyze 16000 *lip* 16,000 units/*pro* 57,500 units/*amyl* 65,000 units del-rel
Ultrase 1-3 tabs just prior to each meal or snack
  Pediatric: same as adult
  Cap: **Ultrase** *lip* 4,500 units/*pro* 20,000 units/*amyl* 25,000 units del-rel
    Ultrase MT *lip* 12,000 units/*pro* 39,000 units/*amyl* 39,000 units del-rel
    Ultrase MT 18 *lip* 18,000 units/*pro* 58,500 units/*amyl* 58,500 units
    del-rel
    Ultrase MT 20 *lip* 20,000 units/*pro* 65,000 units/*amyl* 65,000 units
    del-rel
Viokace initially 500 lip units/kg per meal; max 2,500 lipase units/kg per meal,
or <10,000 lipase units/kg per meal, or <4,000 units/g fat ingested per day
  Pediatric: same as adult
  Tab: **Viokace 8** *lip* 8,000 units/*pro* 30,000 units/*amyl* 30,000 units
    Viokace 16 *lip* 16,000 units/*pro* 60,000 units *amyl* 60,000 units
    Pediatric: not established

Viokace 0440 *lip* 10,440 units/*pro* 39,150 units *amyl* 39,150 units
Viokace 20880 *lip* 20,880 units/*pro* 78,300 units *amyl* 78,300 units
Comment: **Viokace 10440** and **Viokase 20880** should be taken with a daily proton pump inhibitor.
Viokace Powder 1/4 tsp (0.7 g) with meals
Viokace Powder *lip* 16,800 units/*pro* 70,000 units/*amyl* 70,000 units per 1/4 tsp (8 oz)
Zenpep 500 units/kg per meal; max 2,500 units/kg per meal or <10,000 units/kg per day or <4,000 units/g fat ingested per day
 Pediatric: <12 months: 2,000-4,000 units per 120 ml formula or per breast feeding (do not mix directly into formula or breast milk); 12 months-4 years: 1,000 units/kg per meal; max 2,500 units/kg per meal <10,000 units/kg per day; >4 years: same as adult
 Cap: **Zenpep 5000** *lip* 5,000 units/*prot* 17,000 units/*amyl* 27,000 units del-rel
  Zenpep 10000 *lip* 10,000 units/*prot* 34,000 units/*amyl* 55,000 units del-rel
  Zenpep 15000 *lip* 15,000 units/*prot* 51,000 units/*amyl* 82,000 units del-rel
  Zenpep 20000 *lip* 20,000 units/*prot* 68,000 units/*amyl* 109,000 units del-rel
Zymase 1-3 caps just prior to each meal or snack
 Pediatric: not recommended
 Cap: **Zymase** *lip* 12,000 units/*prot* 24,000 units/*amyl* 24,000 units del-rel

◯ PANIC DISORDER

Comment: If possible when considering a benzodiazepine to treat anxiety, a short-acting benzodiazepines should be used only prn to avert intense anxiety and panic for the least time necessary while a different non-addictive anti-anxiety regimen (e.g., SSRI, SNRI, TCA, buspirone, beta-blocker) is established and effective treatment goals achieved. Co-administration of SSRIs with TCAs requires extreme caution. Concomitant use of MAOIs and SSRIs is absolutely contraindicated. Avoid other serotonergic drugs. A potentially fatal adverse event is *serotonin syndrome*, caused by serotonin excess. Milder symptoms require HCP intervention to avert severe symptoms which can be rapidly fatal without urgent/emergent medical care. Symptoms include restlessness, agitation, confusion, hallucinations, tachycardia, hypertension, dilated pupils, muscle twitching, muscle rigidity, loss of muscle coordination, diaphoresis, diarrhea, headache, shivering, piloerection, hyperpyrexia, cardiac arrhythmias, seizures, loss of consciousness, coma, death. Abrupt withdrawal or interruption of treatment with an antidepressant medication is sometimes associated with an *antidepressant discontinuation syndrome* which may be mediated by gradually tapering the drug over a period of two weeks or longer, depending on the dose strength and length of treatment. Common symptoms of the *serotonin discontinuation syndrome* include flu-like symptoms (nausea, vomiting, diarrhea, headaches, sweating), sleep disturbances (insomnia, nightmares, constant sleepiness), mood disturbances (dysphoria, anxiety, agitation), cognitive disturbances (mental confusion, hyperarousal), sensory and movement disturbances (imbalance, tremors, vertigo, dizziness, electric-shock-like sensations in the brain, often described by sufferers as "brain zaps."

SELECTIVE SEROTONIN REUPTAKE INHIBITORS (SSRIs)

➤ *escitalopram* (C)(G) initially 10 mg daily; may increase to 20 mg daily after 1 week; elderly or hepatic impairment, 10 mg once daily

Pediatric: <12 years: not recommended; 12-17 years: initially 10 mg once daily; may increase to 20 mg once daily after 3 weeks

    Lexapro *Tab:* 5, 10*, 20*mg

    Lexapro Oral Solution *Oral soln:* 1 mg/ml (240 ml) (peppermint) (parabens)

▷ *fluoxetine* (C)(G)

    Prozac initially 20 mg daily; may increase after 1 week; doses >20 mg /day should be divided into AM and noon doses; max 80 mg/day

        Pediatric: <7 years: not recommended; 7-17 years: initially 10 mg/day; may increase after 2 weeks to 20 mg/day; range 20-60 mg/day; range for lower weight children 20-30 mg/day

        Cap: 10, 20, 40 mg; *Tab:* 30*, 60*mg; *Oral soln:* 20 mg/5 ml (4 oz) (mint)

    Prozac Weekly following daily *fluoxetine* therapy at 20 mg/day for 13 weeks, may initiate **Prozac Weekly** 7 days after the last 20 mg *fluoxetine* dose

        Pediatric: not recommended

        Cap: 90 mg ent-coat del-rel pellets

▷ *paroxetine maleate* (D)(G)

    Pediatric: not recommended

    Paxil initially 20 mg daily in AM; may increase by 10 mg/day at weekly intervals as needed; max 60 mg/day

        Tab: 10*, 20*, 30, 40 mg

    Paxil CR initially 25 mg daily in AM; may increase by 12.5 mg at weekly intervals as needed; max 62.5 mg/day

        Tab: 12.5, 25, 37.5 mg cont-rel ent-coat

    Paxil Suspension initially 20 mg daily in AM; may increase by 10 mg/day at weekly intervals as needed; max 60 mg/day

        Oral susp: 10 mg/5 ml (250 ml) (orange)

▷ *sertraline* (C) initially 50 mg daily; increase at 1 week intervals if needed; max 200 mg daily

    Pediatric: <6 years: not recommended; 6-12 years: initially 25 mg daily; max 200 mg/day; 13-17 years: initially 50 mg daily; max 200 mg/day

    Zoloft *Tab:* 15*, 50*, 100*mg; *Oral conc:* 20 mg per ml (60 ml, dilute just before administering in 4 oz water, ginger ale, lemon-lime soda, lemonade, or orange juice) (alcohol 12%)

SEROTONIN-NOREPINEPHRINE REUPTAKE INHIBITORS (SNRIs)

▷ *desvenlafaxine* (C) swallow whole; initially 50 mg once daily; max 120 mg/day

    Pediatric: not recommended

    Pristiq *Tab:* 50, 100 mg ext-rel

▷ *venlafaxine* (C)

    Effexor initially 75 mg/day in 2-3 doses; may increase at 4 day intervals in 75 mg increments to 150 mg/day; max 375 mg/day

        Pediatric: <18 years: not recommended

        Tab: 25, 37.5, 50, 75, 100 mg

    Effexor XR initially 75 mg q AM; may start at 37.5 mg daily x 4-7 days, then increase by increments of up to 75 mg/day at intervals of at least 4 days; usual max 375 mg/day

        Pediatric: not recommended

        Cap: 37.5, 75, 150 mg ext-rel

TRICYCLIC ANTIDEPRESSANTS (TCAs)

▷ *doxepin* (C)(G)
  Pediatric: not recommended
    Cap: 10, 25, 50, 75, 100, 150 mg; *Oral conc:* 10 mg/ml (4 oz w. dropper)
▷ *imipramine* (C)(G)
  Pediatric: not recommended
    Tofranil initially 75 mg daily (max 200 mg); *Adolescents:* initially 30-40 mg daily
    (max 100 mg/day); if maintenance dose exceeds 75 mg daily, may switch to
    Tofranil PM for divided <u>or</u> bedtime dose
      Tab: 10, 25, 50 mg
    Tofranil PM initially 75 mg daily 1 hour before HS; max 200 mg
      Cap: 75, 100, 125, 150
    Tofranil Injection 50 mg IM; lower dose for adolescents; switch to oral form as
    soon as possible
      Amp: 25 mg/2 ml (2 ml)

1ST GENERATION ANTIHISTAMINE

▷ *hydroxyzine* (C)(G) 50-100 mg qid; max 600 mg/day
  Pediatric: <6 years: 50 mg/day divided qid; ≥6 years: 50-100 mg/day divided qid
    Atarax *Tab:* 10, 25, 50, 100 mg; *Syr:* 10 mg/5 ml (alcohol 0.5%)
    Vistaril *Cap:* 25, 50, 100 mg; *Oral susp:* 25 mg/5 ml (4 oz) (lemon)

AZASPIRONES

▷ *buspirone* (B) initially 7.5 mg bid; may increase by 5 mg/day q 2-3 days; max 60 mg/day
  Pediatric: <6 years: not recommended; 6-17 years: same as adult
    BuSpar *Tab:* 5, 10, 15*, 30* mg

BENZODIAZEPINES

Short Acting

▷ *alprazolam* (D)(IV)(G)
  Pediatric: <18 years: not recommended
    Niravam initially 0.25-0.5 mg tid; may titrate every 3-4 days; max 4 mg/day
      Tab: 0.25*, 0.5*, 1*, 2*mg orally-disint
    Xanax initially 0.25-0.5 mg tid; may titrate every 3-4 days; max 4 mg/day
      Tab: 0.25*, 0.5*, 1*, 2*mg
    Xanax XR initially 0.5-1 mg once daily, preferably in the AM; increase at in-
    tervals of at least 3-4 days by up to 1 mg/day. Taper no faster than 0.5 mg every
    3 days; max 10 mg/day. When switching from immediate-release *alprazolam*,
    give total daily dose of immediate-release once daily.
      Tab: 0.5, 1, 2, 3 mg ext-rel
▷ *oxazepam* (C)(IV)(G) 10-15 mg tid-qid for moderate symptoms; 15-30 mg tid-qid
  for severe symptoms
  Pediatric: not recommended
    Tab: 15 mg; *Cap:* 10, 15, 30 mg

Intermediate Acting

▷ *lorazepam* (D)(IV)(G) 1-10 mg/day in 2-3 divided doses
  Pediatric: not recommended

Ativan *Tab:* 0.5, 1*, 2*mg
Lorazepam Intensol *Oral conc:* 2 mg/ml (30 ml w. graduated dropper)

Long Acting

▷ *chlordiazepoxide* (D)(IV)(G)
Pediatric: <6 years: not recommended; ≥6 years: 5 mg bid-qid; increase to 10 mg
bid-tid
Librium 5-10 mg tid-qid for moderate symptoms; 20-25 mg tid-qid for severe
symptoms
Cap: 5, 10, 25 mg
Librium Injectable 50-100 mg IM or IV; then 25-50 mg IM tid-qid prn; max
300 mg/day
Inj: 100 mg
▷ *chlordiazepoxide/clidinium* (D)(IV) 1-2 caps tid-qid: max 8 caps/day
Pediatric: not recommended
Librax *Cap: chlor* 5 mg/*clid* 2.5 mg
▷ *clonazepam* (D)(IV)(G) initially 0.25 mg bid; increase to 1 mg/day after 3 days
Pediatric: <18 years: not recommended
Klonopin *Tab:* 0.5*, 1, 2 mg
Klonopin Wafers dissolve in mouth with or without water
Wafer: 0.125, 0.25, 0.5, 1, 2 mg orally-disint
▷ *clorazepate* (D)(IV)(G) 30 mg/day in divided doses; max 60 mg/day
Pediatric: <9 years: not recommended; ≥9 years: same as adult
Tranxene *Tab:* 3.75, 7.5, 15 mg
Tranxene SD do not use for initial therapy
Tab: 22.5 mg ext-rel
Tranxene SD Half Strength do not use for initial therapy
Tab: 11.25 mg ext-rel
Tranxene T-Tab *Tab:* 3.75*, 7.5*, 15*mg
▷ *diazepam* (D)(IV)(G) 2-10 mg bid to qid
Pediatric: not recommended
Diastat *Rectal gel delivery system:* 2.5 mg
Diastat AcuDial *Rectal gel delivery system:* 10, 20 mg
Valium *Tab:* 2*, 5*, 10*mg
Valium Injectable *Vial:* 5 mg/ml (10 ml); *Amp:* 5 mg/ml (2 ml); *Prefilled syringe:*
5 mg/ml (5 ml)
Valium Intensol *Conc oral soln:* 5 mg/ml (30 ml w. dropper) (alcohol 19%)
Valium Oral Solution *Oral soln:* 5 mg/5 ml (500 ml) (wintergreen spice)

PHENOTHIAZINES

▷ *prochlorperazine* (C)(G)
Compazine 5 mg tid-qid
Pediatric: not recommended
Tab: 5 mg; *Syr:* 5 mg/5 ml (4 oz) (fruit); *Rectal supp:* 2.5, 5, 25 mg
Compazine Spansule 15 mg q AM or 10 mg q 12 hours
Pediatric: not recommended
Spansule: 10, 15 mg sust-rel
▷ *trifluoperazine* (C)(G) 1-2 mg bid; max 6 mg/day; max 12 weeks
Pediatric: not recommended
Stelazine *Tab:* 1, 2, 5, 10 mg

PARKINSON'S DISEASE

Parkinson's Disease-associated Dementia, *see Dementia* page 103
Comment: When administering *carbidopa* and *levodopa* separately, administer each at the same time. Titrate daily dose ratio of 1:10 *carbidopa* to *levodopa*. Max daily *carbidopa* 200 mg. Most patients will require *levodopa* 400 to 1600 mg/day in divided doses every 4 to 8 hours. After titrating both drugs to the desired effects without intolerable side effects, switch to a *carbidopa/levodopa* combination form.

DOPAMINE PRECURSOR

▷ *levodopa* (C)(G)
  Tab: 125, 150, 200 mg

DECARBOXYLASE INHIBITOR

▷ *carbidopa* (C)(G)
  Lodosyn *Tab:* 25 mg

DOPAMINE RECEPTOR AGONISTS

▷ *amantadine* (C) initially 100 mg bid; may increase after 1-2 weeks by 100 mg/day; max 400 mg/day in divided doses; for extrapyramidal effects, 100 mg bid; max 300 mg/day in divided doses
  Symmetrel *Cap:* 100 mg; *Syr:* 50 mg/5 ml (16 oz) (raspberry)
▷ *bromocriptine* (B)(G) initially 1.25 mg bid to 2.5 mg tid with meals; increase as needed every 2-4 weeks by 2.5 mg/day; max 100 mg/day
  Parlodel *Tab:* 2.5*mg; *Cap:* 5 mg
▷ *pramipexole* (C) initially 0.125 mg tid; increase at intervals q 5-7 days; max 1.5 mg tid
  Mirapex *Tab:* 0.125, 0.25*, 0.5*, 1*, 1.5*mg
▷ *ropinirole* (C) initially 0.25 mg tid for first week; then 0.5 mg tid for second week; then 0.75 mg tid for third week; then 1 mg tid for fourth week; may increase by 1.5 mg/day at 1 week intervals to 9 mg/day; then increase up to 3 mg/day at 1 week intervals; max 24 mg/day
  Requip *Tab:* 0.25, 0.5, 1, 2, 4, 5 mg
▷ *rotigotine* transdermal patch (C) apply to clean, dry, intact skin on abdomen, thigh, hip, flank, shoulder, or upper arm; rotate sites and allow 14 days before reusing site; if hairy, shave site at least 3 days before application to site; avoid abrupt cessation; taper by 2 mg/24 hours every other day; *Early stage:* initially 2 mg/24 hour patch once daily; may increase weekly by 2 mg/24 hour if needed; max 6 mg/24 hour once daily; *Advanced stage:* initially 4 mg/24 hour patch once daily; may increase weekly by 2 mg/24 hour if needed; max 8 mg/24 hour once daily
  Neupro *Trans patch:* 1 mg/24 hr, 2 mg/24 hr, 3 mg/24 hr, 4 mg/24 hr, 6 mg/24 hr, 8 mg/24 hr (30/carton) (sulfites)

DOPA-DECARBOXYLASE INHIBITORS

Comment: Contraindicated in narrow-angle glaucoma. Use with caution with sympathomimetics and antihypertensive agents.
▷ *carbidopa/levodopa* (C)(G) usually 400-1600 mg *levodopa*/day
  Pediatric: <18 years: not established

Duopa *Ent susp:* carb 4.63 mg/levo 20 mg single-use cassettes for use w. CADD Legacy 1400 Pump
Sinemet 10/100 initially 1 tab tid-qid; increase if needed daily or every other day up to qid
    Tab: carb 10 mg/levo 100 mg* **Sinemet 25/100** initially 1 tab bid-tid; increase if needed daily or every other day up to qid
    Tab: carb 25 mg/lev 100 mg*
Sinemet 25/250 1 tab tid-qid
    Tab: carb 25 mg/lev 250 mg*
Sinemet CR 25/100 initially one 25/100 tab bid; allow 3 days between dosage adjustments
    Tab: carb 25 mg/levo 100 mg cont-rel
Sinemet CR 50/200 initially one 50/200 tab bid; allow 3 days between dosage adjustments
    Tab: carb 50 mg/levo 200 mg cont-rel*

DOPA-DECARBOXYLASE INHIBITOR/DOPAMINE PRECURSOR/COMT INHIBITOR COMBINATION

▷ *carbidopa/levodopa/entacapone* (C) titrate individually with separate components; then switch to corresponding strength **levodopa** and **carbidopa**; max 8 tabs/day
    Tab: **Stalevo 50:** *carb* 12.5 mg/*levo* 50 mg/*enta* 200 mg
          Stalevo 75: *carb* 12.5 mg/*levo* 75 mg/*enta* 200 mg
          Stalevo 100: *carb* 12.5 mg/*levo* 100 mg/ *enta* 200 mg
          Stalevo 125: *carb* 12.5 mg/*levo* 125 mg/*enta* 200 mg
          Stalevo 150: *carb* 12.5 mg/*levo* 150 mg/*enta* 200 mg
          Stalevo 200: *carb* 12.5 mg/*levo* 200 mg/*enta* 200 mg

MONOAMINE OXIDASE INHIBITORS (MAOIs)

▷ *rasagiline* (C)(G) usual maintenance: 0.5-1 mg/day; max: 1 mg/day; initial dose for patients on concomitant **levodopa**: 0.5 mg daily; initial dose for patients not on concomitant **levodopa**: 1 mg daily
    Azilect *Tab:* 0.5, 1 mg
    Comment: Azelect is indicated as monotherapy or as adjunct to **levodopa**. With mild hepatic dysfunction (Child-Pugh 5-6), limit **Azelect** dose to 0.5 mg daily. With moderate to severe hepatic dysfunction (Child-Pugh 7-15), **Azelect** is not recommended. Contraindications include co-administration with *meperidine, methadone, mirtazapine, propoxyphene, tramadol, dextromethorphan, St. John's wort, cyclobenzaprine, methylphenidate, dexmethylphenidate,* or other MAOIs.
▷ *selegiline* (C)(G) 5 mg at breakfast and at lunch; max 10 mg/day
    Tab/Cap: 5 mg
▷ *selegiline* (C)(G) 1.25 mg daily; max 2.5 mg/day
    Zelapar *ODT:* 1.25 mg orally-disint (phenylalanine)

COMT INHIBITORS

▷ *entacapone* (C) 1 tab with each dose of **levodopa** or **carbidopa**; max 8 tabs/day
    Comtan *Tab:* 200 mg

Comment: **Comtan** is an adjunct to *levodopa/carbidopa* in patients with end-of-dose wearing off.

▷ *tolcapone* (C) 100-200 mg tid; max 600 mg/day
Tasmar *Tab:* 100, 200 mg
Comment: Monitor LFTs every 2 weeks. Withdraw **Tasmar** if no substantial improvement in the first 3 weeks of treatment.

CENTRALLY ACTING ANTICHOLINERGICS

▷ *benztropine mesylate* (C) initially 0.5-1 mg q HS, increase if needed; for extrapyramidal disorders 1-4 mg once daily-bid; max 6 mg/day
Cogentin *Tab:* 0.5*, 1*, 2*mg

▷ *biperiden hydrochloride* (C) initially 1 tab tid or qid, then increase as needed; max 8 tabs/day
Akineton *Tab:* 2 mg

▷ *procyclidine* (C) initially 2.5 mg tid; may increase as needed to 5 mg tid-qid every 3-5 days; max 15 mg/day
Kemadrin *Tab:* 5 mg

▷ *trihexyphenidyl* (C)(G) initially 1 mg; increase as needed by 2 mg every 3-5 days; max 15 mg/day
Artane *Tab:* 2*, 5*mg

PSEUDOBULBAR AFFECT (PBA) TREATMENT

▷ *dextromethorphan/quinidine* (C) 1 cap once daily x 7 days; then starting on day 8, 1 cap bid
Nuedexta
Pediatric: not recommended
Cap: dextro 20 mg/*quini* 10 mg
Comment: Pseudobulbar affect (PBA), emotional lability, labile affect, or emotional incontinence refers to a neurologic disorder characterized by involuntary crying or uncontrollable episodes of crying and/or laughing, or other emotional displays. PBA occurs secondary to a neurologic disease or brain injury. Brain injury or neurologic diseases such as traumatic brain injury, stroke, Parkinson's disease, multiple sclerosis, and amyotrophic lateral sclerosis (ALS, or Lou Gehrig's disease).

◯ PARONYCHIA (PERIUNGUAL ABSCESS)

▷ *cephalexin* (B)(G) 500 mg bid x 10 days
Pediatric: 25-50 mg/day in 2 divided doses x 10 days
Keflex *Cap:* 250, 333, 500, 750 mg; *Oral susp:* 125, 250 mg/5 ml (100, 200 ml) (strawberry)

▷ *clindamycin* (B)(G) 150-300 mg q 6 hours x 10 days
Pediatric: 8-16 mg/kg/day in 3-4 divided doses x 10 days
Cleocin *Cap:* 75 (tartrazine), 150 (tartrazine), 300 mg
Cleocin Pediatric Granules *Oral susp:* 75 mg/5 ml (100 ml) (cherry)

▷ *dicloxacillin* (B)(G) 500 mg q 6 hours x 10 days
Pediatric: 12.5-25 mg/kg/day in 4 divided doses x 10 days; *see page* 560 *for dose by weight*
Dynapen *Cap:* 125, 250, 500 mg; *Oral susp:* 62.5 mg/5 ml (80, 100, 200 ml)

▷ *erythromycin base* (B)(G) 500 mg q 6 hours x 10 days
  Pediatric: <45 kg: 30-50 mg in 2-4 doses x 10 days; ≥45 kg: same as adult
    Ery-Tab *Tab:* 250, 333, 500 mg ent-coat
    PCE *Tab:* 333, 500 mg
  Comment: *erythromycin* may increase INR with concomitant *warfarin*, as well as increase serum level of *digoxin*, benzodiazepines and statins.
▷ *erythromycin ethylsuccinate* (B)(G) 400 mg q 6 hours x 10 days
  Pediatric: 30-50 mg/kg/day in 4 divided doses q 6 hours x 10 days; may double dose with severe infection; max 100 mg/kg/day; *see page 563 for dose by weight*
    EryPed *Oral susp:* 200 mg/5 ml (100, 200 ml) (fruit); 400 mg/5 ml (60, 100, 200 ml) (banana); *Oral drops:* 200, 400 mg/5 ml (50 ml) (fruit); *Chew tab:* 200 mg wafer (fruit)
    E.E.S. *Oral susp:* 200, 400 mg/5 ml (100 ml) (fruit)
    E.E.S. Granules *Oral susp:* 200 mg/5 ml (100, 200 ml) (cherry)
    E.E.S. 400 Tablets *Tab:* 400 mg
  Comment: *erythromycin* may increase INR with concomitant *warfarin*, as well as increase serum level of *digoxin*, benzodiazepines and statins.

⃝ PEDICULOSIS: PEDICULOSIS HUMANUS CAPITIS (HEAD LICE) AND PHTHIRUS (PUBIC LICE)

▷ *ivermectin* (C) thoroughly wet hair; leave on for 10 minutes; then rinse off with water; do not re-treat
  Pediatric: <6 months, <33 lbs: not recommended; ≥6 months, ≥33 lbs: same as adult
    Sklice *Lotn:* 0.5% (4 oz, 117 g, laminate tube)
▷ *lindane* (C)(G) apply, leave on for 4 minutes, then thoroughly wash off
  Pediatric: <2 years: not recommended; ≥2 years: same as adult
    Kwell Shampoo *Shampoo:* 1% (60 ml)
▷ *malathion* (B)(G) thoroughly wet hair; allow to dry naturally; shampoo and rinse after 8-12 hours; use a fine tooth comb to remove lice and nits; if lice persist after 7-9 days, may repeat treatment
  Pediatric: same as adult
    Ovide (OTC) *Lotn:* 59% (2 oz)
▷ *permethrin* (B)(G) apply to washed and towel-dried hair; allow to remain on for 10 minutes, then rinse off; repeat after 7 days if needed
  Pediatric: <2 months: not recommended; ≥2 months: same as adult
    Nix (OTC) *Crm rinse:* 1% (2 oz w. comb)
▷ *pyrethrins with piperonyl butoxide* (C)(G) apply and leave on for 10 minutes, then wash off
    A-200 *Shampoo:* pyr 0.33%/*pip but* 3%
    Rid Mousse *Shampoo:* pyr 0.33%/*pip but* 4%
    Rid Shampoo *S hampoo:* pyr 0.33%/*pip but* 3%
  Comment: To remove nits, soak hair in equal parts white vinegar and water for 15-20 minutes.

◯ PELVIC INFLAMMATORY DISEASE (PID)

Comment: The following treatment regimens are published in the **2015 CDC Sexually Transmitted Diseases Treatment Guidelines.** Treatment regimens are presented by generic drug name first, followed by information about brands and dose forms. Treat all sexual partners. Because of the high risk for maternal morbidity and preterm delivery, pregnant women who have suspected PID should be hospitalized and treated with parenteral antibiotics. HIV-infected women with PID respond equally well to standard parenteral and antibiotic regimens as HIV-negative women.

OUTPATIENT REGIMENS

Regimen 1

➤ *ceftriaxone* 250 mg IM in a single dose <u>plus</u>
➤ *doxycycline* 100 mg bid x 14 days <u>with or without</u>
➤ *metronidazole* 500 mg PO bid x 14 days

Regimen 2

➤ *cefoxitin* 2 g IM in a single dose <u>plus</u>
➤ *probenecid* 1 g PO in a single dose administered concurrently <u>plus</u> *doxycycline* 100 mg bid x 14 days <u>with or without</u>
➤ *metronidazole* 500 mg PO bid x 14 days

Regimen 3

➤ Other parenteral third-generation cephalosporin (e.g., *ceftizoxime* <u>or</u> *cefotaxime*) in a single dose <u>plus</u>
➤ *doxycycline* 100 mg bid x 14 days <u>with or without</u>
➤ *metronidazole* 500 mg PO bid x 14 days

DRUG BRANDS AND DOSE FORMS

➤ *cefoxitin* (B)(G)
    Mefoxin *Vial:* 1, 2 g
➤ *ceftriaxone* (B)(G)
    Rocephin Vials 250, 500 mg: 1, 2 g
➤ *doxycycline* (D)(G)
    Actilate *Tab:* 75, 150** mg
    Adoxa *Tab:* 50, 75, 100, 150 mg ent-coat
    Doryx *Tab:* 75, 100, 150 mg del-rel
    Monodox *Cap:* 50, 75, 100 mg
    Oracea *Cap:* 40 mg del-rel
    Vibramycin *Cap:* 50, 100 mg; *Syr:* 50 mg/5 ml (raspberry) (sulfites); *Oral susp:* 25 mg/5 ml (raspberry-apple)
    Vibra-Tab *Tab:* 100 mg film-coat

Comment: *doxycycline* is contraindicated <8 years-of-age, in pregnancy, and lactation (discolors developing tooth enamel). A side effect may be photo-sensitivity (photophobia). Do not give with antacids, calcium supplements, milk or other dairy, or within two hours of taking another drug.

▷ *metronidazole* (not for use in 1st; B in 2nd, 3rd)
   Flagyl *Tab:* 250*, 500*mg
   Flagyl 375 *Cap:* 375 mg
   Flagyl ER *Tab:* 750 mg ext-rel
   Comment: Alcohol is contraindicated during treatment with oral *metronidazole*
   and for 72 hours after therapy due to a possible *disulfiram*-like reaction (nausea,
   vomiting, flushing, headache).
▷ *probenecid* (B)(G)
   Benemid *Tab:* 500*mg; *Cap:* 500 mg

PEPTIC ULCER DISEASE (PUD)

Helicobacter pylori **Eradication Regimens** *see page* 179

H₂ ANTAGONISTS

▷ *cimetidine* (B)(G)
   Pediatric: <16 years: not recommended; ≥16 years: same as adult
   Tagamet 800 mg bid <u>or</u> 400 mg qid; max 2.4 g/day
      Tab: 300, 400*, 800* mg
   Tagamet HB (OTC) *Prophylaxis:* 1 tab ac; *Treatment:* 1 tab bid
      Tab: 200 mg
   Tagamet HB Oral Suspension (OTC) *Prophylaxis:* 1 tsp ac; *Treatment:* 1 tsp bid
      Oral susp: 200 mg/20 ml (12 oz)
   Tagamet Liquid *Liq:* 300 mg/5 ml (mint-peach) (alcohol 2.8%)
▷ *famotidine* (B)(G) 20 mg bid <u>or</u> 40 mg q HS; *max* 6 weeks
   Pediatric: 0.5 mg/kg/day q HS <u>or</u> in 2 divided doses; max 40 mg/day
   Pepcid *Tab:* 20, 40 mg; *Oral susp:* 40 mg/5 ml (50 ml)
   Pepcid AC (OTC) 1 tab ac; max 2 doses/day
      Tab/Rapid dissolving tab: 10 mg
   Pepcid Complete (OTC) 1 tab ac; max 2 doses/day
      Tab: fam 10 mg/*CaCO2* 800 mg/*Mg hydroxide* 165 mg
   Pepcid RPD
      Tab: 20, 40 mg rapid-dissolving
▷ *nizatidine* (B)(G) 150 mg bid; max 12 weeks
   Pediatric: not recommended
   Axid *Cap:* 150, 300 mg
   Axid AR (OTC) 1 tab ac; max 150 mg/day
      Tab: 75 mg
▷ *ranitidine* (B)(G)
   Pediatric: <1 month: not recommended; 1 month-16 years: 2-4 mg/kg/day in 2
   divided doses; max 300 mg/day; *Duodenal/Gastric Ulcer:* 2-4 mg/kg/day divided
   bid; max 300 mg/day; *Erosive Esophagitis:* 5-10 mg/kg/day divided bid; max 300
   mg/day; >16 years: same as adult
   Zantac 150 mg bid <u>or</u> 300 mg q HS
      Tab: 150, 300 mg
   Zantac 75 (OTC) 1 tab ac
      Tab: 75 mg

Zantac EFFERdose dissolve 25 mg tab in 5 ml water; dissolve 150 mg tab in 6-8 oz water

Efferdose: 25, 150 mg effervescent (phenylalanine)

Zantac Syrup *Syr:* 15 mg/ml (peppermint) (alcohol 7.5%)

▷ **ranitidine bismuth citrate** (C) 400 mg bid

Pediatric: not recommended

Tritec *Tab:* 400 mg

PROTON PUMP INHIBITORS (PPIs)

Comment: If hepatic impairment, or if patient is Asian, consider reducing the PPI dosage. Research has demonstrated associations between PPI use and fractures of the hip, wrist, and spine, hypomagnesemia, kidney injuries and chronic kidney disease, possible cardiovascular drug interactions, and infections (e.g., Clostridium difficile and pneumonia). Reducing the acidity of the stomach allows bacteria to thrive and spread to other organs like the lungs and intestines. This risk is increased with high dose and chronic use and greatest in the elderly. (http://www.fda.gov/Drugs/DrugSafety/InformationbyDrugClass/ucm213259.htm)

▷ **dexlansoprazole** (B) 30-60 mg daily for up to 4 weeks

Pediatric: <18 years: not recommended

Dexilant *Cap:* 30, 60 mg ent-coat del-rel granules; may open and sprinkle on applesauce; do not crush or chew granules

▷ **esomeprazole** (B) 20-40 mg daily; max 8 weeks; take 1 hour before food; swallow whole or mix granules with food or juice and take immediately; do not crush or chew granules

Pediatric: <1 year: not recommended; 1-11 years: <20 kg: 10 mg; ≥20 kg: 10-20 mg once daily; 12-17 years: 20-40 mg once daily; max 8 weeks

Nexium *Cap:* 20, 40 mg ent-coat del-rel pellets

Nexium for Oral Suspension *Oral susp:* 10, 20, 40 mg ent-coat del-rel granules/pkt; mix in 2 tblsp water and drink immediately; 30 pkt/carton

▷ **lansoprazole** (B)(OTC)(G) 15-30 mg daily for up to 8 weeks; may repeat course; take before eating

Pediatric: <1 year: not recommended; 1-11, <30 kg: 15 mg once daily; ≥12 years: same as adult

Prevacid *Cap:* 15, 30 mg ent-coat del-rel granules; swallow whole or mix granules with food or juice and take immediately; do not crush or chew granules; follow with water

Prevacid for Oral Suspension *Oral susp:* 15, 30 mg ent-coat del-rel granules/pkt; mix in 2 tblsp water and drink immediately; 30 pkt/ carton (strawberry)

Prevacid SoluTab *ODT:* 15, 30 mg (strawberry) (phenylalanine)

Prevacid 24HR 15 mg ent-coat del-rel granules; swallow whole or mix granules with food or juice and take immediately; do not crush or chew granules; follow with water

▷ **omeprazole** (C)(OTC)(G) 20-40 mg daily; take before eating; swallow whole or mix granules with applesauce and take immediately; do not crush or chew; follow with water

Pediatric: <1 year: not recommended; 5-<10 kg: 5 mg daily; 10-<20 kg: 10 mg daily; ≥20 kg: same as adult

Prilosec *Cap:* 10, 20, 40 mg ent-coat del-rel granules

Pediatric: <18 years: not recommended

> **Prilosec OTC** *Tab:* 20 mg del-rel (regular, wild berry)
▷ *pantoprazole* (B) initially 40 mg bid
  Pediatric: not recommended
> **Protonix** (G) *Tab:* 40 mg ent-coat del-rel
> **Protonix for Oral Suspension** *Oral susp:* 40 mg ent-coat del-rel granules/pkt; mix in 1 tsp apple juice for 5 seconds <u>or</u> sprinkle on 1 tsp apple sauce, and swallow immediately; do not mix in water <u>or</u> any other liquid <u>or</u> food; take approximately 30 minutes prior to a meal; 30 pkt/carton
▷ *rabeprazole* (B)(OTC)(G) initially 20 mg daily; then titrate; may take 100 mg daily in divided doses <u>or</u> 60 mg bid
  Pediatric: <12 years: not recommended; ≥12 years: 20 mg once daily; max 8 weeks
> **AcipHex** *Tab:* 20 mg ent-coat del-rel
> **Antacids** *see GERD page* 150

OTHER

▷ *glycopyrrolate* (B)(G) initially 1-2 mg bid-tid; *Maintenance:* 1 mg bid; max 8 mg/day
  Pediatric: <12 years: not recommended; ≥12 years: same as adult
> **Robinul** *Tab:* 1 mg (dye-free)
> **Robinul Forte** *Tab:* 2 mg (dye-free)

Comment: *glycopyrrolate* is an anticholinergic adjunct to PUD treatment.
▷ *mepenzolate* (B)(G) 25-50 mg divided qid, with meals and at HS
> **Cantil** *Tab:* 25 mg
▷ *sucralfate* (B)(G) **Active ulcer:** 1 g qid; *Maintenance:* 1 g bid
> **Carafate** *Tab:* 1*g; *Oral susp:* 1 g/10 ml (14 oz)

PROPHYLAXIS

▷ *misoprostol* (X) 200 mg qid with food for prevention of NSAID-induced gastric ulcers
> **Cytotec** *Tab:* 100, 200 mg

⬤ PERIPHERAL NEURITIS, DIABETIC NEUROPATHIC PAIN, PERIPHERAL NEUROPATHIC PAIN

▷ **Acetaminophen for IV Infusion** *see Pain page* 296
▷ *acetaminophen* (B)(G) *see Fever page* 144
▷ *aspirin* (D)(G) *see Fever page* 144

Comment: *aspirin*-containing medications are contraindicated with history of allergic-type reaction to *aspirin*, children and adolescents with *Varicella* <u>or</u> other viral illness, and 3rd trimester pregnancy.

α₂-DELTA LIGAND

▷ *pregabalin* (GABA analog) (C)(V) initially 150 mg daily divided bid-tid; may titrate within one week; max 600 mg divided bid-tid; discontinue over one week
  Pediatric: <18 years: not recommended
> **Lyrica** *Cap:* 25, 50, 75, 100, 150, 200, 225, 300 mg; *Oral soln:* 20 mg/ml

SEROTONIN AND NOREPINEPHRINE REUPTAKE INHIBITOR (SNRI)

▷ *duloxetine* (C) swallow whole; 30-60 mg once daily; may increase by 30 mg at 1 week intervals; usual target 60 mg daily; max 120 mg/day
  Pediatric: not recommended
    Cymbalta *Cap:* 20, 30, 60 mg ent-coat pellets
    Comment: Cymbalta is indicated for chronic pain syndromes (e.g., arthritis, fibromyalgia, lowback pain).

TOPICAL/TRANSDERMAL NSAIDs

▷ *capsaicin* (B)(G) apply tid-qid prn to intact skin
  Pediatric: <2 years: not recommended; ≥2 years: apply sparingly tid-qid prn
    Axsain *Crm:* 0.075% (1, 2 oz)
    Capsin *Lotn:* 0.025, 0.075% (59 ml)
    Capzasin-P (OTC) *Crm:* 0.025% (1.5 oz); *Lotn:* 0.025% (2 oz)
    Dolorac *Crm:* 0.025% (28 g)
    Double Cap (OTC) *Crm:* 0.05% (2 oz)
    R-Gel *Gel:* 0.025% (15, 30 g)
    Zostrix (OTC) *Crm:* 0.025% (0.7, 1.5, 3 oz)
    Zostrix HP (OTC) *Emol crm:* 0.075% (1, 2 oz)
▷ *capsaicin* 8% patch (B) apply up to 4 patches for one 60-minute application to clean dry skin; may prep area with topical anesthetic; wear nonlatex gloves; patches may be cut to size/shape; treatment may be repeated every 3 months; remove with cleansing gel after treatment
  Pediatric: <18 years: not recommended
    Qutenza *Patch:* 8% 1640 mcg/cm (179 mg) (1 or 2 patches, each w. 1-50 g tube cleansing gel/carton)
▷ *diclofenac epolamine transdermal patch* (C) apply one patch to affected area bid; remove during bathing; avoid nonintact skin
  Pediatric: not recommended
    Flector Patch *Patch:* 180 mg/patch (30/carton)
▷ *capsaicin* (B)(G) apply tid to qid prn to intact skin
  Pediatric: <2 years: not recommended; ≥2 years: same as adult
    Axsain *Crm:* 0.075% (1, 2 oz)
    Capsin *Lotn:* 0.025, 0.075% (59 ml)
    Capzasin-P (OTC) *Crm:* 0.025% (1.5 oz); *Lotn:* 0.025% (2 oz)
    Dolorac *Crm:* 0.025% (28 g)
    Double Cap (OTC) *Crm:* 0.05% (2 oz)
    R-Gel *Gel:* 0.025% (15, 30 g)
    Zostrix (OTC) *Crm:* 0.025% (0.7, 1.5, 3 oz)
    Zostrix HP (OTC) *Emol crm:* 0.075% (1, 2 oz)
▷ *capsaicin* 8% patch (B) apply up to 4 patches for one 60-minute application to clean dry skin; may prep area with topical anesthetic; wear non-latex gloves; patches may be cut to size/ shape; treatment may be repeated every 3 months; remove with cleansing gel after treatment
  Pediatric: <18 years: not recommended
    Qutenza *Patch:* 8% 1640 mcg/cm (179 mg) (1 or 2 patches w. 1-50 g tube cleansing gel/carton)
▷ *lidocaine* 5% patch (B)(G) apply up to 3 patches at one time for up to 12 hours/24-hour period (12 hours on/12 hours off); patches may be cut into smaller sizes before removal of the release liner; do not re-use

Pediatric: not recommended
    Lidoderm *Patch:* 5% (10x14 cm, 30/carton)

ORAL ANALGESICS

▷ *tramadol* (C)(IV)(G)
    Rybix ODT initially 100 mg once daily; may increase by 100 mg every 5 days; max 300 mg/day; *CrCl <30 mL/min* or *severe hepatic impairment:* not recommended; *Cirrhosis:* max 50 mg q 12 hours
        Pediatric: <17 years: not recommended
        ODT: 50 mg (mint) (phenylalanine)
    Ryzolt initially 100 mg once daily; may increase by 100 mg every; 5 days; max 300 mg/day; *CrCl <30 mL/min* or *severe hepatic impairment:* not recommended
        Pediatric: <16 years: not recommended; ≥16 years: same as adult
        Tab: 100, 200, 300 mg ext-rel
    Ultram 50-100 mg q 4-6 hours prn; max 400 mg/day; *CrCl <30 mL/min:* max 100 mg q 12 hours; *Cirrhosis:* max 50 mg q 12 hours
        Pediatric: <16 years: not recommended; ≥16 years: same as adult
        Tab: 50 mg
    Ultram ER initially 100 mg once daily; may increase by 100 mg every 5 days; max 300 mg/day; *CrCl <30 mL/min* or *severe hepatic impairment:* not recommended
        Pediatric: <18 years: not recommended
        Tab: 100, 200, 300 mg ext-rel
▷ *tramadol/acetaminophen* (C)(IV)(G) 2 tabs q 4-6 hours; max 8 tabs/day; 5 days; *CrCl <30 mL/min:* max 2 tabs q 12 hours; max 4 tabs/day x 5 days
    Pediatric: <16 years: not recommended; ≥16 years: same as adult
    Ultracet *Tab:* tram 37.5/acet 325 mg

MU-OPIOID AGONIST/NOREPINEPHRINE REUPTAKE INHIBITOR

▷ *tapentadol* (C)
    Pediatric: <18 years: not recommended
    Nucynta 50-100 mg q 4-6 hours prn; max 700 mg/day on the first day; 600 mg/day on subsequent days
        Tab: 50, 75, 100 mg
    Nucynta ER *Opioid-naïve:* initially 50 mg q 12 hours, then titrate to optimal dose within therapeutic range; usual therapeutic range 100-250 mg q 12 hours; doses >500 mg not recommended; *Converting from Nucynta:* divide total **Nucynta** daily dose into 2 **Nucynta ER** doses and administer q 12 hours; converting from *oxycodone CR* and other opioids, see mfr recommendations
        Tab: 50, 100, 150, 200, 250 mg ext-rel
    Other Oral Analgesics *see Pain page 298*

PERIPHERAL VASCULAR DISEASE (PVD, ARTERIAL INSUFFICIENCY, INTERMITTENT CLAUDICATION)

ANTIPLATELET THERAPY

▷ *aspirin* (D)(OTC) usually 81 mg once daily; range 75-325 mg once daily
    Ecotrin *Tab/Cap:* 81, 325, 500 mg ent-coat

▷ *cilostazol* (C) 100 mg bid 1/2 hour before <u>or</u> 2 hours after breakfast <u>or</u> dinner; may reduce to 50 mg bid if used with CYP 3A4 (e.g., azole antifungals, macrolides, *diltiazem*, *fluvoxamine*, *fluoxetine*, *nefazodone*, *sertraline*) or CYP 2C19 (e.g., *omeprazole*) inhibitors

    Pletal *Tab:* 50, 100 mg

    Comment: May be used with *aspirin*. Cautious use with other antiplatelet agents and anticoagulants.

▷ *clopidogrel* (B) 75 mg daily

    Plavix *Tab:* 75 mg

▷ *dipyridamole* (B)(G) 25-100 mg tid-qid

    Persantine *Tab:* 25, 50, 75 mg

    Comment: Does not potentiate *warfarin* and may be taken concomitantly. Do not administer *dipyridamole* concomitantly with *aspirin*.

▷ *pentoxifylline* (C) 400 mg tid with food

    PentoPak *Tab:* 400 mg ext-rel

    Trental *Tab:* 400 mg sust-rel

▷ *ticlopidine* (B) 250 mg bid with food

    Ticlid *Tab:* 250 mg

    Comment: Monitor for neutropenia; resolves after discontinuation.

▷ *warfarin* (X) adjust dose to maintain INR in recommended range; *see Anticoagulation Therapy page 515*

    Coumadin *Tab:* 1*, 2*, 2.5*, 5*, 7.5*, 10*mg

    Coumadin for Injection *Vial:* 2 mg/ml (5 mg) pwdr for reconstitution

    Comment: Treatment for over-anticoagulation with *warfarin* is *vitamin K*.

◯ PERTUSSIS (WHOOPING COUGH)

Prophylaxis *see Childhood Immunizations page 466*

POSTEXPOSURE PROPHYLAXIS AND TREATMENT

Comment: Antibiotics do not alter the course of illness, but they do prevent transmission. Infected persons should be isolated until after the fifth day of antibiotic treatment.

▷ *azithromycin* (B)(G) 500 mg x 1 dose on day 1, then 250 mg daily on days 2-5 or 500 mg daily x 3 days

Pediatric: 12 mg/kg/day x 5 days; max 500 mg/day; *see page 548 for dose by weight*

    Zithromax *Tab:* 250, 500, 600 mg; *Oral susp:* 100 mg/5 ml (15 ml); 200 mg/5 ml (15, 22.5, 30 ml) (cherry); *Pkt:* 1 g for reconstitution (cherry-banana)

    Zithromax Tri-pak *Tab:* 3 x 500 mg tabs/pck

    Zithromax Z-pak *Tab:* 6 x 250 mg tabs/pck

    Zmax *Oral susp:* 2 g ext-rel for reconstitution (cherry-banana) (148 mg Na$^+$)

    Comment: *azithromycin* is the drug of choice for infants <1 month-of-age.

▷ *clarithromycin* (C)(G) 250 mg bid or 500 mg ext-rel daily x 10 days

Pediatric: <6 months: not recommended; ≥6 months: 7.5 mg/kg divided bid x 10 days; *see page 558 for dose by weight*

    Biaxin *Tab:* 250, 500 mg

    Biaxin Oral Suspension *Oral susp:* 125, 250 mg/5 ml (50, 100 ml) (fruit-punch)

Biaxin XL *Tab:* 500 mg ext-rel
▷ *erythromycin base* (B)(G) 1 g/day divided qid x 14 days
Pediatric: 40 mg/kg/day in divided doses x 14 days
Ery-Tab *Tab:* 250, 333, 500 mg ent-coat
PCE *Tab:* 333, 500 mg

Comment: *erythromycin* may increase INR with concomitant *warfarin*, as well as increase serum level of *digoxin*, benzodiazepines and statins.

▷ *erythromycin ethylsuccinate* (B)(G) 1 g/day in 4 divided doses x 14 days
Pediatric: 40-50 mg/kg/day in 4 divided doses x 7 days; may double dose with severe infection; max 100 mg/kg/day; *see page 563 for dose by weight*
EryPed *Oral susp:* 200 mg/5 ml (100, 200 ml) (fruit); 400 mg/5 ml (60, 100, 200 ml) (banana); *Oral drops:* 200, 400 mg/5 ml (50 ml) (fruit); *Chew tab:* 200 mg wafer (fruit)
E.E.S. *Oral susp:* 200, 400 mg/5 ml (100 ml) (fruit)
E.E.S. Granules *Oral susp:* 200 mg/5 ml (100, 200 ml) (cherry)
E.E.S. 400 Tablets *Tab:* 400 mg

Comment: *erythromycin* may increase INR with concomitant *warfarin*, as well as increase serum level of *digoxin*, benzodiazepines and statins.

▷ *trimethoprim/sulfamethoxazole* (C)(G)
Pediatric: <2 months: not recommended; ≥2 months: 40 mg/kg/day of *sulfamethox-azole* in 2 doses bid x 10 days; *see page 576 for dose by weight*
Bactrim, Septra 2 tabs bid x 10 days
Tab: trim 80 mg/*sulfa* 400 mg*
Bactrim DS, Septra DS 1 tab bid x 10 days
Tab: trim 160 mg/*sulfa* 800 mg
Bactrim Pediatric Suspension, Septra Pediatric Suspension
Oral susp: trim 40 mg/*sulfa* 200 mg per 5 ml (100 ml) (cherry) (alcohol 0.3%)

Comment: *trimethoprim/sulfamethoxazole* is not recommended in pregnancy or lactation. *CrCl 15-30 mL/min: reduce dose by 1/2; CrCl <15 mL/min: not recommended.*

TREATMENT

Same as Postexposure Prophylaxis

PHARYNGITIS: GONOCOCCAL

Comment: Treat all sexual contacts. Empiric therapy requires concomitant treatment for *Chlamydia*. Post-treatment culture recommended with PMHx history rheumatic fever.

PRIMARY THERAPY

▷ *azithromycin* (B)(G) 1 g x 1 dose
Pediatric: 12 mg/kg/day x 5 days; max 500 mg/day; *see page 548 for dose by weight*
Zithromax *Tab:* 250, 500, 600 mg; *Oral susp:* 100 mg/5 ml (15 ml); 200 mg/5 ml (15, 22.5, 30 ml) (cherry); *Pkt:* 1 g for reconstitution (cherry-banana)
Zithromax Tri-pak *Tab:* 3 x 500 mg tabs/pck
Zithromax Z-pak *Tab:* 6 x 250 mg tabs/pck
Zmax *Oral susp:* 2 g ext-rel for reconstitution (cherry-banana) (148 mg Na⁺)

Comment: Per the CDC 2015 STD Treatment Guidelines, *azithromycin* should be used with ceftriaxone 250mg.
➤ *ceftriaxone* (B)(G) 250 mg IM x 1 dose
Pediatric: <45 kg: 125 mg IM x 1 dose; ≥45 kg: same as adult
   Rocephin *Vial:* 250, 500 mg; 1, 2 g

◯ PHARYNGITIS: STREPTOCOCCAL

➤ *amoxicillin* (B)(G) 500-875 mg bid or 250-500 mg tid x 10 days
Pediatric: <40 kg (88 lb): 20-40 mg/kg/day in 3 divided doses x 10 days or 25-45 mg/kg/day in 2 divided doses x 10 days; ≥40 kg: same as adult; *see page 543 for dose by weight*
   Amoxil *Cap:* 250, 500 mg; *Tab:* 875*mg; *Chew tab:* 125, 200, 250, 400 mg (cherry-banana-peppermint) (phenylalanine); *Oral susp:* 125, 250 mg/5 ml (80, 100, 150 ml) (strawberry); 200, 400 mg/5 ml (50, 75, 100 ml) (bubble gum); *Oral drops:* 50 mg/ml (30 ml) (bubble gum)
   Moxatag *Tab:* 775 mg ext-rel
   Trimox *Tab:* 125, 250 mg; *Cap:* 250, 500 mg; *Oral susp:* 125, 250 mg/5 ml (80, 100, 150 ml) (raspberry-strawberry)
➤ *amoxicillin/clavulanate* (B)(G) 500 mg tid or 875 mg bid x 10 days
   Augmentin *Tab:* 250, 500, 875 mg; *Chew tab:* 125, 250 mg (lemon-lime); 200, 400 mg (cherry-banana) (phenylalanine); *Oral susp:* 125 mg/5 ml (banana), 250 mg/5 ml (75, 100, 150 ml) (orange); 200, 400 mg/5 ml (50, 75, 100 ml) (orange) (phenylalanine)
      Pediatric: 40-45 mg/kg/day divided tid x 10 days or 90 mg/kg/day divided bid x 10 days *see pages 545-546 for dose by weight*
   Augmentin ES-600 *Oral susp:* 600 mg/5 ml (50, 75, 100, 125, 150, 200 ml) (strawberry cream) (phenylalanine) every 12 hours
      Pediatric: <3 months: not recommended; ≥3 months, <40 kg: 90 mg/kg/day in 2 divided doses; ≥40 kg: not recommended
   Augmentin XR 2 tabs q 12 hours x 7-10 days
      Pediatric: <16 years: use other forms; ≥16 years: same as adult
      Tab: 1000*mg ext-rel
➤ *azithromycin* (B)(G) 500 mg x 1 dose on day 1, then 250 mg daily on days 2-5 or 500 mg daily x 3 days
Pediatric: 12 mg/kg/day x 5 days; max 500 mg/day; *see page 548 for dose by weight*
   Zithromax *Tab:* 250, 500, 600 mg; *Oral susp:* 100 mg/5 ml (15 ml); 200 mg/5 ml (15, 22.5, 30 ml) (cherry); *Pkt:* 1 g for reconstitution (cherry-banana)
   Zithromax Tri-pak *Tab:* 3 x 500 mg tabs/pck
   Zithromax Z-pak *Tab:* 6 x 250 mg tabs/pck
   Zmax *Oral susp:* 2 g ext-rel for reconstitution (cherry-banana) (148 mg Na$^+$)
➤ *cefaclor* (B)(G) 250 mg tid or 375 mg bid x 5 days
Pediatric: <1 month: not recommended; 20-40 mg/kg bid or q 12 hours x 10 days; max 1 g/ day; *see page 549 for dose by weight*
   Tab: 500 mg; *Cap:* 250, 500 mg; *Susp:* 125 mg/5 ml (75, 150 ml) (strawberry); 187 mg/5 ml (50, 100 ml) (strawberry); 250 mg/5 ml (75, 150 ml) (strawberry); 375 mg/5 ml (50, 100 ml) (strawberry)
   Cefaclor Extended Release

Pediatric: <16 years: ext-rel not recommended; ≥16 years: same as adult
  Tab: 375, 500 mg ext-rel

▷ *cefadroxil* (B) 1 g in 1-2 doses x 10 days
  Pediatric: 30 mg/kg/day in 2 divided doses x 10 days; *see page 550 for dose by weight*
    Duricef *Cap:* 500 mg; *Tab:* 1 g; *Oral susp:* 250 mg/5 ml (100 ml); 500 mg/5 ml (75, 100 ml) (orange-pineapple)

▷ *cefdinir* (B) 300 mg bid x 10 days
  Pediatric: <6 months: not recommended; 6 months-12 years: 14 mg/kg/day in 1-2 doses x 10 days; >12 years: same as adult; *see page 551 for dose by weight*
    Omnicef *Cap:* 300 mg; *Oral susp:* 125 mg/5 ml (60, 100 ml) (strawberry)

▷ *cefditoren pivoxil* (B) 200 mg bid x 10 days
  Pediatric: not recommended
    Spectracef *Tab:* 200 mg
    Comment: **Spectracef** is contraindicated with milk protein allergy or carnitine deficiency.

▷ *cefixime* (B) 400 mg daily x 5 days
  Pediatric: <6 months: not recommended; 6 months-12 years, <50 kg: 8 mg/kg/day in 1-2 divided doses x 10 days; >12 years, ≥50 kg: same as adult; *see page 552 for dose by weight*
    Suprax *Tab:* 400 mg; *Cap:* 400 mg; *Oral susp:* 100, 200 mg/5 ml (50, 75, 100 ml) (strawberry)

▷ *cefpodoxime proxetil* (B) 100 mg bid x 5-7 days
  Pediatric: <2 months: not recommended; 2 months-12 years: 10 mg/kg/day in 2 divided doses x 5-7 days; >12 years: same as adult; *see page 553 for dose by weight*
    Vantin *Tab:* 100, 200 mg; *Oral susp:* 50, 100 mg/5 ml (50, 75, 100 ml) (lemon creme)

▷ *cefprozil* (B) 500 mg daily x 10 days
  Pediatric: <2 years: not recommended; 2-12 years: 7.5 mg/kg divided bid x 10 days; >12 years: same as adult; *see page 554 for dose by weight*
    Cefzil *Tab:* 250, 500 mg; *Oral susp:* 125, 250 mg/5 ml (50, 75, 100 ml) (bubble gum) (phenylalanine)

▷ *ceftibuten* (B) 400 mg daily x 5 days
  Pediatric: 9 mg/kg daily x 5 days; *see page 555 for dose by weight*
    Cedax *Cap:* 400 mg; *Oral susp:* 90 mg/5 ml (30, 60, 90, 120 ml); 180 mg/5 ml (30, 60, 120 ml) (cherry)

▷ *cefuroxime axetil* (B)(G) 250 mg bid x 10 days
  Pediatric: <3 months: not recommended; ≥3 months: 20 mg/kg/day divided bid x 10 days; *see page 556 for dose by weight*
    Ceftin *Tab:* 250, 500 mg; *Oral susp:* 125, 250 mg/5 ml (50, 100 ml) (tutti-frutti)

▷ *cephalexin* (B)(G) 500 mg bid x 10 days
  Pediatric: 25-50 mg/kg/day in 2 divided doses x 10 days; *see page 557 for dose by weight*
    Keflex *Cap:* 250, 333, 500, 750 mg; *Oral susp:* 125, 250 mg/5 ml (100, 200 ml) (strawberry)

▷ *clarithromycin* (C)(G) 250 mg bid or 500 mg ext-rel daily x 10 days
  Pediatric: <6 months: not recommended; ≥6 months: 7.5 mg/kg divided bid x 10 days; *see page 558 for dose by weight*

Biaxin *Tab:* 250, 500 mg
Biaxin Oral Suspension *Oral susp:* 125, 250 mg/5 ml (50, 100 ml) (fruit-punch)
Biaxin XL *Tab:* 500 mg ext-rel

▷ *dirithromycin* (C)(G) 500 mg daily x 10 days
Pediatric: <12 years: not recommended; ≥12 years: same as adult
Dynabac *Tab:* 250 mg

▷ *erythromycin base* (B)(G) 500 mg qid x 10 days
Pediatric: <45 kg: 30-50 mg divided bid-qid x 10 days; ≥45 kg: same as adult
Ery-Tab *Tab:* 250, 333, 500 mg ent-coat
PCE *Tab:* 333, 500 mg

Comment: *erythromycin* may increase INR with concomitant *warfarin*, as well as increase serum level of *digoxin*, benzodiazepines and statins.

▷ *erythromycin estolate* (B)(G) 250-500 mg qid x 10 days
Pediatric: 20-50 mg/kg divided q 6 hours x 10 days; *see page 562 for dose by weight*
Ilosone *Pulvule:* 250 mg; *Tab:* 500 mg; *Liq:* 125, 250 mg/5 ml (100 ml)

Comment: *erythromycin* may increase INR with concomitant *warfarin*, as well as increase serum level of *digoxin*, benzodiazepines and statins.

▷ *erythromycin ethylsuccinate* (B)(G) 400 mg qid *or* 800 mg bid x 10 days
Pediatric: 30-50 mg/kg/day in 4 divided doses x 7 days; may double dose with severe infection; max 100 mg/kg/day; *see page 563 for dose by weight*
EryPed *Oral susp:* 200 mg/5 ml (100, 200 ml) (fruit); 400 mg/5 ml (60, 100, 200 ml) (banana); *Oral drops:* 200, 400 mg/5 ml (50 ml) (fruit); *Chew tab:* 200 mg wafer (fruit)
E.E.S. *Oral susp:* 200, 400 mg/5 ml (100 ml) (fruit)
E.E.S. Granules *Oral susp:* 200 mg/5 ml (100, 200 ml) (cherry)
E.E.S. 400 Tablets *Tab:* 400 mg

Comment: *erythromycin* may increase INR with concomitant *warfarin*, as well as increase serum level of *digoxin*, benzodiazepines and statins.

▷ *loracarbef* (B) 200 mg bid x 5 days
Pediatric: 15 mg/kg/day in 2 divided doses x 5 days; *see page 570 for dose by weight*
Lorabid *Pulvule:* 200, 400 mg; *Oral susp:* 100 mg/5 ml (50, 100 ml); 200 mg/5 ml (50, 75, 100 ml) (strawberry bubble gum)

▷ *penicillin G (benzathine)* (B)(G) 1.2 million units IM x 1 dose
Pediatric: <60 lb: 300,000-600,000 units IM x 1 dose; ≥60 lb: 900,000 units x 1 dose
Bicillin L-A *Cartridge-needle unit:* 600,000 units (1 ml); 1.2 million units (2 ml)

▷ *penicillin G (benzathine and procaine)* (B)(G) 2.4 million units IM x 1 dose
Pediatric: <30 lb: 600,000 units IM x 1 dose; 30-60 lb: 900,000-1.2 million units IM x 1 dose; >60 mg: same as adult
Bicillin C-R *Cartridge-needle unit:* 600,000 units (1 ml); 1.2 million units; (2 ml); 2.4 million units (4 ml)

▷ *penicillin V potassium* (B)(G) 500 mg bid *or* 250 mg qid x 10 days
Pediatric: 25-50 mg/kg day in 4 divided doses x 10 days; >12 years: same as adult; *see page 572 for dose by weight*
Pen-Vee K *Tab:* 250, 500 mg; *Oral soln:* 125 mg/5 ml (100, 200 ml); 250 mg/5 ml (100, 150, 200 ml)
Veetids *Tab:* 250, 500 mg; *Oral soln:* 125, 250 mg/5 ml (100, 200 ml)

PHEOCHROMOCYTOMA

ALPHA-BLOCKER

▷ *phenoxybenzamine* (C) initially 10 mg bid; increase every other day as needed; usually 20-40 mg bid-tid
  Dibenzyline *Cap:* 10 mg

PINWORM (ENTEROBIUS VERMICULARIS)

Comment: Treatment of all family members is recommended.

ANTIHELMINTICS

▷ *albendazole* (C) 400 mg x 1 dose; may repeat in 2-3 weeks if needed; take after a meal
  Pediatric: <20 kg: 200 mg as a single dose; >20kg: same as adult
  Albenza *Tab:* 200 mg
▷ *mebendazole* (C)(G) 100 mg x 1 dose; may repeat in 2-3 weeks if needed; take after a meal
  Pediatric: same as adult
  Vermox *Chew tab:* 100 mg
▷ *pyrantel pamoate* (C) 11 mg/kg x 1 dose; max 1 g/dose; may repeat in 2-3 weeks if needed; take after a meal
  Pediatric: 25-37 lb: 1/2 tsp x 1 dose; 38-62 lb: 1 tsp x 1 dose; 63-87 lb: 1 tsp x 1 dose; 88-112 lb: 2 tsp x 1 dose; 113-137 lb: 2 tsp x 1 dose; 138-162 lb: 3 tsp x 1 dose; 163-187 lb: 3 tsp x 1 dose; >187 lb: 4 tsp x 1 dose
  Pin-X (OTC); *Cap:* 180 mg; *Liq:* 50 mg/ml (30 ml); 144 mg/ml (30 ml); *Oral susp:* 50 mg/ml (30 ml)
▷ *thiabendazole* (C) 50 mg/kg x 1 dose after a meal; max 3 g; may repeat in 2-3 weeks if needed; take with a meal
  Pediatric: same as adult
  Mintezol *Chew tab:* 500*mg (orange); *Oral susp:* 500 mg/5 ml (120 ml) (orange)
  Comment: *thiabendazole* should not be used as first-line therapy for pinworms. May impair mental alertness.

PITYRIASIS ALBA

Comment: Pityriasis alba is a chronic skin disorder seen in children with a genetic predisposition to atopic disease. Treatment is directed toward controlling roughness and pruritus. There is no known treatment for the associated skin pigment changes. Pityriasis alba resolves spontaneously and permanently in the 2nd or 3rd decade of life.
  Topical Cocorticosteroids *see page 494*

COAL TAR PREPARATIONS

▷ *coal tar* (C)
  Pediatric: same as adult

Scytera (OTC) apply qd-qid; use lowest effective dose
Foam: 2%
T/Gel Shampoo Extra Strength (OTC) use every other day; max 4 x/week; massage into affected area for 5 minutes; rinse; repeat
Shampoo: 1%
T/Gel Shampoo Original Formula (OTC) use every other day; max 7 x/week; massage into affected area for 5 minutes; rinse; repeat
Shampoo: 0.5%
T/Gel Shampoo Stubborn Itch Control (OTC) use every other day; max 7 x/week; massage into affected area for 5 minutes; rinse; repeat
Shampoo: 0.5%

EMOLLIENTS AND OTHER MOISTURIZING AGENTS

see **Dermatitis: Atopic** *page* 110

PITYRIASIS ROSEA

Topical Corticosteroids *see page* 494
Oral Drugs for Allergy, Cough, and Cold *see page* 524

PLAGUE (*YERSINIA PESTIS*)

Comment: *Yersinia pestis* is transmitted via the bite of a flea from an infected rodent or the bite, lick, or scratch of an infected cat. Untreated bubonic plague may progress to secondary pneumonic plague, which may be transmitted via contaminated respiratory droplet spread.

➤ *streptomycin* (C)(G) 15mg/kg IM bid x 10 days
Pediatric: same as adult
Amp: 1 g/2.5 ml or 400 mg/ml (2.5 ml)
Comment: For patients with renal impairment, reduce dose of *streptomycin* to 20 mg/kg/day if mild and 8 mg/kg/day q 3 days if advanced). For patients who are pregnant or who have hearing impairment, shorten the course of treatment to 3 days after fever has resolved.

➤ *moxifloxacin* (C)(G) 400 mg daily x 10 days
Pediatric: <18 years: not recommended
Avelox *Tab:* 400 mg; IV soln: 400 mg/250 mg (latex-free, preservative-free)
Comment: *moxifloxacin* is for prophylaxis as well as treatment for pneumonia and septic plague. *moxifloxacin* is contraindicated <18 years of age and during pregnancy and lactation. Risk of tendonitis or tendon rupture, especially 60 years-of-age and older.

➤ *tetracycline* (D)(G) 500 mg qid or 25-50 mg/kg/day divided q 6 hours x 10 days
Comment: *tetracycline* is contraindicated <8 years-of-age, in pregnancy, and lactation (discolors developing tooth enamel). A side effect may be photo-sensitivity (photophobia). Do not give with antacids, calcium supplements, milk or other dairy, or within two hours of taking another drug.

PNEUMOCYSTIS JIROVECI PNEUMONIA

▷ *atovaquone* (C) take with food; *Treatment:* 750 mg once daily x 21 days; *Prophylaxis:* 1500 mg once daily
Pediatric: see mfr literature
Mepron *Susp:* 750 mg/5 ml (citrus)

▷ *trimethoprim/sulfamethoxazole* (C)(G) *Prophylaxis:* 1 tab 3 x/week; *Treatment:* 1 tab daily x 3 weeks; *Septra* can be given if intolerable to *Bactrim*
Pediatric: <2 months: not recommended; ≥2 months: 40 mg/kg/day of sulfamethoxazole in 2 doses bid x 10 days
Bactrim, Septra 2 tabs bid x 10 days
Tab: trim 80 mg/sulfa 400 mg*
Bactrim DS, Septra DS 1 tab bid x 10 days
Tab: trim 160 mg/sulfa 800 mg*
Bactrim Pediatric Suspension, Septra Pediatric Suspension
Oral susp: trim 40 mg/sulfa 200 mg per 5 ml (100 ml) (cherry) (alcohol 0.3%)
Comment: *trimethoprim/sulfamethoxazole* is not recommended in pregnancy or lactation. *CrCl 15-30 mL/min:* reduce dose by 1/2; *CrCl <15 mL/min:* not recommended

PNEUMONIA: CHLAMYDIAL

RECOMMENDED REGIMEN

▷ *erythromycin base* (B)(G) 500 mg qid hours x 10-14 days
Pediatric: <45 kg: 50 mg in 4 divided doses x 10-14 days; ≥45 kg: same as adult
Ery-Tab *Tab:* 250, 333, 500 mg ent-coat
PCE *Tab:* 333, 500 mg
Comment: *erythromycin* may increase INR with concomitant *warfarin*, as well as increase serum level of *digoxin*, benzodiazepines and statins.

▷ *erythromycin ethylsuccinate* (B)(G) 400 mg qid x 10-14 days
Pediatric: <45 kg: 50 mg/kg/day in 4 divided doses x 10-14 days; ≥45 kg: same as adult; *see page 563 for dose by weight*
EryPed *Oral susp:* 200 mg/5 ml (100, 200 ml) (fruit); 400 mg/5 ml (60, 100, 200 ml) (banana); *Oral drops:* 200, 400/5 ml (50 ml) (fruit); *Chew tab:* 200 mg wafer (fruit)
E.E.S. *Oral susp:* 200, 400 mg/5 ml (100 ml) (fruit)
E.E.S. Granules *Oral susp:* 200 mg/5 ml (100, 200 ml) (cherry)
E.E.S. 400 Tablets *Tab:* 400 mg
Comment: *erythromycin* may increase INR with concomitant *warfarin*, as well as increase serum level of *digoxin*, benzodiazepines and statins.

ALTERNATE REGIMENS

▷ *azithromycin* (B)(G) 500 mg once daily x 10 days
Pediatric: 20 mg/kg per dose once daily x 3 days; max 500 mg/day; *see page 548 for dose by weight*
Zithromax *Tab:* 250, 500, 600 mg; *Oral susp:* 100 mg/5 ml (15 ml); 200 mg/5 ml (15, 22.5, 30 ml) (cherry); *Pkt:* 1 g for reconstitution (cherry-banana)

Zithromax Tri-pak *Tab:* 3 x 500 mg tabs/pck
Zithromax Z-pak *Tab:* 6 x 250 mg tabs/pck
Zmax *Oral susp:* 2 g ext-rel for reconstitution (cherry-banana) (148 mg Na⁺)
▷ *levofloxacin* (C) *Uncomplicated:* 500 mg daily x 7 days; *Complicated:* 750 mg daily x 7 days
Pediatric: <18 years: not recommended

Levaquin *Tab:* 250, 500, 750 mg; *Oral soln:* 25 mg/ml (480 ml) (benzyl alcohol); *Inj conc:* 25 mg/ml for IV infusion after dilution (20, 30 ml single-use vial) (preservative-free); *Premix soln:* 5 mg/ml for IV infusion (50, 100, 150 ml) (preservative-free)

Comment: *levofloxacin* is contraindicated <18 years-of-age, and during pregnancy and lactation. Risk of tendonitis or tendon rupture, especially 60 years-of-age and older. Risk of tendonitis or tendon rupture, especially 60 years-of-age and older.

PNEUMONIA: COMMUNITY ACQUIRED (CAP)/ COMMUNITY ACQUIRED BACTERIAL PNEUMONIA (CABP)

ANTI-INFFECTIVES

Age 3 Months-5 Years

▷ *amoxicillin* (B)(G)
Pediatric: <40 kg (88 lb): 20-40 mg/kg/day in 3 divided doses x 10 days or 25-45 mg/kg/day in 2 divided doses x 10 days; ≥40 kg: same as adult

Amoxil *Cap:* 250, 500 mg; *Tab:* 875 mg; *Chew tab:* 125, 200, 250, 400 mg (cherry-banana-peppermint) (phenylalanine); *Oral susp:* 125, 250 mg/5 ml (80, 100, 150 ml) (strawberry); 200, 400 mg/5 ml (50, 75, 100 ml) (bubble gum); *Oral drops:* 50 mg/ml (30 ml) (bubble gum)

Moxatag *Tab:* 775 mg ext-rel

Trimox *Tab:* 125, 250 mg; *Cap:* 250, 500 mg; *Oral susp:* 125, 250 mg/5 ml (80, 100, 150 ml) (raspberry-strawberry)

▷ *amoxicillin/clavulanate* (B)(G) 500 mg tid or 875 mg bid x 10 days

Augmentin *Tab:* 250, 500, 875 mg; *Chew tab:* 125, 250 mg (lemon-lime); 200, 400 mg/5 ml (cherry-banana) (phenylalanine); *Oral susp:* 125 mg/5 ml (banana), 250 mg/5 ml (75, 100, 150 ml) (orange); 200, 400 mg/5 ml (50, 75, 100 ml) (orange) (phenylalanine)

Pediatric: 40-45 mg/kg/day divided tid x 10 days or 90 mg/kg/day divided bid x 10 days *see pages 545-546 for dose by weight*

Augmentin ES-600 *Oral susp:* 600 mg/5 ml (50, 75, 100, 125, 150, 200 ml) (strawberry cream) (phenylalanine) every 12 hours

Pediatric: <3 months: not recommended; ≥3 months, <40 kg: 90 mg/kg/day in 2 divided doses; ≥40 kg: not recommended

Augmentin XR 2 tabs q 12 hours x 7-10 days

Pediatric: <16 years: use other forms; ≥16 years: same as adult
Tab: 1000*mg ext-rel

▷ *azithromycin* (B)(G)
Pediatric: <6 months: not recommended; ≥6 months: 10 mg/kg x 1 dose on day 1, then 5 mg/kg/day on days 2-5; max 500 mg/day; *see page 548 for dose by weight*

Zithromax *Tab:* 250, 500, 600 mg; *Oral susp:* 100 mg/5 ml (15 ml); 200 mg/5 ml (15, 22.5, 30 ml) (cherry); *Pkt:* 1 g for reconstitution (cherry-banana)

Zithromax Tri-pak *Tab:* 3 x 500 mg tabs/pck

Zithromax Z-pak *Tab:* 6 x 250 mg tabs/pck

Zmax *Oral susp:* 2 g ext-rel for reconstitution (cherry-banana) (148 mg Na$^+$)

▷ *cefaclor* (B)(G) 250 mg tid *or* 375 mg bid x 10 days
Pediatric: <1 month: not recommended; 20-40 mg/kg divided bid *or* q 12 hours x 10 days; max 1 g/day; *see page 549 for dose by weight*
Tab: 500 mg; *Cap:* 250, 500 mg; *Susp:* 125 mg/5 ml (75, 150 ml) (strawberry); 187 mg/5 ml (50, 100 ml) (strawberry); 250 mg/5 ml (75, 150 ml) (strawberry); 375 mg/5 ml (50, 100 ml) (strawberry)

    Cefaclor Extended Release
        Pediatric: <16 years: ext-rel not recommended; ≥16 years: same as adult
        Tab: 375, 500 mg ext-rel

▷ *ceftriaxone*(B)(G)
Pediatric: 50-75 mg/kg IM in 2 divided doses; max 2 g/day
    Rocephin *Vial:* 250, 500 mg; 1, 2 g

▷ *clarithromycin* (C) 500 mg q 12 hours *or* 500 mg ext-rel daily x 10 days
Pediatric: <6 months: not recommended; ≥6 months: 7.5 mg/kg divided bid x 7-14 days; *see page 558 for dose by weight*
    Biaxin *Tab:* 250, 500 mg
    Biaxin Oral Suspension *Oral susp:* 125, 250 mg/5 ml (50, 100 ml) (fruit punch)
    Biaxin XL *Tab:* 500 mg ext-rel

▷ *erythromycin base* (B)(G)
Pediatric: <45 kg: 30-50 mg in 2-4 divided doses x 7-10 days; ≥45 kg: same as adult
    Ery-Tab *Tab:* 250, 333, 500 mg ent-coat
    PCE *Tab:* 333, 500 mg

Comment: *erythromycin* may increase INR with concomitant *warfarin*, as well as increase serum level of *digoxin*, benzodiazepines and statins.

▷ *erythromycin estolate* (B)(G)
Pediatric: 30-50 mg/kg/day in divided doses x 10 days; *see page 562 for dose by weight*
    Ilosone *Pulvule:* 250 mg; *Tab:* 500 mg; *Liq:* 125, 250 mg/5 ml (100 ml)

Comment: *erythromycin* may increase INR with concomitant *warfarin*, as well as increase serum level of *digoxin*, benzodiazepines and statins.

Age 5-18 Years

▷ *amoxicillin* (B)(G) 875 mg bid *or* 500 mg tid x 10 days
Pediatric: <40 kg (88 lb): 20-40 mg/kg/day in 3 divided doses x 10 days *or* 25-45 mg/kg/day in 2 divided doses x 10 days; ≥40 kg: same as adult; *see page 543 for dose by weight*
    Amoxil *Cap:* 250, 500 mg; *Tab:* 875*mg; *Chew tab:* 125, 200, 250, 400 mg (cherry-banana-peppermint) (phenylalanine); *Oral susp:* 125, 250 mg/5 ml (80, 100, 150 ml) (strawberry); 200, 400 mg/5 ml (50, 75, 100 ml) (bubble gum); *Oral drops:* 50 mg/ml (30 ml) (bubble gum)
    Trimox *Tab:* 125, 250 mg; *Cap:* 250, 500 mg; *Oral susp:* 125, 250 mg/5 ml (80, 100, 150 ml) (raspberry-strawberry)

▷ *amoxicillin/clavulanate* (B)(G) 500 mg tid <u>or</u> 875 mg bid x 10 days
    Augmentin *Tab*: 250, 500, 875 mg; *Chew tab*: 125, 250 mg (lemon-lime); 200, 400 mg (cherry-banana) (phenylalanine); *Oral susp*: 125 mg/5 ml (banana), 250 mg/5 ml (75, 100, 150 ml) (orange); 200, 400 mg/5 ml (50, 75, 100 ml) (orange) (phenylalanine)
      Pediatric: 40-45 mg/kg/day divided tid x 10 days <u>or</u> 90 mg/kg/day divided bid x 10 days *see pages 545-546 for dose by weight*
    Augmentin ES-600 *Oral susp*: 600 mg/5 ml (50, 75, 100, 125, 150, 200 ml) (strawberry cream) (phenylalanine) every 12 hours
      Pediatric: <3 months: not recommended; ≥3 months, <40 kg: 90 mg/kg/day in 2 divided doses; ≥40 kg: not recommended
    Augmentin XR 2 tabs q 12 hours x 7-10 days
      Pediatric: <16 years: use other forms; ≥16 years: same as adult
      Tab: 1000*mg ext-rel
▷ *azithromycin* (B)(G) weight-based <u>or</u> 500 mg x 1 dose on day 1, then 250 mg daily on days 2-5 <u>or</u> 500 mg daily x 3 days <u>or</u> **Zmax** 2 g in a single dose
  Pediatric: 10 mg/kg x 1 dose on day 1, then 5 mg/kg/day on days 2-5; max 500 mg/day; *see page 548 for dose by weight*
    Zithromax *Tab*: 250, 500, 600 mg; *Oral susp*: 100 mg/5 ml (15 ml); 200 mg/5 ml (15, 22.5, 30 ml) (cherry); *Pkt*: 1 g for reconstitution (cherry-banana)
    Zithromax Tri-pak *Tab*: 3 x 500 mg tabs/pck
    Zithromax Z-pak *Tab*: 6 x 250 mg tabs/pck
▷ *cefaclor* (B)(G) 250 mg tid <u>or</u> 375 mg bid x 5 days
  Pediatric: <1 month: not recommended; 20-40 mg/kg divided bid <u>or</u> q 12 hours x 10 days; max 1 g/day; *see page 549 for dose by weight*
  Tab: 500 mg; *Cap*: 250, 500 mg; *Susp*: 125 mg/5 ml (75, 150 ml) (strawberry); 187 mg/5 ml (50, 100 ml) (strawberry); 250 mg/5 ml (75, 150 ml) (strawberry); 375 mg/5 ml (50, 100 ml) (strawberry)
    Cefaclor Extended Release
      Pediatric: <16 years: ext-rel not recommended; ≥16 years: same as adult
      Tab: 375, 500 mg ext-rel
▷ *cefdinir* (B) 300 mg bid <u>or</u> 600 mg daily x 10 days
  Pediatric: <6 months: not recommended; 6 months-12 years: 14 mg/kg/day in a single <u>or</u> 2 divided doses x 10 days; >12 years: same as adult; *see page 551 for dose by weight*
    Omnicef
      Cap: 300 mg; *Oral susp*: 125 mg/5 ml (60, 100 ml) (strawberry)
▷ *cefpodoxime proxetil* (B) 200 mg bid x 14 days
  Pediatric: 2 months-12 years: 10 mg/kg/day in 2 doses x 14 days; >12 years: same as adult; *see page 553 for dose by weight*
    Vantin *Tab*: 100, 200 mg; *Oral susp*: 50, 100 mg/5 ml (50, 75, 100 ml) (lemon creme)
▷ *ceftriaxone* (B)
  Pediatric: 50-75 mg/kg IM in 2 divided doses; max 2 g/day
    Rocephin *Vial*: 250, 500 mg; 1, 2 g
▷ *clarithromycin* (C) 7.5 mg/kg divided bid x 7-14 days
  Pediatric: <6 months: not recommended; ≥6 months: 7.5 mg/kg bid x 7-14 days
    Biaxin *Tab*: 250, 500 mg
    Biaxin Oral Suspension *Oral susp*: 125, 250 mg/5 ml (50, 100 ml) (fruit-punch)
    Biaxin XL *Tab*: 500 mg ext-rel

▷ *dirithromycin* (C)(G) 500 mg daily x 14 days
   Pediatric: <12 years: not recommended; ≥12 years: same as adult
     Dynabac *Tab:* 250 mg
▷ *erythromycin base* (B)(G) 500 mg q 6 hours x 10 days
   Pediatric: <45 kg: 30-50 mg in 2-4 divided doses x 10 days; ≥45 kg: same as adult
     Ery-Tab *Tab:* 250, 333, 500 mg ent-coat
     PCE *Tab:* 333, 500 mg
   Comment: *erythromycin* may increase INR with concomitant *warfarin*, as well as increase serum level of *digoxin*, benzodiazepines and statins.
▷ *erythromycin estolate* (B) 250 mg q 6 hours or 500 mg bid x 10 days
   Pediatric: 30-50 mg/kg/day in divided doses x 10 days; *see page 562 for dose by weight*
     Ilosone *Pulvule:* 250 mg; *Tab:* 500 mg; *Liq:* 125, 250 mg/5 ml (100 ml)
   Comment: *erythromycin* may increase INR with concomitant *warfarin*, as well as increase serum level of *digoxin*, benzodiazepines and statins.

Age 18-60 Years Without Comorbidity

▷ *amoxicillin* (B)(G) 500-875 mg bid or 250-500 mg tid x 10 days
     Amoxil *Cap:* 250, 500 mg; *Tab:* 875*mg; *Chew tab:* 125, 200, 250, 400 mg (cherry-banana-peppermint) (phenylalanine); *Oral susp:* 125, 250 mg/5 ml (80, 100, 150 ml) (strawberry); 200, 400 mg/5 ml (50, 75, 100 ml) (bubble gum); *Oral drops:* 50 mg/ml (30 ml) (bubble gum)
     Moxatag *Tab:* 775 mg ext-rel
     Trimox *Tab:* 125, 250 mg; *Cap:* 250, 500 mg; *Oral susp:* 125, 250 mg/5 ml (80, 100, 150 ml) (raspberry-strawberry)
▷ *amoxicillin/clavulanate* (B)(G) 500 mg tid or 875 mg bid x 10 days
     Augmentin *Tab:* 250, 500, 875 mg; *Chew tab:* 125, 250 mg (lemon-lime); 200, 400 mg (cherry-banana) (phenylalanine); *Oral susp:* 125 mg/5 ml (banana), 250 mg/5 ml (75, 100, 150 ml) (orange); 200, 400 mg/5 ml (50, 75, 100 ml) (orange) (phenylalanine)
       Pediatric: 40-45 mg/kg/day divided tid x 10 days or 90 mg/kg/day divided bid x 10 days *see pages 545-546 for dose by weight*
     Augmentin ES-600 *Oral susp:* 600 mg/5 ml (50, 75, 100, 125, 150, 200 ml) (strawberry cream) (phenylalanine) every 12 hours
       Pediatric: <3 months: not recommended; ≥3 months, <40 kg: 90 mg/kg/day in 2 divided doses; ≥40 kg: not recommended
     Augmentin XR 2 tabs q 12 hours x 7-10 days
       Pediatric: <16 years: use other forms; ≥16 years: same as adult
       Tab: 1000*mg ext-rel
▷ *azithromycin* (B)(G) 500 mg x 1 dose on day 1, then 250 mg daily on days 2-5 or 500 mg daily x 3 days or **Zmax** 2 g in a single dose
     Zithromax *Tab:* 250, 500, 600 mg; *Oral susp:* 100 mg/5 ml (15 ml); 200 mg/5 ml (15, 22.5, 30 ml) (cherry); *Pkt:* 1 g for reconstitution (cherry-banana)
     Zithromax Tri-pak *Tab:* 3 x 500 mg tabs/pck
     Zithromax Z-pak *Tab:* 6 x 250 mg tabs/pck
     Zmax *Oral susp:* 2 g ext-rel for reconstitution (cherry-banana) (148 mg Na⁺)

▶ *cefaclor* (B)(G) 250 mg tid <u>or</u> 375 mg bid x 10 days
   Tab: 500 mg; *Cap:* 250, 500 mg; *Susp:* 125 mg/5 ml (75, 150 ml) (strawberry); 187
   mg/5 ml (50, 100 ml) (strawberry); 250 mg/5 ml (75, 150 ml) (strawberry); 375
   mg/5 ml (50, 100 ml) (strawberry)
   Cefaclor Extended Release
       Pediatric: <16 years: ext-rel not recommended; ≥16 years: same as adult
       Tab: 375, 500 mg ext-rel
▶ *cefdinir* (B) 300 mg bid <u>or</u> 600 mg daily x 10 days
   Omnicef *Cap:* 300 mg; *Oral susp:* 125 mg/5 ml (60, 100 ml) (strawberry)
▶ *cefpodoxime proxetil* (B) 200 mg bid x 14 days
   Vantin *Tab:* 100, 200 mg; *Oral susp:* 50, 100 mg/5 ml (50, 75, 100 ml) (lemon creme)
▶ *ceftaroline fosamil* (B) administer by IV infusion after reconstitution every 12 hours
   x 5-7 days; *CrCl ≥50 mL/min:* 600 mg; *CrCl >30-<50 mL/min:* 400 mg; *CrCl: >15-
   <30 mL/min:* 300 mg; ES RD: 200 mg
   Teflaro *Vial:* 400, 600 mg
▶ *ceftriaxone* (B)(G) 1-2 g IM daily; max 4 g
   Rocephin *Vial:* 250, 500 mg; 1, 2 g
▶ *clarithromycin* (C)(G) 500 mg bid <u>or</u> 500 mg ext-rel daily x 7-14 days
   Biaxin *Tab:* 250, 500 mg
   Biaxin Oral Suspension *Oral susp:* 125, 250 mg/5 ml (50, 100 ml) (fruit-punch)
   Biaxin XL *Tab:* 500 mg ext-rel
▶ *dirithromycin* (C)(G) 500 mg daily x 14 days
   Dynabac *Tab:* 250 mg
▶ *doxycycline* (D)(G) 100 mg bid x 7-14 days
   Actilate *Tab:* 75, 150** mg
   Adoxa *Tab:* 50, 75, 100, 150 mg ent-coat
   Doryx *Tab:* 75, 100, 150 mg del-rel
   Monodox *Cap:* 50, 75, 100 mg
   Oracea *Cap:* 40 mg del-rel
   Vibramycin *Cap:* 50, 100 mg; *Syr:* 50 mg/5 ml (raspberry) (sulfites); *Oral susp:*
       25 mg/5 ml (raspberry-apple)
   Vibra-Tab *Tab:* 100 mg film-coat
Comment: *doxycycline* is contraindicated <8 years-of-age, in pregnancy, and
lactation (discolors developing tooth enamel). A side effect may be photo-
sensitivity (photophobia). Do not give with antacids, calcium supplements, milk or
other dairy, or within two hours of taking another drug.
▶ *ertapenem* (B) 1 g daily; *CrCl <30 mL/min:* 500 mg daily x 3-10 days; may switch to
   an oral antibiotic after 3 days if warranted; *IV infusion:* administer over 30 minutes;
   IM injection: reconstitute with lidocaine only
   Ivanz *Vial:* 1 g pwdr for reconstitution
▶ *erythromycin base* (B)(G) 500 mg q 6 hours x 14-21 days; <45 kg: 30-50 mg in 2-4
   doses x 14-21 days; ≥45 kg: same as adult
   Ery-Tab *Tab:* 250, 333, 500 mg ent-coat
   PCE *Tab:* 333, 500 mg
Comment: *erythromycin* may increase INR with concomitant *warfarin*, as well as
increase serum level of *digoxin*, benzodiazepines and statins.
▶ *erythromycin estolate* (B) 500 mg q 6 hours x 14-21 days
   Ilosone *Pulvule:* 250 mg; *Tab:* 500 mg; *Liq:* 125, 250 mg/5 ml (100 ml)
Comment: *erythromycin* may increase INR with concomitant *warfarin*, as well as
increase serum level of *digoxin*, benzodiazepines and statins.

▷ *gemifloxacin* (C) 320 mg daily x 5-7 days
   Pediatric: <18 years: not recommended
      Factive *Tab:* 320* mg
   Comment: *gemifloxacin* is contraindicated <18 years-of-age, and during pregnancy
   and lactation. Risk of tendonitis or tendon rupture, especially 60 years-of-age and older.

▷ *levofloxacin* (C) *Uncomplicated:* 500 mg once daily x 7-14 days; *Complicated:* 750 mg
   once daily x 7-14 days
   Pediatric: <18 years: not recommended
      Levaquin *Tab:* 250, 500, 750 mg; *Oral soln:* 25 mg/ml (480 ml) (benzyl alcohol);
      Inj conc: 25 mg/ml for IV infusion after dilution (20, 30 ml single-use vial)
      (preservative-free); *Premix soln:* 5 mg/ml for IV infusion (50, 100, 150 ml)
      (preservative-free)
   Comment: *levofloxacin* is contraindicated <18 years-of-age, and during pregnancy
   and lactation. Risk of tendonitis or tendon rupture, especially 60 years-of-age and
   older.

▷ *linezolid* (C)(G) 600 mg q 12 hours x 10-14 days
   Pediatric: <5 years: 10 mg/kg q 8 hours x 10-14 days; 5-11 years: 10 mg/kg q 12 hours
   x 10-14 days; >11years: same as adult
      Zyvox *Tab:* 400, 600 mg; *Oral susp:* 100 mg/5 ml (150 ml) (orange) (phenylalanine)
   Comment: *linezolid* is indicated to treat susceptible vancomycin-resistant *E. faecium*
   infections.

▷ *loracarbef* (B) 400 mg bid x 14 days
      Lorabid *Pulvule:* 200, 400 mg; *Oral susp:* 100 mg/5 ml (50, 100 ml); 200 mg/5 ml
      (50, 75, 100 ml) (strawberry bubble gum)

▷ *moxifloxacin* (C)(G) 400 mg daily x 10 days
   Pediatric: <18 years: recommended
      Avelox *Tab:* 400 mg; IV soln: 400 mg/250 mg (latex-free, preservative-free)
   Comment: *moxifloxacin* is contraindicated <18 years of age and during pregnancy
   and lactation. Risk of tendonitis or tendon rupture, especially 60 years-of-age and
   older.

▷ *ofloxacin* (C)(G) 400 mg bid x 10 days
   Pediatric: <18 years: not recommended
      Floxin *Tab:* 200, 300, 400 mg
   Comment: *ofloxacin* is contraindicated <18 years of age and during pregnancy and
   lactation. Risk of tendonitis or tendon rupture, especially 60 years-of-age and older.

▷ *tedizolid phosphate* (B) administer 200 mg once daily x 6 days, via PO or IV infusion
   over 1 hour
   Pediatric: <18 years: not established
      Sivextro *Tab:* 200 mg (6/blister pck)
   Comment: **Sivextro** is indicated for the treatment of adults with community
   acquired bacterial pneumonia (CABP)

▷ *telithromycin* (C) 2 x 400 mg tabs in a singe dose daily x 7-10 days
      Ketek *Tab:* 300, 400 mg
   Comment: *telithromycin* is contraindicated with PMHx hepatitis or jaundice
   associated with macrolide use.

▷ *tigecycline* (D)(G) 100 mg once; then 50 mg q 12 hours x 7-14 days; *Severe hepatic
   impaitment (Child Pugh C):* 100 mg once; then 25 mg q 12 hours
   Pediatric: <18 years: not recommended
      Tygacil *Vial:* 50 mg pwdr for reconstitution and IV infusion (preservative-free)

Comment: **Tygacil** is indicated only for the treatment of adults with community acquired bacterial pneumonia (CABP). *tigecycline* is contraindicated <8 years-of-age, in pregnancy, and lactation (discolors developing tooth enamel). A side effect may be photo-sensitivity (photophobia). Do not give with antacids, calcium supplements, milk or other dairy, or within two hours of taking another drug.

Age Over 60 Years or Presence of Comorbidity

Comment: Consider respiratory quinolone for presence of comorbidity
➤ *amoxicillin/clavulanate* (B)(G) 500 mg tid or 875 mg bid x 10 days
　　Augmentin *Tab:* 250, 500, 875 mg; *Chew tab:* 125, 250 mg (lemon-lime); 200, 400 mg (cherry-banana) (phenylalanine); *Oral susp:* 125 mg/5 ml (banana), 250 mg/5 ml (75, 100, 150 ml) (orange); 200, 400 mg/5 ml (50, 75, 100 ml) (orange) (phenylalanine)
　　　　Pediatric: 40-45 mg/kg/day divided tid x 10 days or 90 mg/kg/day divided bid x 10 days *see page 545 for dose by weight*
　　Augmentin ES-600 *Oral susp:* 600 mg/5 ml (50, 75, 100, 125, 150, 200 ml) (strawberry cream) (phenylalanine) every 12 hours
　　　　Pediatric: <3 months: not recommended; ≥3 months, <40 kg: 90 mg/kg/day in 2 divided doses; ≥40 kg: not recommended
　　Augmentin XR 2 tabs q 12 hours x 7-10 days
　　　　Pediatric: <16 years: use other forms; ≥16 years: same as adult
　　　　Tab: 1000*mg ext-rel
➤ *azithromycin* (B)(G) 500 mg x 1 dose on day 1, then 250 mg daily on days 2-5 or 500 mg daily x 3 days or **Zmax** 2 g in a single dose
　　Zithromax *Tab:* 250, 500, 600 mg; *Oral susp:* 100 mg/5 ml (15 ml); 200 mg/5 ml (15, 22.5, 30 ml) (cherry); *Pkt:* 1 g for reconstitution (cherry-banana)
　　Zithromax Tri-pak *Tab:* 3 x 500 mg tabs/pck
　　Zithromax Z-pak *Tab:* 6 x 250 mg tabs/pck
　　Zmax *Oral susp:* 2 g ext-rel for reconstitution (cherry-banana) (148 mg Na⁺)
➤ *cefaclor* (B)(G) 250 mg tid or 375 mg bid x 7 days
　　Tab: 500 mg; *Cap:* 250, 500 mg; *Susp:* 125 mg/5 ml (75, 150 ml) (strawberry); 187 mg/5 ml (50, 100 ml) (strawberry); 250 mg/5 ml (75, 150 ml) (strawberry); 375 mg/5 ml (50, 100 ml) (strawberry)
　　Cefaclor Extended Release
　　　　Pediatric: <16 years: ext-rel not recommended
　　　　Tab: 375, 500 mg ext-rel
➤ *cefdinir* (B) 300 mg bid or 600 mg daily x 10 days
　　Omnicef *Cap:* 300 mg; *Oral susp:* 125 mg/5 ml (60, 100 ml) (strawberry)
➤ *cefpodoxime proxetil* (B) 200 mg bid x 14 days
　　Vantin *Tab:* 100, 200 mg; *Oral susp:* 50, 100 mg/5 ml (50, 75, 100 ml) (lemon creme)
➤ *ceftriaxone* (B)(G) 1-2 g IM once daily; max 4 g
　　Rocephin *Vial:* 250, 500 mg; 1, 2 g
➤ *clarithromycin* (C)(G) 500 mg bid x 7-14 days
　　Biaxin *Tab:* 250, 500 mg
　　Biaxin Oral Suspension *Oral susp:* 125, 250 mg/5 ml (50, 100 ml) (fruit-punch)
　　Biaxin XL *Tab:* 500 mg ext-rel
➤ *dirithromycin* (C)(G) 500 mg daily x 14 days
　　Dynabac *Tab:* 250 mg

▷ *gemifloxacin* (C) 320 mg daily x 5-7 days
   Pediatric: <18 years: not recommended
      Factive *Tab:* 320* mg
   Comment: *gemifloxacin* is contraindicated <18 years-of-age, and during pregnancy
   and lactation. Risk of tendonitis or tendon rupture, especially 60 years-of-age and
   older.

▷ *levofloxacin* (C)
   Pediatric: <18 years: not recommended; *Uncomplicated:* 500 mg daily x 7-14 days;
   Complicated: 750 mg daily x 7-14 days
      Levaquin *Tab:* 250, 500, 750 mg; *Oral soln:* 25 mg/ml (480 ml) (benzyl alcohol);
      Inj conc: 25 mg/ml for IV infusion after dilution (20, 30 ml single-use vial)
      (preservative-free); *Premix soln:* 5 mg/ml for IV infusion (50, 100, 150 ml)
      (preservative-free)
   Comment: *levofloxacin* is contraindicated <18 years-of-age and during pregnancy
   and lactation. Risk of tendonitis or tendon rupture, especially 60 years-of-age and
   older.

▷ *loracarbef* (B) 400 mg bid x 14 days
      Lorabid *Pulvule:* 200, 400 mg; *Oral susp:* 100 mg/5 ml (50, 100 ml); 200 mg/5
      ml (50, 75, 100 ml) (strawberry bubble gum)

▷ *trimethoprim/sulfamethoxazole* (C)(G)
      Bactrim, Septra 2 tabs bid x 10 days
         Tab: trim 80 mg/*sulfa* 400 mg*
      Bactrim DS, Septra DS 1 tab bid x 10 days
         Tab: trim 160 mg/*sulfa* 800 mg*
   Comment: *trimethoprim/sulfamethoxazole* is not recommended in pregnancy
   or lactation. *CrCl 15-30 mL/min:* reduce dose by 1/2; *CrCl <15 mL/min:* not
   recommended.

▷ *telithromycin* (C) 2 x 400 mg tabs in a singe dose daily x 7-10 days
      Ketek *Tab:* 300, 400 mg
   Comment: *telithromycin* is contraindicated with PMHx hepatitis or jaundice
   associated with macrolide use.

⬤ PNEUMONIA: LEGIONELLA

▷ *ciprofloxacin* (C) 500 mg bid x 14-21 days
   Pediatric: <18 years: not recommended
      Cipro (G) *Tab:* 250, 500, 750 mg; *Oral susp:* 250, 500 mg/5 ml (100 ml) (strawberry)
      Cipro XR *Tab:* 500, 1000 mg ext-rel
      ProQuin XR *Tab:* 500 mg ext-rel
   Comment: *ciprofloxacin* is contraindicated <18 years-of-age, and during pregnancy
   and lactation. Risk of tendonitis or tendon rupture, especially 60 years-of-age and
   older.

▷ *clarithromycin* (C)(G) 500 mg bid or 500 mg ext-rel daily x 14-21 days
      Biaxin *Tab:* 250, 500 mg
      Biaxin Oral Suspension *Oral susp:* 125, 250 mg/5 ml (50, 100 ml) (fruit-punch)
      Biaxin XL *Tab:* 500 mg ext-rel

▷ *dirithromycin* (C)(G) 500 mg once daily x 14-21 days
      Dynabac *Tab:* 250 mg

➤ *erythromycin base* (B)(G) 500 mg qid x 14-21 days
  Pediatric: <45 kg: 30-50 mg in 2-4 divided doses x 14-21 days; ≥45 kg: same as adult
      Ery-Tab *Tab:* 250, 333, 500 mg ent-coat
      PCE *Tab:* 333, 500 mg
  Comment: *erythromycin* may increase INR with concomitant *warfarin*, as well as increase serum level of *digoxin*, benzodiazepines and statins.
➤ *erythromycin estolate* (B)(G) 1-2 g daily in divided doses x 14-21 days
  Pediatric: 30-50 mg/kg/day in divided doses x 14-21 days; *see page 562 for dose by weight*
      Ilosone *Pulvule:* 250 mg; *Tab:* 500 mg; *Liq:* 125, 250 mg/5 ml (100 ml)
  Comment: *erythromycin* may increase INR with concomitant *warfarin*, as well as increase serum level of *digoxin*, benzodiazepines and statins.
➤ *trimethoprim/sulfamethoxazole* (C)(G)
  Pediatric: <2 months: not recommended; ≥2 months: 40 mg/kg/day of *sulfamethoxazole* in 2 doses bid x 10 days
      Bactrim, Septra 2 tabs bid x 10 days
      Tab: trim 80 mg/*sulfa* 400 mg*
      Bactrim DS, Septra DS 1 tab bid x 10 days
      Tab: trim 160 mg/*sulfa* 800 mg*
      Bactrim Pediatric Suspension, Septra Pediatric Suspension
      Oral susp: trim 40 mg/*sulfa* 200 mg per 5 ml (100 ml) (cherry) (alcohol 0.3%)
  Comment: *trimethoprim/sulfamethoxazole* is not recommended in pregnancy or lactation. *CrCl 15-30 mL/min:* reduce dose by 1/2; *CrCl <15 mL/min:* not recommended.

⬤ PNEUMONIA: MYCOPLASMA

ANTI-INFECTIVES

➤ *azithromycin* (B)(G) 500 mg x 1 dose on day 1, then 250 mg daily on days 2-5 or 500 mg daily x 3 days or **Zmax** 2 g in a single dose
  Pediatric: 12 mg/kg/day x 5 days; max 500 mg/day; *see page 548 for dose by weight*
      Zithromax *Tab:* 250, 500, 600 mg; *Oral susp:* 100 mg/5 ml (15 ml); 200 mg/5 ml (15, 22.5, 30 ml) (cherry); *Pkt:* 1 g for reconstitution (cherry-banana)
      Zithromax Tri-pak *Tab:* 3 x 500 mg tabs/pck
      Zithromax Z-pak *Tab:* 6 x 250 mg tabs/pck
      Zmax *Oral susp:* 2 g ext-rel for reconstitution (cherry-banana) (148 mg Na⁺)
➤ *clarithromycin* (C)(G) 500 mg bid or 500 mg ext-rel daily x 14-21 days
  Pediatric: <6 months: not recommended; ≥6 months: 7.5 mg/kg bid x 7 days; *see page 558 for dose by weight*
      Biaxin *Tab:* 250, 500 mg
      Biaxin Oral Suspension *Oral susp:* 125, 250 mg/5 ml (50, 100 ml) (fruit-punch)
      Biaxin XL *Tab:* 500 mg ext-rel
➤ *erythromycin base* (B)(G) 500 mg q 6 hours x 14-21 days
  Pediatric: <45 kg: 30-50 mg in 2-4 doses x 14-21 days; ≥45 kg: same as adult
      Ery-Tab *Tab:* 250, 333, 500 mg ent-coat
      PCE *Tab:* 333, 500 mg

Comment: *erythromycin* may increase INR with concomitant *warfarin*, as well as increase serum level of *digoxin*, benzodiazepines and statins.

▶ *erythromycin ethylsuccinate* (B)(G) 400 mg qid x 14-21 days
Pediatric: 30-50 mg/kg/day in 4 divided doses x 14-21 days; may double dose with severe infection; max 100 mg/kg/day; *see page 563 for dose by weight*
   EryPed *Oral susp:* 200 mg/5 ml (100, 200 ml) (fruit); 400 mg/5 ml (60, 100, 200 ml) (banana); *Oral drops:* 200, 400 mg/5 ml (50 ml) (fruit); *Chew tab:* 200 mg wafer (fruit)
   E.E.S. *Oral susp:* 200, 400 mg/5 ml (100 ml) (fruit)
   E.E.S. Granules *Oral susp:* 200 mg/5 ml (100, 200 ml) (cherry)
   E.E.S. 400 Tablets *Tab:* 400 mg

Comment: *erythromycin* may increase INR with concomitant *warfarin*, as well as increase serum level of *digoxin*, benzodiazepines and statins.

▶ *tetracycline* (D)(G) 500 mg qid
Pediatric: <8 years: not recommended; ≥8 years, <100 lb: 25-50 mg/kg/day in 2-4 divided doses; ≥8 years, ≥100 lb: same as adult; *see page 574 for dose by weight*
   Achromycin V *Cap:* 250, 500 mg
   Sumycin *Tab:* 250, 500 mg; *Cap:* 250, 500 mg; *Oral susp:* 125 mg/5 ml (100, 200 ml) (fruit) (sulfites)

Comment: *tetracycline* is contraindicated <8 years-of-age, in pregnancy, and lactation (discolors developing tooth enamel). A side effect may be photosensitivity (photophobia). Do not give with antacids, calcium supplements, milk or other dairy, or within two hours of taking another drug.

 PNEUMONIA: PNEUMOCOCCAL

PROPHYLAXIS

▶ *pneumococcal* vaccine (C) 0.5 ml IM or SC in deltoid x 1 dose
   Pneumovax
      Pediatric: <2 years: not recommended; ≥2 years: same as adult
      Vial: 25 mcg/0.5 ml (0.5 ml single-dose, 10/pck; 2.5 ml)
   Pnu-Imune 23
      Pediatric: <2 years: not recommended; ≥2 years: same as adult
      Vial: 25 mcg/0.5 ml (0.5 ml single-dose, 5/pck; 2.5 ml)
   Prevnar 13 for adults ≥50 years of age
      Pediatric: total 4 doses: 2, 4, 6, and 12-15 months-of-age; may start at 6 weeks of age; administer first 3 doses 4-8 weeks apart and the 4th dose at least 2 months after the 3rd dose
      Vial: 25 mcg/0.5 ml (2.5 ml multi-dose; *Prefilled syringe:* (0.5 ml single-dose 10/pck)

Comment: Pneumococcal vaccine contains 23 polysaccharide isolates representing approximately 85-90% of common U.S. isolates. Administer the pneumococcal vaccine in the anterolateral aspect of the thigh for infants and the deltoid for toddlers, children, and adults.

TREATMENT

see **CAP/CABP** page 330

POLIOMYELITIS

PROPHYLAXIS

▷ **trivalent poliovirus vaccine, inactivated (type 1, 2, and 3)** (C)
  Pediatric: <6 weeks: not recommended; ≥6 weeks: one dose at 2, 4, 6-18 months
  and 4-6 years of age
    Ipol 0.5 ml SC <u>or</u> IM in deltoid area

POLYARTICULAR JUVENILE IDIOPATHIC ARTHRITIS (PJIA)

Acetaminophen for IV Infusion *see Pain page* 296
Oral Prescription NSAIDs *see page* 489
Other Oral Analgesics *see Pain page* 298
Topical/Transdermal NSAIDs *see Pain page* 297
Parenteral Corticosteroids *see page* 499
Oral Corticosteroids *see page* 497
Topical Analgesic and Anesthetic Agents *see page* 330

TOPICAL ANALGESICS

▷ **capsaicin** (B)(G) apply tid <u>or</u> qid prn to intact skin
  Pediatric: <2 years: not recommended; ≥2 years: same as adult
    Axsain *Crm:* 0.075% (1, 2 oz)
    Capsin *Lotn:* 0.025, 0.075% (59 ml)
    Capzasin-P (OTC) *Crm:* 0.025% (1.5 oz); *Lotn:* 0.025% (2 oz)
    Dolorac *Crm:* 0.025% (28 g)
    Double Cap (OTC) *Crm:* 0.05% (2 oz)
    R-Gel *Gel:* 0.025% (15, 30 g)
    Zostrix (OTC) *Crm:* 0.025% (0.7, 1.5, 3 oz)
    Zostrix HP (OTC) *Emol crm:* 0.075% (1, 2 oz)
  Comment: Provides some relief by 1-2 weeks; optimal benefit may take 4-6 weeks.

ORAL SALICYLATES

▷ **indomethacin** (C) initially 25 mg bid <u>or</u> tid, increase as needed at weekly intervals by
  25-50 mg/day; max 200 mg/day
  Pediatric: <14 years: usually not recommended; >2 years, if risk warranted: 1-2 mg/
  kg/day in divided doses; max 3-4 mg/kg/day (<u>or</u> 150-200 mg/day, whichever is less;
  <14 years, ER cap not recommended
  Cap: 25, 50 mg; *Susp;* 25 mg/5 ml (pineapple-coconut, mint) (alcohol 1%); *Supp:* 50
  mg; *ER Cap:* 75 mg ext-rel
  Comment: **indomethacin** is indicated only for acute painful flares. Administer with
  food <u>and/or</u> antacids. Use lowest effective dose for shortest duration.
▷ **methotrexate** (X) 7.5 mg x 1 dose per week <u>or</u> 2.5 mg x 3 at 12 hour intervals once a
  week; max 20 mg/week; therapeutic response begins in 3-6 weeks; administer **methotrexate** injection SC only into the abdomen <u>or</u> thigh
  Pediatric: <2 years: not recommended; ≥2 years: 10 mg/m² once weekly; max 20 mg/m²

Rasuvo *Autoinjector:* 7.5 mg/0.15 ml, 10 mg/0.20 ml, 12.5 mg/ 0.25 ml, 15 mg/0.30 ml, 17.5 mg/0.35 ml, 20 mg/0.40 ml, 22.5 mg/0.45 ml, 25 mg/0.50 ml, 27.5 mg/0.55 ml, 30 mg/0.60 ml (solution concentration for SC injection is 50 mg/ml)

Rheumatrex *Tab:* 2.5*mg (5, 7.5, 10, 12.5, 15 mg/week, 4/card unit dose pack)

Trexall *Tab:* 5*, 7.5*, 10*, 15*mg (5, 7.5, 10, 12.5, 15 mg/week, 4/card unit dose pack)

Comment: *methotrexate* (MTX) is contraindicated with immunodeficiency, blood dyscrasias, alcoholism, and chronic liver disease.

POLYCYSTIC OVARIAN SYNDROME (STEIN-LEVENTHAL DISEASE)

See **Contraceptives** *page* 474
See **Type 2 Diabetes Mellitus** *page* 421

POLYMYALGIA RHEUMATICA

Comment: Initial treatment is low-dose prednsone at 12-25 mg/day. May attempt a very slow tapering regimen after 2-4 weeks. If relapse occurs, increase the daily dose of corticosteroid to the previous effective dose. Most people with polymyalgia rheumatica need to continue corticosteroid treatment for at least a year. Approximately 30-60% of people will have at least one relapse during corticosteroid tapering. Joint guidelines from the American Academy of Rheumatology (AAR) and the European League Against Rheumatism (ELAR) suggest using concomitant methotrexate (MTX) along with corticosteroids in some patients. It may be useful early in the course of treatment or later, if the patient relapses or does not respond to corticosteroids. The American Academy of Rheumatology (AAR) recommends the following daily doses for anyone on a chronic oral corticosteroid regimen: Calcium 1,200-1,500 mg/day and vitamin D 800-1,000 IU/day.

Oral Corticosteroids *see page* 497

For calcium and vitamin D supplementation, see **Hypocalcemia** *page* 218

➤ *methotrexate* (X) 7.5 mg x 1 dose per week or 2.5 mg x 3 at 12 hour intervals once a week; max 20 mg/week; therapeutic response begins in 3-6 weeks; administer methotrexate injection SC only into the abdomen or thigh

Pediatric: <2 years: not recommended; ≥2 years: 10 mg/m2 once weekly; max 20 mg/m2

Rasuvo *Autoinjector:* 7.5 mg/0.15 ml, 10 mg/0.20 ml, 12.5 mg/ 0.25 ml, 15 mg/0.30 ml, 17.5 mg/0.35 ml, 20 mg/0.40 ml, 22.5 mg/0.45 ml, 25 mg/0.50 ml, 27.5 mg/0.55 ml, 30 mg/0.60 ml (solution concentration for SC injection is 50 mg/ml)

Rheumatrex *Tab:* 2.5*mg (5, 7.5, 10, 12.5, 15 mg/week, 4/card unit dose pack)

TrexallR *Tab:* 5*, 7.5*, 10*, 15*mg (5, 7.5, 10, 12.5, 15 mg/week, 4/card unit dose pack)

Comment: *methotrexate* (MTX) is contraindicated with immunodeficiency, blood dyscrasias, alcoholism, and chronic liver disease.

◯ POSTHERPETIC NEURALGIA

GAMMA AMINOBUTYRIC ACID ANALOG

▷ *gabapentin* (C) *CrCl 30-60 mL/min:* 600-1800 mg; *CrCl <30 mL/min* or *on hemodialysis:* not recommended

Comment: Avoid abrupt cessation of *gabapentin* and *gabapentin enacarbil.* To discontinue, withdraw gradually over 1 week or longer.

Pediatric: <18 years: not recommended

Gralise initially 300 mg on Day 1; then 600 mg on Day 2; then 900 mg on Days 3-6; then 1200 mg on Days 7-10; then 1500 mg on Days 11-14; titrate up to 1800 mg on Day 15; take entire dose once daily with the evening meal; do not crush, split, or chew

Tab: 300, 600 mg

Neurontin (G) 300mg daily x 1 day, then 300 mg bid x 1 day, then 300 mg tid continuously; max 1,800 mg/day in 3 divided doses; taper over 7 days

Pediatric: <3 years: not recommended; 3-12 years: initially 10-15 mg/kg/day in 3 divided doses; max 12 hours between doses; titrate over 3 days; 3-4 years: titrate to 40 mg/kg/day; 5-12 years: titrate to 25-35 mg/kg/day; max 50 mg/kg/day;

Tab: 600*, 800* mg; *Cap:* 100, 300, 400 mg; *Oral soln:* 250 mg/5 ml (480 ml) (strawberry-anise) >12 years: same as adult

▷ *gabapentin enacarbil* (C) 600 mg once daily at about 5:00 PM; if dose not taken at recommended time, next dose should be taken the following day; swallow whole; take with food; *CrCl 30-59 mL/min:* 600 mg on Day 1, Day 3, and every day thereafter; *CrCl <30 mL/min:* or on hemodialysis: not recommended

Pediatric: not recommended

Horizant *Tab:* 600 ext-rel

Tricyclic Antidepressants (TCAs)

Comment: Co-administration of SSRIs and TCAs requires extreme caution.

▷ *amitriptyline* (C)(G) initially 75 mg/day in divided doses of 50-100 mg/day q HS; max 300 mg/day

Pediatric: not recommended

Tab: 10, 25, 50, 75, 100, 150 mg

▷ *amoxapine* (C) initially 50 mg bid-tid; after 1 week may increase to 100 mg bid-tid; usual effective dose 200-300 mg/day; if total dose exceeds 300 mg/day, give in divided doses (max 400 mg/day); may give as a single bedtime dose (max 300 mg q HS)

Pediatric: not recommended

Tab: 25, 50, 100, 150 mg

▷ *desipramine* (C)(G) 100-200 mg/day in single or divided doses; max 300 mg/day

Pediatric: not recommended

Norpramin *Tab:* 10, 25, 50, 75, 100, 150 mg

▷ *doxepin* (C)(G) 75 mg/day; max 150 mg/day

Pediatric: not recommended

Cap: 10, 25, 50, 75, 100, 150 mg; *Oral conc:* 10 mg/ml (4 oz w. dropper)

▷ *imipramine* (C)(G)

Pediatric: not recommended

Tofranil initially 75 mg daily (max 200 mg); adolescents initially 30-40 mg daily (max 100 mg/day); if maintenance dose exceeds 75 mg daily, may switch to **Tofranil PM** for divided or bedtime dose

Tab: 10, 25, 50 mg

Tofranil PM initially 75 mg daily 1 hour before HS; max 200 mg

Cap: 75, 100, 125, 150 mg

Tofranil Injection 50 mg IM; lower dose for adolescents; switch to oral form as soon as possible

Amp: 25 mg/2 ml (2 ml)

▷ *nortriptyline* **(D)(G)** initially 25 mg tid-qid; max 150 mg/day
Pediatric: not recommended

Pamelor *Cap:* 10, 25, 50, 75 mg; *Oral soln:* 10 mg/5 ml (16 oz)

▷ *protriptyline* **(C)** initially 5 mg tid; usual dose 15-40 mg/day in 3-4 divided doses; max 60 mg/day
Pediatric: <12 years: not recommended

Vivactyl *Tab:* 5, 10 mg

▷ *trimipramine* **(C)** initially 75 mg/day in divided doses; max 200 mg/day
Pediatric: not recommended

Surmontil *Cap:* 25, 50, 100 mg

α₂-DELTA LIGAND

▷ *pregabalin (GABA analog)* **(C)(V)** initially 150 mg daily divided bid-tid and may titrate within one week; max 600 mg divided bid-tid; discontinue over one week
Pediatric: <18 years: not recommended

Lyrica *Cap:* 25, 50, 75, 100, 150, 200, 225, 300 mg; *Oral soln:* 20 mg/ml

TOPICAL/TRANSDERMAL ANALGESICS

▷ *capsaicin* **(B)(G)** apply tid-qid prn to intact skin; avoid mucus membranes
Pediatric: <2 years: not recommended; ≥2 years: same as adult

Double Cap (OTC) *Crm:* 0.05% (2 oz)
Qutenza *Patch:* 8% (1-2, both with 50 g tube of cleansing gel)
Zostrix (OTC) *Crm:* 0.025% (0.7, 1.5, 3 oz)
Zostrix HP (OTC) *Emol crm:* 0.075% (1, 2 oz)

Comment: Provides some relief by 1-2 weeks; optimal benefit may take 4-6 weeks.

▷ *diclofenac epolamine* **(C)** apply one patch to affected area bid; remove during bathing; avoid non-intact skin; do not re-use
Pediatric: not recommended

Flector Patch *Patch:* 180 mg/patch (30/carton)

Comment: *diclofenac* is contraindicated with *aspirin* allergy and late pregnancy.

▷ *doxepin* **(B)** cream apply to affected area qid at intervals of at least 3-4 hours; max 8 days
Pediatric: not recommended

Prudoxin *Crm:* 5% (45 g)
Zonalon *Crm:* 5% (30, 45 g)

▷ *tacrolimus* **(C)** apply to affected area bid; continue for 1 week after clearing
Pediatric: <2 years: not recommended; 2-15 years: use 0.03% strength

Protopic *Oint:* 0.03, 0.1% (30, 60 g)

TOPICAL/TRANSDERMAL ANESTHETICS

▷ *lidocaine* cream (B)
  Pediatric: not recommended
        LidaMantle *Crm:* 3% (1, 2 oz)
        Lidoderm *Crm:* 3% (85 g)
▷ *lidocaine* lotion (B)
  Pediatric: not recommended
        LidaMantle *Lotn:* 3% (177 ml)
▷ *lidocaine* 5% patch (B)(G) apply up to 3 patches at one time for up to 12 hours/24-hour period (12 hours on/12 hours off); patches may be cut into smaller sizes before removal of the release liner; do not re-use
  Pediatric: not recommended
        Lidoderm *Patch:* 5% (10x14 cm; 30/carton)
▷ *lidocaine/dexamethasone* (B)
        Decadron Phosphate with Xylocaine *dexa* 4 mg/*lido* 10 mg per ml (5 ml)
▷ *lidocaine/hydrocortisone* (B)(G)
  Pediatric: not recommended
        LidaMantle HC *Crm: lido* 3%/*hydro* 0.5% (1, 3 oz); *Lotn:* (177 ml)
        Acetaminophen for IV Infusion see *Pain* page 296

ORAL ANALGESICS

▷ *acetaminophen* (B)(G) see **Fever** page 144
▷ *aspirin* (D)(G) see **Fever** page 144
  Comment: *aspirin*-containing medications are contraindicated with history of allergic-type reaction to *aspirin*, children and adolescents with *Varicella* or other viral illness, and 3rd trimester pregnancy.
▷ *tramadol* (C)(IV)(G)
        Rybix ODT initially 100 mg once daily; may increase by 100 mg every 5 days; max 300 mg/day; *CrCl <30 mL/min or severe hepatic impairment:* not recommended; *Cirrhosis:* max 50 mg q 12 hours
        Pediatric: <17 years: not recommended
        ODT: 50 mg (mint) (phenylalanine)
        Ryzolt initially 100 mg once daily; may increase by 100 mg every 5 days; max 300 mg/day; *CrCl <30 mL/min or severe hepatic impairment:* not recommended
        Pediatric: <16 years: not recommended; ≥16 years: same as adult
        Tab: 100, 200, 300 mg ext-rel
        Ultram 50-100 mg q 4-6 hours prn; max 400 mg/day; *CrCl <30 mL/min:* max 100 mg q 12 hours; *Cirrhosis:* max 50 mg q 12 hours
        Pediatric: <16 years: not recommended; ≥16 years: same as adult
        Tab: 50*mg
        Ultram ER initially 100 mg once daily; may increase by 100 mg every 5 days; max 300 mg/day; *CrCl <30 mL/min: or severe hepatic impairment:* not recommended
        Pediatric: <18 years: not recommended
        Tab: 100, 200, 300 mg ext-rel
▷ *tramadol/acetaminophen* (C)(IV)(G) 2 tabs q 4-6 hours; max 8 tabs/day; 5 days; *CrCl <30 mL/min:* max 2 tabs q 12 hours; max 4 tabs/day x 5 days
  Pediatric: <16 years: not recommended; ≥16 years: same as adult
        Ultracet *Tab: tram* 37.5/*acet* 325 mg
Other Oral Analgesics see *Pain* page 298

TRICYCLIC ANTIDEPRESSANTS (TCAs)

Comment: Co-administration of TCAs with SSRIs requires extreme caution.

▷ *amitriptyline* (C)(G) titrate to achieve pain relief; max 300 mg/day
 Pediatric: not recommended
  Tab: 10, 25, 50, 75, 100, 150 mg

▷ *amoxapine* (C) titrate to achieve pain relief; if total dose exceeds 300 mg/day, give in divided doses; max 400 mg/day
 Pediatric: not recommended
  Tab: 25, 50, 100, 150 mg

▷ *desipramine* (C)(G) titrate to achieve pain relief; max 300 mg/day
 Pediatric: not recommended
  Norpramin *Tab:* 10, 25, 50, 75, 100, 150 mg

▷ *doxepin* (C)(G) titrate to achieve pain relief; max 150 mg/day
 Pediatric: not recommended
  Cap: 10, 25, 50, 75, 100, 150 mg; *Oral conc:* 10 mg/ml (4 oz w. dropper)

▷ *imipramine* (C)(G)
 Pediatric: not recommended
  Tofranil titrate to achieve pain relief; max 200 mg/day; adolescents max 100 mg/day; if maintenance dose exceeds 75 mg/day, may switch to **Tofranil PM** at bedtime
   Tab: 10, 25, 50 mg
  Tofranil PM titrate to achieve pain relief; initially 75 mg at HS; max 200 mg at HS
   Cap: 75, 100, 125, 150 mg
  Tofranil Injection 50 mg IM; lower dose for adolescents; switch to oral form as soon as possible
   Amp: 25 mg/2 ml (2 ml)

▷ *nortriptyline* (D)(G) titrate to achieve pain relief; initially 10-25 mg tid-qid; max 150 mg/day; lower doses for elderly and adolescents
 Pediatric: not recommended
  Pamelor titrate to achieve pain relief; max 150 mg/day
   Cap: 10, 25, 50, 75 mg; *Oral soln:* 10 mg/5 ml (16 oz)

▷ *protriptyline* (C) titrate to achieve pain relief; initially 5 mg tid; max 60 mg/day
 Pediatric: <12 years: not recommended
  Vivactyl *Tab:* 5, 10 mg

▷ *trimipramine* (C) titrate to achieve pain relief; max 200 mg/day
 Pediatric: not recommended
  Surmontil *Cap:* 25, 50, 100 mg

 POST-TRAUMATIC STRESS DISORDER (PTSD)

Comment: No one pharmacological agent has emerged as the best treatment for PTSD. A combination of pharmacological agents (e.g., antidepressants, nonadrenergic agents, antipsychosis drugs) may comprise an individualized treatment plan to successfully manage core symptoms of PTSD as well as associated anxiety, depression, sleep disturbances, and co-occurring psychiatric disorders.

SELECTIVE SEROTONIN REUPTAKE INHIBITORS (SSRIs)

Comment: The FDA has approved two SSRIs for the treatment of PTSD: *paroxetine* and *sertraline*. However, the safety and efficacy of other SSRIs (*fluoxetine*, *citalopram, escitalopram, fluvoxamine*) have been tested in clinical practice. Co-administration of SSRIs with TCAs requires extreme caution. Concomitant use of MAOIs and SSRIs is absolutely contraindicated. Avoid St. John's wort and other serotonergic agents. A potentially fatal adverse event is *serotonin syndrome*, caused by serotonin excess. Milder symptoms require HCP intervention to avert severe symptoms which can be rapidly fatal without urgent/emergent medical care. Symptoms include restlessness, agitation, confusion, hallucinations, tachycardia, hypertension, dilated pupils, muscle twitching, muscle rigidity, loss of muscle coordination, diaphoresis, diarrhea, headache, shivering, piloerection, hyperpyrexia, cardiac arrhythmias, seizures, loss of consciousness, coma, death. Abrupt withdrawal or interruption of treatment with an antidepressant medication is sometimes associated with an *Antidepressant Discontinuation Syndrome* which may be mediated by gradually tapering the drug over a period of two weeks or longer, depending on the dose strength and length of treatment. Common symptoms of the *serotonin discontinuation Syndrome* include flu-like symptoms (nausea, vomiting, diarrhea, headaches, sweating), sleep disturbances (insomnia, nightmares, constant sleepiness), mood disturbances (dysphoria, anxiety, agitation), cognitive disturbances (mental confusion, hyperarousal), sensory and movement disturbances (imbalance, tremors, vertigo, dizziness, electric-shock-like sensations in the brain, often described by sufferers as "brain zaps."

▶ *paroxetine maleate* (D)(G)
  Pediatric: not recommended
    Paxil initially 20 mg daily in AM; may increase by 10 mg/day at weekly intervals as needed; max 60 mg/day
      Tab: 10*, 20*, 30, 40 mg
    Paxil CR initially 25 mg daily in AM; may increase by 12.5 mg at weekly intervals as needed; max 62.5 mg/day
      Tab: 12.5, 25, 37.5 mg cont-rel ent-coat
    Paxil Suspension initially 20 mg daily in AM; may increase by 10 mg/day at weekly intervals as needed; max 60 mg/day
      Oral susp: 10 mg/5 ml (250 ml; orange)
▶ *sertraline* (C) initially 50 mg daily; increase at 1 week intervals if needed; max 200 mg daily
  Pediatric: <6 years: not recommended; 6-12 years: initially 25 mg daily; max 200 mg/day; 13-17 years: initially 50 mg daily; max 200 mg/day
    Zoloft *Tab:* 15*, 50*, 100*mg; *Oral conc:* 20 mg per ml (60 ml [dilute just before administering in 4 oz water, ginger ale, lemon-lime soda, lemonade, or orange juice]) (alcohol 12%)

ATYPICAL ANTIPSYCHOSIS DRUGS

▶ *olanzapine* (C)(G) initially 2.5-5 mg once daily at HS; increase by 5 mg every week to 20 mg at HS; usual maintenance 10-20 mg /day
    Zyprexa *Tab:* 2.5, 5, 7.5, 10, 15, 20 mg
    Zyprexa Zydis *ODT:* 5, 10, 15, 20 mg (phenylalanine)
▶ *quetiapine* (C)(G) initially 25 mg bid; increase total daily dose by 50 mg, as needed and tolerated, to max 300-600 mg/day
    Seroquel *Tab:* 25, 100, 200, 300 mg
    Seroquel XR *Tab:* 50, 150, 200, 300, 400 mg ext-rel

▷ *risperidone* (C)(G) initially 0.5-1 mg bid; titrate to 3 mg bid by the end of the first week; usual maintenance 4-6 mg/day

> **Risperdal** *Tab:* 0.25, 0.5, 1, 2, 3, 4 mg; *Soln:* 1 mg/ml (30 ml w. pipette); *Consta (Inj):* 25, 37.5, 50 mg
> **Risperdal M-Tabs** *M-tab:* 0.5, 1, 2, 3, 4 mg orally-disint (phenylalanine)

NONADRENERGIC AGENTS

ALPHA-1 ANTAGONISTS

Comment: *prazosin* is useful in reducing combat-trauma nightmares, normalizing dreams for combat veterans, and mediating other sleep disturbances.

▷ *prazosin* (C)(G) first dose at HS, 1 mg bid-tid; increase dose slowly; usual range 6-15 mg/ day in divided doses; max 20-40 mg/day

Pediatric: not recommended

> **Minipress** *Cap:* 1, 2, 5 mg

CENTRAL ALPHA-2 AGONISTS

Comment: *clonidine* is useful to reduce nightmares, hypervigilance, startle reactions, and outbursts of rage.

▷ *clonidine* (C)

Pediatric: <12 years: not recommended; ≥12 years: same as adult

> **Catapres** initially 0.1 mg bid; usual range 0.2-0.6 mg/day in divided doses; max 2.4 mg/day *Tab:* 0.1*, 0.2*, 0.3*mg
> **Catapres-TTS** initially 0.1 mg patch weekly; increase after 1-2 weeks if needed; max 0.6 mg/day
>> *Patch:* 0.1, 0.2 mg/day (12/carton); 0.3 mg/day (4/carton)
> **Kapvay** (G) initially 0.1 mg bid; usual range 0.2-0.6 mg/day in divided doses; max 2.4 mg/ day *Tab:* 0.1, 0.2 mg
> **Nexiclon XR** initially 0.18 mg (2 ml) suspension or 0.17 mg tab once daily; usual max 0.52 mg (6 ml suspension) once daily
>> *Tab:* 0.17, 0.26 mg ext-rel; *Oral susp:* 0.09 mg/ml ext-rel (4 oz)

BETA-ADRENERGIC BLOCKER (NON-CARDIOSELECTIVE)

Comment: *propranolol* is useful to mediate hyperarousal. For other non-cardioselective beta-adrenergic blockers, *see* **Hypertension**, *page 200*

▷ *propranolol* (C)(G) 40-240 mg daily

Pediatric: not recommended

> **Inderal** *Tab:* 10*, 20*, 40*, 60*, 80*mg
> **Inderal LA** initially 80 mg daily in a single dose; increase q 3-7 days; usual range 120-160 mg/day; max 320 mg/day in a single dose

SEROTONIN AND NOREPINEPHRINE REUPTAKE INHIBITORS (SNRIs)

▷ *desvenlafaxine* (C)(G) swallow whole; initially 50 mg once daily; max 120 mg/day

Pediatric: not recommended

> **Pristiq** *Tab:* 50, 100 mg ext-rel

▷ *duloxetine* (C)(G) swallow whole; initially 30 mg once daily x 1 week; then increase to 60 mg once daily; max 120 mg/day

Pediatric: not recommended

Cymbalta *Cap:* 20, 30, 40, 60 mg del-rel
▷ *venlafaxine* (C)(G)
Effexor initially 75 mg/day in 2-3 divided doses; may increase at 4-day intervals in 75 mg increments to 150 mg/day; max 225 mg/day
Pediatric: <18 years: not recommended
Tab: 37.5, 75, 150, 225 mg
Effexor XR initially 75 mg q AM; may start at 37.5 mg daily x 4-7 days, then increase by increments of up to 75 mg/day at intervals of at least 4 days; usual max 375 mg/day
Pediatric: not recommended
Tab/Cap: 37.5, 75, 150 mg ext-rel

5HT2/3 RECEPTOR BLOCKERS

▷ *mirtazapine* (C) initially 15 mg q HS; increase at intervals of 1-2 weeks; 1-2 weeks; usual range 15-60 mg/day; max 60 mg/day
Pediatric: not recommended
Remeron *Tab:* 15*, 30*, 45*mg
Remeron SolTab *ODT:* 15, 30, 45 mg (orange) (phenylalanine)

SEROTONIN/ACETYLCHOLINE/NOREPINEPHRINE/DOPAMINE BLOCKER

▷ *trazodone* (C)(G) initially 150 mg/day in divided doses with food; increase by 50 mg/day q 3-4 days; max 400 mg/day in divided doses <u>or</u> 50-400 mg at HS
Pediatric: <18 years: not recommended
Oleptro *Tab:* 50, 100*, 150*, 200, 250, 300 mg

TRICYCLIC ANTIDEPRESSANTS (TCAs)

▷ *amitriptyline* (C)(G) 10-20 mg at HS
Pediatric: not recommended
Tab: 10, 25, 50, 75, 100, 150 mg
▷ *doxepin* (C)(G) 10-200 mg at HS
Pediatric: not recommended
Cap: 10, 25, 50, 75, 100, 150 mg; *Oral conc:* 10 mg/ml (4 oz w. dropper)
▷ *imipramine* (C)(G) 10-200 mg q HS
Tofranil 100-300 mg at HS <u>or</u> divided bid <u>or</u> tid
Pediatric: <6 years: not recommended; 6-12 years: initially 25 mg; >12 years: 50 mg max 2.5 mg/kg/day
Tab: 10, 25, 50 mg
Tofranil PM initially 75 mg daily 1 hour before HS; max 200 mg
Cap: 75, 100, 125, 150 mg
Tofranil Injection 50 mg IM; lower dose for adolescents; switch to oral form as soon as possible
Amp: 25 mg/2 ml (2 ml)
▷ *nortriptyline* (D)(G) 10-150 mg q HS
Pediatric: not recommended
Pamelor *Cap:* 10, 25, 50, 75 mg; *Oral soln:* 10 mg/5 ml

MONOAMINE OXIDASE INHIBITORS (MAOIs)

Comment: Many drug and food interactions with this class of drugs, use cautiously. MOAIs should be reserved for refractory depression that has not responded to other classes of antidepressants. Concomitant use of MAOIs and SSRIs is contraindicated. See mfr literature for drug and food interactions. MAOIs have been used to reduce recurrent recollections of the trauma, nightmares, flashbacks, numbing, sleep disturbances, and social withdrawal in PTSD.

▷ *phenelzine* (C)(G) initially 15 mg tid; max 90 mg/day
   Pediatric: <16 years: not recommended; ≥16 years: same as adult
   Nardil
      Tab: 15 mg
▷ *selegiline* (C) initially 10 mg tid; max 60 mg/day
   Pediatric: <12 years: not recommended; ≥12 years: same as adult
      Emsam *Transdermal patch:* 6 mg/24 hrs, 9 mg/24 hrs, 12 mg/24 hrs
      Comment: At the **Emsam** transdermal patch 6 mg/24 hrs dose, the dietary restrictions commonly required when using nonselective MAOIs are not necessary.

PREGNANCY

see **Appendix Z: Prescription Prenatal Vitamins** *page* 520
Comment: Prenatal vitamins should have at least 1 mg folic acid content. Take one dose once daily. It is recommended that prenatal vitamins be started at least 3 months prior to conception to improve preconception nutritional status, and continued throughout pregnancy and the postnatal period, in lactating and nonlactating women, and throughout the childbearing years.

NAUSEA/VOMITING

▷ *doxyalamine succinate/pyridoxine* (A) do not crush or chew; take on an empty stomach with water; initially 2 tabs at HS on day 1; may increase to 1 tab AM and 2 tabs at HS day 2; may increase to 1 tab AM, 1 tab mid-afternoon, 2 tabs at HS; max 4 tabs/day
      Diclegis *Tab: doxyl* 10 mg/*pyri* 10 mg del-rel
▷ *promethazine* (C)(G) 12.5-50 mg po/IM/rectally q 4-6 hours prn
      Phenergan *Tab:* 12.5*, 25*, 50 mg; *Plain syr:* 6.25 mg/5 ml; *Fortis syr:* 25 mg/5 ml; *Rectal supp:* 12.5, 25, 50 mg; *Amp:* 25, 50 mg/ml (1 ml)
▷ *ondansetron* (C)(G) 4-8 mg bid prn
      Zofran *Tab:* 4, 8, 24 mg
      Zofran Injection *Vial:* 2 mg/ml (2 ml single-dose); 2 mg/ml (20 ml multi-dose) for IV or IM administration
      Zofran ODT *ODT:* 4, 8 mg (strawberry) (phenylalanine)
      Zofran Oral Solution *Oral soln:* 4 mg/5 ml (50 ml) (strawberry)
      Zuplenz Oral Soluble Film: 4, 8 mg orally-disint (10/carton) (peppermint)

PREMENSTRUAL DYSPHORHIC DISORDER (PMDD)/ PREMENSTRUAL SYNDROME (PMS)

Oral Prescription NSAIDs *see page* 489
Other Oral Analgesics *see* **Pain** *page* 298
Oral Contraceptives *see page* 474

▷ *ethinyl estradiol/drospirenone* (X)(G) 1 tab once daily x 28 days; repeat cyclical; start on start on first Sunday after menses begins <u>or</u> on first day of next menses
  Pediatric: same as adult
    Yaz *Tab:* ethin estra 20 mcg/*drospir* 3 mg

DIURETICS

▷ *spironolactone* (D)(G) initially 50-100 mg once daily <u>or</u> in divided doses; titrate at 2-week intervals
  Pediatric: not recommended
    Aldactone *Tab:* 25, 50*, 100*mg

ANTIDEPRESSANTS

▷ *fluoxetine* (C)(G)
    Prozac initially 20 mg daily; may increase after 1 week; doses >20 mg/day should be divided into AM and noon doses; max 80 mg/day
      Pediatric: <8 years: not recommended; 8-17 years: initially 10 <u>or</u> 20 mg/day; start lower weight children at 10 mg/day; if starting at 10 mg/day, may increase after 1 week to 20 mg /day
      Tab: 10*mg; *Cap:* 10, 20, 40 mg; *Oral soln:* 20 mg/5 ml (4 oz) (mint)
    Prozac Weekly following daily *fluoxetine* therapy at 20 mg/day for 13 weeks, may initiate **Prozac Weekly** 7 days after the last 20 mg *fluoxetine* dose
      Pediatric: not recommended
      Cap: 90 mg ent-coat del-rel pellets
    Sarafem administer daily <u>or</u> 14 days before expected menses and through first full day of menses; initially 20 mg/day; max 80 mg/day
      Tab: 10, 15, 20 mg; *Cap:* 20 mg
▷ *paroxetine maleate* (D)(G)
  Pediatric: not recommended
    Paxil initially 20 mg daily in AM; may increase by 10 mg/day at weekly intervals as needed; max 60 mg/day
      Tab: 10*, 20*, 30, 40 mg
    Paxil CR initially 25 mg daily in AM; may increase by 12.5 mg at weekly intervals as needed; max 62.5 mg/day; may start 14 days before and continue through day one of menses
      Tab: 12.5, 25, 37.5 mg cont-rel ent-coat
    Paxil Suspension initially 20 mg daily in AM; may increase by 10 mg/day at weekly intervals as needed; max 60 mg/day
      Oral susp: 10 mg/5 ml (250 ml) (orange)
▷ *sertraline* (C)
    For 2 weeks prior to onset of menses: initially 50 mg daily x 3; then increase to 100 mg daily for remainder of the cycle; *For full cycle:* initially 50 mg daily; then may increase by 50 mg/day each cycle to max 150 mg/day
      Pediatric: not recommended
    Zoloft *Tab:* 25*, 50*, 100*mg; *Oral conc:* 20 mg per ml (60 ml) (alcohol 12%); dilute just before administering in 4 oz water, ginger ale, lemon-lime soda, lemonade, <u>or</u> orange juice
▷ *nortriptyline* (D)(G) initially 25 mg tid-qid; max 150 mg/day
  Pediatric: not recommended
    Pamelor *Cap:* 10, 25, 50, 75 mg; *Oral soln:* 10 mg/5 ml
Contraceptives see page 474

CALCIUM SUPPLEMENTS

▷ *calcium* (C) 1200 mg/day
see Osteoporosis page 283

 PRIMARY IMMUNODEFICIENCY IN ADULTS

▷ *recombinant human hyaluronidase (human normal immunoglobulin)* (C)
   HyQvia see mfr literature for dose by weight table and dose schedule table
      Vial: 10%; 2.5 g/200 u, 5 g/400 u, 10 g/800 u, 20 g/1600 u, 30 g/2400 u (2
      single-use/dual-vial unit (preservative-free)

   Comment: HyQvia is an immune globulin with a recombinant human
   hyaluronidase indicated for the treatment of primary immunodeficiency
   (PI) in adults. This includes, but is not limited to, common variable
   immunodeficiency (CVID), X-linked agammaglobulinemia, congenital
   agammaglobulinemia, Wiskott-Aldrich syndrome, and severe combined
   immunodeficiencies. **HyQvia** contains IgG antibodies, collected from human
   plasma donated by healthy people. **HyQvia** is a dual vial unit with one vial of
   immune globulin infusion 10% (Human) and one vial of recombinant human
   hyaluronidase. The hyaluronidase part of **HyQvia** helps more of the immune
   globulin get absorbed into the body. HyQvia is a ready-for-use sterile,
   liquid preparation of highly purified, concentrated, broad spectrum IgG
   antibodies. The distribution of the IgG subclasses is similar to that of normal
   plasma. Contains 100 mg/ml protein. **HyQvia** is collected only at FDA
   approved blood establishments and is tested by FDA licensed serological
   tests for Hepatitis B Surface Antigen (HBsAg), and for antibodies to Human
   Immunodeficiency Virus (HIV-1/HIV-2) and Hepatitis C Virus (HCV)
   in accordance with U.S. regulatory requirements. As an additional safety
   measure, mini-pools of the plasma are tested for the presence of HIV-1 and
   HCV by FDA licensed Nucleic Acid Testing (NAT). Protect from light. Use
   within 3 months after removal to room temperature but within the expiration
   date on the carton and vial labels. Do not return vials to the refrigerator after
   being stored at room temperature.

PROCTITIS: ACUTE (PROCTOCOLITIS/ENTERITIS)

Comment: The following regimen for the treatment of proctitis, proctocolitis, and
enteritis is published in the **2015 CDC Sexually Transmitted Diseases Treatment
Guidelines**.

RECOMMENDED REGIMEN

▷ *ceftriaxone* (B)(G) 250 mg IM in a single dose
   Rocephin *Vial:* 250, 500 mg; 1, 2 g
      plus
▷ *doxycycline* 100 mg bid x 7 days
   Actilate *Tab:* 75, 150** mg
   Adoxa *Tab:* 50, 75, 100, 150 mg ent-coat
   Doryx *Tab:* 75, 100, 150 mg del-rel

Monodox *Cap:* 50, 75, 100 mg
Oracea *Cap:* 40 mg del-rel
Vibramycin *Cap:* 50, 100 mg; *Syr:* 50 mg/5 ml (raspberry) (sulfites); *Oral susp:* 25 mg/5 ml (raspberry-apple)
Vibra-Tab *Tab:* 100 mg film-coat

Comment: *doxycycline* is contraindicated <8 years-of-age, in pregnancy, and lactation (discolors developing tooth enamel). A side effect may be photo-sensitivity (photophobia). Do not give with antacids, calcium supplements, milk or other dairy, or within two hours of taking another drug.

PROSTATITIS: ACUTE

ANTI-INFECTIVES

▷ *ciprofloxacin* (C) 500 mg bid x 4-6 weeks
Pediatric: <18 years: not recommended
   Cipro (G) *Tab:* 250, 500, 750 mg; *Oral susp:* 250, 500 mg/5 ml (100 ml) (strawberry)
   Cipro XR *Tab:* 500, 1000 mg ext-rel
   ProQuin XR *Tab:* 500 mg ext-rel

Comment: *ciprofloxacin* is contraindicated <18 years-of-age, and during pregnancy and lactation. Risk of tendonitis or tendon rupture, especially 60 years-of-age and older.

▷ *norfloxacin* (C) 400 mg bid x 28 days
   Noroxin *Tab:* 400 mg

Comment: *norfloxacin* is contraindicated <18 years-of-age, and during pregnancy and lactation. Risk of tendonitis or tendon rupture, especially 60 years-of-age and older.

▷ *ofloxacin* (C)(G) 300 mg x bid x 6 weeks
   Floxin *Tab:* 200, 300, 400 mg

Comment: *ofloxacin* is contraindicated <18 years-of-age, and during pregnancy and lactation. Risk of tendonitis or tendon rupture, especially 60 years-of-age and older.

▷ *trimethoprim/sulfamethoxazole* (C)(G)
   Bactrim, Septra 2 tabs bid x 10 days
      Tab: trim 80 mg/*sulfa* 400 mg*
   Bactrim DS, Septra DS 1 tab bid x 10 days
      Tab: trim 160 mg/*sulfa* 800 mg*
   Bactrim Pediatric Suspension, Septra Pediatric Suspension
      Oral susp: trim 40 mg/*sulfa* 200 mg per 5 ml (100 ml) (cherry) (alcohol 0.3%)

Comment: *CrCl 15-30 mL/min:* reduce dose by 1/2; *CrCl <15 mL/min:* not recommended

PROSTATITIS: CHRONIC

ANTI-INFECTIVES

▷ *carbenicillin* (B) 2 tabs qid x 4-12 weeks
   Geocillin *Tab:* 382 mg

▷ *ciprofloxacin* (C) 500 mg bid x 3 or more months
  Pediatric: <18 years: not recommended
    Cipro (G) *Tab:* 250, 500, 750 mg; *Oral susp:* 250, 500 mg/5 ml (100 ml) (strawberry)
    Cipro XR *Tab:* 500, 1000 mg ext-rel
    ProQuin XR *Tab:* 500 mg ext-rel
  Comment: *ciprofloxacin* is contraindicated <18 years-of-age, and during pregnancy
  and lactation. Risk of tendonitis or tendon rupture, especially 60 years-of-age and
  older.
▷ *ofloxacin* (C)(G) 300 mg bid x 4-12 weeks
    Floxin *Tab:* 200, 300, 400 mg
  Comment: *ofloxacin* is contraindicated <18 years-of-age, and during pregnancy and
  lactation. Risk of tendonitis or tendon rupture, especially 60 years-of-age and older.
▷ *norfloxacin* (C) 400 mg bid x 4-12 weeks
    Noroxin *Tab:* 400 mg
  Comment: *norfloxacin* contraindicated <18 years-of-age, and during pregnancy
  and lactation. Risk of tendonitis or tendon rupture, especially 60 years-of-age and
  older.
▷ *trimethoprim/sulfamethoxazole* (C)(G)
    Bactrim, Septra 2 tabs bid x 10 days
      Tab: trim 80 mg/*sulfa* 400 mg*
    Bactrim DS, Septra DS 1 tab bid x 10 days
      Tab: trim 160 mg/*sulfa* 800 mg
    Bactrim Pediatric Suspension, Septra Pediatric Suspension 20 ml bid x 10 days
      Oral susp: trim 40 mg/*sulfa* 200 mg per 5 ml (100 ml) (cherry) (alcohol 0.3%)
  Comment: *CrCl 15-30 mL/min:* reduce dose by 1/2; *CrCl <15 mL/min:* not
  recommended

SUPPRESSION THERAPY

▷ *trimethoprim/sulfamethoxazole* (C)(G)
    Bactrim, Septra 2 tabs bid x 10 days
      Tab: trim 80 mg/*sulfa* 400 mg*
    Bactrim DS, Septra DS 1 tab bid x 10 days
      Tab: trim 160 mg/*sulfa* 800 mg*
    Bactrim Pediatric Suspension, Septra Pediatric Suspension 20 ml bid x 10 days
      Oral susp: trim 40 mg/*sulfa* 200 mg per 5 ml (100 ml) (cherry) (alcohol 0.3%)
  Comment: *CrCl 15-30 mL/min:* reduce dose by 1/2; *CrCl <15 mL/min:* not
  recommended

 PRURITUS

Oral Drugs for Allergy, Cough, and Cold *see page* 524
Topical Corticosteroids *see page* 494
Parenteral Corticosteroids *see page* 499
Oral Corticosteroids *see page* 497
Eucerin Products (OTC)
Lac-Hydrin Products (OTC)
Lubriderm Products (OTC)
Aveeno Products (OTC)

TOPICAL OIL

▷ *fluocinolone acetamide* 0.01% topical oil **(C)**
  Pediatric: <6 years: not recommended; ≥6 years: apply sparingly bid for up to 4 weeks
    Derma-Smoothe/FS Topical Oil apply sparingly tid
      Topical oil: 0.01% (4 oz) (peanut oil)

TOPICAL ANALGESICS

▷ *capsaicin* **(B)(G)** apply tid-qid prn to intact skin
  Pediatric: <2 years: not recommended; ≥2 years: same as adult
    Double Cap (OTC) *Crm:* 0.05% (2 oz)
    Qutenza (B) *Patch:* 8% (1-2, both with 50 g tube of cleansing gel)
    Zostrix (OTC) *Crm:* 0.025% (0.7, 1.5, 3 oz)
    Zostrix HP (OTC) *Emol crm:* 0.075% (1, 2 oz)
Comment: Provides some relief by 1-2 weeks; optimal benefit may take 4-6 weeks.
▷ *doxepin* **(B)** cream apply to affected area qid at intervals of at least 3-4 hours; max 8 days
  Pediatric: not recommended
    Prudoxin *Crm:* 5% (45 g)
    Zonalon *Crm:* 5% (30, 45 g)
▷ *tacrolimus* **(C)** apply to affected area bid; continue for 1 week after clearing
  Pediatric: <2 years: not recommended; 2-15 years: use 0.03% strength; apply to affected area bid; continue for 1 week after clearing
    Protopic *Oint:* 0.03, 0.1% (30, 60 g)

⬤ PSEUDOBULBAR AFFECT (PBA) DISORDER

Comment: Pseudobulbar affect (PBA), emotional lability, labile affect, or emotional incontinence refers by to a neurologic disorder characterized involuntary crying or uncontrollable episodes of crying and/or laughing, or other emotional displays. PBA occurs secondary to a neurologic disease or brain injury. Brain injury or neurologic diseases such as traumatic brain injury, stroke, Parkinson's disease, multiple sclerosis, and amyotrophic lateral sclerosis (ALS, or Lou Gehrig's disease).
▷ *dextromethorphan/quinidine* **(C)** 1 cap once daily x 7 days; then starting on day 8, 1 cap bid
    Nuedexta apply bid to lesions and gently rub in completely
      Pediatric: not recommended
      Cap: dextro 20 mg/quini 10 mg

⬤ PSEUDOGOUT

Injectable Acetaminophen *see Pain page 296*
Oral Prescription NSAIDs *see page 489*
Other Oral Analgesics *see Pain page 298*
Topical/Transdermal NSAIDs *see Pain page 297*
Parenteral Corticosteroids *see page 499*
Oral Corticosteroids *see page 497*
Topical Analgesic and Anesthetic Agents *see page 487*

PSEUDOMEMBRANOUS COLITIS

Comment: Staphylococcal enterocolitis and antibiotic-associated pseudomembranous colitis caused by *C. difficile*.

ANTI-INFECTIVES

▷ *vancomycin* (B, caps; C, susp) 500 mg to 2 g in 3-4 doses x 7-10 days; max 2 g/day
    Pediatric: 40 mg/kg/day in 3-4 doses x 7-10 days; max 2 g/day
▷ *metronidazole* (not for use in 1st; B in 2nd, 3rd)(G) 500 mg tid x 14 days
        Flagyl *Tab:* 250*, 500*mg
        Flagyl 375 *Cap:* 375 mg
        Flagyl ER *Tab:* 750 mg ext-rel
    Comment: Alcohol is contraindicated during treatment with oral *metronidazole* and for 72 hours after therapy due to a possible *disulfiram*-like reaction (nausea, vomiting, flushing, headache).

 PSITTACOSIS

ANTI-INFECTIVES

▷ *tetracycline* (D)(G) 250 mg qid <u>or</u> 500 mg tid x 7-14 days
    Pediatric: <8 years: not recommended; ≥8 years, <100 lb: 25-50 mg/kg/day in 4 doses x 7-14 days; ≥8 years, ≥100 lb: same as adult
        Achromycin V *Cap:* 250, 500 mg
        Sumycin *Tab:* 250, 500 mg; *Cap:* 250, 500 mg; *Oral susp:* 125 mg/5 ml (100, 200 ml) (fruit) (sulfites)
    Comment: *tetracycline* is contraindicated <8 years-of-age, in pregnancy, and lactation (discolors developing tooth enamel). A side effect may be photo-sensitivity (photophobia). Do not give with antacids or calcium supplements within two hours of another drug.

 PSEUDOBULBAR AFFECT (PBA)

Comment: Pseudobulbar affect (PBA), emotional lability, labile affect, <u>or</u> emotional incontinence refers to a neurologic disorder characterized by involuntary crying <u>or</u> uncontrollable episodes of crying <u>and/or</u> laughing, <u>or</u> other emotional displays. PBA occurs secondary to a neurologic disease <u>or</u> brain injury. Brain injury <u>or</u> neurologic diseases such as traumatic brain injury, stroke, Parkinson's disease, multiple sclerosis, and amyotrophic lateral sclerosis (ALS, <u>or</u> Lou Gehrig's disease).

▷ *dextromethorphan/quinidine* (C) 1 cap once daily x 7 days; then starting on day 8, 1 cap bid
        Nuedexta
        Pediatric: not recommended
        Cap: dextro 20 mg/*quini* 10 mg

PSORIASIS

Emollients *see* ***Dermatitis: Atopic*** *page* 110
Topical Corticosteroids *see page* 494

VITAMIN D-3 DERIVATIVES

➤ *calcipotriene* (C)
   Dovonex apply bid to lesions and gently rub in completely
      Pediatric: not recommended
      Crm: 0.005% (30, 120 g)

VITAMIN D-3 DERIVATIVE/CORTICOSTEROID COMBINATIONS

➤ *calcipotriene/betamethasone dipropionate* (C)
   Pediatric: <18 years: not recommended
      Enstilar apply to affected area and gently rub in once daily x up to 4 weeks; limit
      treatment area to 30% of body surface area; do not occlude; do not use on face,
      axillae, groin, or atrophic skin; max 100 g/week
         Foam: calci 0.005%/*beta* 0.064% (60 g spray can)
      Taclonex apply to affected area and gently rub in once daily as needed, up to 4 weeks
      Taclonex Ointment apply bid to lesions and gently rub in completely; limit
      treatment area to 30% of body surface area; do not occlude; do not use on face,
      axillae, groin, or atrophic skin; max 100 g/week
         Oint: calci 0.005%/*beta* 0.064% (60, 100 g)
      Taclonex Scalp Topical Suspension apply to affected area and gently rub in once
      daily x 2 weeks or until cleared; max 8 weeks; limit treatment area to 30% of
      body surface area; do not occlude; do not use on face, axillae, groin, or atrophic
      skin; max 100 g/week
         Bottle: (30, 60 g; 120 g [2x60 g])
➤ *Calcitrol* (C)
   Vectical apply bid to lesions and gently rub in completely; max weekly dose
   should not exceed 200 g
      Pediatric: <18 years: not recommended
      Oint: 3 mcg/g (100 g)

IMMUNOSUPPRESSANTS

➤ *alefacept* (B) 7.5 mg IV bolus or 15 mg IM once weekly x 12 weeks; may re-treat x
   12 weeks
   Pediatric: not recommended
      Amevive *IV dose pack:* 7.5 mg single-use (w. 10 ml sterile water diluents [use
      0.6 ml]; 1, 4/pck); *IM dose pack:* 15 mg single-use (w. 10 ml sterile water diluent
      [use 0.6 ml]; 1, 4/pck)
   Comment: CD4+ and T-lymphycyte count should be checked prior to initiating
   treatment with *alefacept* and then monitored. Treatment should be withheld if
   CD4+ T-lymphocyte counts are below 250 cells/mcl.
➤ *cyclosporine* (C) 1.25 mg/kg bid; may increase after 4 weeks by 0.5mg /kg/day; then
   adjust at 2-week intervals; max 4 mg/kg/day; administer with meals
   Pediatric: <18 years: not recommended

Neoral *Cap:* 25, 100 mg (alcohol)
Neoral Oral Solution *Oral soln:* 100 mg/ml (50 ml) may dilute in room temperature apple juice or orange juice (alcohol)

ANTIMITOTICS

▷ *anthralin* (C) apply once daily
  Pediatric: not recommended
    Zithranol-RR *Crm:* 1.2% (15, 45 g)

RETINOIDS

▷ *acitretin* (X) 25-50 mg once daily with main meal
  Pediatric: not recommended
    Soriatane *Cap:* 10, 25 mg
▷ *tazarotene* (X)(G) apply once daily at HS
  Pediatric: not recommended
    Avage Cream *Crm:* 0.1% (30 g)
    Tazorac Cream *Crm:* 0.05, 0.1% (15, 30, 60 g)
    Tazorac Gel *Gel:* 0.05, 0.1% (30, 100 g)

COAL TAR PREPARATIONS

▷ *coal tar* (C)(G)
  Pediatric: same as adult
    Scytera (OTC) apply qd-qid; use lowest effective dose
      Foam: 2%
    T/Gel Shampoo Extra Strength (OTC) use every other day; max 4 x/week; massage into affected areas for 5 minutes; rinse; repeat *Shampoo:* 1%
    T/Gel Shampoo Original Formula (OTC) use every other day; max 7 x/week; massage into affected areas for 5 minutes; rinse; repeat *Shampoo:* 0.5%
    T/Gel Shampoo Stubborn Itch Control (OTC) use every other day; max 7 x/week; massage into affected areas for 5 minutes; rinse; repeat *Shampoo:* 0.5%

INTERLEUKIN-17A ANTAGONIST

▷ *secukinumab* (B) inject SC into the upper arm, abdomen, or thigh; rotate sites; administer 300 mg SC (as two separate 150 mg SC inject-ions) at weeks 0, 1, 2, 3, and 4; then 300 mg every 4 weeks; for some patients, 150 mg/dose may be sufficient
  Pediatric: <18 years: not recommended
    Cosentyx *Vial:* 150 mg/ml pwdr for SC inj after reconstitution single-use (preservative-free)
    Comment: **Cosentyx** may be used as monotherapy or in combination with *methotrexate* (MTX).

INTERLEUKIN-12/INTERLEUKIN-23 ANTAGONIST

▷ *ustekinumab* (B) inject SC; rotate sites; <100 kg: 45 mg once; then 4 weeks later; then every 12 weeks; ≥100 kg: 90 mg once; then 4 weeks later; then every 12 weeks
  Pediatric: <18 years: not recommended
    Stelara *Vial:* 45 mg/0.5 ml single-use (preservative-free)

Comment: **Stelara** may be used as monotherapy <u>or</u> in combination with *metho-trexate* (MTX).

TUMOR NECROSIS FACTOR (TNF) BLOCKERS

▷ *etanercept* (B) inject SC into thigh, abdomen, <u>or</u> upper arm; rotate sites; initially 50 mg twice weekly (3-4 days apart) for 3 months; then 50 mg/week maintenance <u>or</u> 25 mg <u>or</u> 50 mg per week for 3 months; then 50 mg/week maintenance
Pediatric: <18 years: not recommended
Enbrel *Vial:* 25 mg pwdr for SC injection after reconstitution (4/ carton w. supplies) (preservative-free, diluent contains benzyl alcohol); *Prefilled syringe:* 50 mg/ml (preservative-free); *SureClick autoinjector: 50 mg/ml (preservative-free)*
▷ *adalimumab* (B) initially 80 mg SC once followed by 40 mg once every other week starting one week after initial dose; inject into thigh <u>or</u> abdomen; rotate sites
Pediatric: <18 years: not recommended
Humira *Prefilled syringe:* 20 mg/0.4 ml; 40 mg/0.8 ml single-dose (2/pck; 2, 6/ starter pck) (preservative-free)
▷ *golimumab* (B) administer SC <u>or</u> IV infusion (in combination with *methotrexate [MTX]*)
Pediatric: <18 years: not established
Simponi 50 mg SC once monthly; rotate sites
Prefilled syringe, SmartJect autoinjector: 50 mg/0.5 ml, single-use (preservative-free)
Simponi Aria 2 mg/kg IV infusion week 0 and week 4; then every 8 weeks thereafter
Vial: 50 mg/4 ml, single-use, soln for IV infusion after dilution (latex-free, preservative-free)
▷ *infliximab* (B) administer by IV infusion over 2 hours; 5 mg/kg weeks 0, 2, 6; then once every 8 weeks
Pediatric: <6 years: not recommended; ≥6 years: same as adult
Remicade *Vial:* 100 mg pwdr for reconstitution for IV infusion (preservative-free)

MOISTURIZING AGENTS

Aquaphor Healing Ointment (OTC) *Oint:* (1.75, 3.5, 14 oz) (alcohol)
Eucerin Daily Sun Defense (OTC) *Lotn:* 6 oz (fragrance-free)
Comment: **Eucerin Daily Sun Defense** is a moisturizer with SPF 15.
Eucerin Facial Lotion (OTC) *Lotn:* 4 oz
Eucerin Light Lotion (OTC) *Lotn:* 8 oz
Eucerin Lotion (OTC) *Lotn:* 8, 16 oz
Eucerin Original Creme (OTC) *Crm:* 2, 4, 16 oz (alcohol)
Eucerin Plus Creme *Crm:* 4 oz
Eucerin Plus Lotion (OTC) *Lotn:* 6, 12 oz
Eucerin Protective Lotion (OTC) *Lotn:* 4 oz (alcohol)
Comment: **Eucerin Protective Lotion** is a moisturizer with SPF 25.
Lac-Hydrin Cream (OTC) *Crm:* 280, 385 g
Lac-Hydrin Lotion (OTC) *Lotn:* 225, 400 g
Lubriderm Dry Skin Scented (OTC) *Lotn:* 6, 10, 16, 32 oz
Lubriderm Dry Skin Unscented (OTC) *Lotn:* 3.3, 6, 10, 16 oz (fragrance-free)
Lubriderm Sensitive Skin Lotion (OTC) *Lotn:* 3.3, 6, 10, 16 oz (lanolin-free)

Lubriderm Dry Skin (OTC) *Lotn (scented):* 2.5, 6, 10, 16 oz;
Lotn (fragrance-free): 1, 2.5, 6, 10, 16 oz
Lubriderm Bath 1-2 capfuls in bath <u>or</u> rub onto wet skin as needed; then rinse
Oil: 8 oz

 PSORIATIC ARTHRITIS

Injectable Acetaminophen *see Pain page* 296
Oral Prescription NSAIDs *see Pain page* 489
Other Oral Analgesics *see Pain page* 298
Topical/Transdermal NSAIDs *see Pain page* 297
Parenteral Corticosteroids *see page* 499
Oral Corticosteroids *see page* 497
Topical Analgesic and Anesthetic Agents *see page* 487

TOPICAL ANALGESICS

▷ *capsaicin* (B)(G) apply tid-qid prn to intact skin
Pediatric: <2 years: not recommended; >2 years: same as adult
Axsain *Crm:* 0.075% (1, 2 oz)
Capsin *Lotn:* 0.025, 0.075% (59 ml)
Capzasin-P (OTC) *Crm:* 0.025% (1.5 oz); *Lotn:* 0.025% (2 oz)
Dolorac *Crm:* 0.025% (28 g)
Double Cap (OTC) *Crm:* 0.05% (2 oz)
R-Gel *Gel:* 0.025% (15, 30 g)
Zostrix (OTC) *Crm:* 0.025% (0.7, 1.5, 3 oz)
Zostrix HP (OTC) *Emol crm:* 0.075% (1, 2 oz)
Comment: Provides some relief by 1-2 weeks; optimal benefit may take 4-6 weeks.
▷ *trolamine salicylate* (NR)
Mobisyl apply tid-qid
Crm: 10%
Comment: Provides some relief by 1-2 weeks; optimal benefit may take 4-6 weeks.
▷ *diclofenac sodium* (C; D ≥30 wks) apply qid prn to intact skin
Pediatric: not established
Pennsaid 1.5% in 10 drop increments, dispense and rub into front, side, and
back of knee: usually; 40 drops (40 mg) qid
Topical soln: 1.5% (150 ml)
Pennsaid 2% apply 2 pump actuations (40 mg) and rub into front, side, and
back of knee bid
Topical soln: 2% (20 mg/pump actuation, 112 g)
Comment: **Pennsaid** is indicated for the treatment of pain associated with
osteoarthritis of the knee.
Pennsaid 2% apply 2 pump actuations (40 mg) and rub into front, side, and
back of knee bid
Topical soln: 2% (20 mg/pump actuation; 112 g)
Voltaren Gel (G) *Gel:* 1% (100 g)
Comment: Contraindicated with *aspirin* allergy. As with other NSAIDs,
Voltaren Gel should be avoided in late pregnancy (≥30 weeks) because it may
cause premature closure of the ductus arteriosus.

ORAL SALICYLATE

➤ *indomethacin* (C) initially 25 mg bid-tid, increase as needed at weekly intervals by 25-50 mg/day; max 200 mg/day
Pediatric: <14 years: usually not recommended; >2 years, if risk warranted: 1-2 mg/kg/day in divided doses; max 3-4 mg/kg/day or 150-200 mg/day, whichever is less; <14 years, ER cap not recommended
Cap: 25, 50 mg; *Susp:* 25 mg/5 ml (pineapple-coconut, mint; alcohol 1%); *Supp:* 50 mg; *ER Cap:* 75 mg ext-rel
Comment: *indomethacin* is indicated only for acute painful flares. Administer with food and/or antacids. Use lowest effective dose for shortest duration.

ORAL NSAIDs

See more **Oral NSAIDs** page 489

➤ *diclofenac sodium* (C)
Voltaren 50 mg bid-qid or 75 mg bid or 25 mg qid with an additional 25 mg at HS if necessary
Tab: 25, 50, 75 mg ent-coat
Voltaren XR 100 mg once daily; rarely, 100 mg bid may be used
Tab: 100 mg ext-rel

NSAID PLUS PPI

➤ *esomeprazole/naproxen* (C) 1 tab bid; use lowest effective dose for the shortest duration swallow whole; take at least 30 minutes before a meal
Pediatric: <18 years: not recommended
Vimovo *Tab: nap* 375 mg/*eso* 20 mg ext-rel; *nap* 500 mg/*eso* 20 mg ext-rel
Comment: **Vimovo** is indicated to improve signs/symptoms, and risk of gastric ulcer in patients at risk of developing NSAID-associated gastric ulcer.

COX-2 INHIBITORS

Comment: Cox-2 inhibitors are contraindicated with history of asthma, urticaria, and allergic-type reactions to *aspirin*, other NSAIDs, and sulfonamides, 3rd trimester of pregnancy, and coronary artery bypass graft (CABG) surgery.
➤ *celecoxib* (C)(G) 50-400 mg once daily-bid; max 800 mg/day
Pediatric: <18 years: not recommended
Celebrex *Cap:* 50, 100, 200, 400 mg
➤ *meloxicam* (C)(G) initially 7.5 mg once daily; max 15 mg once daily
Pediatric: <2 years: not recommended; ≥2 years: 0.125 mg/kg; max 7.5 mg once daily
Mobic *Tab:* 7.5, 15 mg; *Oral susp:* 7.5 mg/5 ml (100 ml) (raspberry)
Vivlodex *Cap:* 5, 10 mg

PHOSPHODIESTERASE 4 (PDE4) INHIBITOR

➤ *apremilast* (C) swallow whole; initial titration over 5 days; maintenance 30 mg bid; *Day 1:* 10 mg in AM; *Day 2:* 10 mg AM and 10 mg PM; *Day 3:* 10 mg AM and 20 mg PM; *Day 4:* 20 mg AM and 20 mg PM; *Day 5:* 20 mg AM and 30 mg PM; *Day 6 and ongoing:* 30 mg AM and 30 mg PM
Pediatric: <18 years: not established
Otezla *Tab:* 10, 20, 30 mg; *2-Week Starter Pack*

Comment: Register pregnant patients exposed to by calling 877-311-8972.

INTERLEUKIN-12/INTERLEUKIN-23 ANTAGONIST

▷ *ustekinumab* (B) inject SC; rotate sites; <100 kg: 45 mg once; then 4 weeks later; then every 12 weeks; ≥100 kg: 90 mg once; then 4 weeks later; then every 12 weeks
Pediatric: <18 years: not recommended
   Stelara *Vial:* 45 mg/0.5 ml single-use (preservative-free)
   Comment: **Stelara** may be used as monotherapy or in combination with *methohtrexate* (MTX).

TUMOR NECROSIS FACTOR (TNF) BLOCKERS

▷ *adalimumab* (B) 40 mg SC once every other week; may increase to once weekly without *methotrexate* (MTX); administer in abdomen or thigh; rotate sites; 2-17 years, supervise first dose
Pediatric: <2 years: not recommended; 10-<15 kg: 10 mg every other week; 15-<30 kg: 20 mg every other week; 30 kg: 40 mg every other week
   Humira *Prefilled syringe:* 20 mg/0.4 ml; 40 mg/0.8 ml single-dose (2/pck) (2, 6/ starter pck) (preservative-free)
   Comment: **Humira** may use with *methotrexate* (MTX), DMARDS, corticoids, salicylates, NSAIDs, or analgesics.
▷ *etanercept* (B) 25 mg SC twice weekly, 72-96 hours apart or 50 mg SC weekly; rotate sites
Pediatric: <4 years: not recommended; 4-17 years: 0.4 mg/kg SC twice weekly, 72-96 hours apart (max 25 mg/dose) or 0.8 mg/kg SC weekly (max 50 mg/dose)
   Enbrel *Vial:* 25 mg pwdr for SC injection after reconstitution (4/ carton w. supplies) (preservative-free; diluent contains benzyl alcohol); *Prefilled syringe:* 50 mg/ml (preservative-free); *SureClick*
      autoinjector: 50 mg/ml (preservative-free)
   Comment: *etanercept* reduces pain, morning stiffness, and swelling. May be administered in combination with *methotrexate*. Live vaccines should not be administered concurrently. Do not administer with active infection.
▷ *golimumab* (B) administer SC or IV infusion (in combination with *methotrexate* [MTX])
Pediatric: <18 years: not established
   Simponi 50 mg SC once monthly; rotate sites
      Prefilled syringe, SmartJect autoinjector: 50 mg/0.5 ml, single-use (preservative-free)
   Simponi Aria 2 mg/kg IV infusion week 0 and week 4; then every 8 weeks thereafter
      Vial: 50 mg/4 ml, single-use, soln for IV infusion after dilution (latex-free, preservative-free)
   Comment: Corticosteroids, nonbiologic DMARDs, and/or NSAIDs may be continued during treatment with *golimumab*.
▷ *infiximab* (B) administer SC or IV infusion (in combination with *methotrexate* [MTX]) administer by IV infusion over at least 2 hours; 5 mg/kg once weekly at weeks 0, 2, 6, and then every 8 weeks
Pediatric: <18 years: not established
   Remicade *Vial:* 100 mg pwdr for reconstitution and dilution; (preservative-free)

PULMONARY ARTERIAL HYPERTENSION (PAH) (WHO GROUP I)

PROSTACYCLIN RECEPTOR AGONIST

▶ *selexipag* (X) initially 200 mcg bid; increase by 200 mcg bid to highest tolerated dose up to 1600 mcg bid; *Moderate hepatic impairment (Child-Pugh B):* initially 200 mcg once daily; increase by 200 mcg once daily at weekly intervals as tolerated; swallow whole; may take with food to improve tolerability
Pediatric: not established

> **Uptravi**
> *Tab:* 200, 400, 600, 800, 1000, 1200, 1400, 1600 mcg; *Titration pck:* 140 x 200 mcg + 60 x 800 mcg)
> **Comment:** Discontinue **Uptravi** if pulmonary veno-occlusive disease is confirmed <u>or</u> severe hepatic impairment (Child-Pugh C). May be potentiated by concomitant strong CYP2C8 inhibitors (e.g., gemfibrozil); *Nursing mothers:* not recommended. Discontinue breastfeeding <u>or</u> discontinue the drug.

GUANYLATE CYCLASE STIMULATOR

▶ *riociguat* (X) initially 0.5-1 mg tid; titrate every 2 weeks as tolerated (SBP ≥95 and absence of hypotensive symptoms) to highest tolerated dose; max 2.5 mg tid
Pediatric: not recommended

> **Adempas**
> *Tab:* 0.5, 1, 1.5, 2, 2.5 mg
> **Comment:** If **Adempas** is interrupted for ≥3 days, re-titrate. Consider titrating to dosage higher than 2.5 mg tid, if tolerated, in patients who smoke. Consider a starting dose of 0.5 mg tid when initiating **Adempas** in patients receiving strong cytochrome P450 (CYP) and P-glycoprotein/ breast cancer resistance protein (P-gp/BCRP) inhibitors such as azole antimycotics (e.g., *ketoconazole*, *itraconazole*) <u>or</u> HIV protease inhibitors (e.g., *ritonavir*). Monitor for signs and symptoms of hypotension with strong CYP and P-gp/ BCRP inhibitors. Obtain pregnancy tests prior to initiation and monthly during treatment. **Adempas** has consistently shown to have teratogenic effects when administered to animals. Females can only receive **Adempas** through the Adempas Risk Evaluation and Mitigation Strategy (REMS) Program, a restricted distribution program: **www .AdempasREMS.com** <u>or</u> **855-4 ADEMPAS**. It is not known if **Adempas** is present in human milk; however, *riociguat* <u>or</u> its metabolites were present in the milk of rats. Because of the potential for serious adverse reactions in nursing infants from *riociguat*, discontinue nursing <u>or</u> **Adempas**. In placebo-controlled clinical trials, serious bleeding has occurred (including hemoptysis, hematemesis, vaginal hemorrhage, catheter site hemorrhage, subdural hematoma, and intra-abdominal hemorrhage). Safety and efficacy have not been demonstrated in patients with creatinine clearance <15 mL/min <u>or</u> on dialysis <u>or</u> severe hepatic impairment (Child-Pugh C).
> Endothelin Receptor Antagonist, Selective for the Endothelin Type-A (ETA) Receptor

▶ *ambrisentan* (X) 20 mg once daily; at 4-week intervals, either the dose of **Letairis Le-taris** initially 5 mg once daily, with <u>or</u> without <u>or</u> **tadalafil** can be increased, as needed and tolerated, to **Letairis** 10 mg <u>or</u> *tadalafil* 40 mg; do not split, crush, <u>or</u> chew.

Pediatric: not recommended
Letairis
  Tab: 5, 10 mg *film-coat*
  Comment: In patients with PAH, plasma ET-1 concentrations are increased
  as much as 10-fold and correlate with increased mean right atrial pressure
  and disease severity. ET-1 and ET-1 mRNA concentrations are increased
  as much as 9-fold in the lung tissue of patients with PAH, primarily in the
  endothelium of pulmonary arteries. These findings suggest that ET-1 may play
  a critical role in the pathogenesis and progression of PAH. When taken with
  tadalafil, **Letairis** is indicated to reduce the risk of disease progression and
  hospitalization, to reduce the risk of hospitalization due to worsening PAH,
  and to improve exercise tolerance. **Letaris** is contraindicated in idiopathic
  pulmonary fibrosis (IPF). Exclude pregnancy before the initiation of treatment
  with **Letairis.** Females of reproductive potential must use acceptable methods
  of contraception during treatment with **Letairis** and for one month after
  treatment. Obtain monthly pregnancy tests during treatment and 1 month after
  discontinuation of treatment. Females can only receive **Letairis** through the
  Letairis Risk Evaluation and Mitigation Strategy (REMS) Program, a restricted
  distribution program, because of the risk of embryo-fetal toxicity: **www.
  Letairisrems.com** or 1-866-664-5327.

PHOSPHODIESTERASE TYPE 5 (PDE5) INHIBITORS, CGMP-SPECIFIC DRUGS

▷ *sildenafil citrate* (B) *Orally:* initially 5 or 20 mg tid, 4-6 hours apart; max 20 mg tid;
  IV bolus: 2.5 mg or 10 mg bolus injection tid, 4-6 hours apart; max 10 mg tid; the
  dose does not need to be adjusted for body weight.
  Pediatric: not recommended
  Revatio
    Tab: 20 mg film-coat; *Oral susp:* 10 mg/ml pwdr for reconstitution (1.12 g,
    112 ml) (grape) (sorbitol); *Vial:* 10 mg/12.5 ml (0.8 mg/ml)
    Comment: A 10 mg IV dose is predicted to provide pharmacological effect
    equivalent to the 20 mg oral dose. **Revatio** is contraindicated with concomitant
    nitrate drugs including *nitroglycerin, isosorbide dinitrate,* isosorbide
    mononitrate, and some recreational drugs such as "poppers." Taking **Revatio**
    with a nitrate can cause a sudden and serious decrease in blood pressure. **Revatio**
    is contraindicated with concomitant guanylate cyclase stimulator drugs such as
    riociguat (**Adempas**). Avoid the use of grapefruit products while taking **Revatio.**
    Stop **Revatio** and get emergency medical help if sudden vision loss. **Revatio**
    is contraindicated with other phosphodiesterase type 5 (PDE5) Inhibitors,
    cGMP-specific drugs such as *avanafil* (**Stendra**), *tadalafil* (**Cialis**) or *vardenafil*
    (**Levitra**). Caution with history of recent MI, stroke, life-threatening arrhythmia,
    hypotension, hypertension, cardiac failure, unstable angina, retinitis pigmentosa,
    CYP3A4 inhibitors (e.g., *cimetidine,* the azoles, *erythromycin,* protease inhibitors
    (e.g., *ritonavir*), CYP3A4 inducers (e.g., *rifampin, carbamazepine, phenytoin,
    phenobarbital*), alcohol, antihypertensive agents. Side effects include headache,
    flushing, nasal congestion, rhinitis, dyspepsia, and diarrhea. Use **Revatio** with
    caution in patients with anatomical deformation of the penis (e.g., angulation,
    cavernosal fibrosis, or Peyronie's disease) or in patients who have conditions,
    which may predispose them to priapism (e.g., sickle cell anemia, multiple
    myeloma, or leukemia). In the event of an erection that persists longer than 4

hours, the patient should seek immediate medical assistance. If priapism (painful erection greater than 6 hours in duration) is not treated immediately, penile tissue damage and permanent loss of potency could result.

➤ *tadalafil* (B) 40mg once daily; *CrCl 31-80 mL/min:* initially 20 mg once daily; increase to 40mg once daily if tolerated; *CrCl <30 mL/min:* not recommended; *Mild* or *moderate hepatic cirrhosis (Child Pugh Class A* or *B):* initially 20 mg once daily. *Severe hepatic cirrhosis (Child Pugh Class C):* not recommended; *use with* **ritonavir**; *Receiving ritonavir for at least 1 week:* initiate *tadalafil* at 20 mg once daily; may increase to 40mg once daily if tolerated; *Already on tadalafil:* stop *tadalafil* at least 24 hours prior to initiating **ritonavir**; resume *tadalafil* at 20 mg once daily after at least 1 week; may increase to 40mg once daily if tolerated
Pediatric: not established
    Adcirca
Comment: Contraindicated with concomitant organic nitrates and guanylate cyclase stimulators (e.g., *riociguat*).

➤ *treprostinil* (B) swallow whole; take with food
    Orenitram
      Tab: 0.125, 0.25, 1, 2.5 mg ext-rel
    Comment: **Orenitram** is indicated to improve exercise capacity. It is contraindicated with severe hepatic impairment (Child-Pugh C). **Orenitram** inhibits platelet aggregation and increases the risk of bleeding. Concomitant administration of **Orenitram** with diuretics, antihypertensive agents or other vasodilators increases the risk of symptomatic hypotension.

⬤ PYELONEPHRITIS: ACUTE

URINARY TRACT ANALGESIA

➤ *phenazopyridine* (B)(G) 95-200 mg q 6 hours prn; max 2 days
Pediatric: not recommended
    AZO Standard, Prodium, Uristat (OTC) *Tab:* 95 mg
    AZO Standard Maximum Strength (OTC) *Tab:* 97.5 mg
    Pyridium, Urogesic *Tab:* 100, 200 mg

OUTPATIENT ANTI-INFECTIVE TREATMENT

Comment: Acute pyelonephritis can be treated with a single IM antibiotic administration followed by a PO antibiotic regimen and close follow up. Example: **Rocephin** 1 g IM followed by **Bactrim DS**, *cephalexin*, *ciprofloxacin*, *levofloxacin*, or *loracarbef*.

➤ *cephalexin* (B)(G) 1-4 g/day in 4 divided doses x 10-14 days
Pediatric: 25-50 mg/kg/day in 4 divided doses x 10-14 days; *see page 557 for dose by weight*
    Keflex *Cap:* 250, 333, 500, 750 mg; *Oral susp:* 125, 250 mg/5 ml (100, 200 ml) (strawberry)

➤ *ciprofloxacin* (C) 500 mg bid or 1000 mg XR once daily x 3-14 days
Pediatric: <18 years: not recommended
    Cipro (G) *Tab:* 250, 500, 750 mg; *Oral susp:* 250, 500 mg/5 ml (100 ml) (strawberry)
    Cipro XR *Tab:* 500, 1000 mg ext-rel
    ProQuin XR *Tab:* 500 mg ext-rel

Comment: *ciprofloxacin* is contraindicated <18 years-of-age, and during pregnancy and lactation. Risk of tendonitis or tendon rupture, especially 60 years-of-age and older.

▶ *levofloxacin* (C) *Uncomplicated:* 500 mg once daily x 10 days; *Complicated:* 750 mg once daily x 10 days

Pediatric: <18 years: not recommended

    Levaquin *Tab:* 250, 500, 750 mg; *Oral soln:* 25 mg/ml (480 ml) (benzyl alcohol); *Inj conc:* 25 mg/ml for IV infusion after dilution for IV infusion (50, 100, 150 ml) (preservative-free)

Comment: *levofloxacin* is contraindicated <18 years-of-age, and during pregnancy and lactation. Risk of tendonitis or tendon rupture, especially 60 years-of-age and older.

▶ *loracarbef* (B) 400 mg bid x 14 days

Pediatric: 15 mg/kg/day in 2 divided doses x 14 days; *see page 570 for dose by weight*

    Lorabid *Pulvule:* 200, 400 mg; *Oral susp:* 100 mg/5 ml (50, 100 ml); 200 mg/5 ml (50, 75, 100 ml) (strawberry bubble gum)

▶ *trimethoprim/sulfamethoxazole* (D)(G) bid x 10 days

Pediatric: <2 months: not recommended; ≥2 months: 40 mg/kg/day of *sulfamethoxazole* in 2 divided doses x 10 days; *see page 576 for dose by weight*

    Bactrim, Septra 2 tabs bid x 10 days
       Tab: trim 80 mg/*sulfa* 400 mg*
    Bactrim DS, Septra DS 1 tab bid x 10 days
       Tab: trim 160 mg/*sulfa* 800 mg*
    Bactrim Pediatric Suspension, Septra Pediatric Suspension
       Oral susp: trim 40 mg/*sulfa* 200 mg per 5 ml (100 ml) (cherry) (alcohol 0.3%)

Comment: *trimethoprim/sulfamethoxazole* is not recommended in pregnancy or lactation. *CrCl 15-30 mL/min:* reduce dose by 1/2; *CrCl <15 mL/min:* not recommended

RABIES

PRE-EXPOSURE PROPHYLAXIS

Comment: Postpone pre-exposure prophylaxis during acute febrile illness or infection. Have *epinephrine* 1:1000 readily available.

▶ *rabies immune globulin, human (HRIG)* (C) 3 injections of 1 ml IM each on day 0, 7, and either day 21 or 28; booster doses 1 ml IM every 2 years

Pediatric: same as adult (except for infants administer in the vastus lateralis muscle)

    Imovax *Vial:* 2.5 u/ml (1 ml, single dose)

POSTEXPOSURE PROPHYLAXIS

Comment: Have *epinephrine* 1:1000 readily available.

▶ *rabies immune globulin, human (HRIG)* (C) 20 IU/kg infiltrated into wound area as much as feasible, then remaining dose administered IM at site remote from vaccine administration

Pediatric: same as adult

    BayRab, Imogam Rabies *Vial:* 150 IU/ml (2, 10 ml)

▷ *rabies vaccine, human diploid cell* (C) *Not previously immunized:* administer first dose 1 ml in the deltoid as soon as possible after exposure; then repeat on days 3, 7, 14, 28 *or* 30, and 90; administer 1st dose with rabies immune globulin; *Previously immunized:* only 2 doses are administered, immediately after exposure and again 3 days later; no rabies immune globulin is needed.
Pediatric: same as adult (except for infants administer in vastus lateralis muscle)
    Imovax, RabAvert *Vial:* 2.5 IU/ml (2.5 IU of freeze-dried vaccine w. diluent)

TETANUS PROPHYLAXIS

see *Tetanus* page 398 for patients not previously immunized

RESPIRATORY SYNCYTIAL VIRUS (RSV)

PROPHYLAXIS

▷ *palivizumab* 15 mg/kg IM administered monthly throughout the RSV season
    Synagis *Vial:* 100 mg/ml
    Treatment see *Bronchiolitis* page 58

RESTLESS LEGS SYNDROME (RLS)

GAMMA AMINOBUTYRIC ACID ANALOGS

▷ *gabapentin* (C)(G) 100 mg once daily x 1 day; then 100 mg bid x 1 day; then 100 mg tid thereafter; max 900 mg tid
Pediatric: not recommended
    Gralise (C) initially 300 mg on Day 1; then 600 mg on Day 2; then 900 mg on Days 3-6; then 1200 mg on Days 7-10; then 1500 mg on Days 11-14; titrate up to 1800 mg on Day 15; take entire dose once daily with the evening meal; do not crush, split, *or* chew
    Tab: 300, 600 mg
    Neurontin (G) 100 mg daily x 1 day, then 100 mg bid x 1 day, then 100 mg tid continuously; max 900 mg tid
    Pediatric: <3 years: not recommended; 3-12 years: initially 10-15 mg/kg/day in 3 divided doses; max 12 hours between doses; titrate over 3 days; 3-4 years: titrate to 40 mg/kg/day; 5-12 years: titrate to 25-35 mg/kg/day; max 50 mg/kg/day;
▷ *gabapentin enacarbil* (C) 600 mg once daily at about 5:00 PM; if dose not taken at recommended time, next dose should be taken the following day; swallow whole; take with food; *CrCl 30-59 mL/min:* 600 mg on Day 1, Day 3, and every day thereafter; *CrCl <30 mL/min or* on hemodialysis: not recommended
Pediatric: not recommended
    Horizant *Tab:* 600 ext-rel
Comment: Avoid abrupt cessation of *gabapentin* and *gabapentin enacarbil*. To discontinue, withdraw gradually over 1 week *or* longer.

DOPAMINE RECEPTOR AGONISTS

▷ *pramipexole dihydrochloride* (C) initially 0.125 mg once daily 2-3 hours before bedtime; may double dose every 4-7 days; max 0.75 mg/day

Pediatric: not recommended

> **Mirapex** *Tab:* 0.125, 0.25*, 0.5*, 0.75*, 1*, 1.5* mg

▷ *ropinirole* (C) take once daily 1-3 hours prior to bedtime; initially 0.25 mg on days 1 and 2; then 0.5 mg on days 3-7; increase by 0.5 mg/day at 1 week intervals to 3 mg; max 4 mg/day

Pediatric: not recommended

> **Requip** *Tab:* 0.25, 0.5, 1, 2, 3, 4, 5 mg

▷ *rotigotine* transdermal patch (C) apply to clean, dry, intact skin on abdomen, thigh, hip, flank, shoulder, or upper arm; initially 1mg/24 hour patch once daily; may increase weekly by 1mg/24 hour if needed; max 3mg/24 hour once daily; rotate sites and allow 14 days before reusing site; if hairy, shave site at least 3 days before application to site; avoid abrupt cessation; reduce by 1 mg/24 hour every other day

Pediatric: not recommended

> **Neupro** *Trans patch:* 1mg/24hrs, 2mg/24hrs, 3mg/24hrs, 4mg/24 hrs, 6mg/24hrs, 8mg/24hrs (30/carton) (sulfites)

◯ RETINITIS: CYTOMEGALOVIRUS (CMV)

Comment: *cidofovir and valganciclovir* are nucleoside analogues and prodrugs of *ganciclovir* indicated for the treatment of AIDS-related *cytomegalovirus* (CMV) retinitis and prevention of CMV disease in adult kidney, heart, and kidney-pancreas transplant patients at high risk, and for prevention of CMV disease in pediatric kidney and heart transplant patients at high risk.

▷ *cidofovir* (C) administer via IV infusion over 1 hour; pre-treat with oral *probenecid* (2 g, 3 hours prior to starting the *cidofovir* infusion and 1 g, 2 and 8 hours after the infusion is ended) and 1 liter of IV NaCl should be infused immediately before each dose of *cidofovir* (a 2nd liter of NaCl should also be infused either during or after each dose of *cidofovir* if a fluid load is tolerable); *Induction:* 5 mg/kg once weekly for 2 consecutive weeks; *Maintenance:* 5 mg/kg once every 2 weeks; reduce to 3 mg/kg if serum Cr increases 0.3-0.4 mg/dL above baseline; discontinue if serum Cr increases to >0.5 mg/dL above baseline or if >3+ proteinuria develops

Pediatric: not recommended

> **Vistide** *Vial:* 75 mg/ml (5 ml) (preservative-free)

Comment: *cidofovir* is a nucleoside analogue indicated for treatment of AIDS-related *cytomegalovirus* (CMV) retinitis.

▷ *valganciclovir* (C)(G) take with food; *Induction:* 900 mg bid x 21 days; *Maintenance:* 900 mg daily; *CrCl <60 mL/min:* reduce dose (see mfr literature; hemodialysis or *CrCl <10 mL/min* not recommended (use *ganciclovir*)

Pediatric: <4 months: not recommended; 4 months-16 years: see mfr literature for dosing calculation equation

> **Valcyte** *Tab:* 450 mg (preservative-free); *Oral pwdr for reconstitution:* 50 mg/ml (tutti-frutti)

◯ RHEUMATOID ARTHRITIS (RA)

Injectable Acetaminophen *see Pain page 296*
Oral Prescription NSAIDs *see page 489*
Other Oral Analgesics *see Pain page 298*

Topical/Transdermal NSAIDs *see* **Pain** *page* 297
Parenteral Glucocorticosteroids *see page* 499
Oral Glucocorticosteroids *see page* 497
Topical Analgesic and Anesthetic Agents *see page* 487

TOPICAL ANALGESICS

▷ *capsaicin* (B)(G) apply tid-qid prn to intact skin
  Pediatric: <2 years: not recommended; ≥2 years: same as adult
    Axsain *Crm:* 0.075% (1, 2 oz)
    Capsin *Lotn:* 0.025, 0.075% (59 ml)
    Capzasin-P (OTC) *Crm:* 0.025% (1.5 oz); *Lotn:* 0.025% (2 oz)
    Dolorac *Crm:* 0.025% (28 g)
    Double Cap (OTC) *Crm:* 0.05% (2 oz)
    R-Gel *Gel:* 0.025% (15, 30 g)
    Zostrix (OTC) *Crm:* 0.025% (0.7, 1.5, 3 oz)
    Zostrix HP (OTC) *Emol crm:* 0.075% (1, 2 oz)
▷ *trolamine salicylate* (NR)
    Mobisyl apply tid-qid
      Crm: 10%
  Comment: Provides some relief by 1-2 weeks; optimal benefit may take 4-6 weeks.

ORAL SALICYLATE

▷ *indomethacin* (C) initially 25 mg bid-tid, increase as needed at weekly intervals by
  25-50 mg/day; max 200 mg/day
  Pediatric: <14 years: usually not recommended; >2 years, if risk warranted: 1-2 mg/
  kg/day in divided doses; max 3-4 mg/kg/day (<u>or</u> 150-200 mg/day, whichever is less;
  <14 years, ER cap not recommended
  Cap: 25, 50 mg; *Susp;* 25 mg/5 ml (pineapple-coconut, mint; alcohol 1%); *Supp:*
  50 mg; *ER Cap:* 75 mg ext-rel
  Comment: *indomethacin* is indicated only for acute painful flares. Administer with
  food <u>and/or</u> antacids. Use lowest effective dose for shortest duration.

NSAID

See more Oral NSAIDs *page* 489

▷ *diclofenac sodium* (C)(G)
    Voltaren 50 mg bid-qid <u>or</u> 75 mg bid <u>or</u> 25 mg qid with an additional 25 mg at
    HS if necessary
      Tab: 25, 50, 75 mg ent-coat
    Voltaren XR 100 mg once daily; rarely, 100 mg bid may be used
      Tab: 100 mg ext-rel

NSAID PLUS PPI

▷ *esomeprazole/naproxen* (C) 1 tab bid; use lowest effective dose for the shortest duration swallow whole; take at least 30 minutes before a meal
  Pediatric: <18 years: not recommended
    Vimovo *Tab: nap* 375 mg/*eso* 20 mg ext-rel; *nap* 500 mg/*eso* 20 mg ext-rel

Comment: Vimovo is indicated to improve signs/symptoms, and risk of gastric ulcer in patients at risk of developing NSAID-associated gastric ulcer.

COX-2 INHIBITORS

Comment: Cox-2 inhibitors are contraindicated with history of asthma, urticaria, and allergic-type reactions to *aspirin*, other NSAIDs, and sulfonamides, 3rd trimester of pregnancy, and coronary artery bypass graft (CABG) surgery.

▷ celecoxib (C)(G) 50-400 mg once daily-bid; max 800 mg/day
  Pediatric: <18 years: not recommended
    Celebrex Cap: 50, 100, 200, 400 mg
▷ meloxicam (C)(G) initially 7.5 mg once daily; max 15 mg once daily
  Pediatric: <2 years: not recommended; ≥2 years: 0.125 mg/kg; max 7.5 mg once daily
    Mobic Tab: 7.5, 15 mg; Oral susp: 7.5 mg/5 ml (100 ml) (raspberry)
    Vivlodex Cap: 5, 10 mg

JANUS KINASE (JAK) INHIBITOR

▷ tofacitinib (C) 5 mg twice daily; reduce to 5 mg once daily for moderate-to-severe renal impairment <u>or</u> moderate hepatic impairment, concomitant potent CYP3A4 inhibitors, <u>or</u> drugs that result in both CYP3A4 and potent CYP2C19 inhibition
  Pediatric: not established
    Xeljanz Tab: 5 mg
    Xeljanz XR Tab: 11 mg ext-rel
    Comment: Xeljanz is indicated for moderate-to-severe RA as monotherapy in patients who have inadequate response <u>or</u> intolerance to *methotrexate* (MTX) <u>and/or</u> in combination with other non-biologic DMARDs.

DISEASE MODIFYING ANTI-RHEUMATIC DRUGS (DMARDs)

Comment: DMARDs are first-line treatment options for RA. DMARDs include penicillamine, gold salts (*auranofin, aurothio-glucose*), immunosuppressants, and *hydroxychloroquine*. The DMARDs reduce ESR, reduce RF, and favorably affect the outcome of RA. Immunosuppressants may require 6 weeks to affect benefits and 6 months for full improvement.

▷ auranofin (gold salt) (C) 3 mg bid <u>or</u> 6 mg once daily; if inadequate response after 6 months, increase to 3 mg tid
  Pediatric: not recommended
    Ridaura Vial: 100 mg/20 ml
▷ azathioprine (D) 1 mg/kg/day in a single <u>or</u> divided doses; may increase by 0.5 mg/kg/day q 4 weeks; max 2.5 mg/kg/day; minimum trial to ascertain effectiveness is 12 weeks
  Pediatric: not recommended
    Azasan Tab 75*, 100*mg
    Imuran Tab 50*mg
▷ cyclosporine (immunosuppressant) (C) 1.25 mg/kg bid; may increase after 4 weeks by 0.5 mg/kg/day; then adjust at 2 week intervals; max 4 mg/kg/day; administer with meals
  Pediatric: not recommended
    Neoral Cap: 25, 100 mg (alcohol)

Neoral Oral Solution *Oral soln:* 100 mg/ml (50 ml) may dilute in room temperature apple juice or orange juice (alcohol)

Comment: **Neoral** is indicated for RA unresponsive to *methotrexate* (MTX).

▷ *hydroxychloroquine* (C) 400-600 mg/day
Pediatric: not recommended
  Plaquenil *Tab:* 200 mg
  Comment: May require several weeks to achieve beneficial effects. If no improvement in 6 months, discontinue.

▷ *leflunomide* (X)(G) initially 100 mg once daily x 3 days; maintenance dose 20 mg once daily; max 20 mg daily
Pediatric: <18 years: not recommended
  Arava *Tab:* 10, 20, 100 mg
  Comment: **Arava** is contraindicated with breastfeeding.

▷ *methotrexate* (X) 7.5 mg x 1 dose per week or 2.5 mg x 3 at 12 hour intervals once a week; max 20 mg/week; therapeutic response begins in 3-6 weeks; administer *methotrexate* injection SC only into the abdomen or thigh
Pediatric: <2 years: not recommended; ≥2 years: 10 mg/m^2 once weekly; max 20 mg/m^2
  Rasuvo *Autoinjector:* 7.5 mg/0.15 ml, 10 mg/0.20 ml, 12.5 mg/ 0.25 ml, 15 mg/0.30 ml, 17.5 mg/0.35 ml, 20 mg/0.40 ml, 22.5 mg/0.45 ml, 25 mg/0.50 ml, 27.5 mg/0.55 ml, 30 mg/0.60 ml (solution concentration for SC injection is 50 mg/ml)
  Rheumatrex *Tab:* 2.5*mg (5, 7.5, 10, 12.5, 15 mg/week, 4/card unit-of-use dose pack)
  Trexall *Tab:* 5*, 7.5*, 10*, 15*mg (5, 7.5, 10, 12.5, 15 mg/week, 4/card unit-of-use dose pack)
  Comment: *methotrexate* (MTX) is contraindicated with immunodeficiency, blood dyscrasias, alcoholism, and chronic liver disease.

▷ *penicillamine* (D) 125-250 mg once daily initially; may increase by 125-250 mg/day q 1-3 months; max 1.5 g/day
Pediatric: not recommended
  Cuprimine *Cap:* 125, 250 mg
  Depen *Tab:* 250 mg

▷ *sulfasalazine* (C; D in 2nd, 3rd)(G) initially 0.5 g once daily bid; gradually increase every 4 days; usual maintenance 2-3 g/day in equally divided doses at regular intervals; max 4 g/day
Pediatric: <6 years: not recommended; 6-16 years: initially 1/4 to 1/3 of maintenance dose; increase weekly; maintenance 30-50 mg/kg/day in 2 divided doses at regular intervals; max 2 g/day
  Azulfidine *Tab:* 500 mg
  Azulfidine EN *Tab:* 500 mg ent-coat

TUMOR NECROSIS FACTOR (TNF) BLOCKERS

▷ *adalimumab* (B) 40 mg SC once every other week; may increase to once weekly without *methotrexate* (MTX); administer in abdomen or thigh; rotate sites; 2-17 years, supervise first dose
Pediatric: <2 years, <10 kg: not recommended; 10-<15 kg: 10 mg every other week; 15-<30 kg: 20 mg every other week; ≥30 kg: 40 mg every other week

Humira *Prefilled syringe:* 20 mg/0.4 ml; 40 mg/0.8 ml single-dose (2/pck; 2, 6/ starter pck) (preservative-free)
Comment: **Humira** may use with *methotrexate* (MTX), DMARDs, corticosteroids, salicylates, NSAIDs, or analgesics.

➤ *certolizumab pegol* (B) 400 mg SC on day 1, at week 2, and at week 4; then 200 mg every other week; rotate sites
Pediatric: not recommended
Cimzia *Vial:* 200 mg single-dose w. supplies (2/pck, 2, 6/starter pck); *Prefilled syringe:* 200 mg single-dose w. supplies (2/pck, 2, 6/starter pck) (preservative-free)

➤ *etanercept* (B) 25 mg SC twice weekly, 72-96 hours apart or 50 mg SC weekly; rotate sites
Pediatric: <4 years: not recommended; 4-17 years: 0.4 mg/kg SC twice weekly, 72-96 hours apart (max 25 mg/dose) or 0.8 mg/kg SC weekly (max 50 mg/dose)
Enbrel *Vial:* 25 mg pwdr for SC injection after reconstitution (4/ carton w. supplies) (preservative-free; diluent contains benzyl alco hol); *Prefilled syringe:* 50 mg/ml (preservative-free); *SureClick autoinjector:* 50 mg/ml (preservative-free)
Comment: *etanercept* reduces pain, morning stiffness, and swelling. May be administered in combination with *methotrexate*. Live vaccines should not be administered concurrently. Do not administer with active infection.

➤ *golimumab* (B) administer SC or IV infusion (in combination with *methotrexate* [MTX])
Pediatric: <18 years: not established
Simponi 50 mg SC once monthly; rotate sites
Prefilled syringe, SmartJect autoinjector: 50 mg/0.5 ml, single-use (preservative-free)
Simponi Aria 2 mg/kg IV infusion week 0 and week 4; then every 8 weeks thereafter
Vial: 50 mg/4 ml, single-use, soln for IV infusion after dilution (latex-free, preservative-free)
Comment: corticosteroids, non-biologic DMARDs, and/or NSAIDs may be continued during treatment with *golimumab*.

➤ *infliximab* (B) administer SC or IV infusion (in combination with *methotrexate* [MTX]) administer by IV infusion over at least 2 hours; 3 mg/kg once weekly at weeks 0, 2, 6, and then every 8 weeks; may increase to 10 mg/kg or *administer* every 4 weeks
Pediatric: <18 years: not established
Remicade *Vial:* 100 mg pwdr for reconstitution and dilution; (preservative-free)
Comment: Use *infliximab* concomitantly with *methotrexate* when there has been insufficient response to *methotrexate* alone.

Interleukin-1 Receptor Antagonist

➤ *anakinra (interleukin-1 receptor antagonist)* (B) 100 mg SC once daily; discard any unused portion
Pediatric: not recommended
Kineret *Prefilled syringe:* 100 mg/single-dose syringe (7, 28/pk) (preservative-free)

Interleukin-6 Receptor Antagonist

➤ *tocilizumab* (B) administer as an IV infusion over 60 minutes once every 4 weeks; initially 4 mg/kg; may increase to 8 mg/kg based on clinical response

Pediatric: not recommended
> **Actemra** *Vial:* 80 mg/4 ml, 200 mg/10 ml, 400 mg/20 ml for IV infusion after dilution

Selective Costimulation Modulator

▷ *abatacept* (C) administer as an IV infusion over 30 minutes at weeks 0, 2, and 4; then every 4 weeks thereafter; <60 kg, administer 500 mg/ dose; 60-100 kg, administer 750 mg/dose; >100 kg, administer 1 g/dose; 60-100 kg, administer 750 mg/dose; >100 kg, administer 1 g/dose
Pediatric: <6 years: not recommended; 6-17 years: administer as an IV infusion over 30 minutes at weeks 0, 2, and 4; then every 4 weeks thereafter; <75 kg, administer 10 mg/kg; same as adult (max 1 g)
> **Orencia** *Vial:* 250 mg pwdr for IV infusion after reconstitution (silicone-free) (preservative-free); *Prefilled syringe:* 125 mg/ml soln for SC injection (preservative-free)

CD20 ANTIBODY

▷ *rituximab* (C) administer glucocorticoid 30 minutes prior to each infusion; concomitant *methotrexate* therapy, administer a 1000 mg IV infusion at 0 and 2 weeks; then every 24 weeks <u>or</u> based on response, but not sooner than every 16 weeks.
Pediatric: <6 years: not recommended; >6 years: same as adult
> **Rituxan** *Vial:* 10 mg/ml (10, 50 ml) (preservative-free)

INTRA-ARTICULAR INJECTION

▷ *sodium hyaluronate* 20 mg as intra-articular injection weekly x 5 weeks
Pediatric: not recommended
> **Hyalgan** *Prefilled syringe:* 20 mg/2 ml
> **Comment:** Remove joint effusion and inject with *lidocaine* if possible before injecting **Hyalgan**.

 RHINITIS/SINUSITIS: ALLERGIC

Oral Prescription Drugs for the Management of Allergy, Cough, and Cold Symptoms
see page 524
Parenteral Corticosteroids *see page 499*
Oral Corticosteroids *see page 497*

ALLERGEN EXTRACTS

Comment: Allergen extracts (**Grastek, Oralair, Ragwitek**) are not for immediate relief of allergic symptoms. Contraindicated with severe, unstable, and uncontrolled asthma, history of eosinophilic esophagitis, and severe local <u>or</u> systemic reaction. First dose under supervision HCP and observe ≥30 minutes. Subsequent doses may be taken at home.
▷ *short ragweed pollen allergen extract* (C) one SL tab once daily
Pediatric: <18 years: not established
> **Ragwitek** *SL tab:* Amerosia artemisiifolia 12 amb a 1-unit (30, 90/blister pck)

Comment: Initiate **Ragwitek** at least 12 weeks before onset of ragweed pollen season and continue throughout season.

▷ *sweet vernal, orchard, perennial rye, timothy, Kentucky blue grass mixed pollen allergen extract* (C) 300 IR once daily
  Pediatric: <10 years: not established; 10-17 years: Day 1: 100 IR; Day 2: 200 IR; Day 3 and thereafter: 300 IR once daily
  Oralair *SL tab:* 100, 300 IR (index of reactivity) (30/blister pck)
  Comment: **Oralair** is indicated for grass pollen-induced allergic rhinitis with or without conjunctivitis confirmed by positive skin test. Initiate **Orlair** at least 4 months before onset of grass pollen season and continue throughout season.

▷ *timothy grass pollen allergen extract* (C) one SL tab once daily
  Pediatric: <5 years: not established; ≥5 years: same as adult
  Grastek *SL tab:* 2800 bioequivalent allergy units (BAUS) (30/blister pck)
  Comment: **Grastek** is indicated for grass pollen-induced allergic rhinitis with or without conjunctivitis confirmed by positive skin test. Initiate **Grastek** at least 12 weeks before onset of grass pollen season and continue throughout season.

NASAL DECONGESTANT

▷ *tetrahydrozoline* (C)
  Tyzine 2-4 drops or 3-4 sprays in each nostril q 3-8 hours prn
    Pediatric: <6 years: not recommended; ≥6 years: same as adult
    Nasal spray: 0.1% (15 ml); *Nasal drops:* 0.1% (30 ml)
  Tyzine Pediatric Nasal Drops 2-3 sprays or drops in each nostril q 3-6 hours prn
    Nasal drops: 0.05% (15 ml)

LEUKOTRIENE RECEPTOR ANTAGONISTS

Comment: For prophylaxis and chronic treatment only. Not for primary (rescue) treatment of acute asthma attack.

▷ *montelukast* (B)(G) 10 mg once daily in the PM; for EIB, take at least 2 hours before exercise; max 1 dose/day
  Pediatric: <12 months: not recommended; 12-23 months: one 4 mg granule pkt daily; 2-5 years: one 4 mg chew tab or granule pkt daily; 6-14 years: one 5 mg chew tab daily daily; >15 years: same as adult
    Singulair *Tab:* 10 mg
    Singulair Chewable *Chew tab:* 4, 5 mg (cherry, phenylalanine)
    Singulair Oral Granules: 4 mg/pkt; take within 15 minutes of opening pkt; may mix with applesauce, carrots, rice, or ice cream

▷ *zafirlukast* (B)(G) 20 mg bid, 1 hour ac or 2 hours pc
  Pediatric: <7 years: not recommended; 7-11 years: 10 mg bid 1 hour ac or 2 hours pc; >11 years: same as adult
    Accolate *Tab:* 10, 20 mg

▷ *zileuton* (C) 1 tab qid
  Pediatric: <12 years: not recommended; ≥12 years: same as adult
    Zyflo *Tab:* 600 mg

NASAL GLUCOCORTICOSTEROIDS

▷ *beclomethasone dipropionate* (C)

Beconase 1 spray in each nostril bid-qid
Pediatric: <6 years: not recommended; 6-12 years: 1 spray in each nostril tid; >12 years: same as adult
Nasal spray: 42 mcg/actuation (6.7 g, 80 sprays; 16.8 g, 200 sprays)
Beconase AQ 1-2 sprays in each nostril bid
Pediatric: <6: not recommended; ≥6 years: same as adult
Nasal spray: 42 mcg/actuation (25 g, 180 sprays)
Beconase Inhalation Aerosol 1-2 sprays in each nostril bid to qid
Pediatric: <6: not recommended; 6-12 years: 1 spray in each nostril tid; >12 years: same as adult
Nasal spray: 42 mcg/actuation (6.7 g, 80 sprays; 16.8 g, 200 sprays)
Vancenase AQ 1-2 sprays in each nostril bid
Pediatric: <6 years: not recommended; ≥6 years: same as adult
Nasal spray: 84 mcg/actuation (25 g, 200 sprays)
Vancenase AQ DS 1-2 sprays in each nostril once daily
Pediatric: <6 years: not recommended; ≥6 years: same as adult
Nasal spray: 84, 168 mcg/actuation (19 g, 120 sprays)
Vancenase Pockethaler 1 spray in each nostril bid <u>or</u> qid
Pediatric: <6: not recommended; ≥6 years: 1 spray in each nostril tid
Pockethaler: 42 mcg/actuation (7 g, 200 sprays)
QNASL Nasal Aerosol 2 sprays, 80 mcg/spray, in each nostril once daily
Pediatric: <12 years: 2 sprays, 40 mcg/spray, in each nostril once daily; ≥12 years: same as adult
Nasal spray: 40 mcg/actuation (4.9 g, 60 sprays); 80 mcg/actuation (8.7 g, 120 sprays)

▷ *budesonide* (C)
Rhinocort initially 2 sprays in each nostril bid in the AM and PM, <u>or</u> 4 sprays in each nostril in the AM; max 4 sprays each nostril/day; use lowest effective dose
Pediatric: <6 years: not recommended; >6 years: same as adult
Nasal spray: 32 mcg/actuation (7 g, 200 sprays)
Rhinocort Aqua Nasal Spray initially 1 spray in each nostril once daily; max 4 sprays in each nostril once daily
Pediatric: <6 years: not recommended; ≥6-12 years: initially 1 spray in each nostril once daily; max 2 sprays in each nostril once daily
Nasal spray: 32 mcg/actuation (10 ml, 60 sprays)

▷ *ciclesonide* (C)
Pediatric: <6 years: not recommended; ≥6 years: same as adult
Omnaris 2 sprays in each nostril once daily
Nasal spray: 50 mcg/actuation (12.5 g, 120 sprays)
Zetonna 1-2 sprays in each nostril once daily
Nasal spray: 37 mcg/actuation (6.1 g, 60 sprays) (HFA)

▷ *dexamethasone* (C) 2 sprays in each nostril bid-tid; max 12 sprays/day; maintain at lowest effective dose
Pediatric: <6 years: not recommended; ≥6-12 years: 1-2 sprays in each nostril bid; max 8 sprays/day; maintain at lowest effective dose; >12 years: same as adult
Dexacort Turbinaire *Nasal spray:* 84 mcg/actuation (12.6 g, 170 sprays)

▷ *fluticasone furoate* (C) 2 sprays in each nostril once daily; may reduce to 1 spray each nostril once daily

Pediatric: <2 years: not recommended; ≥2-11 years: 1 spray in each nostril once daily; ≥12 years: same as adult
    Veramyst *Nasal spray:* 27.5 mcg/actuation (10 g, 120 sprays) (alcohol-free)

▶ *fluticasone propionate* (C)(OTC)(G) initially 2 sprays in each nostril once daily or 1 spray bid; maintenance 1 spray once daily
Pediatric: <4 years: not recommended; >4 years: initially 1 spray in each nostril once daily; may increase to 2 sprays in each nostril once daily; maintenance 1 spray in each nostril once daily; max 2 sprays in each nostril/day
    Flonase *Nasal spray:* 50 mcg/actuation (16 g, 120 sprays)

▶ *flunisolide* (C) 2 sprays in each nostril bid; may increase to 2 sprays in each nostril tid; max 8 sprays/nostril/day
Pediatric: <6 years: not recommended; 6-14 years: initially 1 spray in each nostril tid or 2 sprays in each nostril bid; max 4 sprays/nostril/day; >14 years: same as adult
    Nasalide *Nasal spray:* 25 mcg/actuation (25 ml, 200 sprays)
    Nasarel *Nasal spray:* 25 mcg/actuation (25 ml, 200 sprays)

▶ *mometasone furoate* (C)(G) 2 sprays in each nostril once daily
Pediatric: <2 years: not recommended; 2-11 years: 1 spray in each nostril once daily; max 2 sprays in each nostril once daily; >11 years: same as adult
    Nasonex *Nasal spray:* 50 mcg/actuation (17 g, 120 sprays)

▶ *olopatadine* (C) 2 sprays in each nostril bid
Pediatric: <6 years: not recommended; 6-11 years: 1 spray each nostril bid; >11 years: same as adult
    Patanase *Nasal spray:* 0.6%; 665 mcg/actuation (30.5 g, 240 sprays) (benzalkonium chloride)

▶ *triamcinolone acetonide* (C)(G) initially 2 sprays in each nostril once daily; max 4 sprays in each nostril once daily or 2 sprays in each nostril bid or 1 spray in each nostril qid; maintain at lowest effective dose
Pediatric: <6 years: not recommended; ≥6 years: 1 spray in each nostril once daily; max 2 sprays in each nostril once daily
    Nasacort Allergy 24HR (OTC) *Nasal spray:* 55 mcg/actuation (10 g, 120 sprays)
    Tri-Nasal *Nasal spray:* 50 mcg/actuation (15 ml, 120 sprays)

NASAL MAST CELL STABILIZERS

▶ *cromolyn sodium* (B)(OTC) 1 spray in each nostril tid-qid; max 6 sprays in each nostril/day
Pediatric: <2 years: not recommended; ≥2 years: same as adult
    Children's NasalCrom, NasalCrom *Nasal spray:* 5.2 mg/spray (13 ml, 100 sprays; 26 ml, 200 sprays)
Comment: Begin 1-2 weeks before exposure to known allergen. May take 2-4 weeks to achieve maximum effect.

NASAL ANTIHISTAMINES

▶ *azelastine* (C)
Pediatric: <5 years: not recommended; ≥5-12 years: 1 spray in each nostril bid; >12 years: same as adult
    Astelin Ready Spray 2 sprays in each nostril bid
      Nasal spray: 137 mcg/actuation (30 ml, 200sprays) (benzalkonium chloride)
    Astepro 0.15% Nasal Spray 1 or 2 sprays each nostril once daily bid

Pediatric: not recommended
Nasal spray: 205.5 mcg/actuation (17 ml, 106 sprays; 30 ml, 200 sprays) (ben-zalkonium chloride)

NASAL ANTIHISTAMINE/GLUCOCORTICOID COMBINATION

▷ *azelastine/fluticasone* (C) 1 spray in each nostril bid
  Pediatric: <6 years: not recommended; ≥6 years: same as adult
    Dymista *Nasal spray:* azel 137 mcg/*flutic* 50 mcg per actuation (23 g, 120 sprays) (benzalkonium chloride)

NASAL ANTICHOLINERGICS

▷ *ipratropium bromide* (B)(G)
    Atrovent Nasal Spray 0.03% 2 sprays in each nostril bid-tid
      Pediatric: <6 years: not recommended; ≥6 years: same as adult
      Nasal spray: 21 mcg/actuation (30 ml, 345 sprays)
    Atrovent Nasal Spray 0.06% 2 sprays in each nostril tid-qid; max 5-7 days
      Pediatric: <5 years: not recommended; ≥5-11 years: 2 sprays in each nostril tid; >11 years: same as adult
      Nasal spray: 42 mcg/actuation (15 ml, 165 sprays)
  Comment: Avoid use with narrow-angle glaucoma, prostate hyperplasia, and bladder neck obstruction.

⬤ RHINITIS MEDICAMENTOSA

Comment: The nasal/oral regimen selected should be instituted with concurrent weaning from the nasal decongestant.
Oral Prescription Drugs for the Management of Allergy, Cough, and Cold Symptoms *see page 524*
Nasal Glucocorticosteroids *see Allergic Rhinitis page 372*
Oral Corticosteroids *see page 497*
Parenteral Corticosteroids *see page 499*

NASAL ANTICHOLINERGICS

▷ *ipratropium bromide* (B)(G)
    Atrovent Nasal Spray 0.03% stop nasal decongestant; 2 sprays in each nostril bid-tid with progressive weaning as tolerated
      Pediatric: <6 years: not recommended; ≥6 years: same as adult
      Nasal spray: 21 mcg/actuation (30 ml, 345 sprays)
    Atrovent Nasal Spray 0.06% stop nasal decongestant; 2 sprays in each nostril tid-qid with progressive weaning as tolerated
      Pediatric: <5 years: not recommended; ≥5-11 years: 2 sprays in each nostril tid; ≥11 years: same as adult
      Nasal spray: 42 mcg/actuation (15 ml, 165 sprays)
  Comment: Avoid use with narrow-angle glaucoma, prostate hyperplasia, and bladder neck obstruction

NASAL ANTIHISTAMINE

▷ *azelastine* (C) 2 sprays in each nostril bid
  Pediatric: <5 years: not recommended; ≥5-12 years: 1 spray in each nostril bid
    Astelin Ready Spray
      Nasal spray: 137 mcg/actuation (30 ml, 200 sprays)

RHINITIS: VASOMOTOR

NASAL ANTICHOLINERGICS

▷ *ipratropium bromide* (B)(G)
    Atrovent Nasal Spray 0.03% stop nasal decongestant; 2 sprays in each nostril
    bid-tid with progressive weaning as tolerated
      Pediatric: <6 years: not recommended; ≥6 years: same as adult
      Nasal spray: 21 mcg/actuation (30 ml, 345 sprays)
    Atrovent Nasal Spray 0.06% stop nasal decongestant; 2 sprays in each nostril
    tid-qid with progressive weaning as tolerated
      Pediatric: <5 years: not recommended; ≥5-11 years: 2 sprays in each nostril
      tid; >11 years: same as adult
      Nasal spray: 42 mcg/actuation (15 ml, 165 sprays)
Comment: Avoid use with narrow-angle glaucoma, prostate hyperplasia, and bladder
neck obstruction

ROSEOLA (EXANTHEM SUBITUM)

Antipyretics *see Fever page 143*

ROCKY MOUNTAIN SPOTTED FEVER (*RICKETTSIA RICKETTSII*)

ANTI-INFECTIVES

▷ *doxycycline* (D)(G) 200 mg on first day; then 100 mg bid x 7-10 days
  Pediatric: <8 years: not recommended; ≥8 years, <100 lb: 2-2.5 mg/kg q 12 hours x
  7-10 days; ≥8 years, >100 lb: same as adult
    Adoxa *Tab:* 50, 75, 100, 150 mg ent-coat
    Doryx *Tab:* 75, 100, 150 mg del-rel
    Monodox *Cap:* 50, 75, 100 mg
    Oracea *Cap:* 40 mg del-rel
    Vibramycin *Cap:* 50, 100 mg; *Syr:* 50 mg/5 ml (raspberry; sulfites); *Oral susp:*
    25 mg/5 ml (raspberry-apple)
    Vibra-Tab *Tab:* 100 mg film-coat
Comment: *doxycycline* contraindicated <8 years-of-age, in pregnancy, and lactation
(discolors developing tooth enamel). A side effect may be photo-sensitivity
(photophobia). Do not give with antacids, calcium supplements, milk or other
dairy, or within two hours of taking another drug.

▷ *tetracycline* (D)(G) 500 mg q 6 hours x 7-10 days
  Pediatric: <8 years: not recommended; ≥8 years, <100 lb: 10 mg/kg/day q 6 hours x 7-10 days; ≥8 years, >100 lb: same as adult
    Achromycin V *Cap:* 250, 500 mg
    Sumycin *Tab:* 250, 500 mg; *Cap:* 250, 500 mg; *Oral susp:* 125 mg/5 ml (100, 200 ml) (fruit) (sulfites)
  Comment: *tetracycline* is contraindicated <8 years-of-age, in pregnancy, and lactation (discolors developing tooth enamel). A side effect may be photo-sensitivity (photophobia). Do not give with antacids, calcium supplements, milk or other dairy, or within two hours of taking another drug.

● ROTAVIRUS GASTROENTERITIS

PROPHYLAXIS

Comment: RotaTeq targets the most common strains of rotavirus (G1, G2, G3, G4), which are responsible for more than 90% of rotavirus disease in the United States.
▷ *rotavirus vaccine, live* not recommended for adults
  Pediatric: <6 weeks or >32 weeks: not recommended; >6 weeks and <32 weeks: administer 1st dose at 6-12 weeks of age; administer 2nd and 3rd doses at 4-10-week intervals for a total of 3 doses; if an incomplete dose is administered, do not administer a replacement dose, but continue with the remaining doses in the recommended series
    RotaTeq *Oral susp:* 2 ml single-use tube (fetal bovine serum [trace], preservative-free, thimerosal-free)

● ROUNDWORM (ASCARIASIS)

ANTIHELMINTICS

▷ *albendazole* (C) 400 mg once daily x 7 days; take with a meal
  Pediatric: <2 years: 200 mg once daily x 3 days; may repeat in 3 weeks; ≥2-12 years: 400 mg once daily x 3 days; may repeat in 3 weeks
    Albenza *Tab:* 200 mg
▷ *mebendazole* (C)(G) 100 mg bid x 3 days; may repeat in 2-3 weeks if needed; take after a meal
  Pediatric: same as adult (chew or crush and mix with food)
    Vermox *Chew tab:* 100 mg
▷ *pyrantel pamoate* (C) 11 mg/kg once daily x 3 days; max 1 g/dose; take after a meal
  Pediatric: 25-37 lb: 1/2 tsp x 1 dose; 38-62 lb: 1 tsp x 1 dose; 63-87 lb: 1 tsp x 1 dose; 88-112 lb: 2 tsp x 1 dose; 113-137 lb: 2 tsp x 1 dose; 138-162 lb: 3 tsp x 1 dose; 163-187 lb: 3 tsp x 1 dose; >187 lb: 4 tsp x 1 dose
    Pin-X (OTC) *Cap:* 180 mg; *Liq:* 50 mg/ml (30 ml); 144 mg/ml (30 ml); *Oral susp:* 50 mg/ml (30 ml)
▷ *thiabendazole* (C) 25 mg/kg bid x 7 days; max 1.5 g/dose; max 3000 mg/day; take after a meal
  Pediatric: same as adult
    Mintezol *Chew tab:* 500*mg (orange); *Oral susp:* 500 mg/5 ml (120 ml) (orange)
  Comment: *thiabendazole* is not for prophylaxis. May impair mental alertness.

RUBELLA (GERMAN MEASLES)

PROPHYLAXIS

▷ *rubella virus, live, attenuated/neomycin* vaccine (C)
Pediatric: <12 months: not recommended (if vaccinated <12 months, revaccinate at 12 months); ≥12 months: 25 mcg SC
    Meruvax II 25 mcg SC
▷ *measles, mumps, rubella, live, attenuated, neomycin vaccine* (C)
    MMR II 25 mcg SC (preservative-free)
Comment: Contraindications: hypersensitivity to *neomycin* <u>or</u> eggs, primary <u>or</u> acquired immune deficiency, immunosuppressant therapy, bone marrow <u>or</u> lymphatic malignancy, and pregnancy (within 3 months following vaccination).
    see Childhood Immunizations page 466

TREATMENT

▷ *immune globulin* (Ig) 0.25 ml/kg IM (0.5 mg/kg in immunocompromised children)
Antipyretics see Fever page 143

 RUBEOLA (RED MEASLES)

PROPHYLAXIS

▷ *measles, mumps, rubella, live, attenuated, neomycin vaccine* (C)
    MMR II 25 mcg SC (preservative-free)
Comment: Contraindications: hypersensitivity to *neomycin* <u>or</u> eggs, primary <u>or</u> acquired immune deficiency, immunosuppressant therapy, bone marrow <u>or</u> lymphatic malignancy, and pregnancy (within 3 months following vaccination).
    see Childhood Immunizations page 466

TREATMENT

▷ *immune globulin* (Ig) 0.25 ml/kg IM (0.5 mg/kg in immunocompromised children)
    Antipyretics see Fever page 143

 SALMONELLOSIS

▷ *ciprofloxacin* (C) 500 mg bid x 3-5 days
Pediatric: <18 years: not recommended
    Cipro (G) *Tab:* 250, 500, 750 mg; *Oral susp:* 250, 500 mg/5 ml (100 ml) (strawberry)
    Cipro XR *Tab:* 500, 1000 mg ext-rel
    ProQuin XR *Tab:* 500 mg ext-rel
Comment: *ciprofloxacin* is contraindicated <18 years-of-age, and during pregnancy and lactation. Risk of tendonitis or tendon rupture, especially 60 years-of-age and older.

▷ *trimethoprim/sulfamethoxazole* (D)(G)
Pediatric: <2 months: not recommended; ≥2 months: 40 mg/kg/day of *sulfamethox-azole* in 2 divided doses bid x 10 days; *see page 576 for dose by weight*
   Bactrim, Septra 2 tabs bid x 10 days
      Tab: trim 80 mg/*sulfa* 400 mg*
   Bactrim DS, Septra DS 1 tab bid x 10 days
      Tab: trim 160 mg/*sulfa* 800 mg*
   Bactrim Pediatric Suspension, Septra Pediatric Suspension
      Oral susp: trim 40 mg/*sulfa* 200 mg per 5 ml (100 ml) (cherry) (alcohol 0.3%)
Comment: *trimethoprim/sulfamethoxazole* is not recommended in pregnancy or lactation. *CrCl 15-30 mL/min:* reduce dose by 1/2; *CrCl <15 mL/min:* not recommended

SCABIES (*SARCOPTES SCABIEI*)

Comment: This section presents treatment regimens for scabies infestation published in the 2015 CDC Sexually Transmitted Diseases Treatment Guidelines, as well as other available treatments.

RECOMMENDED REGIMEN

▷ *permethrin* (B)(G) massage into skin from head to soles of feet; leave on x 8-14 hours, then rinse off
Pediatric: <2 months: not recommended; ≥2 months: same as adult
   Acticin, Elimite *Crm:* 5% (60 g)

ALTERNATIVE REGIMEN

▷ *lindane* (B)(G) 1 oz of lotion or 30 g of cream apply to all skin surfaces from neck down to the soles of the feet; leave on x 8 hours, then wash off thoroughly; may repeat if needed in 14 days
Pediatric: <2 months: not recommended; ≥2 months: same as adult
   Kwell *Lotn:* 1% (60, 473 ml); *Crm:* 1% (60 g); *Shampoo:* 1% (60, 473 ml)

OTHER TOPICAL TREATMENTS

▷ *crotamiton* (C) massage into skin from chin down; repeat in 24 hours
Pediatric: not recommended
   Eurax *Lotn:* 10% (60 g); *Crm:* 10% (60 g)

SCARLET FEVER (SCARLATINA)

Comment: Microorganism responsible for scarlet fever is Group A beta-hemolytic *Streptococcus* (GABHS). Strep cultures and screens will be positive.
▷ *azithromycin* (B) 500 mg x 1 dose on day 1, then 250 mg once daily on days 2-5 or 500 mg once daily x 3 days
Pediatric: 12 mg/kg/day x 5 days; max 500 mg/day; *see page 548 for dose by weight*
   Zithromax *Tab:* 250, 500, 600 mg; *Oral susp:* 100 mg/5 ml (15 ml); 200 mg/5 ml (15, 22.5, 30 ml) (cherry); *Pkt:* 1 g for reconstitution (cherry-banana)
   Zithromax Tri-pak *Tab:* 3 x 500 mg tabs/pck

Zithromax Z-pak *Tab:* 6 x 250 mg tabs/pck
Zmax *Oral susp:* 2 g ext-rel for reconstitution (cherry-banana) (148 mg Na⁺)

▷ *cefadroxil* (B)
  Pediatric: 15-30 mg/kg/day in 2 divided doses x 10 days; *see page 550 for dose by weight*
    Duricef *Cap:* 500 mg; *Tab:* 1 g; *Oral susp:* 250 mg/5 ml (100 ml); 500 mg/5 ml (75, 100 ml) (orange-pineapple)

▷ *cephalexin* (B)(G)
  Pediatric: 25-50 mg/kg/day in 2 divided doses x 10 days; *see page 557 for dose by weight*
    Keflex *Cap:* 250, 333, 500, 750 mg; *Oral susp:* 125, 250 mg/5 ml (100, 200 ml) (strawberry)

▷ *clarithromycin* (C)(G) 250 mg bid <u>or</u> 500 mg ext-rel once daily x 10 days
  Pediatric: <6 months: not recommended; ≥6 months: 7.5 mg/kg bid x 10 days; *see page 558 for dose by weight*
    Biaxin *Tab:* 250, 500 mg
    Biaxin Oral Suspension *Oral susp:* 125, 250 mg/5 ml (50, 100 ml) (fruit punch)
    Biaxin XL *Tab:* 500 mg ext-rel

▷ *clindamycin* (B)(G) 150-300 mg q 6 hours x 10 days
  Pediatric: 8-16 mg/kg/day in 3-4 divided doses x 10 days
    Cleocin *Cap:* 75 (tartrazine), 150 (tartrazine), 300 mg
    Cleocin Pediatric Granules *Oral susp:* 75 mg/5 ml (100 ml) (cherry)

▷ *erythromycin estolate* (B)(G) 250 mg q 6 hours x 10 days
  Pediatric: 20-50 mg/kg q 6 hours x 10 days; *see page 562 for dose by weight*
    Ilosone *Pulvule:* 250 mg; *Tab:* 500 mg; *Liq:* 125, 250 mg/5 ml (100 ml)
  Comment: *erythromycin* may increase INR with concomitant *warfarin*, as well as increase serum level of *digoxin*, benzodiazepines and statins.

▷ *erythromycin ethylsuccinate* (B)(G) 400 mg qid <u>or</u> 800 mg bid x 10 days
  Pediatric: 30-50 mg/kg/day in 4 divided doses x 10 days; may double dose with severe infection; max 100 mg/kg/day; *see page 563 for dose by weight*
    EryPed *Oral susp:* 200 mg/5 ml (100, 200 ml) (fruit); 400 mg/5 ml (60, 100, 200 ml) (banana); *Oral drops:* 200, 400 mg/5 ml (50 ml) (fruit); *Chew tab:* 200 mg wafer (fruit)
    E.E.S. *Oral susp:* 200, 400 mg/5 ml (100 ml) (fruit)
    E.E.S. Granules *Oral susp:* 200 mg/5 ml (100, 200 ml) (cherry)
    E.E.S. 400 Tablets *Tab:* 400 mg

Comment: *erythromycin* may increase INR with concomitant *warfarin*, as well as increase serum level of *digoxin*, benzodiazepines and statins.

▷ *penicillin G (benzathine and procaine)* (B)(G) 2.4 million units IM x 1 dose
  Pediatric: <30 lb: 600,000 units IM x 1 dose; 30-60 lb: 900,000-1.2 million units IM x 1 dose
    Bicillin C-R Cartridge-needle unit: 600,000 units (1 ml); 1.2 million units; (2 ml); 2.4 million units (4 ml)

▷ *penicillin V potassium* (B) 250 mg tid x 10 days
  Pediatric: 25-50 mg/kg day in 4 divided doses x 10 days; ≥12 years: same as adult; *see page 572 for dose by weight*
    Pen-Vee K *Tab:* 250, 500 mg; *Oral soln:* 125 mg/5 ml (100, 200 ml); 250 mg/5 ml (100, 150, 200 ml)

⬤ SEIZURE DISORDER

Status Epilepticus *see Status Epilepticus page* 393
Anticonvulsant Drugs *see page* 508

⬤ SEXUAL ASSAULT (STD EXPOSURE)

Comment: The following treatment regimens for victims of sexual assault are
published in the **2015 CDC Sexually Transmitted Diseases Treatment Guidelines.**

RECOMMENDED PROPHYLAXIS REGIMEN

▷ *ceftriaxone* 250 mg IM in a single dose <u>plus</u> *metronidazole* 2 g in a single dose <u>plus</u>
azithromycin 1 g in a single dose

ALTERNATE PROPHYLAXIS REGIMENS

Regimen 1

▷ *ceftriaxone* 250 mg IM in a single dose <u>plus</u> *metronidazole* 2 g in a single dose <u>plus</u>
doxycycline 100 mg bid x 7 days

Regimen 2

▷ *cefixime* 400 mg in a single dose <u>plus</u> *metronidazole* 2 g in a single dose <u>plus</u> *azith-romycin* 1 g in a single dose

Regimen 3

▷ *cefixime* 400 mg in a single dose <u>plus</u> *metronidazole* 2 g in a single dose <u>plus</u> *doxycy-cline* 100 mg bid x 7 days

Regimen 4

▷ *azithromycin* (B) 1 g as a single dose <u>plus</u> *metronidazole* 2 g in a single dose

DRUG BRANDS AND DOSE FORMS

▷ *azithromycin* (B)
    Zithromax *Tab:* 250, 500, 600 mg; *Oral susp:* 100 mg/5 ml (15 ml); 200 mg/5 ml
    (15, 22.5, 30 ml) (cherry); *Pkt:* 1 g for reconstitution (cherry-banana)
    Zithromax Tri-pak *Tab:* 3 x 500 mg tabs/pck
    Zithromax Z-pak *Tab:* 6 x 250 mg tabs/pck
    Zmax *Oral susp:* 2 g ext-rel for reconstitution (cherry-banana) (148 mg Na+)
▷ *cefixime* (B)
    Suprax *Tab:* 400 mg; *Cap:* 400 mg; *Oral susp:* 100, 200 mg/5 ml (50, 75, 100 ml)
    (strawberry)
▷ *ceftriaxone* (B)(G)
    Rocephin *Vial:* 250, 500 mg; 1, 2 g
▷ *doxycycline* (D)(G)
    Adoxa *Tab:* 50, 75, 100, 150 mg ent-coat
    Doryx *Tab:* 75, 100, 150 mg del-rel
    Monodox *Cap:* 50, 75, 100 mg
    Oracea *Cap:* 40 mg del-rel

Vibramycin *Cap:* 50, 100 mg; *Syr:* 50 mg/5 ml (raspberry; sulfites); *Oral susp:* 25 mg/5 ml (raspberry-apple)
Vibra-Tab *Tab:* 100 mg film-coat

Comment: *Doxycycline* is contraindicated <8 years-of-age, in pregnancy, and lactation (discolors developing tooth enamel). A side effect may be photo-sensitivity (photophobia). Do not give with antacids, calcium supplements, milk or other dairy, or within two hours of taking another drug.

▷ *metronidazole* **(not for use in 1st; B in 2nd, 3rd)(G)**
Flagyl *Tab:* 250*, 500*mg
Flagyl 375 *Cap:* 375 mg
Flagyl ER *Tab:* 750 mg ext-rel

Comment: Alcohol is contraindicated during treatment with oral *metronidazole* and for 72 hours after therapy due to a possible *disulfiram*-like reaction (nausea, vomiting, flushing, headache).

◯ SHIGELLOSIS

ANTI-INFECTIVES

▷ *azithromycin* **(B)** 500 mg x 1 dose on day 1, then 250 mg once daily on days 2-5 or 500 mg once daily x 3 days or **Zmax** 2 g in a single dose
Pediatric: <6 months: not recommended; >6 months: 10 mg/kg x 1 dose on day 1; then 5 mg/kg/day on days 2-5; max 500 mg/day; *see page 548 for dose by weight*
Zithromax *Tab:* 250, 500, 600 mg; *Oral susp:* 100 mg/5 ml (15 ml); 200 mg/5 ml (15, 22.5, 30 ml) (cherry); *Pkt:* 1 g for reconstitution (cherry-banana)
Zithromax Tri-pak *Tab:* 3 x 500 mg tabs/pck
Zithromax Z-pak *Tab:* 6 x 250 mg tabs/pck
Zmax *Oral susp:* 2 g ext-rel for reconstitution (cherry-banana) (148 mg Na$^+$)

▷ *ciprofloxacin* **(C)** 500 mg bid x 3 days
Pediatric: <18 years: not recommended
Cipro (G) *Tab:* 250, 500, 750 mg; *Oral susp:* 250, 500 mg/5 ml (100 ml) (strawberry)
Cipro XR *Tab:* 500, 1000 mg ext-rel
ProQuin XR *Tab:* 500 mg ext-rel

Comment: *ciprofloxacin* is contraindicated <18 years-of-age, and during pregnancy and lactation. Risk of tendonitis or tendon rupture, especially 60 years-of-age and older.

▷ *ofloxacin* **(C)(G)** 400 mg bid x 3 days
Pediatric: <18 years: not recommended
Floxin *Tab:* 200, 300, 400 mg

Comment: *ofloxacin* is contraindicated <18 years-of-age, and during pregnancy and lactation. Risk of tendonitis or tendon rupture, especially 60 years-of-age and older.

▷ *tetracycline* **(D)(G)** 250-500 mg qid x 5 days
Pediatric: <8 years: not recommended; ≥8 years, <100 lb: 25-50 mg/kg/day in 4 divided doses x 5 days; ≥8 years, >100 lb: same as adult; *see page 574 for dose by weight*
Achromycin V *Cap:* 250, 500 mg
Sumycin *Tab:* 250, 500 mg; *Cap:* 250, 500 mg; *Oral susp:* 125 mg/5 ml (100, 200 ml) (fruit) (sulfites)

Comment: *tetracycline* is contraindicated <8 years-of-age, in pregnancy, and lactation (discolors developing tooth enamel). A side effect may be photo-sensitivity (photophobia). Do not give with antacids, calcium supplements, milk or other dairy, or within two hours of taking another drug.

▷ *trimethoprim/sulfamethoxazole* (D)(G)
    Bactrim, Septra 2 tabs bid x 10 days
      Tab: trim 80 mg/*sulfa* 400 mg*
    Bactrim DS, Septra DS 1 tab bid x 10 days
      Tab: trim 160 mg/*sulfa* 800 mg*
    Bactrim Pediatric Suspension, Septra Pediatric Suspension 20 ml bid x 10 days
      Oral susp: trim 40 mg/*sulfa* 200 mg per 5 ml (100 ml) (cherry) (alcohol 0.3%)
    Comment: *trimethoprim/sulfamethoxazole* is not recommended in pregnancy or lactation. *CrCl 15-30 mL/min:* reduce dose by 1/2; *CrCl <15 mL/min:* not recommended

⬤ SINUSITIS/RHINOSINUSITIS: ACUTE BACTERIAL

ANTI-INFECTIVES

▷ *amoxicillin* (B)(G) 500-875 mg bid or 250-500 mg tid x 10 days
Pediatric: <40 kg (88 lb): 20-40 mg/kg/day in 3 divided doses x 10 days or 25-45 mg/kg/day in 2 divided doses x 10 days; *see page 543 for dose by weight*
    Amoxil *Cap:* 250, 500 mg; *Tab:* 875*mg; *Chew tab:* 125, 200, 250, 400 mg (cherry-banana-peppermint) (phenylalanine); *Oral susp:* 125, 250 mg/5 ml (80, 100, 150 ml) (strawberry); 200, 400 mg/5 ml (50, 75, 100 ml) (bubble gum); *Oral drops:* 50 mg/ml (30 ml) (bubble gum)
    Moxatag *Tab:* 775 mg ext-rel
    Trimox *Tab:* 125, 250 mg; *Cap:* 250, 500 mg; *Oral susp:* 125, 250 mg/5 ml (80, 100, 150 ml) (raspberry-strawberry)
▷ *amoxicillin/clavulanate* (B)(G) 500 mg tid or 875 mg bid x 10 days
    Augmentin *Tab:* 250, 500, 875 mg; *Chew tab:* 125, 250 mg (lemon-lime); 200, 400 mg (cherry-banana) (phenylalanine); *Oral susp:* 125 mg/5 ml (banana), 250 mg/5 ml (75, 100, 150 ml) (orange); 200, 400 mg/5 ml (50, 75, 100 ml) (orange) (phenylalanine)
      Pediatric: 40-45 mg/kg/day divided tid x 10 days or 90 mg/kg/day divided bid x 10 days *see pages 545-546 for dose by weight*
    Augmentin ES-600 *Oral susp:* 600 mg/5 ml (50, 75, 100, 125, 150, 200 ml) (strawberry cream) (phenylalanine) every 12 hours
      Pediatric: <3 months: not recommended; ≥3 months, <40 kg: 90 mg/kg/day in 2 divided doses; ≥40 kg: not recommended
    Augmentin XR 2 tabs q 12 hours x 7-10 days
      Pediatric: <16 years: use other forms; ≥16 years: same as adult
      Tab: 1000*mg ext-rel
▷ *cefaclor* (B)(G) 250-500 mg q 8 hours x 10 days; max 2 g/day
Pediatric: <1 month: not recommended; 20-40 mg/kg bid or q 12 hours x 10 days; max 1 g/day; *see page 549 for dose by weight*
Tab: 500 mg; *Cap:* 250, 500 mg; *Susp:* 125 mg/5 ml (75, 150 ml) (strawberry); 187 mg/5 ml (50, 100 ml) (strawberry); 250 mg/5 ml (75, 150 ml) (strawberry); 375 mg/5 ml (50, 100 ml) (strawberry)
Pediatric: <16 years: ext-rel not recommended; ≥16 years: same as adult
    Cefaclor Extended Release *Tab:* 375, 500 mg ext-rel

▷ *cefdinir* (B) 300 mg bid or 600 mg once daily x 10 days
Pediatric: <6 months: not recommended; 6 months-12 years: 14 mg/kg/day in a single or 2 divided doses x 10 days; 12 years: same as adult; *see page 551 for dose by weight*
Omnicef *Cap:* 300 mg; *Oral susp:* 125 mg/5 ml (60, 100 ml) (strawberry)

▷ *cefixime* (B) 400 mg once daily x 10 days
Pediatric: <6 months: not recommended; 6 months-12 years, <50 kg: 8 mg/kg/day in 1-2 divided doses x 10 days; >12 years, >50 kg: same as adult; *see page 552 for dose by weight*
Suprax *Tab:* 400 mg; *Cap:* 400 mg; *Oral susp:* 100, 200 mg/5 ml (50, 75, 100 ml) (strawberry)

▷ *cefpodoxime proxetil* 200 mg bid x 10 days
Pediatric: <2 months: not recommended; 2 months-12 years: 10 mg/kg/day (max 400 mg/ dose) or 5 mg/kg/day bid (max 200 mg/dose) x 10 days; *see page 553 for dose by weight*
Vantin *Tab:* 100, 200 mg; *Oral susp:* 50, 100 mg/5 ml (50, 75, 100 mg) (lemon creme)

▷ *cefprozil* (B) 250-500 mg bid x 10 days
Pediatric: <6 months: not recommended; 6 months-12 years: *Mild:* 7.5 mg/kg bid x 10 days; *Moderate/Severe:* 15 mg/kg q 12 hours x 10 days; >12 years: same as adult; *see page 554 for dose by weight*
Cefzil *Tab:* 250, 500 mg; *Oral susp:* 125, 250 mg/5 ml (50, 75, 100 ml) (bubble gum) (phenylalanine)

▷ *ceftibuten* (B) 400 mg once daily x 10 days
Pediatric: 9 mg/kg once daily x 10 days; max 400 mg/day; *see page 555 for dose by weight*
Cedax *Cap:* 400 mg; *Oral susp:* 90 mg/5 ml (30, 60, 90, 120 ml); 180 mg/5 ml (30, 60, 120 ml) (cherry)

▷ *cefuroxime axetil* (B)(G) 250 mg bid x 10 days
Pediatric: <3 months: not recommended; 3 months-12 years: 20-30 mg/kg/day in 2 divided doses x 10 days; >12 years: same as adult; *see page 556 for dose by weight*
Ceftin *Tab:* 250, 500 mg; *Oral susp:* 125, 250 mg/5 ml (50, 100 ml) (tutti-frutti)

▷ *ciprofloxacin* (C) 500 mg bid x 10 days
Pediatric: <18 years: not recommended
Cipro (G) *Tab:* 250, 500, 750 mg; *Oral susp:* 250, 500 mg/5 ml (100 ml) (strawberry)
Cipro XR *Tab:* 500, 1000 mg ext-rel
ProQuin XR *Tab:* 500 mg ext-rel
Comment: *ciprofloxacin* is contraindicated <18 years-of-age, and during pregnancy and lactation. Risk of tendonitis or tendon rupture, especially 60 years-of-age and older.

▷ *clarithromycin* (C)(G) 500 mg bid or 1000 mg ext-rel once daily x 10 days
Pediatric: <6 months: not recommended; ≥6 months: 7.5 mg/kg bid x 10 days; *see page 558 for dose by weight*
Biaxin *Tab:* 250, 500 mg
Biaxin Oral Suspension *Oral susp:* 125, 250 mg/5 ml (50, 100 ml) (fruit punch)
Biaxin XL *Tab:* 500 mg ext-rel

▷ *levofloxacin* (C) *Uncomplicated:* 500 mg once daily x 10-14 days; *Complicated:* 750 mg once daily x 10-14 days
Pediatric: <18 years: not recommended

Levaquin *Tab:* 250, 500, 750 mg; *Oral soln:* 25 mg/ml (480 ml) (benzyl alcohol); *Inj conc:* 25 mg/ml for IV infusion after dilution (20, 30 ml single-use vial) (preservative-free); *Premix soln:* 5 mg/ml for IV infusion (50, 100, 150 ml) (preservative-free)

Comment: *levofloxacin* is contraindicated <18 years-of-age, and during pregnancy and lactation. Risk of tendonitis or tendon rupture, especially 60 years-of-age and older.

▷ *loracarbef* (B) 400 mg bid x 10 days
Pediatric: 15 mg/kg/day in 2 divided doses x 10 days; *see page* 570 *for dose by weight*

Lorabid *Pulvule:* 200, 400 mg; *Oral susp:* 100 mg/5 ml (50, 100 ml);
200 mg/5 ml (50, 75, 100 ml) (strawberry bubble gum)

▷ *moxifloxacin* (C)(G) 400 mg once daily x 10 days
Pediatric: <18 years: not recommended

Avelox *Tab:* 400 mg

Comment: *moxifloxacin* is contraindicated <18 years of age, and during pregnancy and lactation. Risk of tendonitis or tendon rupture, especially 60 years-of-age and older.

▷ *trimethoprim/sulfamethoxazole* (D)(G)
Pediatric: <2 months: not recommended; ≥2 months: 40 mg/kg/day of *sulfamethoxazole* in 2 divided doses bid x 10 days; *see page* 576 *for dose by weight*

Bactrim, Septra 2 tabs bid x 10 days
Tab: trim 80 mg/*sulfa* 400 mg*

Bactrim DS, Septra DS 1 tab bid x 10 days
Tab: trim 160 mg/*sulfa* 800 mg*

Bactrim Pediatric Suspension, Septra Pediatric Suspension
Oral susp: trim 40 mg/*sulfa* 200 mg per 5 ml (100 ml) (cherry) (alcohol 0.3%)

Comment: *trimethoprim/sulfamethoxazole* is not recommended in pregnancy or lactation. *CrCl 15-30 mL/min:* reduce dose by 1/2; *CrCl <15 mL/min:* not recommended

⬤ SJOGRENS SYNDROME (CHRONIC DRY MOUTH)

CHOLINERGIC/MUSCARINIC AGONIST COMBINATION

▷ *cevimeline* (C)(G) 30 mg tid
Evoxac *Cap:* 30 mg

Comment: *cevimeline* is contraindicated in acute iritis, narrow angle glaucoma, and uncontrolled asthma.

▷ *pilocarpine* (C)(G) 5 mg qid or 7.5 mg tid
Salagen *Tab:* 5, 7.5 mg

ORAL ENZYME RINSE

▷ *xylitol/solazyme/selectobac* (NR) swish 5 ml for 30 seconds bid-tid
Orazyme Dry Mouth Rinse *Oral soln:* 1.5, 16 oz

⬤ SKIN: CALLOUSED

KERATOLYTICS

▷ *salicylic acid* (C)(OTC) apply lotion, cream <u>or</u> gel to affected area once daily-bid; apply patch to affected area and leave on x 48 hours with max 5 applications/14 days
Pediatric: <12 years: not recommended; ≥12 years: same as adult
▷ *urea* (C)
Pediatric: <12 years: not recommended; ≥12 years: same as adult
Carmol 40 apply to affected area with applicator stick provided once daily-tid; smooth over until cream is absorbed; protect surrounding tissue; may cover with adhesive bandage <u>or</u> gauze secured with adhesive tape
Crm/Gel: 40% (30 g)
Keratol 40 apply to affected area with applicator stick provided once daily-tid; smooth over until cream is absorbed; protect surrounding tissue; may cover with adhesive bandage <u>or</u> gauze secured with adhesive tape
Crm: 40% (1, 3, 7 oz); *Gel:* 40% (15 ml); *Lotn:* 40% (8 oz)

Comment: The moisturizing effect of **Carmol 40** and **Keratol 40** is enhanced by applying while the skin is still moist (after washing <u>or</u> bathing).

⬤ SKIN INFECTION: BACTERIAL (CARBUNCLE, FOLLICULITIS, FURUNCLE)

Comment: Abscesses usually require surgical incision and drainage.

ANTIBACTERIAL SKIN CLEANSERS

Dial soap (OTC) bid
Lever 2000 Antibacterial soap (OTC) bid
▷ *hexachlorophene* (C)
pHisoHex dispense 5 ml into wet hand, work up into lather; then apply to area to be cleansed; rinse thoroughly
Liq clnsr: 5, 16 oz

TOPICAL ANTI-INFECTIVES

▷ *mupirocin* (B)(G) apply to lesions bid
Pediatric: same as adult
Bactroban *Oint:* 2% (22 g); *Crm:* 2% (15, 30 g)
Centany *Oint:* 2% (15, 30 g)
▷ *polymyxin B/neomycin* (C) oint apply once daily-tid
Neosporin (OTC) *Oint:* 15 g

ORAL ANTI-INFECTIVES

▷ *amoxicillin* (B)(G) 500-875 mg bid <u>or</u> 250-500 mg tid x 10 days
Pediatric: <40 kg (88 lb): 20-40 mg/kg/day in 3 divided doses x 10 days <u>or</u> 25-45 mg/kg/day in 2 divided doses x 10 days; *see page 543 for dose by weight*

Amoxil *Cap:* 250, 500 mg; *Tab:* 875*mg; *Chew tab:* 125, 200, 250, 400 mg (cherry-banana-peppermint) (phenylalanine); *Oral susp:* 125, 250 mg/5 ml (80, 100, 150 ml) (strawberry); 200, 400 mg/5 ml (50, 75, 100 ml) (bubble gum); *Oral drops:* 50 mg/ml (30 ml) (bubble gum)

Moxatag *Tab:* 775 mg ext-rel

Trimox *Tab:* 125, 250 mg; *Cap:* 250, 500 mg; *Oral susp:* 125, 250 mg/5 ml (80, 100, 150 ml) (raspberry-strawberry)

▷ *azithromycin* (B) 500 mg x 1 dose on day 1, then 250 mg once daily on days 2-5 or 500 mg once daily x 3 days or **Zmax** 2 g in a single dose

Pediatric: 12 mg/kg/day x 5 days; max 500 mg/day; *see page 548 for dose by weight*

Zithromax *Tab:* 250, 500, 600 mg; *Oral susp:* 100 mg/5 ml (15 ml); 200 mg/5 ml (15, 22.5, 30 ml) (cherry); *Pkt:* 1 g for reconstitution (cherry-banana)

Zithromax Tri-pak *Tab:* 3 x 500 mg tabs/pck

Zithromax Z-pak *Tab:* 6 x 250 mg tabs/pck

Zmax *Oral susp:* 2 g ext-rel for reconstitution (cherry-banana) (148 mg Na⁺)

▷ *cefaclor* (B)(G) 250-500 mg q 8 hours x 10 days; max 2 g/day

Pediatric: <1 month: not recommended; 20-40 mg/kg bid or q 12 hours x 10 days; max 1 g/ day; *see page 549 for dose by weight*

Tab: 500 mg; *Cap:* 250, 500 mg; *Susp:* 125 mg/5 ml (75, 150 ml) (strawberry); 187 mg/5 ml (50, 100 ml) (strawberry); 250 mg/5 ml (75, 150 ml) (strawberry); 375 mg/5 ml (50, 100 ml) (strawberry)

Cefaclor Extended Release

Pediatric: <16 years: ext-rel not recommended

Tab: 375, 500 mg ext-rel

▷ *cefadroxil* (B) 1-2 g in a single or 2 divided doses x 10 days

Pediatric: 15-30 mg/kg/day in 2 divided doses x 10 days; *see page 550 for dose by weight*

Duricef *Cap:* 500 mg; *Tab:* 1 g; *Oral susp:* 250 mg/5 ml (100 ml); 500 mg/5 ml (75, 100 ml) (orange-pineapple)

▷ *cefdinir* (B) 300 mg bid x 10 days

Pediatric: <6 months: not recommended; 6 months-12 years: 14 mg/kg/day in 1-2 divided doses x 10 days; *see page 551 for dose by weight*

Omnicef *Cap:* 300 mg; *Oral susp:* 125 mg/5 ml (60, 100 ml) (strawberry)

▷ *cefditoren pivoxil* (B) 200 mg bid x 10 days

Pediatric: not recommended

Spectracef *Tab:* 200 mg

Comment: Contraindicated with milk protein allergy or carnitine deficiency.

▷ *cefpodoxime* (B) *proxetil* 400 mg bid x 7-14 days

Pediatric: <2 months: not recommended; 2 months-12 years: 10 mg/kg/day (max 400 mg/dose) or 5 mg/kg/day bid (max 200 mg/dose) x 7-14 days; *see page 553 for dose by weight*

Vantin *Tab:* 100, 200 mg; *Oral susp:* 50, 100 mg/5 ml (50, 75, 100 mg) (lemon creme)

▷ *cefprozil* (B) 250-500 mg bid or 500 mg once daily x 10 days

Pediatric: 2-12 years: 7.5 mg/kg bid x 10 days; >12 years: same as adult; *see page 554 for dose by weight*

Cefzil *Tab:* 250, 500 mg; *Oral susp:* 125, 250 mg/5 ml (50, 75, 100 ml) (bubble gum) (phenylalanine)

▷ *ceftriaxone* (B)(G) 1-2 g IM once daily; max 4 g/day

Rocephin

Pediatric: 50-75 mg/kg IM in 1-2 divided doses; max 2 g/day
Vial: 250, 500 mg; 1, 2 g

▷ *cefuroxime axetil* (B)(G) 250-500 mg bid x 10 days
Pediatric: <3 months: not recommended; 3 months-12 years: 20-30 mg/kg/day in 2 divided doses x 10 days; >12 years: same as adult; *see page 556 for dose by weight*
    Ceftin *Tab:* 250, 500 mg; *Oral susp:* 125, 250 mg/5 ml (50, 100 ml) (tutti-frutti)

▷ *cephalexin* (B)(G) 500 mg bid x 10 days
Pediatric: 25-50 mg/kg/day in 4 divided doses x 10 days; *see page 557 for dose by weight*
    Keflex *Cap:* 250, 333, 500, 750 mg; *Oral susp:* 125, 250 mg/5 ml (100, 200 ml) (strawberry)

▷ *clarithromycin* (C)(G) 250-500 mg bid or 500-1000 mg ext-rel once daily x 7-14 days
Pediatric: <6 months: not recommended; >6 months: 7.5 mg/kg bid x 7-14 days; *see page 558 for dose by weight*
    Biaxin *Tab:* 250, 500 mg
    Biaxin Oral Suspension *Oral susp:* 125, 250 mg/5 ml (50, 100 ml) (fruit punch)
    Biaxin XL *Tab:* 500 mg ext-rel

▷ *dicloxacillin* (B) 500 mg qid x 10 days
Pediatric: 12.5-25 mg/kg/day in 4 divided doses x 10 days; *see page 560 for dose by weight*
    Dynapen *Cap:* 125, 250, 500 mg; *Oral susp:* 62.5 mg/5 ml (80, 100, 200 ml)

▷ *dirithromycin* (C)(G) 500 mg once daily x 5-7 days
Pediatric: <12 years: not recommended; ≥12 years: same as adult
    Dynabac *Tab:* 250 mg

▷ *doxycycline* (D)(G) 100mg bid x 9 days
Pediatric: <8 years: not recommended; ≥8 years, <100 lb: 1 mg/lb in a single dose once daily x 9 days x 9 days; ≥8 years, >100 lb: same as adult; *see page 561 for dose by weight*
    Adoxa *Tab:* 50, 75, 100, 150 mg ent-coat
    Doryx *Tab:* 75, 100, 150 mg del-rel
    Monodox *Cap:* 50, 75, 100 mg
    Oracea *Cap:* 40 mg del-rel
    Vibramycin *Cap:* 50, 100 mg; *Syr:* 50 mg/5 ml (raspberry; sulfites); *Oral susp:* 25 mg/5 ml (raspberry-apple)
    Vibra-Tab *Tab:* 100 mg film-coat
Comment: *Doxycycline* is contraindicated <8 years-of-age, in pregnancy, and lactation (discolors developing tooth enamel). A side effect may be photo-sensitivity (photophobia). Do not give with antacids, calcium supplements, milk or other dairy, or within two hours of taking another drug.

▷ *erythromycin base* (B)(G) 250-500 mg tid x 10 days
Pediatric: 30-50 mg/kg/day in 2-4 divided doses x 10 days
    Ery-Tab *Tab:* 250, 333, 500 mg ent-coat
    PCE *Tab:* 333, 500 mg
Comment: *erythromycin* may increase INR with concomitant **warfarin**, as well as increase serum level of **digoxin**, benzodiazepines and statins.

▷ *erythromycin estolate* (B)(G) 250-500 mg q 6 hours x 10 days
Pediatric: 20-50 mg/kg q 6 hours x 10 days; *see page 562 for dose by weight*
    Ilosone *Pulvule:* 250 mg; *Tab:* 500 mg; *Liq:* 125, 250 mg/5 ml (100 ml)

Comment: *erythromycin* may increase INR with concomitant ***warfarin***, as well as increase serum level of ***digoxin***, benzodiazepines and statins.

▷ ***erythromycin ethylsuccinate*** (B)(G) 400 mg qid x 10 days
Pediatric: 30-50 mg/kg/day in 4 divided doses x 10 days; may double dose with severe infection; max 100 mg/kg/day; *see page 563 for dose by weight*
    EryPed *Oral susp:* 200 mg/5 ml (100, 200 ml) (fruit); 400 mg/5 ml (60, 100, 200 ml) (banana); *Oral drops:* 200, 400 mg/5 ml (50 ml) (fruit); *Chew tab:* 200 mg wafer (fruit)
    E.E.S. *Oral susp:* 200, 400 mg/5 ml (100 ml) (fruit)
    E.E.S. Granules *Oral susp:* 200 mg/5 ml (100, 200 ml) (cherry)
    E.E.S. 400 Tablets *Tab:* 400 mg

Comment: *erythromycin* may increase INR with concomitant ***warfarin***, as well as increase serum level of ***digoxin***, benzodiazepines and statins.

▷ ***gemifloxacin*** (C) 320 mg once daily x 5-7 days
Pediatric: <18 years: not recommended
    Factive *Tab:* 320*mg

Comment: ***gemifloxacin*** is contraindicated <18 years-of-age, and during pregnancy and lactation. Risk of tendonitis or tendon rupture, especially 60 years-of-age and older.

▷ ***levofloxacin*** (C) *Uncomplicated:* 500 mg once daily x 7-10 days; *Complicated:* 750 mg once daily x 7-10 days
Pediatric: <18 years: not recommended
    Levaquin *Tab:* 250, 500, 750 mg; *Oral soln:* 25 mg/ml (480 ml) (benzyl alcohol); *Inj conc:* 25 mg/ml for IV infusion after dilution (20, 30 ml single-use vial) (preservative-free); *Premix soln:* 5 mg/ml for IV infusion (50, 100, 150 ml) (preservative-free)

Comment: *levofloxacin* is contraindicated <18 years-of-age, and during pregnancy and lactation. Risk of tendonitis or tendon rupture, especially 60 years-of-age and older.

▷ ***linezolid*** (C)(G) 400-600 mg q 12 hours x 10-14 days
Pediatric: <5 years: 10 mg/kg q 8 hours x 10-14 days; 5-11 years: 10 mg/kg q 12 hours x 10-14 days; >11 years: same as adult
    Zyvox *Tab:* 400, 600 mg; *Oral susp:* 100 mg/5 ml (150 ml) (orange) (phenylalanine)

Comment: *linezolid* is indicated to treat susceptible vancomycin-resistant *E. faecium* infections.

▷ ***loracarbef*** (B) 200 mg bid x 7 days
Pediatric: 15 mg/kg/day in 2 divided doses x 7 days; *see page 570 for dose by weight*
    Lorabid *Pulvule:* 200, 400 mg; *Oral susp:* 100 mg/5 ml (50, 100 ml); 200 mg/5 ml (50, 75, 100 ml) (strawberry bubble gum)

▷ ***minocycline*** (D)(G) 200 mg on first day; then 100 mg q 12 hours x 9 more days
Pediatric: <8 years: not recommended; ≥8 years, <100 lb: 2 mg/lb on first day in 2 divided doses, followed by 1 mg/lb q 12 hours x 9 more days; ≥8 years, >100 lb: same as adult
    Dynacin *Cap:* 50, 100 mg
    Minocin *Cap:* 50, 75, 100 mg; *Oral susp:* 50 mg/5 ml (60 ml) (custard) (sulfites, alcohol 5%)

Comment: *minocycline* is contraindicated <8 years-of-age, in pregnancy, and lactation (discolors developing tooth enamel). A side effect may be photosensitivity (photophobia). Do not give with antacids, calcium supplements, milk or other dairy, or within two hours of taking another drug.

▷ *moxifloxacin* (C)(G) 400 mg once daily x 10 days
  Pediatric: <18 years: not recommended
    Avelox *Tab:* 400 mg
  Comment: *moxifloxacin* is contraindicated <18 years-of-age, and during pregnancy and lactation. Risk of tendonitis or tendon rupture, especially 60 years-of-age and older.
▷ *ofloxacin* (C)(G) 400 mg bid x 10 days
  Pediatric: <18 years: not recommended
    Floxin *Tab:* 200, 300, 400 mg
  Comment: *ofloxacin* is contraindicated <18 years-of-age, and during pregnancy and lactation. Risk of tendonitis or tendon rupture, especially 60 years-of-age and older.
▷ *tetracycline* (D)(G) 500 mg qid x 10 days
  Pediatric: <8 years: not recommended; ≥8 years, <100 lb: 25-50 mg/kg/day in 4 divided doses x 10 days; ≥8 years, >100 lb: same as adult; *see page 574 for dose by weight*
    Achromycin V *Cap:* 250, 500 mg
    Sumycin *Tab:* 250, 500 mg; *Cap:* 250, 500 mg; *Oral susp:* 125 mg/5 ml (100, 200 ml) (fruit) (sulfites)
  Comment: *tetracycline* is contraindicated <8 years-of-age, in pregnancy, and lactation (discolors developing tooth enamel). A side effect may be photo-sensitivity (photophobia). Do not give with antacids, calcium supplements, milk or other dairy, or within two hours of taking another drug.

 ## SLEEP APNEA (HYPOPNEA SYNDROME)

ANTI-NARCOLEPTIC AGENTS

▷ *armodafinil* (C)(IV) *OSAHS:* 150-250 mg once daily in the AM; *SWSD:* 150 mg 1 hour before starting shift; reduce dose with severe hepatic impairment hepatic impairment
  Pediatric: <17 years: not recommended
    Nuvigil *Tab:* 50, 150, 200, 250 mg
▷ *modafinil* (C)(IV) 100-200 mg q AM; max 400 mg/day
  Pediatric: <16 years: not recommended; ≥16 years: same as adult
    Provigil *Tab:* 100, 200*mg
  Comment: *modafinil* promotes wakefulness in patients with excessive sleepiness due to obstructive sleep apnea/hypopnea syndrome.

SLEEPINESS: EXCESSIVE/SHIFT WORK SLEEP DISORDER (SWSD)

ANTI-NARCOLEPTIC AGENT

▷ *armodafinil* (C)(IV) *OSAHS:* 150-250 mg once daily in the AM; *SWSD:* 150 mg 1 hour before starting shift; reduce dose with severe hepatic impairment hepatic impairment
  Pediatric: <17 years: not recommended
    Nuvigil *Tab:* 50, 150, 200, 250 mg

▷ *modafinil* (C)(IV) 100-200 mg q AM; max 400 mg/day
  Pediatric: <16 years: not recommended; ≥16 years: same as adult
    Provigil *Tab:* 100, 200*mg
    Comment: **Provigil** promotes wakefulness in patients with narcolepsy, shift work sleep disorder, and excessive sleepiness due to obstructive sleep apnea/hypopnea syndrome.

◯ SMALLPOX (VARIOLA MAJOR)

PROPHYLAXIS

▷ *vaccina virus* vaccine *(dried, calf lymph type)* (C)
  Pediatric: <12 months: not recommended; 12 months-18 years, non-emergency: not recommended
    DRYvax
      Kit: vial dried smallpox vaccine (1), 0.25 ml diluent in syringe (1), vented needle (1), 100 individually wrapped bifurcated needles (5 needles/strip, 20 strips) (polymyxin B sulfate, dihydrostreptomycin sulfate, chlortetracycline HCL, neomycin sulfate, glycerin, phenol)
    Comment: **DRYvax** is a dried live vaccine with approximately 100 million *Infectious vaccina* viruses (pock-forming units [pfu] per ml). Contact with immunosuppressed individuals should be avoided until the scab has separated from the skin (2 to 3 weeks) and/or a protective occlusive dressing covers the inoculation site. Scarification only. Do not inject IV, IM, or SC. Revaccination is recommended every 10 years.

◯ SPRAIN

Comment: RICE: Rest; Ice; Compression; Elevation.
Injectable Acetaminophen *see Pain page* 296
Oral Prescription NSAIDs *see page* 489
Other Oral Analgesics *see Pain page* 298
Topical/Transdermal NSAIDs *see Pain page* 297
Parenteral Corticosteroids *see page* 499
Oral Corticosteroids *see page* 497
Topical Analgesic and Anesthetic Agents *see page* 487

◯ STATUS ASTHMATICUS

Inhaled Beta-Agonists (Bronchodilators) *see Asthma page* 32
Oral Beta-Agonists (Bronchodilators) *see Asthma page* 35
Inhaled Anticholinergics *see Asthma page* 29
Inhaled Anticholinergic/Beta-Agonist Combination *see Asthma page* 33
Methylxanthines *see Asthma page* 36
Parenteral Corticosteroids *see page* 499
Oral Corticosteroids *see page* 497

EPINEPHRINE

▷ *epinephrine* (C)(G) 0.3-0.5 mg (0.3-0.5 ml of a 1:1000 soln) SC q 20-30 minutes as needed up to 3 doses
   Pediatric: <2 years: 0.05-0.1 ml; 2-6 years: 0.1 ml; 6-12 years: 0.2 ml; All: q 20-30 minutes as needed up to 3 doses; >12 years: same as adult

ANAPHYLAXIS EMERGENCY TREATMENT KITS

▷ *epinephrine* (C) 0.3 ml IM or SC in thigh; may repeat if needed
   Pediatric: 0.01 mg/kg SC or IM in thigh; may repeat if needed; <15 kg: not recommended; 15-30 kg: 0.15 mg; >30 kg: same as adult
      AdrenaClick *Auto-injector:* 0.15, 0.3 mg (1 mg/ml; 2/carton) (sulfites)
      Auvi-Q *Auto-injector:* 0.15, 0.3 mg (1 mg/ml; 2/carton w. 1 nonactive training device) (sulfites)
      EpiPen *Autoinjector 0.3 mg* (*epi* 1:1000, 0.3 ml (2/carton) (sulfites)
      EpiPen Jr *Autoinjector 0.15 mg* (*epi* 1:2000, 0.3 ml (2/carton) (sulfites)
      Twinject *Autoinjector: 0.15, 0.3 mg* (epi 1:1000, 2/carton) (sulfites)
▷ *epinephrine/chlorpheniramine* (C) epinephrine 0.3 ml SC or IM plus 4 tabs *chlorpheniramine* by mouth
   Pediatric: infants-2 years: 0.05-0.1 ml SC or IM; 2-6 years: 0.15 ml SC or IM plus 1 tab *chlor;* 6-12 years: 0.2 ml SC or IM plus 2 tabs *chlor;* >12 years: same as adult
      Ana-Kit: 0.3 ml syringes of *epi* 1:1000 (2/carton) for self-injection plus *chlor* 2 mg chewable tabs x 4

◯ STATUS EPILEPTICUS

Anticonvulsant Drugs *see page 508*
▷ *diazepam* injectable (D)(IV) initially 5-10 mg IV in large vein; may repeat q 10-15 minutes; max 30 mg; may repeat in 2-4 hours if needed; do not dilute; may give IM if IV not accessible
   Pediatric: 1 month-5 years: 0.2-0.5 mg IV q 2-5 minutes; max 5 mg; >5 years: 1 mg IV q 2-5 minutes; max 10 mg; may repeat in 2-4 hours if needed
      Diastat *Rectal gel delivery system:* 2.5 mg
      Diastat AcuDial *Rectal gel delivery system:* 10, 20 mg
      Valium Injectable *Vial:* 5 mg/ml (10 ml); *Amp:* 5 mg/ml (2 ml); *Prefilled syringe:* 5 mg/ml (5 ml)
      Valium Intensol *Conc oral soln:* 5 mg/ml (30 ml w. dropper) (alcohol 19%)
      Valium Oral Solution *Oral soln:* 5 mg/5 ml (500 ml) (wintergreen-spice)
▷ *lorazepam* injectable (D)(IV) 4 mg IV over 2 minutes (dilute first); may repeat in 10-15 minutes; may give IM if needed (undiluted)
   Pediatric: <18 years: not recommended
      Ativan Injectable *Vial:* 2 mg/ml (1, 10 ml); *Tubex:* 2 mg/ml (0.5 ml); *Cartridge:* 2, 4 mg/ml (1 ml)
▷ *phenytoin (injectable)* (D)(G) 10-15 mg/kg IV, not to exceed 50 mg/ minute; follow with 100 mg orally or IV q 6-8 hours; do not dilute in IV fluid
   Pediatric: 15-20 mg/kg IV, not to exceed 1-2 mg/kg/minute
      Dilantin *Vial:* 50 mg/ml (2, 5 ml); *Amp:* 50 mg/ml (2 ml)
   Comment: Monitor *phenytoin* serum levels. Therapeutic serum level: 10-20 g/ml. Side effects include gingival hyperplasia.

STYE (HORDEOLUM)

OPHTHALMIC ANTI-INFECTIVES

➤ *erythromycin* ophthalmic ointment (B) 1 cm up to 6 times/day
  Pediatric: same as adult
    Ilotycin Ophthalmic Ointment *Ophth oint:* 5 mg/g (1/8 oz)
➤ *erythromycin* ophthalmic solution (B) initially 1-2 drops q 1-2 hours; may then increase dose interval
  Pediatric: same as adult
    Isopto Cetamide Ophthalmic Solution *Ophth soln:* 15% (15 ml)
➤ *gentamicin* ophthalmic ointment (C) 1 cm bid-tid
  Pediatric: same as adult
    Garamycin Ophthalmic Ointment *Ophth oint:* 3 mg/g (3.5 g)
    Genoptic Ophthalmic Ointment *Ophth oint:* 3 mg/g (3.5 g)
    Gentacidin Ophthalmic Ointment *Ophth oint:* 3 mg/g (3.5 g)
➤ *polymyxin B/bacitracin* ophthalmic ointment (C) apply 1/2 inch q 3-4 hours
  Pediatric: same as adult
    Polysporin *Ophth oint:* poly 10,000 U/bac 500 units per g (3.75 g)
➤ *polymyxin B/bacitracin/neomycin* ophthalmic ointment (C)(G) apply 1/2 inch q 3-4 hours
  Pediatric: same as adult
    Neosporin Ophthalmic Ointment *Ophth oint:* poly B 10,000 U/bac 400 U/
    neo 3.5 mg/g (3.75 g)
➤ *polymyxin B/neomycin/gramicidin* ophthalmic solution (C) 1-2 drops 2-3 times q 1 hour; then 1-2 drops bid-qid x 7-10 days
  Pediatric: same as adult
    Neosporin Ophthalmic Solution
      Ophth soln: poly 10,000 U/neo 1.75 mg/gram 0.025 mg/ml (10 ml)
➤ *sodium sulfacetamide* ophthalmic solution and ointment (C)
    Bleph-10 Ophthalmic Solution 2 drops q 4 hour x 7-14 days
      Pediatric: <2 years: not recommended; ≥2 years: 1-2 drops q 2-3 hours
      during the day
      Ophth soln: 10% (2.5, 5, 15 ml; benzalkonium chloride)
    Bleph-10 Ophthalmic Ointment apply 1/2 inch qid and HS
      Pediatric: <2 years: not recommended; ≥2 years: apply 1/4-1/3 inch qid and HS
      Ophth oint: 10% (3.5 g) (phenylmercuric acetate)

SUNBURN

➤ *prednisone* (C)(G) 10 mg qid x 4-6 days if severe and extensive
➤ *silver sulfadiazine* (C)(G) apply topically to burn once daily-bid
  Pediatric: not recommended
    Silvadene *Crm:* 1% (20, 50, 85, 400, 1000 g jar; 20 g tube)

SYPHILIS (*TREPONEMA PALLIDUM*)

Comment: The following treatment regimens for *T. pallidum* are published in the **2015 CDC Sexually Transmitted Diseases Treatment Guidelines**. Treat all sexual contacts.

Consider testing for other STDs. *Penicillin G*, administered parenterally, is the preferred drug for treating all stages of syphilis. The preparation used (i.e., benzathine, aqueous procaine, or aqueous crystalline), the dosage, and the length of treatment depend on the stage and clinical manifestations of the disease. Combinations of *benzathine penicillin*, *procaine penicillin*, and oral penicillin preparations are not appropriate (e.g., **Bicillin C-R**). All women should be screened serologically for syphilis early in pregnancy. There are no proven alternatives to penicillin for the treatment of syphilis during pregnancy. Pregnant patients who are allergic to penicillin should be desensitized and treated with *penicillin*. Sexual transmission of *T. pallidum* is thought to occur only when mucotaneous syphilis at any stage should be evaluated clinically and serologically and treated with a recommended regimen according to CDC guidelines.

PRIMARY, SECONDARY, AND EARLY LATENT (<1 YEAR) SYPHILIS

Regimen 1

▷ *penicillin G (benzathine)* 2.4 million units IM in a single dose

LATE LATENT, LATENT SYPHILIS OF UNKNOWN DURATION, AND TERTIARY SYPHILIS

Regimen 1

▷ *penicillin G (benzathine)* 7.2 million units total administered in 3 divided doses of 2.4 million units each IM at 1 week intervals

REGIMEN: ADULT, NEUROSYPHILIS

Regimen 1

▷ *aqueous crystalline penicillin G* 18-24 million units per day, administered as 3-4 million units IV every 4 hours or continuous IV infusion, for 10-14 days

ALTERNATIVE REGIMEN: ADULT, NEUROSYPHILIS

Regimen 1

▷ *penicillin G (procaine)* 2.4 million units IM once daily x 10-14 days plus *probenecid* 500 mg qid x 10-14 days

PRIMARY AND SECONDARY SYPHILIS IN HIV-INFECTED PERSONS

Regimen 1

▷ *penicillin G (benzathine)* 2.4 million units IM in a single dose

LATENT SYPHILIS AMONG HIV-INFECTED PERSONS

Comment: Treatment is the same as for HIV-negative persons.

CONGENITAL SYPHILIS

Regimen 1

▷ *aqueous crystalline penicillin G* 100,000-150,000 units/kg/day, administered as 50,000 units IV every 12 hours during the first 7 days of life and every 8 hours thereafter for a total of 10 days

ALTERNATE REGIMEN

Regimen 1

▷ *penicillin G (benzathine)* 50,000 units/kg IM in a single dose

Regimen 2

▷ *penicillin G (procaine)* 50,000 units/kg/dose IM, administered in a single daily dose x 10 days

OLDER INFANTS AND CHILDREN

Regimen 1

▷ *aqueous crystalline penicillin G* 200,000-300,000 units/kg/day, administered as 50,000 units IV every 12 hours during the first 7 days of life and every 4-6 hours thereafter for a total of 10 days

DRUG BRANDS AND DOSE FORMS

▷ *aqueous crystalline penicillin G* (B)(G)
▷ *penicillin G (benzathine)* (B)(G)
   Bicillin L-A *Cartridge-needle unit:* 600,000 million units (1 ml); 1.2 million units (2 ml); 2.4 million units (4 ml)
▷ *penicillin G (procaine)* (B)(G)
   Bicillin C-R Cartridge-needle unit: 600,000 units (1 ml); 1.2 mill- ion units; (2 ml); 2.4 million units (4 ml)
▷ *probenecid* (B)(G)
   Benemid *Tab:* 500*mg; *Cap:* 500 mg

 TEMPORAL ARTERITIS

Parenteral Corticosteroids *see page* 499
Oral Corticosteroids *see page* 497

 TEMPOROMANDIBULAR JOINT (TMJ) DISORDER

Injectable Acetaminophen *see Pain page* 296
Oral Prescription NSAIDs *see page* 489
Other Oral Analgesics see *Pain page* 298
Topical/Transdermal NSAIDs *see Pain page* 297
Parenteral Corticosteroids *see page* 499
Oral Corticosteroids *see page* 497
Topical Analgesic and Anesthetic Agents *see page* 487

 TESTOSTERONE DEFICIENCY, HYPOTESTOSTERONEMIA, HYPOGONADISM

Comment: *testosterone* is contraindicated in male breast cancer and prostate cancer. *testosterone* replacement therapy is indicated in males with primary hypogonadism

(congenital or acquired due to cryptorchidism, bilateral torsion, orchitis, vanishing testis syndrome, or orchidectomy), or hypogonadotropic hypogonadism (congenital or acquired), and delayed puberty not secondary to a pathological disorder (x-ray of the hand and wrist to determine bone age should be obtained every 6 months to assess the effect of treatment on the epiphyseal centers).

ORAL ANDROGENS

▷ *fluoxymesterone* (X)(III) *Hypogonadism:* 5-20 mg once daily; *Delayed puberty:* use low dose and limit duration to 4-6 months
Pediatric: use by specialist only
Halotestin *Tab:* 2*, 5*, 10*mg (tartrazine)

▷ *methyltestosterone* (X)(III) usually 10-50 mg once daily; for delayed puberty, use low dose and limit duration to 4-6 months
Android *Cap:* 10 mg
Methitest *Tab:* 10*mg
Testred *Cap:* 10 mg

▷ *testosterone* (X)(III) 30 mg q 12 hours to gum region, just above the incisor tooth on either side of the mouth; hold system in place for 30 seconds; rotate sites with each application
Striant *Buccal tab:* 30 mg (6 blister pks; 10 buccal systems/blister pck)
Comment: Serum total *testosterone* concentrations may be checked 4 to 12 weeks after initiating treatment with **Striant**. To capture the maximum serum concentration, an early morning sample (just prior to applying the AM dose) is recommended.

TOPICAL ANDROGENS

Comment: Wash hands after application. Allow solution to dry before it touches clothing. Do not wash site for at least 2 hours after application. Pregnant and nursing women, and children, must avoid skin contact with application sites on men. If there is contact, wash the area as soon as possible with soap and water.

▷ *testosterone* (X)(III)
Pediatric: <18 years: not recommended
AndroGel 1% initially apply 5 g once daily in the AM to clean, dry, intact skin of the shoulders, upper arms, and/or abdomen; do not apply to scrotum; may increase to 7.5 g/day and then to 10 g/day if needed
Gel: 2.5, 5 g (30 pkts); 75 g (60 metered 1.25 g doses)
AndroGel 1.62% initially apply 2.5 g (2 pump actuations) once daily in the AM to clean, dry, skin of the shoulders and upper arms intact skin of the upper arms; do not apply to abdomen or genitals; may adjust dose between 1 and 4 pump actuations based on the pre-dose morning serum testosterone concentration at approximately 14 and 28 days after starting treatment or adjusting dose
Gel: 2.25 mg pump actuation (75 g, 60 metered 1.25 g doses)
Axiron apply to clean dry intact skin of the axillae; do not apply to the scrotum, penis, abdomen, shoulders, or upper arms; initially apply 60 mg (30 mg/axilla) once daily in the AM; adjust dose based on serum testosterone concentration 2 to 8 hours after applying and at least 14 days after starting therapy or following dose adjustment; may increase dose in 30 mg increments if serum testosterone <300 ng/dL up to 120 mg; reduce dose to 30 mg if levels >1050 ng/dL; discontinue if serum testosterone remains at >1050 ng/dL

Soln: 30 mg/1.5 ml pump actuation (90 ml; 60 metered actuations) (alcohol, latex-free)

Fortesta (G) initially 40 mg of testosterone (4 pump actuations) applied to the thighs once daily in the AM; may adjust between 10 mg minimum and 70 mg maximum.

Gel: 10 mg/0.5 g pump actuation (120 actuations)

Comment: The **Fortesta** dose should be based on the serum *testosterone* concentration 2 hours after applying **Fortesta** and at approximately 14 days and 35 days after starting treatment or following dose adjustment. Dose adjustment criteria: ≤500 ng/dL, increase daily dose by 10 mg; 500-≤1250 ng/dL, no change; 1250-≤2500 ng/dL, decrease daily dose by 10 mg; ≥2500 ng/dL, decrease daily dose by 20 mg.

Gel: 10 mg (0.5 g)/pump actuation (60 g; 120 metered dose actuations) (ethanol)

Testim (G) initially apply 5 g once daily in the AM to clean, dry, intact skin of the shoulders and/or upper arms; do not apply to the genitals or abdomen; may increase to 10 g after 2 weeks

Gel: 1%, clear, hydroalcoholic (5 mg/5 g, 5 single-use tube)

Vogelxo Gel (G) 1% initially apply 5 g once daily in the AM to clean, dry, intact skin of the shoulders, upper arms, and/or abdomen; do not apply to scrotum; may increase to 7.5 g/day and then to 10 g/day if needed

Gel: 5 g/pkt (30 pkts); 5 g/tube (30 tubes); metered dose pumps (2 x 75 g, 1.25 g actuation)

INTRANASAL ANDROGENS

▷ *testosterone (nasal gel)* **(X)(III)** initially one pump actuation each nostril (33 mg) 3x/day, at least 6-8 hours apart, at the same times each day max: 6 pump actuation/day
Pediatric: <18 years: not established

    Natesto

    Gel: 5.5 mg/actuation, metered dose pump (11 g, 60 actuations)

TRANSDERMAL ANDROGEN

▷ *testosterone* **(X)(III)**
    Androderm initially apply 4 mg nightly at approximately 10 PM to clean, dry area of the arm, back, or upper buttocks; leave on x 24 hours; may increase to 7.5 mg or decrease to 2.5 mg based on confirmed AM serum testosterone concentrations
    Pediatric: <15 years: not recommended
    Transdermal patch: 2, 4 mg/24hr

 TETANUS

PROPHYLAXIS

see **Childhood Immunizations** *page 466*

POSTEXPOSURE PROPHYLAXIS IN PREVIOUSLY NONIMMUNIZED PERSONS

▷ *tetanus immune globulin, human* **(C)** 250 mg deep IM in a single dose

Pediatric: >7 years: same as adult
> **BayTET, Hyper-TET**
> > *Vial:* 250 units single dose; *Prefilled syringe:* 250 units
▷ *tetanus toxoid* **vaccine (C)** 0.5 ml IM x 3 dose series
> > *Vial:* 5 Lf units/0.5 ml (0.5, 5 ml); *Prefilled syringe:* 5 Lf units/0.5 ml (0.5 ml)

Comment: Dose of **BayTET/HyperTET** S/D is calculated as 4 units/kg. However, it may be advisable to administer the entire contents of the syringe of **BayTET/ HyperTET** S/D (250 units) regardless of the child's size, since theoretically the same amount of toxin will be produced in the child's body by the infecting tetanus organism as it will in an adult's body. At the same time but in a different extremity and with a different syringe, administer Diphtheria and Tetanus Toxoids and Pertussis Vaccine Adsorbed (DTP) or Diphtheria and Tetanus Toxoids Adsorbed (For Pediatric Use) (DT), if pertussis vaccine is contraindicated, should be administered per mfr package insert. Tetanus Immune globulin may interact with live viral vaccines such as measles, mumps, rubella, and polio. It is also unknown if **BayTET/HyperTET** can cause fetal harm when administered to a pregnant woman or can affect reproduction capacity. The single injection of tetanus toxoid only initiates the series for producing active immunity in the recipient. Impress upon the patient the need for further toxoid injections in 1 month and 1 year, otherwise the active immunization series is incomplete. If a contraindication to using tetanus toxoid-containing preparations exists for a person who has not completed a primary series of tetanus toxoid immunization, and that person has a wound that is neither clean nor minor, only passive immunization should be given using tetanus immune globulin.

⬤ THREADWORM (STRONGYLOIDIASIS)

ANTIHELMINTICS

▷ *albendazole* **(C)** 400 mg bid x 7 days; take after a meal
> *Pediatric:* <2 years: 200 mg once daily x 3 days; may repeat in 3 weeks; ≥2-12 years: 400 mg once daily x 3 days; may repeat in 3 weeks; >12 years: same as adult
> > **Albenza** *Tab:* 200 mg
▷ *mebendazole* **(C)(G)** 100 mg bid x 3 days; may repeat in 2-3 weeks if needed; take after a meal
> *Pediatric:* same as adult (chew or crush and mix with food)
> > **Vermox** *Chew Tab:* 100 mg
▷ *pyrantel pamoate* **(C)** 11 mg/kg x 1 dose; max 1 g/dose; take after a meal
> *Pediatric:* 25-37 lb: 1/2 tsp x 1 dose; 38-62 lb: 1 tsp x 1 dose; 63-87 lb: 1 tsp x 1 dose; 88-112 lb: 2 tsp x 1 dose; 113-137 lb: 2 tsp x 1 dose; 138-162 lb: 3 tsp x 1 dose; 163-187 lb: 3 tsp x 1 dose; >187 lb: 4 tsp x 1 dose
> > **Pin-X (OTC)** *Cap:* 180 mg; *Liq:* 50 mg/ml (30 ml); 144 mg/ml (30 ml); *Oral susp:* 50 mg/ml (30 ml)
▷ *thiabendazole* **(C)** 25 mg/kg dosed bid x 7 days; max 1.5 g/dose; take with meals
> *Pediatric:* same as adult; <30 lb: consult mfr literature; >30 lb: 25 mg/kg/dose bid with meals; 30-50 lb: 250 mg bid with meals; >50 lb: 10 mg/lb/dose bid with meals; max 3g/day Mintezol *Chew tab:* 500*mg (orange); *Oral susp:* 500 mg/5 ml (120 ml) (orange)

Comment: *thiabendazole* is not for prophylaxis. May impair mental alertness.

⬤ TINEA CAPITIS

Comment: Tinea capitis must be treated with an oral anti-fungal.

FOR SEVERE KERION PRURITUS

▷ *prednisone* (C) 1 mg/kg/day for 7-14 days
see **Oral Corticosteroids** *page* 497

SYSTEMIC ANTI-FUNGALS

▷ *griseofulvin, microsize* (C)(G) 500 mg once daily x 4-6 weeks <u>or</u> longer; max 1 g/day
Pediatric: <30 lb: 5 mg/lb/day; 30-50 lb: 125-250 mg/day; >50 lb: 250-500 mg/day;
5 mg/lb/day x 4-6 weeks <u>or</u> longer; *see page* 568 *for dose by weight*
    Grifulvin V *Tab:* 250, 500 mg; *Oral susp:* 125 mg/5 ml (120 ml; alcohol 0.02%)
▷ *griseofulvin, ultramicrosize* (C)(G) 375 mg/day in a single <u>or</u> divided doses x 4-6
weeks <u>or</u> longer
Pediatric: <2 years: not recommended; ≥2 years: 3.3 mg/lb/day in a single <u>or</u> divided
doses x 4-6 weeks <u>or</u> longer
    Gris-PEG *Tab:* 125, 250 mg
Comment: *griseofulvin* should be taken with fatty foods (e.g., milk, ice cream).
Liver enzymes should be monitored.
▷ *ketoconazole* (C)(G) initially 200 mg once daily; max 400 mg/day x 4 weeks
Pediatric: <2 years: not recommended; ≥2 years: 3.3-6.6 mg/kg once daily x 4 weeks
    Nizoral *Tab:* 200 mg
Comment: Caution with *ketoconazole* due to concerns about potential for
hepatotoxicity.

⬤ TINEA CORPORIS (RINGWORM)

TOPICAL ANTI-FUNGALS

▷ *butenafine* (C)(G) apply bid x 1 week <u>or</u> once daily x 4 weeks
Pediatric: <12 years: not recommended; ≥12 years: same as adult
    Lotrimin Ultra (OTC) *Crm:* 1% (12, 24 g)
    Mentax *Crm:* 1% (15, 30 g)
Comment: *butenafine* is a benzylamine, not an azole. Fungicidal activity continues
for at least 5 weeks after last application.
▷ *ciclopirox* (B)
    Loprox Cream apply bid; max 4 weeks
      Pediatric: <10 years: not recommended; ≥10 years: same as adult
      Crm: 0.77% (15, 30, 90 g)
    Loprox Lotion apply bid; max 4 weeks
      Pediatric: <10 years: not recommended; ≥10 years: same as adult
      Lotn: 0.77% (30, 60 ml)
    Loprox Gel apply bid; max 4 weeks
      Pediatric: <16 years: not recommended
      Gel: 0.77% (30, 45 g)
▷ *clotrimazole* (B)(G) apply to affected area bid x 7 days
Pediatric: same as adult
    Lotrimin *Crm:* 1% (15, 30, 45 g)

> **Lotrimin AF (OTC)** *Crm:* 1% (12 g); *Lotn:* 1% (10 ml); *Soln:* 1% (10 ml)
> ► *econazole* (C) apply once daily x 14 days
>> *Pediatric:* same as adult
>>> **Spectazole** *Crm:* 1% (15, 30, 85 g)
> ► *ketoconazole* (C) apply once daily x 14 days
>> *Pediatric:* not recommended
>>> **Nizoral Cream** *Crm:* 2% (15, 30, 60 g)
> ► *miconazole* **2%** (C) apply once daily-bid x 2 weeks
>> *Pediatric:* same as adult
>>> **Lotrimin AF Spray Liquid (OTC)** *Spray liq:* 2% (113 g) (alcohol 17%)
>>> **Lotrimin AF Spray Powder (OTC)** *Spray pwdr:* 2% (90 g) (alcohol 10%)
>>> **Monistat-Derm** *Crm:* 2% (1, 3 oz); *Spray liq:* 2% (3.5 oz); *Spray pwdr:* 2% (3 oz)
> ► *naftifine* (B)
>> *Pediatric:* not recommended
>>> **Naftin Cream** apply once daily x 14 days
>>>> *Crm:* 1% (15, 30, 60 g)
>>> **Naftin Gel** apply bid x 14 days
>>>> *Gel:* 1% (20, 40, 60 g)
> ► *oxiconazole nitrate* (B) apply once daily-bid x 2 weeks
>> *Pediatric:* same as adult
>>> **Oxistat** *Crm:* 1% (15, 30, 60 g); *Lotn:* 1% (30 ml)
> ► *sulconazole* (C) apply once daily-bid x 3 weeks
>> *Pediatric:* not recommended
>>> **Exelderm** *Crm:* 1% (15, 30, 60 g); *Lotn:* 1% (30 mg)
> ► *terbinafine* (B)(G)
>> *Pediatric:* <12 years: not recommended
>>> **Lamisil Cream (OTC)** apply to affected and surrounding area once daily-bid x 1-4 weeks until significantly improved
>>>> *Crm:* 1% (15, 30 g)
>>> **Lamisil AT Cream (OTC)** apply to affected and surrounding area once daily-bid x 1-4 weeks until significantly improved
>>>> *Crm:* **1% (15, 30 g)**
>>> **Lamisil Solution (OTC)** apply to affected and surrounding area once daily x 1 week
>>>> *Soln:* 1% (30 ml spray bottle)

TOPICAL ANTIFUNGAL/STEROID COMBINATION

> ► *clotrimazole/betamethasone* (C)(G) apply bid x 2 weeks; max 4 weeks
>> *Pediatric:* <12 years: not recommended; >12 years: same as adult
>>> **Lotrisone** *Crm:* clotrim 1 mg/*beta* 0.5 mg (15, 45 g); *Lotn:* clotrim 1 mg/*beta* 0.5 mg (30 ml)

SYSTEMIC ANTIFUNGALS

> ► *griseofulvin, microsize* (C)(G) 500 mg/day x 2-4 weeks; max 1 g/day
>> *Pediatric:* <30 lb: 5 mg/lb/day; 30-50 lb: 125-250 mg/day; >50 lb: 250-500 mg/day; *see page 568 for dose by weight*
>>> **Grifulvin V** *Tab:* 250, 500 mg; *Oral susp:* 125 mg/5 ml (120 ml) (alcohol 0.02%)
> ► *griseofulvin, ultramicrosize* (C)(G) 375 mg/day in a single <u>or</u> divided doses x 2-4 weeks
>> *Pediatric:* <2 years: not recommended; ≥2 years: 3.3 mg/lb/day in a single <u>or</u> divided doses

Gris-PEG *Tab:* 125, 250

Comment: *griseofulvin* should be taken with fatty foods (e.g., milk, ice cream). Liver enzymes should be monitored.

➤ *ketoconazole* (C) initially 200 mg once daily; max 400 mg/day x 4 weeks
   Pediatric: <2 years: not recommended; >2 years: 3.3-6.6 mg/kg/day x 4 weeks
      Nizoral *Tab:* 200 mg

Comment: Caution with *ketoconazole* due to concerns about potential for hepatotoxicity.

◯ TINEA CRURIS (JOCK ITCH)

TOPICAL ANTIFUNGALS

➤ *butenafine* (B)(G) apply bid x 1 week <u>or</u> once daily x 4 weeks
   Pediatric: <12 years: not recommended; ≥12 years: same as adult
      Lotrimin Ultra (C)(OTC) *Crm:* 1% (12, 24 g)
      Mentax *Crm:* 1% (15, 30 g)

Comment: *butenafine* is a benzylamine, not an azole. Fungicidal activity continues for at least 5 weeks after last application.

➤ *ciclopirox* (B)
      Loprox Cream apply bid; max 4 weeks
         Pediatric: <10 years: not recommended; ≥10 years: same as adult
         Crm: 0.77% (15, 30, 90 g)
      Loprox Lotion apply bid; max 4 weeks
         Pediatric: <10 years: not recommended; ≥10 years: same as adult
         Lotn: 0.77% (30, 60 ml)
      Loprox Gel apply bid; max 4 weeks
         Pediatric: <16 years: not recommended; ≥16 years: same as adult
         Gel: 0.77% (30, 45 g)

➤ *clotrimazole* (B)(G) apply to affected area bid x 7 days
   Pediatric: same as adult
      Lotrimin *Crm:* 1% (15, 30, 45 g)
      Lotrimin AF (OTC) *Crm:* 1% (12 g); *Lotn:* 1% (10 ml); *Soln:* 1% (10 ml)

➤ *econazole* (C) apply once daily x 2 weeks
   Pediatric: same as adult
      Spectazole *Crm:* 1% (15, 30, 85 g)

➤ *ketoconazole* (C)(G) apply bid x 4 weeks
   Pediatric: not recommended
      Nizoral Cream *Crm:* 2% (15, 30, 60 g)

➤ *miconazole* **2%** (C)(G) apply once daily-bid x 2 weeks
   Pediatric: same as adult
      Lotrimin AF Spray Liquid (OTC) *Spray liq:* 2% (113 g) (alcohol 17%)
      Lotrimin AF Spray Powder (OTC) *Spray pwdr:* 2% (90 g) (alcohol 10%)
      Monistat-Derm *Crm:* 2% (1, 3 oz); *Spray liq:* 2% (3.5 oz); *Spray pwdr:* 2% (3 oz)

➤ *naftifine* (B)
   Pediatric: not recommended
      Naftin Cream apply once daily x 2 weeks
         Crm: 1% (15, 30, 60 g)
      Naftin Gel apply bid x 2 weeks
         Gel: 1% (20, 40, 60 g)

▷ *oxiconazole nitrate* (B) apply once daily-bid x 2 weeks
 Pediatric: same as adult
  Oxistat *Crm:* 1% (15, 30, 60 g); *Lotn:* 1% (30 ml)
▷ *sulconazole* (C) apply once daily-bid x 3 weeks
 Pediatric: not recommended
  Exelderm *Crm:* 1% (15, 30, 60 g); *Lotn:* 1% (30 mg)
▷ *terbinafine* (B)(G)
 Pediatric: <12 years: not recommended; ≥12 years: same as adult
  Lamisil Cream (OTC) apply bid x 1-4 weeks
   Crm: 1% (15, 30 g)
  Lamisil AT Cream (OTC) apply to affected and surrounding area once daily-bid
  x 1-4 weeks until significantly improved
   Crm: 1% (15, 30 g)
  Lamisil Solution (OTC) apply to affected and surrounding area once daily x 1 week
   Soln: 1% (30 ml spray bottle)
▷ *tolnaftate* (C)(OTC)(G) apply sparingly bid x 2-4 weeks
 Pediatric: <2 years: not recommended; ≥2 years: same as adult
  Tinactin *Crm:* 1% (15, 30 g); *Pwdr:* 1% (45, 90 g); *Soln:* 1% (10 ml); *Aerosol liq:* 1% (4 oz); *Aerosol pwdr:* 1% (3.5, 5 oz)
▷ *undecylenate acid* (NR) apply bid x 4 weeks
 Pediatric: same as adult
  Desenex (OTC) *Pwdr:* 25% (1.5, 3 oz); *Spray pwdr:* 25% (2.7 oz); *Oint:* 25% (0.5, 1 oz)

TOPICAL ANTIFUNGAL/ANTI-INFLAMMATORY AGENTS

▷ *clotrimazole/betamethasone* (C)(G) apply bid x 4 weeks; max 4 weeks
 Pediatric: <12 years: not recommended; ≥12 years: same as adult
 Crm: clotrim 10 mg/*beta* 0.5 mg (15, 45 g); *Lotn: clotrim* 10 mg/*beta* 0.5 mg (30 ml)

SYSTEMIC ANTIFUNGALS

▷ *griseofulvin, microsize* (C)(G) 1 g once daily x 2 weeks
 Pediatric: <30 lb: 5 mg/lb/day; 30-50 lb: 125-250 mg/day; >50 lb: 250-500 mg/day;
 5 mg/lb/day x 4-6 weeks or longer; *see page 568 for dose by weight*
  Grifulvin V *Tab:* 250, 500 mg; *Oral susp:* 125 mg/5 ml (120 ml) (alcohol 0.02%)
▷ *griseofulvin, ultramicrosize* (C) 375 mg/day in a single or divided doses x 2 weeks
 Pediatric: <2 years: not recommended; ≥2 years: 3.3 mg/lb/day in a single or divided doses
  Gris-PEG *Tab:* 125, 250 mg
Comment: *griseofulvin* should be taken with fatty foods (e.g., milk, ice cream). Liver
enzymes should be monitored.
▷ *ketoconazole* (C) initially 200 mg once daily; max 400 mg once daily x 4 weeks
 Pediatric: <2 years: not recommended; ≥2 years: 3.3-6.6 mg/kg/day
  Nizoral *Tab:* 200 mg
Comment: Caution with *ketoconazole* due to concerns about potential for
hepatotoxicity.

◯ TINEA PEDIS (ATHLETE'S FOOT)

TOPICAL ANTIFUNGALS

▷ *butenafine* (B)(G) apply bid x 1 week or once daily x 4 weeks
 Pediatric: <12 years: not recommended; ≥12 years: same as adult

       Lotrimin Ultra (C)(OTC) *Crm:* 1% (12, 24 g)

       Mentax *Crm:* 1% (15, 30 g)

Comment: *butenafine* is a benzylamine, not an azole. Fungicidal activity continues for at least 5 weeks after last application.

▷ *Burrows solution* (NR) wet dressings

▷ *ciclopirox* (B)

       Loprox Cream apply bid; max 4 weeks

          Pediatric: <10 years: not recommended; ≥10 years: same as adult

          Crm: 0.77% (15, 30, 90 g)

       Loprox Lotion apply bid; max 4 weeks

          Pediatric: <10 years: not recommended; ≥10 years: same as adult

          Lotn: 0.77% (30, 60 ml)

       Loprox Gel apply bid; max 4 weeks

          Pediatric: <16 years: not recommended; ≥16 years: same as adult

          Gel: 0.77% (30, 45 g)

▷ *clotrimazole* (C)(G) apply bid to affected area x 4 weeks

  Pediatric: same as adult

       Desenex *Crm:* 1% (0.5 oz)

       Lotrimin *Crm:* 1% (15, 30, 45, 90 g); *Lotn:* 1% (30 ml); *Soln:* 1% (10, 30 ml)

       Lotrimin AF (OTC) *Crm:* 1% (15, 30, 45, 90 g); *Lotn:* 1% (20 ml); *Soln:* 1% (20 ml)

▷ *econazole* (C) apply once daily x 4 weeks

  Pediatric: same as adult

       Spectazole *Crm:* 1% (15, 30, 85 g)

▷ *ketoconazole* (C) apply once daily x 6 weeks

  Pediatric: not recommended

       Nizoral Cream *Crm:* 2% (15, 30, 60 g)

▷ *miconazole* 2% (C)(G) apply bid x 4 weeks

  Pediatric: same as adult

       Lotrimin AF Spray Liquid (OTC) *Spray liq:* 2% (113 g) (alcohol 17%)

       Lotrimin AF Spray Powder (OTC) *Spray pwdr:* 2% (90 g; alcohol 10%)

       Monistat-Derm *Crm:* 2% (1, 3 oz); *Spray liq:* 2% (3.5 oz); *Spray pwdr:* 2% (3 oz)

▷ *naftifine* (B)

  Pediatric: not recommended

       Naftin Cream apply once daily x 4 weeks

          Crm: 1% (15, 30, 60 g)

       Naftin Gel apply bid x 4 weeks

          Gel: 1% (20, 40, 60 g)

▷ *oxiconazole nitrate* (B) apply once daily-bid x 4 weeks

  Pediatric: same as adult

       Oxistat *Crm:* 1% (15, 30, 60 g); *Lotn:* 1% (30 ml)

▷ *sertaconazole* (C) apply once daily-bid x 4 weeks

  Pediatric: <12 years: not recommended; ≥12 years: same as adult

       Ertaczo *Crm:* 2% (15, 30 g)

▷ *sulconazole* (C) apply once daily-bid x 4 weeks

  Pediatric: not recommended

       Exelderm *Crm:* 1% (15, 30, 60 g); *Lotn:* 1% (30 mg)

▷ *terbinafine* (B)(G)

  Pediatric: <12 years: not recommended; ≥12 years: same as adult

> **Lamisil Cream (OTC)** apply bid x 1-4 weeks
>   *Crm:* 1% (15, 30 g)
> **Lamisil AT Cream (OTC)** apply to affected and surrounding area once daily-bid x 1-4 weeks until significantly improved
>   *Crm:* 1% (15, 30 g)
> **Lamisil Solution (OTC)** apply to affected and surrounding area bid x 1 week
>   *Soln:* 1% (30 ml spray bottle)

▷ *tolnaftate* (C)(OTC)(G) apply sparingly bid x 2-4 weeks
    Pediatric: <2 years: not recommended; ≥2 years: same as adult
        Tinactin *Crm:* 1% (15, 30 g); *Pwdr:* 1% (45, 90 g); *Soln:* 1% (10 ml); *Aerosol liq:* 1% (4 oz); *Aerosol pwdr:* 1% (3.5, 5 oz)

TOPICAL ANTIFUNGAL/ANTI-INFLAMMATORY COMBINATION

▷ *clotrimazole/betamethasone* (C)(G) apply bid x 4 weeks; max 4 weeks
    Pediatric: <12 years: not recommended; ≥12 years: same as adult
        Lotrisone *Crm: clotrim* 1 mg/*beta* 0.5 mg (15, 45 g); *Lotn: clotrim* 1 mg/*beta* 0.5 mg (30 ml)

SYSTEMIC ANTIFUNGALS

▷ *griseofulvin, microsize* (C)(G) 1 g once daily x 4-8 weeks
    Pediatric: <30 lb: 5 mg/lb/day; 30-50 lb: 125-250 mg/day; >50 lb: 250-500 mg/day; 5 mg/lb/day x 4-6 weeks or longer; *see page 568 for dose by weight*
        Grifulvin V *Tab:* 250, 500 mg; *Oral susp:* 125 mg/5 ml (120 ml) (alcohol 0.02%)
▷ *griseofulvin, ultramicrosize* (C) 750 mg/day in a single or divided doses x 4-6 weeks
    Pediatric: <2 years: not recommended; ≥2 years: 3.3 mg/lb/day in a single or divided doses
        Gris-PEG *Tab:* 125, 250
    Comment: *griseofulvin* should be taken with fatty foods (e.g., milk, ice cream). Liver enzymes should be monitored.
▷ *ketoconazole* (C) initially 200 mg once daily; max 400 mg/day x 4 weeks
    Pediatric: <2 years: not recommended; ≥2 years: 3.3-6.6 mg/kg once daily x 4 weeks
        Nizoral *Tab:* 200 mg
    Comment: Caution with *ketoconazole* due to concerns about potential for hepatotoxicity.

 TINEA VERSICOLOR

Comment: Resolution may take 3-6 months.

TOPICAL ANTIFUNGALS

▷ *butenafine* (G) apply once daily x 2 weeks
    Pediatric: <12 years: not recommended; ≥12 years: same as adult
        Lotrimin Ultra (C)(OTC) *Crm:* 1% (12, 24 g)
        Mentax (B) *Crm:* 1% (15, 30 g)
    Comment: *butenafine* is a benzylamine, not an azole. Fungicidal activity continues for at least 5 weeks after last application.

➤ *ciclopirox* (B)
    Loprox Cream apply bid; max 4 weeks
      Pediatric: <10 years: not recommended; ≥10 years: same as adult
      Crm: 0.77% (15, 30, 90 g)
    Loprox Lotion apply bid; max 4 weeks
      Pediatric: <10 years: not recommended; ≥10 years: same as adult
      Lotn: 0.77% (30, 60 ml)
    Loprox Gel apply bid; max 4 weeks
      Pediatric: <16 years: not recommended; ≥16 years: same as adult
      Gel: 0.77% (30, 45 g)
➤ *clotrimazole* (B)(G) apply bid x 7 days
  Pediatric: same as adult
    Lotrimin *Crm:* 1% (15, 30, 45 g)
    Lotrimin AF (OTC) *Crm:* 1% (12 g); *Lotn:* 1% (10 ml); *Soln:* 1% (10 ml)
➤ *econazole* (C) apply once daily x 2 weeks
  Pediatric: same as adult
    Spectazole *Crm:* 1% (15, 30, 85 g)
➤ *miconazole 2%* (C)(G) apply once daily x 2 weeks
  Pediatric: same as adult
    Lotrimin AF Spray Liquid (OTC) *Spray liq:* 2% (113 g) (alcohol 17%)
    Lotrimin AF Spray Powder (OTC) *Spray pwdr:* 2% (90 g) alcohol 10%)
    Monistat-Derm *Crm:* 2% (1, 3 oz); *Spray liq:* 2% (3.5 oz); *Spray pwdr: 2% (3 oz)*
➤ *ketoconazole* (C)(G)
  Pediatric: not recommended
    Nizoral Cream apply once daily x 2 weeks
      Crm: 2% (15, 30, 60 g)
    Nizoral Shampoo lather into area and leave on 5 minutes x 1 application
      Shampoo: 2% (4 oz)
➤ *oxiconazole nitrate* (B) apply once daily x 2 weeks
  Pediatric: same as adult
    Oxistat *Crm:* 1% (15, 30, 60 g); *Lotn:* 1% (30 ml)
➤ *selenium sulfide* shampoo (C)(G) apply after shower, allow to dry, leave on overnight; then scrub off vigorously in AM; repeat in 1 week and again q 3 months until resolution occurs
  Pediatric: same as adult
    Selsun Blue *Shampoo:* 1% (120, 210, 240, 330 ml); 2.5% (120 ml)
➤ *sulconazole* (C) apply once daily-bid x 3 weeks
  Pediatric: not recommended
    Exelderm *Crm:* 1% (15, 30, 60 g); *Lotn:* 1% (30 mg)
➤ *terbinafine* (B) apply bid to affected and surrounding area x 1 week
  Pediatric: <12 years: not recommended; ≥12 years: same as adult
    Lamisil Solution (OTC) *Soln:* 1% (30 ml spray bottle)

ORAL ANTI-FUNGALS

➤ *ketoconazole* (C) initially 200 mg once daily; max 400 mg/day x 4 weeks
  Pediatric: <2 years: not recommended; ≥2 years: 3.3-6.6 mg/kg once daily x 4 weeks
    Nizoral *Tab:* 200 mg

TOBACCO DEPENDENCE/NICOTINE WITHDRAWAL SYNDROME

NON-NICOTINE PRODUCTS

Alpha₄-Beta₂ Nicotinic Acetylcholine Receptor Partial Agonist

▷ *varenicline* (C)

Pediatric: <18 years: not recommended

Chantix set target quit date; begin therapy 1 week prior to target quit date; take after eating with a full glass of water; initially 0.5 mg once daily for 3 days; then 0.5 mg bid x 4 days; then 1 mg bid; treat x 12 weeks; may continue treatment for 12 more weeks

Tab: 0.5, 1 mg; *Starting Month Pak:* 0.5 mg x 11 tabs + 1 mg x 42 tabs; *Continuing Month Pak:* 1 mg x 56 tabs

Comment: Caution with **Chantix** due to potential risk for anxiety or suicidal ideation.

AMINOKETONES

▷ *bupropion HBr* (C)(G)

Pediatric: <18 years: not recommended

Aplenzin initially 100 mg bid for at least 3 days; may increase to 375 <u>or</u> 400 mg/day after several weeks; then after at least 3 more days, 450 mg in 4 divided doses; max 450 mg/day, 174 mg/single dose

Tab: 174, 348, 522 mg

▷ *bupropion HCl* (B)(G)

Pediatric: <18 years: not recommended

Wellbutrin initially 100 mg bid for at least 3 days; may increase to 375 <u>or</u> 400 mg/day after several weeks; then after at least 3 more days, 450 mg in 4 divided doses; max 450 mg/day, 150 mg/single dose

Tab: 75, 100 mg

Wellbutrin SR initially 150 mg in AM for at least 3 days; may increase to 150 mg bid if well tolerated; usual dose 300 mg/day; max 400 mg/day

Tab: 100, 150 mg sust-rel

Wellbutrin XL initially 150 mg in AM for at least 3 days; increase to 150 mg bid if well tolerated; usual dose 300 mg/day; max 400 mg/day

Tab: 150, 300 mg sust-rel

Zyban 150 mg once daily x 3 days; then 150 mg bid x 7-12 weeks; max 300 mg/day

Pediatric: <18 years: not recommended

Tab: 150 mg sust-rel

Comment: Contraindications to *bupropion* include seizure disorder, eating disorder, concurrent MAOI and alcohol use. Smoking should be discontinued after the 7th day of therapy with *bupropion*. Avoid bedtime dose.

TRANSDERMAL NICOTINE SYSTEMS (D)

Habitrol (OTC) initially one 21 mg/24 hour patch/day x 4-6 weeks; then one 14 mg/24 hour patch/day x 2-4 weeks; then one 7 mg/24 hour patch/day x 2-4 weeks; then discontinue

Pediatric: not recommended
Transdermal patch: 7, 14, 21 mg/24 hour
Nicoderm CQ (OTC) initially one 21 mg/24 hour patch/day x 6 weeks, then one 14 mg/24 hour patch/day x 2 weeks; then one 7 mg/24 hour patch/day x 2 weeks
Pediatric: not recommended
Transdermal patch: 7, 14, 21 mg/24 hour
Comment: Nicoderm CQ is available as a clear patch.
Nicotrol Step-down Patch (OTC) 1 patch/day x 6 weeks
Pediatric: not recommended
Transdermal patch: 5, 10, 15 mg/16 hour (7/pck)
Nicotrol Transdermal (OTC) 1 patch/day x 6 weeks
Pediatric: not recommended
Transdermal patch: 15 mg/16 hour (7/pck)
Prostep initially one 22 mg/24 hour patch/day x 4-8 weeks; then discontinue <u>or</u> one 11 mg/24 hour patch/day x 2-4 additional weeks
Pediatric: not recommended
Transdermal patch: 11, 22 mg/24 hour (7/pck)

NICOTINE GUM

➤ *nicotine polacrilex* **(D)** chew one piece of gum slowly and intermittently over 30 minutes q 1-2 hours x 6 weeks; then q 2-4 hours x 3 weeks; then q 4-8 hours x 3 weeks; max 24 pieces/day; 2 mg if smoked <25 cigarettes/day; 4 mg if smoked >24 cigarettes/day
Pediatric: not recommended
Nicorette (OTC) *Gum squares:* 2, 4 mg (108 piece starter kit and 48 piece refill) (orange, mint, <u>or</u> original, sugar-free)

NICOTINE LOZENGE

➤ *nicotine polacrilex* **(X)(OTC)(G)** dissolve over 20-30 minutes; minimize swallowing; do not eat <u>or</u> drink for 15 min before and during use; Use 2 mg lozenge if first cigarette smoked >30 minutes after waking; Use 4 mg lozenge if first cigarette smoked within 30 min of waking; 1 lozenge q 1-2 hours (at lest 9/day) x 6 weeks; then q 2-4 hours x 3 weeks; then q 4-8 hours x 3 weeks; then stop; max 5 lozenges/6 hours and 20 lozenges/day
Pediatric: <18 years: not recommended
Commit Lozenge *Loz:* 2, 4 mg (72/pck) (phenylalanine)
Nicorette Mini Lozenge (G) *Loz:* 2, 4 mg (72/pck) (mint; phenylalanine)

NICOTINE INHALATION PRODUCTS

➤ *nicotine* 0.5 mg aqueous nasal spray **(D)**
Pediatric: not recommended
Nicotrol NS 1-2 doses/hour nasally; max 5 doses/hour <u>or</u> 40 doses/day; usual max 3 months
Nasal spray: 0.5 mg/spray; 10 mg/ml (10 ml, 200 doses)
➤ *nicotine* 10 mg inhalation system **(D)**
Pediatric: not recommended
Nicotrol Inhaler individualize therapy; at least 6 cartridges/day x 3-6 weeks; max 16 cartridges/day x first 12 weeks; then reduce gradually over 12 more weeks

Inhaler: 10 mg/cartridge, 4 mg delivered (42 cartridge/pck) (menthol)

Comment: **Nicotrol Inhaler** is a smoking replacement; to be used with decreasing frequency. Smoking should be discontinued before starting therapy. Side effects include cough, nausea, mouth, or throat irritation. This system delivers nicotine, but no tars or carcinogens. Each cartridge lasts about 20 minutes with frequent continuous puffing and provides nicotine equivalent to 2 cigarettes.

ⓞ TONSILLITIS: ACUTE

▷ *amoxicillin* **(B)(G)** 500-875 mg bid or 250-500 mg tid x 10 days
Pediatric: <40 kg (88 lb): 20-40 mg/kg/day in 3 divided doses x 10 days or 25-45 mg/kg/day in 2 divided doses x 10 days; *see page 543 for dose by weight*
    Amoxil *Cap:* 250, 500 mg; *Tab:* 875*mg; *Chew tab:* 125, 200, 250, 400 mg (cherry-banana-peppermint) (phenylalanine); *Oral susp:* 125, 250 mg/5 ml (80, 100, 150 ml) (strawberry); 200, 400 mg/5 ml (50, 75, 100 ml) (bubble gum); *Oral drops:* 50 mg/ml (30 ml) (bubble gum)
    Moxatag *Tab:* 775 mg ext-rel
    Trimox *Tab:* 125, 250 mg; *Cap:* 250, 500 mg; *Oral susp:* 125, 250 mg/5 ml (80, 100, 150 ml) (raspberry-strawberry)
▷ *azithromycin* **(B)** 500 mg x 1 dose on day 1, then 250 mg once daily on days 2-5 or 500 mg once daily x 3 days or **Zmax** 2 g in a single dose
Pediatric: 12 mg/kg/day x 5 days; max 500 mg/day; *see page 548 for dose by weight*
    Zithromax *Tab:* 250, 500, 600 mg; *Oral susp:* 100 mg/5 ml (15 ml); 200 mg/5 ml (15, 22.5, 30 ml) (cherry); *Pkt:* 1 g for reconstitution (cherry-banana)
    Zithromax Tri-pak *Tab:* 3 x 500 mg tabs/pck
    Zithromax Z-pak *Tab:* 6 x 250 mg tabs/pck
    Zmax *Oral susp:* 2 g ext-rel for reconstitution (cherry-banana) (148 mg Na$^+$)
▷ *cefaclor* **(B)(G)** 250-500 mg q 8 hours x 10 days; max 2 g/day
Pediatric: <1 month: not recommended; 20-40 mg/kg bid or q 12 hours x 10 days; max 1 g/ day; *see page 549 for dose by weight*
Tab: 500 mg; *Cap:* 250, 500 mg; *Susp:* 125 mg/5 ml (75, 150 ml) (strawberry); 187 mg/5 ml (50, 100 ml) (strawberry); 250 mg/5 ml (75, 150 ml) (strawberry); 375 mg/5 ml (50, 100 ml) (strawberry)
    Pediatric: <16 years: ext-rel not recommended; ≥16 years; same as adult
    Cefaclor Extended Release *Tab:* 375, 500 mg ext-rel
▷ *cefadroxil* **(B)** 1 g once daily or divided bid x 10 days
Pediatric: 30 mg/kg/day in 2 divided doses x 10 days; *see page 550 for dose by weight*
    Duricef *Cap:* 500 mg; *Tab:* 1 g; *Oral susp:* 250 mg/5 ml (100 ml); 500 mg/5 ml (75, 100 ml) (orange-pineapple)
▷ *cefdinir* **(B)** 300 mg bid x 5-10 days or 600 mg once daily x 10 days
Pediatric: <6 months: not recommended; 6 months-12 years: 14 mg/kg/day in a single or 2 divided doses x 10 days; >12 years: same as adult; *see page 551 for dose by weight*
    Omnicef *Cap:* 300 mg; *Oral susp:* 125 mg/5 ml (60, 100 ml) (strawberry)
▷ *cefditoren pivoxil* **(B)** 200 mg bid x 10 days
Pediatric: <12 years: not recommended
    Spectracef *Tab:* 200 mg

Comment: Contraindicated with milk protein allergy or carnitine deficiency.
▷ *ceftibuten* (B) 200 mg once daily x 10 days
   Pediatric: 9 mg/kg once daily x 10 days; max 400 mg/day; *see page 555 for dose by weight*
      Cedax *Cap:* 400 mg; *Oral susp:* 90 mg/5 ml (30, 60, 90, 120 ml); 180 mg/5 ml (30, 60, 120 ml) (cherry)
▷ *cefixime* (B) 400 mg once daily x 10 days
   Pediatric: <6 months: not recommended; 6 months-12 years, <50 kg: 8 mg/kg/day in a single or 2 divided doses x 10 days; >12 years, >50 kg: same as adult; *see page 552 for dose by weight*
      Suprax *Tab:* 400 mg; *Cap:* 400 mg; *Oral susp:* 100, 200 mg/5 ml (50, 75, 100 ml) (strawberry)
▷ *cefpodoxime proxetil* (B) 200 mg bid x 5-7 days
   Pediatric: <2 months: not recommended; 2 months-12 years: 10 mg/kg/day (max 400 mg/dose) or 5 mg/kg/day bid (max 200 mg/dose) x 5-7 days; *see page 553 for dose by weight*
      Vantin *Tab:* 100, 200 mg; *Oral susp:* 50, 100 mg/5 ml (50, 75, 100 mg) (lemon creme)
▷ *cefprozil* (B) 500 mg once daily x 10 days
   Pediatric: 2-12 years: 7.5 mg/kg bid x 10 days; >12 years: same as adult; *see page 554 for dose by weight*
      Cefzil *Tab:* 250, 500 mg; *Oral susp:* 125, 250 mg/5 ml (50, 75, 100 ml) (bubble gum) (phenylalanine)
▷ *cephalexin* (B)(G) 250 mg tid x 10 days
   Pediatric: 25-50 mg/kg/day in 4 divided doses x 10 days; *see page 557 for dose by weight*
      Keflex *Cap:* 250, 333, 500, 750 mg; *Oral susp:* 125, 250 mg/5 ml (100, 200 ml) (strawberry)
▷ *clarithromycin* (C)(G) 250 mg bid or 500 mg ext-rel once daily 10 days
   Pediatric: <6 months: not recommended; ≥6 months: 7.5 mg/kg bid x 10 days; *see page 558 for dose by weight*
      Biaxin *Tab:* 250, 500 mg
      Biaxin Oral Suspension *Oral susp:* 125, 250 mg/5 ml (50, 100 ml) (fruit punch)
      Biaxin XL *Tab:* 500 mg ext-rel
▷ *dirithromycin* (C)(G) 500 mg once daily x 10 days
   Pediatric: <12 years: not recommended; ≥12 years: same as adult
      Dynabac *Tab:* 250 mg
▷ *erythromycin base* (B)(G) 300-400 mg tid x 10 days
   Pediatric: 30-50 mg/kg/day in 2-4 divided doses x 10 days
      Ery-Tab *Tab:* 250, 333, 500 mg ent-coat
      PCE *Tab:* 333, 500 mg
Comment: *erythromycin* may increase INR with concomitant *warfarin*, as well as increase serum level of *digoxin*, benzodiazepines and statins.
▷ *erythromycin ethylsuccinate* (B)(G) 400 mg qid x 7 days
   Pediatric: 30-50 mg/kg/day in 4 divided doses x 7 days; may double dose with severe infection; max 100 mg/kg/day; *see page 563 for dose by weight*
      EryPed *Oral susp:* 200 mg/5 ml (100, 200 ml) (fruit); 400 mg/5 ml (60, 100, 200 ml) (banana); *Oral drops:* 200, 400 mg/5 ml (50 ml) (fruit); *Chew tab:* 200 mg wafer (fruit)

E.E.S. *Oral susp:* 200, 400 mg/5 ml (100 ml) (fruit)
E.E.S. **Granules** *Oral susp:* 200 mg/5 ml (100, 200 ml) (cherry)
E.E.S. **400 Tablets** *Tab:* 400 mg

Comment: *erythromycin* may increase INR with concomitant *warfarin*, as well as increase serum level of *digoxin*, benzodiazepines and statins.

▷ *loracarbef* (B) 200 mg bid x 10 days
Pediatric: 15 mg/kg/day in 2 divided doses x 10 days; *see page* 570 *for dose by weight*
Lorabid *Pulvule:* 200, 400 mg; *Oral susp:* 100 mg/5 ml (50, 100 ml); 200 mg/5 ml (50, 75, 100 ml) (strawberry bubble gum)

▷ *penicillin V potassium* (B)(G) 250 mg tid x 10 days
Pediatric: 25-50 mg/kg day in 4 divided doses x 10 days; ≥12 years: same as adult; *see page 572 for dose by weight*
Pen-Vee K *Tab:* 250, 500 mg; *Oral soln:* 125 mg/5 ml (100, 200 ml); 250 mg/5 ml (100, 150, 200 ml)

TRICHINOSIS

ANTIHELMINTICS

▷ *albendazole* (C) 400 mg as bid x 15 days; take after a meal
Pediatric: <2 years: 200 mg once daily x 3 days; may repeat in 3 weeks; 2-12 years: 400 mg once daily x 3 days; may repeat in 3 weeks; >12 years: same as adult
Albenza *Tab:* 200 mg

▷ *mebendazole* (C)(G) 200-400 mg tid x 3 days; then 400-500 mg tid x 10 days; take with food
Pediatric: same as adult (chew or crush and mix with food)
Vermox *Chew tab:* 100 mg

▷ *pyrantel pamoate* (C) 11 mg/kg x 1 dose; max 1 g/dose; take after a meal
Pediatric: 25-37 lb: 1/2 tsp x 1 dose; 38-62 lb: 1 tsp x 1 dose; 63-87 lb: 1 tsp x 1 dose; 88-112 lb: 2 tsp x 1 dose; 113-137 lb: 2 tsp x 1 dose; 138-162 lb: 3 tsp x 1 dose; 163-187 lb: 3 tsp x 1 dose; >187 lb: 4 tsp x 1 dose
Pin-X (OTC) *Cap:* 180 mg; *Liq:* 50 mg/ml (30 ml); 144 mg/ml (30 ml); *Oral susp:* 50 mg/ml (30 ml)

▷ *thiabendazole* (C) 25 mg/kg bid x 7 days; max 1.5 g/dose; take after a meal
Pediatric: same as adult; <30 lb: consult mfr literature; ≥30 lb: 25 mg/kg in 2 divided doses/day with meals; 30-50 lbs: 250 mg bid with meals; >50 lb: 10 mg/lb/dose bid with meals; max 3g/day
Mintezol *Chew tab:* 500*mg (orange); *Oral susp:* 500 mg/5 ml (120 ml) (orange)
Comment: *thiabendazole* is not for prophylaxis.

TRICHOMONIASIS (TRICHOMONAS VAGINALIS)

Comment: The following treatment regimens for *Trichomoniasis* are published in the **2015 CDC Sexually Transmitted Diseases Treatment Guidelines**. Treat all sexual contacts. A multi-dose treatment regimen should be considered in HIV-positive women.

RECOMMENDED REGIMENS (NON-PREGNANT)

Regimen 1

▷ *metronidazole* 2 g once in a single dose

Regimen 2

▷ *tinidazole* 2 g once in a single dose

RECOMMENDED ALTERNATE REGIMEN

Regimen 1

▷ *metronidazole* 500 mg bid x 7 days

DRUG BRANDS AND DOSE FORMS

▷ *metronidazole* (not for use in 1st; B in 2nd, 3rd)(G)
  Flagyl *Tab:* 250*, 500*mg
  Flagyl 375 *Cap:* 375 mg
  Flagyl ER *Tab:* 750 mg ext-rel
  Comment: Alcohol is contraindicated during treatment with oral *metronidazole* and for 72 hours after therapy due to a possible *disulfiram*-like reaction (nausea, vomiting, flushing, headache).
▷ *tinidazole* (not for use in 1st; B in 2nd, 3rd)
  Tindamax *Tab:* 250*, 500*mg
  Comment: Alcohol is contraindicated during treatment with oral *tinidazole* and for 72 hours after therapy due to a possible *disulfiram*-like reaction (nausea, vomiting, flushing, headache).

RECOMMENDED REGIMENS: PREGNANCY/LACTATION

Comment: All pregnant women should be considered for treatment. Women can be treated with 2 g *metronidazole* in a single dose at any stage of pregnancy. Lactating women who are administered *metronidazole* should be instructed to interrupt breastfeeding for 12-24 hours after receiving the 2 g dose of *metronidazole*.

⭕ TRIGEMINAL NEURALGIA (TIC DOULOUREUX)

▷ *baclofen* (C)(G) initially 5-10 mg tid with food; usual dose 10-80 mg/day
  Pediatric: not recommended
  Lioresal *Tab:* 10*, 20*mg
  Tab: 10, 20 mg
  Comment: Potential for seizures or hallucinations on abrupt withdrawal of *baclofen*.
▷ *carbamazepine* (C)
  Carbatrol initially 200 mg bid; may increase weekly as needed by 200 mg/day; usual maintenance 800 mg-1.2 g/day
    Pediatric: <12 years: max <35 mg/kg/day; use ext-rel form above 400 mg/day; 12-15 years: max 1 g/day in 2 divided doses; >15 years: usual maintenance 1.2 g/day in 2 divided doses
    Cap: 200, 300 mg ext-rel
  Tegretol initially 100 mg bid or 1/2 tsp susp qid; may increase dose by 100 mg q 12 hours or by 1/2 tsp susp q 6 hours; usual maintenance 400-800 mg/day; max 1200 mg/day

Pediatric: <6 years: initially 10-20 mg/kg/day in 2 divided doses; increase weekly as needed in 3-4 divided doses; max 35 mg/kg/day in 3-4 divided doses; ≥6 years: initially 100 mg bid; increase weekly as needed by 100 mg/ day in 3-4 divided doses; max 1 g/day in 3-4 divided doses

> *Tab:* 200*mg; *Chew tab:* 100*mg; *Oral susp:* 100 mg/5 ml (450 ml; citrus-vanilla)

Tegretol XR initially 200 mg bid; may increase weekly by 200 mg/day in 2 divided doses

Pediatric: <6 years: use other forms; ≥6 years: initially 100 mg bid; may increase weekly by 100 mg/day in 2 divided doses; max 1 g/day

> *Tab:* 100, 200, 400 mg ext-rel

▷ *clonazepam* (D)(IV)(G) initially 0.25 mg bid; increase to 1 mg/day after 3 days
Pediatric: <10 years, <30 kg: initially 0.1-0.3 mg/kg/day; may increase up to 0.05 mg/kg/day bid-tid; usual maintenance 0.1-0.2 mg/kg/day tid

> **Klonopin** *Tab:* 0.5*, 1, 2 mg

> **Klonopin Wafers** dissolve in mouth with <u>or</u> without water

> *Wafer:* 0.125, 0.25, 0.5, 1, 2 mg orally-disint

▷ *divalproex sodium* (D) initially 250 mg bid; gradually increase to max 1000 mg/day if needed
Pediatric: <10 years: not recommended; ≥10 years: same as adult

> **Depakene** *Cap:* 250 mg; *Syr:* 250 mg/5 ml

> **Depakote** *Tab:* 125, 250 mg

> **Depakote ER** *Tab:* 250, 500 mg ext-rel

> **Depakote Sprinkle** *Cap:* 125 mg

▷ *phenytoin* (D) 400 mg/day in divided doses

> **Dilantin** *Cap:* 30, 100 mg; *Oral susp:* 125 mg/5 ml (8 oz); *Infatab:* 50 mg

Comment: Monitor *phenytoin* serum levels. Therapeutic serum level: 10-20 g/ml. Side effects include gingival hyperplasia.

▷ *valproic acid* (D) initially 15 mg/kg/day; may increase weekly by 5-10 mg/kg/day; max 60 mg/kg/day <u>or</u> 250 mg/day

> **Depakene** *Cap:* 250 mg; *Syr:* 250 mg/5 ml

TRICYCLIC ANTIDEPRESSANTS (TCAs)

Comment: Co-administration of TCAs with SSRIs requires extreme caution.

▷ *amitriptyline* (C)(G) titrate to achieve pain relief; max 300 mg/day
Pediatric: not recommended

> *Tab:* 10, 25, 50, 75, 100, 150 mg

▷ *amoxapine* (C) titrate to achieve pain relief; if total dose exceeds 300 mg/day, give in divided doses; max 400 mg/day
Pediatric: not recommended

> *Tab:* 25, 50, 100, 150 mg

▷ *desipramine* (C)(G) titrate to achieve pain relief; max 300 mg/day
Pediatric: not recommended

> **Norpramin** *Tab:* 10, 25, 50, 75, 100, 150 mg

▷ *doxepin* (C)(G) titrate to achieve pain relief; max 150 mg/day
Pediatric: not recommended

> *Cap:* 10, 25, 50, 75, 100, 150 mg; *Oral conc:* 10 mg/ml (4 oz w. dropper)

▷ *imipramine* (C)(G)
Pediatric: not recommended

Tofranil titrate to achieve pain relief; max 200 mg/day; adolescents max 100 mg/day; if maintenance dose exceeds 75 mg/day, may switch to **Tofranil PM** at bedtime

Tab: 10, 25, 50 mg

Tofranil PM titrate to achieve pain relief; initially 75 mg at HS; max 200 mg at HS

Cap: 75, 100, 125, 150 mg

Tofranil Injection 50 mg IM; lower dose for adolescents; switch to oral form as soon as possible

Amp: 25 mg/2 ml (2 ml)

▷ *nortriptyline* **(D)(G)** titrate to achieve pain relief; initially 10-25 mg tid-qid; max 150 mg/day; lower doses for elderly and adolescents
Pediatric: not recommended

Pamelor titrate to achieve pain relief; max 150 mg/day

Cap: 10, 25, 50, 75 mg; *Oral soln:* 10 mg/5 ml (16 oz)

▷ *protriptyline* **(C)** titrate to achieve pain relief; initially 5 mg tid; max 60 mg/day
Pediatric: <12 years: not recommended

Vivactyl *Tab:* 5, 10 mg

▷ *trimipramine* **(C)** titrate to achieve pain relief; max 200 mg/day
Pediatric: not recommended

Surmontil *Cap:* 25, 50, 100 mg

PULMONARY TUBERCULOSIS (TB) (MYCOBACTERIUM TUBERCULOSIS)

SCREENING

▷ *purified protein derivative (PPD)* **(C)** 0.1 ml intradermally; examine inoculation site for induration at 48 to 72 hours.
Pediatric: same as adult

Aplisol, Tubersol *Soln:* 5 US units/0.1 ml (1, 5 ml)

ANTI-TUBERCULAR AGENTS

Comment: Avoid *streptomycin* in pregnancy. *pyridoxine* (*vitamin B-6*) 25 mg once daily x 6 months should be administered concomitantly with *INH* for prevention of side effects. *rifapentine* produces red-orange discoloration of body tissues and body fluids and may stain contact lenses.

▷ *bedaquiline* **(B)(G)**

Sirturo *Tab:* 100 mg

Comment: *bedaquiline* is a diarylquinoline antimycobacterial ATP synthase for the treatment of pulmonary multi-drug resistant TB (MDR-TB).

▷ *ethambutol (EMB)* **(B)(G)**

Myambutol *Tab:* 100, 400*mg

▷ *isoniazid (INH)* **(C)** *Tab:* 300*mg

▷ *pyrazinamide (PZA)* **(C)** *Tab:* 500*mg

▷ *rifampin (RIF)* **(C)(G)**

Rifadin, Rimactane *Cap:* 150, 300 mg

▷ *rifapentine* **(C)**

Priftin *Tab:* 150 mg (24, 32 ct pck)

Comment: The 32-count packs of **Priftin** are intended for patients with active tuberculosis infection (TB). The 24-count packs are are intended for patients with latent tuberculosis infection (LTBI) who are at high risk for progression to tuberculosis disease. **Priftin** for active TB is indicated for patients ≥12 years-of-age. **Priftin** for LTBI is indicated for patients ≥2 years-of-age.

▷ *rilipivirine* (C) *Tab:* 25 mg
  Rifabutin *Cap:* 150 mg
▷ *streptomycin (SM)* (C)(G) *Amp:* 1 g/2.5 ml <u>or</u> 400 mg/ml (2.5 ml)

COMBINATION AGENTS

▷ *rifampin/isoniazid* (C)
  Rifamate *Cap:* rif 300 mg/*iso* 150 mg
▷ *rifampin/isoniazid/pyrazinamide* (C)
  Rifater *Tab:* rif 120 mg/*iso* 50 mg/*pyr* 300 mg

PROPHYLAXIS AFTER EXPOSURE TO TUBERCULOSIS, WITH NEGATIVE PPD

▷ *isoniazid* (C) 300 mg once daily in a single dose x at least 6 months
  Pediatric: 10-20 mg/kg/day x 9 months

PROPHYLAXIS AFTER EXPOSURE, WITH NEW PPD CONVERSION

▷ *isoniazid* (C) 300 mg once daily in a single dose x 12 months
  Pediatric: 10-20 mg/kg/day x 9 months
  Tab: 100, 300*mg; *Syr:* 50 mg/5 ml; *Inj:* 100 mg/ml
▷ *rifampin* (C) 600 mg once daily + *isoniazid* (C) 300 mg once daily x 4 months
  Pediatric: *rifampin* (C) 10-20 mg/kg + *isoniazid* (C) 10-20 mg/kg once daily x 4 months
▷ *rifapentine* (C) 600 mg once weekly + *isoniazid* (C) 300 mg once weekly x 12 weeks
  Pediatric: ≤12 years: Treat x 12 weeks; 10-14 kg: *rifapentine* (C) 300 mg once weekly
  + *isoniazid* (C) 25 mg/kg (max 900 mg) once weekly; 14.1-25 kg: *rifapentine* (C)
  450 mg once weekly + *isoniazid* (C) 25 mg/kg (max 900 mg) once weekly; 25.1-32
  kg: *rifapentine* (C) 600 mg once weekly + *isoniazid* (C) 25 mg/kg (max 900 mg)
  once weekly; 32.1-50 kg: *rifapentine* (C) 750 mg once weekly + *isoniazid* (C) 25
  mg/kg (max 900 mg) once weekly; >50 kg: *rifapentine* (C) 900 mg once weekly +
  isoniazid (C) 25 mg/kg (max 900 mg) once weekly; >12 years: same as adult

ADULT TREATMENT REGIMENS (>12 YEARS)

Regimen 1

▷ *rifampin* (C) 600 mg + *isoniazid* (C) 300 mg + *pyrazinamide* (C) 2 g + *ethambutol*
  (C) 15-25 mg/kg <u>or</u> *streptomycin* (C) 1 g once daily x 8 weeks; then *isoniazid* (C)
  300 mg + *rifampin* (C) 600 mg once daily x 16 weeks <u>or</u> *isoniazid* 900 mg + *rifampin*
  (C) 600 mg 2-3 times/week x 16 weeks

Regimen 2

▷ *rifampin* 600 mg + *isoniazid* 300 mg + *pyrazinamide* 2 g + *ethambutol* 15-25 mg/kg
  <u>or</u> *streptomycin* 1 g once daily x 2 weeks; then *rifampin* 600 mg + *isoniazid* 900 mg
  + *pyrazinamide* 4 g + *ethambutol* 50 mg/kg <u>or</u> *streptomycin* 1.5 g 2 times/week x 6
  weeks; then *isoniazid* 300 mg + *rifampin* 600 mg once daily x 16 weeks <u>or</u> 2 times/
  week x 16 weeks *rifampin* 600 mg once daily x 16 weeks <u>or</u> 2 times/week x 16 weeks

Regimen 3

▷ *rifampin* 600 mg + *isoniazid* 900 mg + *pyrazinamide* 3 g + *ethambutol* 25-30 mg/kg or *streptomycin* 1.5 g 3 times/week x 6 months

Regimen 4 (for smear and culture negative for pulmonary TB in adult)

▷ Options 1, 2, or 3 x 8 weeks; then *isoniazid* 300 mg + *rifampin* 600 mg once daily x 16 weeks; then *rifampin* 600 mg + *isoniazid* 300 mg + *pyrazinamide* 2 g + *ethambutol* 15-25 mg/kg or *streptomycin* 1 g once daily x 8 weeks or 2-3 times/week x 8 weeks

Regimen 5 (for smear and culture negative for pulmonary TB in adult)

▷ *rifanpentine* 600 mg twice weekly x 2 months (at least 72 hours between doses) + once daily *isoniazid* 300 mg, *ethambutol* 15-25 mg/kg + *pyrazinamide* 2 g; then *rifanpentine* 600 mg once weekly x 4 months + once daily *isoniazid* 300 mg + another appropriate anti-tuberculosis agent for susceptible organisms

Regimen 6 (when pyrazinamide is contraindicated)

▷ *rifampin* 600 mg + *isoniazid* 300 mg + *ethambutol* 15-25 mg/kg + *streptomycin* 1 g once daily x 4-8 weeks; then *isoniazid* 300 mg + *rifampin* 600 mg once daily x 24 weeks or 2 x/week x 24 weeks

PEDIATRIC TREATMENT REGIMENS

Regimen 1

▷ *rifampin* 10-20 mg/kg + *isoniazid* 10-20 mg/kg + *pyrazinamide* 15-20 mg/kg + *ethambutol* 15-25 mg/kg or *streptomycin* 20-40 mg/kg once daily x 8 weeks; then *isoniazid* 10-20 mg/kg + *rifampin* 10-20 mg/kg once daily x 16 weeks or *isoniazid* 20-40 mg/kg + *rifampin* 10-20 mg/kg 2-3 times/week x 16 weeks

Regimen 2

▷ *rifampin* 10-20 mg/kg + *isoniazid* 10-20 mg/kg + *pyrazinamide* 15-30 mg/kg + *ethambutol* 15-25 mg/kg or *streptomycin* 20-40 mg/kg once daily x 2 weeks; then *rifampin* 10-20 mg/kg + *isoniazid* 20-40 mg/kg + *pyrazinamide* 50-70 mg/kg + *ethambutol* 50 mg/kg or *streptomycin* 25-30 mg/kg 2 times/week x 6 weeks; then *isoniazid* 10-20 mg/kg + *rifampin* 10-20 mg/kg once daily x 16 weeks or *rifampin* 10-20 mg/kg + *isoniazid* 20-40 mg/kg 2 times/week x 16 weeks

Regimen 3

▷ *rifampin* 10-20 mg/kg + *isoniazid* 20-40 mg/kg + *pyrazinamide* 50-70 mg/kg + *ethambutol* 25-30 mg/kg or *streptomycin* 25-30 mg/kg 3 times/week x 6 months

Regimen 4 (when pyrazinamide is contraindicated)

▷ *rifampin* 10-20 mg/kg + *isoniazid* 10-20 mg/kg + *ethambutol* 15-25 mg/ kg + *streptomycin* 20-40 mg/kg once daily x 4-8 weeks; then *isoniazid* 10-20 mg/kg + *rifampin* 10-20 mg/kg once daily x 24 weeks or *rifampin* 10-20 mg/ kg + *isoniazid* 20-40 mg/ kg 2 x/week x 24 weeks

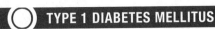

TYPE 1 DIABETES MELLITUS

Comment: Target glycosylated hemoglobin (HbA1c) is <7%. Addition of daily ACE-I <u>and/or</u> ARB therapy is strongly recommended for renal protection. Insulin may be indicated in the management of Type 2 diabetes with <u>or</u> without concomitant oral anti-diabetic agents.

TREATMENT FOR ACUTE HYPOGLYCEMIA

➤ *glucagon (recombinant)* (B) administer SC, IM, <u>or</u> IV; if patient does not respond in 15 minutes, may administer a single dose <u>or</u> 2 divided doses; <20 kg: 0.5 mg <u>or</u> 20-30 mg/kg; ≥20 kg: 1 mg
Pediatric: same as adult

INHALED INSULIN

Rapid-Acting Inhalation Powder Insulin

➤ *insulin human (inhaled)* (C) one inhaler may be used for up to 15 days, then discard; dose at meal times as follows: *Insulin naïve:* initially 4 units at each meal; adjust according to blood glucose monitoring
Conversion from SC to inhaled mealtime insulin:
SC 1-4 units: inhal 4 units
SC 5-8 units: inhal 8 units
SC 9-12 units: inhal 12 units
SC 13-16 units: inhal 16 units
SC 17-20 units: inhal 20 units
SC 21-24 units: inhal 24 units
Pediatric: <18 years: not established

Afrezza Inhalation Powder administer at the beginning of the meal; *Mealtime insulin naïve:* initially 4 units at each meal; *Using SC prandial insulin:* convert dose to **Afrezza** using a conversion table (see mfr literature); *Using SC pre-mixed:* divide 1/2 of total daily injected pre-mixed insulin equally among 3 meals of the day; administer 1/2 total injected pre-mixed dose as once daily injected basal insulin dose
Inhal: 4, 8, 12 unit single-inhalation color-coded cartridges (30, 60, 90/pkg w. 2 disposable inhalers)

Comment: Afrezza is not a substitute for long-acting insulin. **Afrezza** must be used in combination with long-acting insulin in patients with T1DM. **Afrezza** is not recommended for the treatment of diabetic ketoacidosis. **Afrezza** is contraindicated with chronic lung disease because of the risk of acute bronchospasm. The use of **Afrezza** is not recommended in patients who smoke <u>or</u> who have recently stopped smoking. Each card contains 5 blister strips with 3 cartridges each (total 15 cartridges). The doses are color-coded. **Afrezza** is contraindicated with chronic respiratory disease (e.g., asthma, COPD) and patients prone to episodes of hypoglycaemia.

INJECTABLE INSULINS

Rapid-Acting Insulins

➤ *insulin aspart (recombinant)* (B) onset <15 minutes; peak 1-3 hours; duration 3-5 hours; administer 5-10 minutes prior to a meal; SC <u>or</u> infusion pump <u>or</u> IV infusion

Pediatric: <3 years: not recommended; ≥3 years: same as adult

    NovoLog *Vial:* 100 U/ml (10 ml); *PenFill cartridge:* 100 U/ml (3 ml, 5/pk) (zinc, m-cresol)

▶ ***insulin glulisine (rDNA origin)* (C)** onset <15 minutes; peak 1 hour; duration 2-4 hours; administer up to 15 minutes before, <u>or</u> within 20 minutes after starting a meal; use with an intermediate <u>or</u> long-acting insulin; SC only; may administer via insulin pump; do not dilute <u>or</u> mix with other insulin in pump

Pediatric: <4 years: not recommended; ≥4 years: same as adult

    Apidra *Vial:* 100 U/ml (10 ml); *Cartridge:* 100 U/ml (3 ml, 5/pck; m-cresol)

▶ ***insulin lispro (recombinant)* (B)** onset <15 minutes; peak 1 hour; duration 3.5-4.5 hours; administer up to 15 minutes before, <u>or</u> immediately after, a meal; SC <u>or</u> IV infusion pump only

Pediatric: <3 years: not recommended; ≥3 years: same as adult

    Humalog

        Vial: 100 U/ml (10 ml); *Prefilled disposable KwikPen:* 100 U/ml (3 ml, 5/pck) (zinc, m-cresol); *HumaPen Memoir* and *HumaPen Luxura* HD inj device for *Humulog cartridges* (100 U/ml, 3 ml 5/pck) (zinc, m-cresol)

▶ ***insulin regular* (B)**

    Humulin R U-100 *(human, recombinant)* **(OTC)** onset 30 minutes; peak 2-4 hours; duration up to 6-8 hours; SC <u>or</u> IV <u>or</u> IM

        Vial: 100 U/ml (10 ml)

    Humulin R U-500 *(human, recombinant)* onset 30 minutes; peak 1.75-4 hours; duration up to 24 hours; SC only; for in-hospital use only

        Vial: 500 U/ml (20 ml); *KwikPen:* 3 ml (2, 5/carton)

    Comment: Humulin R U-500 formulation is 5 times more concentrated than standard U-100 concentration, indicated for adults and children who require ≥200 units of insulin/day, allowing patients to inject 80% less liquid to receive the desired dose.

    Iletin II Regular *(pork)* **(OTC)** onset 30 minutes; peak 2-4 hours; duration 6-8 hours; SC, IV <u>or</u> IM

        Vial: 100 U/ml (10 ml)

    Novolin R *(human)* **(OTC)** onset 30 minutes; peak 2.5-5 hours; duration 8 hours; SC, IV, <u>or</u> IM

        Vial: 100 U/ml (10 ml); *PenFill cartridge:* 100 U/ml (1.5 ml, 5/pck); *Prefilled syringe:* 100 U/ml (1.5 ml, 5/pck)

▶ ***pramlintide* (amylin analogue/amylinomimetic) (C)** administer immediately before major meals (≥250 kcal <u>or</u> ≥30 g carbohydrates); initially 15 mcg; titrate in 15 mcg increments for 3 days if no significant nausea occurs; if nausea occurs at 45 <u>or</u> 60 mcg, reduce to 30 mcg; if not tolerated, consider discontinuing therapy; *Maintenance:* 60 mcg (30 mcg *only* if 60 mcg not tolerated)

    Symlin *Vial:* 0.6 mg/ml (5 ml; m-cresol, mannitol)

    Comment: Symlin is indicated as adjunct to mealtime insulin with <u>or</u> without a sulfonylurea <u>and/or</u> metformin when blood glucose control is suboptimal despite optimal insulin therapy. Do not mix with insulin. When initiating **Symlin**, reduce preprandial short/rapid-acting insulin dose by 50% and monitor pre- and post-prandial and bedtime blood glucose. Do not use in patients with poor compliance, HgbA1c is >9%, recurrent hypoglycemia requiring assistance in the previous 6 months, <u>or</u> if taking a prokinetic drug. With Type 2 DM, initial therapy is 60 mcg/dose and max is 120 mcg/dose.

RAPID-ACTING AND INTERMEDIATE-ACTING INSULIN

Insulin Aspart Protamine Suspension/Insulin Aspart Combinations

▷ *insulin aspart protamine suspension 70%/insulin aspart 30% (recombinant)* **(B)** onset 15 min; peak 2.4 hours; duration up to 24 hours; SC only
Pediatric: not recommended
> **NovoLog Mix 70/30 (OTC)** *Vial:* 100 U/ml (10 ml)
> **NovoLog Mix 70/30 FlexPen (OTC)** *Prefilled disposable pen:* 100 U/ml (3 ml, 5/pck); *PenFill cartridge:* 100 U/ml (3 ml, 5/pck)

LONG-ACTING INSULINS

▷ *insulin detemir (human)* **(B)** administer once daily with evening meal or at HS as basal insulin; may administer twice daily (AM/PM); onset 1 hour; no peak; duration 24 hours; switching from another basal insulin, dose should be the same on a unit-to-unit basis; may need more *insulin detemir* when switching from **NPH**; SC only; *Type 1:* starting dose 1/3 of total daily insulin requirements; rapid-acting or short-acting, pre-meal insulin should be used to satisfy the remainder of daily insulin requirements; *Type 2 (inadequately controlled on oral antidiabetic agents):* initially 10 units or 0.1-0.2 units/kg, once daily in the evening or divided twice daily (AM/PM)
Pediatric: <2 years: not recommended; ≥2 years: same as adult
> **Levemir** *Vial:* 100 U/ml (10 ml); *FlexPen:* 100 U/ml (3 ml, 5/pck); (zinc, m-cresol)
Comment: Do not mix or dilute *insulin detemir* with other insulins.
▷ *insulin isophane suspension (NPH)* **(B)**
> **Humulin N** *(human, recombinant)* **(OTC)** onset 1-2 hours; peak 6-12 hours; duration 18-24 hours; SC only
>> *Vial:* 100 U/ml (10 ml); *Prefilled disposable pen:* 100 U/ml (3 ml, 5/pck)
> **Novolin N** *(recombinant)* **(OTC)** onset 1.5 hours; peak 4-12 hours; duration 24 hours; SC only
>> *Vial:* 100 U/ml (10 ml); *PenFill cartridge:* 1.5 ml (5/pck); *KwikPens:* 1.5 ml (5/pck)
> **Iletin II NPH** *(pork)* **(OTC)** onset 1-2 hours; peak 6-12 hours; duration 18-26 hours; SC only
>> *Vial:* 100 U/ml (10 ml)
▷ *insulin glargine (recombinant)* **(C)**
Comment: Do not mix or dilute *insulin glargine* with other insulins.
> **Basaglar** administer SC once daily, at the same time each day, in the deltoid, abdomen, or thigh; *T1DM:* initially 1/3 of total daily insulin dose give the remainder of the total dose as short- or rapid-acting preprandial insulin; *T2DM:* initially 2 units/kilogram or up to 10 units once daily; *Switching from once daily insulin glargine 300 units/ml:* initially 80% of the insulin glargine 300 units/ml; *Switching from twice daily NPH:* initially 80% of the total daily NPH dose
>> *Pediatric:* <6 years: not established; ≥6 years: individualize and adjust as needed
>> *Prefilled* **Basaglar** *KwikPen (disposable),* 100 U/ml (3 ml) (5/carton)
Comment: Basaglar has not pronounced peak; duration 24 hours or longer. Basaglar has an amino acid sequence identical to insulin glargine, **Lantus.**
Lantus administer once daily at HS as basal insulin; onset 1.1 hrs, no pronounced peak, duration 24 hours or longer; initial average starting dose 10 units for insulin-naïve patients; when switching from once daily *NPH or Ultralente*

insulin, initial dose of *insulin glargine* should be on a unit-for-unit basis; when switching from twice daily *NPH* insulin, start at 20% lower than the previous total daily *NPH* dose; SC only

> *Pediatric:* <6 years: not recommended; ≥6 years: same as adult
> *Vial:* 100 U/ml (10 ml); *Cartridge:* 100 U/ml (3 ml, for use in the *OptiPen One Insulin Delivery Device*) (5/carton) (m-cresol); *SoloStar pen (disposable):* 100 U/ml (3 ml) (5/carton)

Toujeo administer daily at the same time each day; SC in the upper arm, abdomen, or thigh; onset of action 6 hours; duration of action 24 hours-5 days; *T2DM, insulin naïve:* initially 0.2 units/kg; titrate every 3-4 days; *T1DM, insulin naïve:* initially 1/3-1/2 total daily insulin dose; remainder as short-acting insulin divided between each meal; *Switch from once daily long- or intermediate-acting insulin:* on a unit-for-unit basis; *Switching from Lantus:* a higher daily dose is expected; *Switching from twice daily NPH:* reduce initial dose by 20% of total daily NPH dose

> *Pediatric:* <18 years: not established
> *Soln for SC injection:* 300 units/ml prefilled disposable SoloStar Pen (1.5 ml, 3-5/carton)

▷ *insulin zinc suspension (lente)* (B)

> *Pediatric:* <18 years: not recommended
>> **Humulin L *(human)*** (OTC) onset 1-3 hours; peak 6-12 hours; duration 18-24 hours; SC only
>>> *Vial:* 100 U/ml (10 ml)
>> **Iletin II Lente *(pork)*** (OTC) onset 1-3 hours; peak 6-12 hours; duration 18-26 hours; SC only
>>> *Vial:* 100 U/ml (10 ml)
>> **Novolin L *(human)*** (OTC) onset 2.5 hours; peak 7-15 hours; duration 22 hours; SC only
>>> *Vial:* 100 U/ml (10 ml)

Ultra Long-Acting Insulin

▷ *insulin extended zinc suspension (Ultralente) (human)* (B) onset 4-6 hours; peak 8-20 hours; duration 24-48 hours; SC only

> *Pediatric:* <18 years: not recommended
>> **Humulin U** (OTC) *Vial:* 100 U/ml (10 ml)

Insulin Lispro Protamine/Insulin Lispro Combinations

▷ *insulin lispro protamine75%/insulin lispro 25%* (B)

> *Pediatric:* <18 years: not recommended
>> **Humalog Mix 75/25 *(human)*** onset 15 minutes; peak 30 minutes to 1 hour; duration 24 hours; SC only
>>> *Vial:* 100 U/ml (10 ml); *Prefilled disposable KwikPen:* 100 U/ml (3 ml, 5/pck) (zinc, m-cresol); *HumaPen Memoir* and *HumaPen Luxura* HD inj device for *Humalog cartridges* (100 U/ml, 3 ml, 5/pck) (zinc, m-cresol)

▷ *insulin lispro protamine 50%/insulin lispro 50%* (B)

> *Pediatric:* <18 years: not recommended
>> **Humalog Mix 50/50 *(recombinant)*** (B) onset 15 minutes; peak 2.3 hours; range 1-5 hours; SC only

Vial: 100 U/ml (10 ml); *Prefilled disposable KwikPen:* 100 U/ml (3 ml, 5/pck) (zinc, m-cresol); *HumaPen Memoir* and *Huma-Pen Luxura* HD inj device for *Humalog cartridges* (100 U/ml, 3 ml, 5/pck) (zinc, m-cresol)

Insulin Isophane Suspension (NPH)/Insulin Regular Combinations

▷ *NPH 70%/regular 30%* **(B)**
  Pediatric: same as adult
   Humulin 70/30 *(human, recombinant)* **(OTC)** onset 30 minutes; peak 2-12 hours; duration up to 24 hours; SC only
   Vial: 100 U/ml (10 ml)
   Novolin 70/30 *(recombinant)* **(OTC)** onset 30 minutes; peak 2-12 hours; duration up to 24 hours; SC only
   Vial: 100 U/ml (10 ml)
▷ *NPH 50%/regular 50%* **(B)**
   Pediatric: <18 years: not recommended
   Humulin 50/50 *(human)* **(OTC)** onset 30 minutes; peak 3-5 hours; duration up to 24 hours; SC only
   Vial: 100 U/ml (10 ml)

Insulin Lispro Protamine/Insulin Lispro Combinations

▷ *insulin lispro protamine 75%/insulin lispro 25%* **(B)**
  Pediatric: <18 years: not recommended
   Humalog Mix 75/25 *(recombinant)* onset 15 minutes; peak 30-90 minutes; duration 24 hours; SC only
   Vial: 100 U/ml (10 ml); *Prefilled disposable KwikPen:* 100 U/ ml (3 ml, 5/pck) (zinc, m-cresol); *HumaPen Memoir* and *Huma-Pen Luxura* HD inj device for *Humalog cartridges* (100 U/ml, 3 ml 5/pck) (zinc, m-cresol)
▷ *insulin lispro protamine 50%/insulin lispro 50%* **(B)**
  Pediatric: <18 years: not recommended
   Humalog Mix 50/50 *(recombinant)* onset 15 minutes; peak 1 hour; duration up to 16 hours; SC only
   Vial: 100 U/ml (10 ml); *Prefilled disposable KwikPen:* 100 U/ml (3 ml, 5/pck) (zinc, m-cresol); *HumaPen Memoir* and *HumaPen LUXURA* HD inj device for *Humalog cartridges* (100 U/ml, 3 ml 5/pck) (zinc, m-cresol); U/ml (3 ml, 5/pck) (zinc, m-cresol); *HumaPen Memoir* and *HumaPen LUXURA* HD inj device for *Humalog cartridges* (100 U/ml, 3 ml 5/pck) (zinc, m-cresol); (100 U/ml, 3 ml 5/pck (zinc, m-cresol)

TYPE 2 DIABETES MELLITUS

Comment: Normal fasting glucose is <100 mg/dL. Impaired glucose tolerance is a risk factor for type 2 diabetes and a marker for cardiovascular disease risk; it occurs early in the natural history of these two diseases. Impaired fasting glucose is >100 mg/dL and <125 mg/dL. Impaired glucose tolerance is OGTT, 2 hour post-load 75 g glucose >140 mg/dL and <200 mg/dL. Target preprandial glucose is 80 mg/dL to 120 mg/dL. Target bedtime glucose is 100mg/dL to 140 mg/dL. Target glycosylated hemoglobin (HbA1c) is <7.0%. Addition of daily ACE-I <u>and/or</u> ARB therapy is strongly recommended for renal protection. Consider diabetes screening at age 25 years for persons in high-risk groups (non-Caucasian, positive family history for DM, obesity). Hypertension and hyperlipidemia are common comorbid conditions. Macrovascular complications include cerebral vascular disease, coronary artery disease, and peripheral vascular disease. Microvascular complications include retinopathy, nephropathy, neuropathy, and cardiomyopathy. Oral hypoglycemics are contraindicated in pregnancy.

Insulins *see Type 1 Diabetes Mellitus page* 417

TREATMENT FOR ACUTE HYPOGLYCEMIA

▷ *glucagon (recombinant)* (B) administer SC, IM, <u>or</u> IV; if patient does not respond in 15 minutes, may administer a single <u>or</u> 2 divided doses
Adults and Children: <20 kg: 0.5 mg <u>or</u> 20-30 mg/kg; >20 kg: 1 mg

SULFONYLUREAS

Comment: Sulfonylureas are secretagogues (i.e., stimulate pancreatic insulin secretion); therefore, the patient taking a sulfonylurea should be alerted to the risk for hypoglycemia. Action is dependent on functioning beta cells in the pancreatic islets.

1st Generation Sulfonylureas

▷ *chlorpropamide* (C)(G) initially 250 mg/day with breakfast; max 750 mg
Pediatric: not recommended
Diabinese *Tab:* 100*, 250*mg
▷ *tolazamide* (C)(G) initially 100-250 mg/day with breakfast; increase by 100-250 mg/day at weekly intervals; maintenance 100 mg 1 g/day; max 1 g/day
Pediatric: not recommended
Tolinase *Tab:* 100, 250, 500 mg
▷ *tolbutamide* (C) initially 1-2 g in divided doses; max 2 g/day
Pediatric: not recommended
Tab: 500 mg

2nd Generation Sulfonylureas

▷ *glimepiride* (C) initially 1-2 mg once daily with breakfast; after reaching dose of 2 mg, increase by 2 mg at 1-2 week intervals as needed; usual maintenance 1-4 mg once daily; max 8 mg/day
Pediatric: not recommended
Amaryl *Tab:* 1*, 2*, 4*mg
▷ *glipizide* (C)(G)
Pediatric: not recommended
Glucotrol initially 5 mg before breakfast; increase by 2.5-5 mg every few days if needed; max 15 mg/day; max 40 mg/day in divided doses
Tab: 5*, 10* mg
Glucotrol XL initially 5 mg with breakfast; usual range 5-10 mg/day; max 20 mg/day
Tab: 2.5, 5, 10 mg ext-rel
▷ *glyburide* (C)(G) initially 2.5-5 mg/day with breakfast; increase by 2.5 mg at weekly intervals; maintenance 1.25-20 mg/day in a single <u>or</u> 2 divided doses; max 20 mg/day
Pediatric: not recommended
DiaBeta, Micronase *Tab:* 1.25*, 2.5*, 5*mg
▷ *glyburide, micronized* (B)
Pediatric: not recommended

Glynase PresTab initially 1.5-3 mg/day with breakfast; increase by 1.5 mg at weekly intervals if needed; usual maintenance 0.75-12 mg/day in single or divided doses; max 12 mg/day
  Tab: 1.5*, 3*, 6*mg

ALPHA-GLUCOSIDASE INHIBITORS

Comment: Alpha-glucosidase inhibitors block the enzyme that breaks down carbohydrates in the small intestine, delaying digestion and absorption of complex carbohydrates, and lowering peak post-prandial glycemic concentrations. Use as monotherapy or in combination with a sulfonylurea. Contraindicated in inflammatory bowel disease, colon ulceration, and intestinal obstruction. Side effects include flatulence, diarrhea, and abdominal pain.

▷ *acarbose* (B) initially 25 mg tid ac, increase at 4-8 week intervals; or initially 25 mg once daily, increase gradually to 25 mg tid; usual range 50-100 mg tid; max 100 mg tid
  Pediatric: not recommended
    Precose *Tab:* 25, 50, 100 mg
▷ *miglitol* (B) initially 25 mg tid at the start of each main meal, titrated to 50 mg tid at the start of each main meal; max 100 mg tid
  Pediatric: not recommended
    Glyset *Tab:* 25, 50, 100 mg

BIGUANIDE

Comment: The biguanides decrease gluconeogenesis by the liver in the presence of insulin. Action is dependent on the presence of circulating insulin. Lower hepatic glucose production leads to lower overnight, fasting, and pre-prandial plasma glucose levels. Common side effects include GI distress, nausea, vomiting, bloating, and flatulence which usually eventually resolve. May be used as monotherapy (in adults only) or with a sulfonylurea or insulin.

▷ *metformin* (B)(G) take with meals
  Comment: *metformin* is contraindicated with renal impairment, metabolic acidosis, ketoacidosis. Suspend *metformin*, prior to, and for 48 hours after, surgery or receiving IV iodinated contrast agents.
    Fortamet initially 1000 mg once daily; may increase by 500 mg/day at 1 week intervals; max 2.5 g/day
      Pediatric: <17 years: not recommended
      Tab: 500, 1000 mg ext-rel
    Glucophage initially 500 mg bid; may increase by 500 mg/day at 1 week intervals; max 1 g bid or 2.5 g in 3 divided doses; or initially 850 mg once daily in AM; may increase by 850 mg/day in divided doses at 2 week intervals; max 2000 mg/day; take with meals
      Pediatric: <10 years: not recommended; ≥10-16 years: use only as monotherapy; dose same as adult
      Tab: 500, 850, 1000*mg
    Glucophage XR initially 500 mg by mouth every evening; may increase by 500 mg/day at 1 week intervals; max 2 g/day
      Pediatric: <10 years: not recommended; ≥10-16 years: use immediate release form; >16 years: same as adult
      Tab: 500, 750 mg ext-rel

Glumetza ER (G) initially 1000 mg once daily; may increase by 500 mg/day at week intervals; max 2 g/day
   Pediatric: <18 years: not recommended
   Tab: 500, 1000 mg ext-rel
Riomet XR initially 500 mg once daily; may increase by 500 mg/day at 1 week intervals; max 2 g/day in divided doses; take with meals
   Pediatric: <10 years: not recommended; ≥10 years: monotherapy only
   Oral soln: 500 mg/ml (4 oz; cherry)

MEGLITINIDES

Comment: Meglitinides are secretagogues (i.e., stimulate pancreatic insulin secretion) in response to a meal. Action is dependent on functioning beta cells in the pancreatic islets. Use as monotherapy or in combination with *metformin*.
▷ *nateglinide* (C) 60-120 mg tid ac 1-30 minutes prior to start of the meal
   Pediatric: not recommended
      Starlix *Tab:* 60, 120 mg
▷ *repaglinide* (C)(G) initially 0.5 mg with 2-4 meals/day; take 30 minutes ac; titrate by doubling dose at intervals of at least 1 week; range 0.5-4 mg with 2-4 meals/day; max 16 mg/day
   Pediatric: not recommended
      Prandin *Tab:* 0.5, 1, 2 mg

THIAZOLIDINEDIONES (TZDs)

Comment: The TZDs decrease hepatic gluconeogenesis and reduce insulin resistance (i.e., increase glucose uptake and utilization by the muscles). Liver function tests are indicated before initiating these drugs. Do not start if ALT more than 3 times greater than normal. Recheck ALT monthly for the first six months of therapy; then every two months for the remainder of the first year and periodically thereafter. Liver function tests should be obtained at the first symptoms suggestive of hepatic dysfunction (nausea, vomiting, fatigue, dark urine, anorexia, abdominal pain).

▷ *pioglitazone* (C)(G) initially 15-30 mg once daily; max 45 mg/day as a monotherapy; usual max 30 mg/day in combination with *metformin*, insulin, or a sulfonylurea
   Pediatric: <18 years: not recommended
      Actos *Tab:* 15, 30, 45 mg
▷ *rosiglitazone* (C) initially 4 mg/day in a single or 2 divided doses; may increase after 8-12 weeks; max 8 mg/day as a monotherapy or combination therapy with *metformin* or a sulfonylurea; not for use with *insulin*
   Pediatric: <18 years: not recommended
      Avandia *Tab:* 2, 4, 8 mg

DIPEPTIDYL PEPTIDASE-4 (DPP-4) INHIBITOR/THIAZOLIDINEDIONE COMBINATION

Comment: The FDA has reported that alogliptin-containing drugs may increase the risk of heart failure, especially in patients who already have cardiovascular or renal disease. The drug Oseni (*alogliptin/pioglitazone*) is in this risk group.
▷ *alogliptin/pioglitazone* (C) take 1 dose once daily with first meal of the day; max: *rosiglitazone* 8 mg and max *glimepiride* per day; Same precautions as *alogliptin* and *pioglitazone*

Pediatric: <18 years: not recommended
> **Oseni**
>> *Tab:* **Oseni 12.5/15:** *alo* 12.5 mg/*pio* 15 mg;
>> **Oseni 12.5/30:** *alo* 12.5 mg/*pio* 30 mg
>> **Oseni 12.5/45:** *alo* 12.5 mg/*pio* 45 mg
>> **Oseni 25/15:** *alo* 25/*pio* 15 mg
>> **Oseni 25/30:** *alo* 25/*pio* 30 mg
>> **Oseni 25/45:** *alo* 25 mg/*pio* 45 mg

2ND GENERATION SULFONYLUREA/BIGUANIDE COMBINATIONS

Comment: *Metaglip* and *Glucovance* are combination secretagogues (sulfonylureas) and insulin sensitizers (biguanides). *Sulfonylurea:* Action is dependent on functioning beta cells in the pancreatic islets; patient should be alerted to the risk for hypoglycemia. Common side effects of the biguanide include GI distress, nausea, vomiting, bloating, and flatulence which usually eventually resolve. Take with food. *metformin* is contraindicated with renal impairment, metabolic acidosis, ketoacidosis. Suspend *metformin*, prior to, and for 48 hours after, surgery or receiving IV iodinated contrast agents.

▷ *glipizide/metformin* (C) take with meals; *Primary therapy:* 2.5/250 once daily or if FBS is 280-320 mg/dL, may start at 2.5/250 bid; may increase by 1 tab/day every 2 weeks; max 10/2000 per day in 2 divided doses; *Second Line Therapy:* 2.5/500 or 5/500 bid; may increase by up to 5/500 every 2 weeks; max: 20/2000 per day; Same precautions as *glipizide* and *metformin*
Pediatric: not recommended
> **Metaglip**
>> *Tab:* **Metaglip 2.5/250:** *glip* 2.5 mg/*met* 250 mg
>> **Metaglip 2.5/500:** *glip* 2.5 mg/*met* 500 mg
>> **Metaglip 5/500:** *glip* 5 mg/*met* 500 mg

▷ *glyburide/metformin* (B) take with meals; *Primary therapy (initial therapy if HgbA1c <9.0%):* initially 1.25/250 once daily; max *glyburide* 20 mg and *metformin* 2000 mg per day; *Primary therapy (initial therapy if HbA1c >9.0% or FBS >200):* initially 1.25/250 bid; max *glyburide* 20 mg and *metformin* 2000 mg per day; *Second line therapy (initial therapy if HbA1c >7.0%):* initially 2.5/500 or 5/500 bid; max *glyburide* 20 mg and *metformin* 2000 mg per day; *Previously treated with a sulfonylurea and metformin:* dose to approximate total daily doses of *glyburide* and *metformin* already being taken; max: *glyburide* 20 mg and *metformin* 2000 mg per day; Same precautions as *glyburide* and *metformin*
Pediatric: not recommended
> **Glucovance**
>> *Tab:* **Glucovance 1.25/250:** *glyb* 1.25 mg/*met* 250 mg
>> **Glucovance 2.5/500:** *glyb* 2.5 mg/*met* 500 mg
>> **Glucovance 5/500:** *glyb* 5 mg/*met* 500 mg

Comment: *metformin* is contraindicated with renal impairment, metabolic acidosis, ketoacidosis. Suspend *metformin*, prior to, and for 48 hours after, surgery or receiving IV iodinated contrast agents.

THIAZOLIDINEDIONE/BIGUANIDE COMBINATION

▷ *pioglitazone/metformin* (C) take in divided doses with meals; *Previously on metformin alone:* initially 15mg/500mg or 15mg/850 mg once or twice daily; *Previously on pioglitazone alone:* initially 15mg/500mg bid; *Previously on pioglitazone and metformin:*

switch on a mg/mg basis; may increase after 8-12 weeks; max: *pioglitazone* 45 mg and *metformin* 2000 mg per day; Same precautions as *pioglitazone* and *metformin*
Pediatric: not recommended

> **Actoplus Met, Actoplis Met R (G)**
>> *Tab:* **Actoplus Met 15/500:** *pio* 15 mg/*met* 500 mg
>> **Actoplus Met 15/850:** *pio* 15 mg/*met* 850 mg
>> **Actoplus Met XR 15/1000:** *pio* 15 mg/*met* 1000 mg
>> **Actoplus Met XR 30/1000:** *pio* 30 mg/*met* 1000 mg

Comment: *metformin* is contraindicated with renal impairment, metabolic acidosis, ketoacidosis. Suspend *metformin*, prior to, and for 48 hours after, surgery <u>or</u> receiving IV iodinated contrast agents.

➤ **rosiglitazone/metformin** (C) take in divided doses with meals; *Previously on metformin alone:* add **rosiglitazone** 4 mg/day; may increase after 8-12 weeks; *Previously on rosiglitazone alone:* add **metformin** 1000 mg/day; may increase after 1-2 weeks; *Previously on* **rosiglitazone** *and* **metformin:** switch on a mg/mg basis; may increase **rosiglitazone** by 4 mg <u>and/or</u> **metformin** by 500 mg per day; max: **rosiglitazone** 8 mg and **metformin** 2000 mg per day; Same precautions as **rosiglitazone** and **metformin**
Pediatric: not recommended

> **Avandamet**
>> *Tab:* **Avandamet 2/500:** *rosi* 2 mg/*met* 500 mg
>> **Avandamet 2/1000:** *rosi* 2 mg/*met* 1000 mg
>> **Avandamet 4/500:** *rosi* 4 mg/*met* 500 mg
>> **Avandamet 4/1000:** *rosi* 4 mg/*met* 1000 mg

Comment: *rosiglitazone* has been withdrawn from retail pharmacies. In order to enroll and receive **rosiglitazone**, healthcare providers and patients must enroll in the *Avandia-Rosiglitazone Medicines Access Program.* The program limits the use of **rosiglitazone** to patients already being treated successfully, and those whose blood sugar cannot be controlled with other antidiabetic medicines. **metformin** is contraindicated with renal impairment, metabolic acidosis, ketoacidosis. Suspend **metformin**, prior to, and for 48 hours after, surgery <u>or</u> receiving IV iodinated contrast agents.

THIAZOLIDINEDIONE/SULFONYLUREA COMBINATIONS

➤ **pioglitazone/glimepiride** (C) take 1 dose daily with first meal of the day; *Previously on sulfonylurea alone:* initially 30mg/2mg; *Previously on* **pioglitazone** *and* **glimepiride:** switch on a mg/mg basis; max: **pioglitazone** 30 mg and **glimepiride** 4 mg per day; Same precautions as **pioglitazone** and **glimepiride**
Pediatric: <18 years: not recommended

> **Duetact**
>> *Tab:* **Duetact 30/2:** *pio* 30 mg/*glim* 2 mg
>> **Duetact 304:** *pio* 30 mg/*glim* 4 mg

➤ **rosiglitazone/glimepiride** (C) take 1 dose daily with first meal of the day; max: **rosiglitazone** 8 mg and **glimepiride** 4 mg per day; Same precautions as **rosiglitazone** and **glimepiride**
Pediatric: <18 years: not recommended

> **Avandaryl**
>> *Tab:* **Avandaryl 4/1:** *rosi* 4 mg/*glim* 1 mg
>> **Avandaryl 4/2:** *rosi* 4 mg/*glim* 2 mg
>> **Avandaryl 4/4:** *rosi* 4 mg/*glim* 4 mg

Avandaryl 8/2: *rosi* 8 mg/*glim* 2 mg
Avandaryl 8/4: *rosi* 8 mg/*glim* 4 mg

GLUCAGON-LIKE PEPTIDE-1 (GLP-1) RECEPTOR AGONISTS

Comment: GLP-1 receptor agonists act as an agonist at the GLP-1 receptors. They have a longer half-life than the native protein allowing them to be dosed once daily. They increase intracellular cAMP resulting in *insulin* release in the presence of increased serum concentration, decrease *glucagon* secretion, and delay gastric emptying, thus, reducing fasting, premeal, and post-prandial glucose throughout the day. GLP-1 receptor agonists are not a substitute for *insulin*, not for treatment of DKA, and not for post-prandial administration.

▶ *albiglutide* (C) administer by SC injection into the upper arm, abdomen, or thigh once daily; initially 30 mg once weekly on the same day; may increase to max 50 mg once weekly
  Pediatric: <18 years: not established
    Tanzeum *Prefilled pen/syringe:* 30, 50 mg/pen pwdr for injection after reconstitution (4/pck) (preservative-free)
▶ *dulaglutide* (C) administer by SC injection into the upper arm, abdomen, or thigh once daily; initially 0.6 mg/day for 1 week; then 1.2 mg/day; may increase to max 1.8 mg/day; if more than 3 days since last dose, restart at 0.6 mg/day and titrate as before
  Pediatric: <18 years: not established
    Trulicity *Prefilled pen/syringe:* 0.75, 1.5 mg/0.5 ml single-dose (4/pck)
▶ *exenatide* (C) administer by SC injection into the upper arm, abdomen, or thigh
  Pediatric: not recommended
    Bydureon administer 2 mg weekly (every 7 days); inject immediately after mixing; if changing from *Byetta*, discontinue and start *Vial:* 2 mg pwdr for reconstitution (1 vial pwdr and 1 syringe prefilled w. diluents, vial connector, and needles, 4/pck)
    Byetta inject within 60 minutes before AM and PM meals; initially 5 mcg/dose; may increase to 10 mcg/dose after one month
      Prefilled pen: 250 mcg/ml (5, 10 mcg/dose; 60 doses, needles not included) (m-cresol, mannitol)
▶ *liraglutide* (C) administer by SC injection into the upper arm, abdomen, or thigh once daily; initially 0.6 mg/day for 1 week; then 1.2 mg/day; may increase to 1.8 mg/day
  Pediatric: <18 years: not recommended
    Victoza *Prefilled pen:* 6 mg/ml (3 ml; needles not included)

SODIUM-GLUCOSE CO-TRANSPORTER 2 (SGLT2) INHIBITORS

Comment: SGLT2 inhibitors block the SGLT2 protein involved in 90% of glucose reabsorption in the proximal renal tubule, resulting in increased renal glucose excretion (typically >2000 mg/dL), and lower blood glucose levels (low risk of hypoglycemia), modest weight loss, and mild reduction in blood pressure (probably due to sodium loss). These agents probably also increase insulin sensitivity, decrease gluconeogenesis, and improve *insulin* release from pancreatic beta cells. SGLT2 inhibitors are contraindicated in T1DM, and are decreased or contraindicated with decreased eGFR, increased SCr, renal failure, ESRD, renal dialysis, metabolic acidosis, or diabetic ketoacidosis. The most commen side effects are UTI, female genital mycotic infection, and increased urination. These effects may be managed with adequate hydration and genital hygiene. The SGLT2 inhibitors are not recommended in nursing women. There is potential for a hypersensitivity reaction to include angioedema and anaphylaxis. Caution with SGLT2 use due to reports of increased risk of treatment-emergent bone fractures.

▶ *canagliflozin* (C) take one tab before the first meal of the day; initially 100 mg; may titrate up to max 300 mg once daily; *eGFR <45:* do not initiate
Pediatric: <18 years: not established
 Invokana *Tab:* 100, 300 mg
 Comment: **Invokana** is contraindicated with eGFR <45; If eGFR 45-≤60, max 100 mg once daily or consider other antihyperglycemic

▶ *dapagliflozin* (C) take one tab before the first meal of the day; initially 5 mg; may increase to max 10 mg once daily
Pediatric: <18 years: not established
 Farxiga *Tab:* 5, 10 mg
 Comment: **Farxiga** is contraindicated with eGFR <60.

▶ *empagliflozin* (C) take one tab before the first meal of the day; initially 10 mg; may increase to max 25 mg once daily
Pediatric: <18 years: not established
 Jardiance *Tab:* 10, 25 mg
 Comment: **Jardiance** is contraindicated with eGFR <45.

SODIUM-GLUCOSE CO-TRANSPORTER 2 (SGLT2) INHIBITOR/BIGUANIDE COMBINATIONS

Comment: Caution with **SGLT2** use due to reports of increased risk of treatment-emergent bone fractures. *metformin* is contraindicated with renal impairment, metabolic acidosis, ketoacidosis. Suspend *metformin*, prior to, and for 48 hours after, surgery or receiving IV iodinated contrast agents.

▶ *canagliflozin/metformin* (C) take 1 dose twice daily with meals; max daily dose 300/2000; *eGFR 45-≤60: canagliflozin* max 100 mg once daily or consider other antihyperglycemic; *eGFR <45:* do not initiate
Pediatric: <18 years: not established
 Invokamet
  Tab: **Invokamet 50/500:** *cana* 50 mg/*met* 500 mg
   Invokamet 50/1000: *cana* 50 mg/*met* 1000 mg
   Invokamet 150/500: *cana* 150 mg/*met* 500 mg
   Invokamet 150/1000: *cana* 150 mg/*met* 1000 mg

▶ *dapagliflozin/metformin* (C) swall whole; do not crush or chew; take once daily first meal of the day; max daily dose 10/2000
Pediatric: <18 years: not established
 Xigduo XR
  Tab: **Xigduo XR 5/500:** *dapa* 5 mg/*met* 500 mg ext-rel
   Xigduo XR 5/1000: *dapa* 5 mg/*met* 1000 mg ext-rel
   Xigduo XR 10/500: *dapa* 10 mg/*met* 500 mg ext-rel
   Xigduo XR 10/1000: *dapa* 10 mg/*met* 1000 mg ext-rel
 Comment: **Xigduo** is contraindicated with eGFR <60, SCr >1.5 (men), or SCr >1.4 (women)

▶ *empagliflozin/metforman* (C) take 1 dose twice daily with meals; max daily dose 25/2000

Pediatric: <18 years: not established
> **Synjardy**
> *Tab:* **Synjardy 5/500:** *invo* 5 mg/*met* 500 mg
> **Synjardy 5/1000:** *invo* 5 mg/*met* 1000 mg
> **Synjardy 12.5/500:** *invo* 12.5 mg/*met* 500 mg
> **Synjardy 12.5/1000:** *invo* 12.5 mg/*met* 1000 mg
> Comment: **Synjardy** is contraindicated with eGFR <45, SCr >1.5 (men), <u>or</u> SCr >1.4 (women).

SODIUM-GLUCOSE CO-TRANSPORTER 2 (SGLT2) INHIBITOR/DIPEPTIDYL PEPTIDASE-4 (DPP-4) INHIBITOR COMBINATION

Comment: Caution with **SGLT2** use due to reports of increased risk of treatment-emergent bone fractures.

▷ *empagliflozin/linagliptin* (C) initially 10/5 once daily with the first meal of the day; max daily dose 25/5
Pediatric: <18 years: not established
> **Glyxambi**
> *Tab:* **Glyxambi 10/5:** *empa* 10 mg/*lina* 5 mg
> **Glyxambi 25/5:** *empa* 25 mg/*lina* 5 mg
> Comment: **Glyxambi** is contraindicated with eGFR <45.

DIPEPTIDYL PEPTIDASE-4 (DPP-4) INHIBITOR

Comment: DPP-4 is an enzyme that degrades incretin hormones glucagon-like peptide-1 (GLP-1) and glucose-dependent insulinotropic polypeptide (GIP). Thus, DPP-4 inhibitors increase the concentration of active incretin hormones, stimulating the release of *insulin* in a glucose-dependent manner and decreasing the levels of circulating *glucagon*. The FDA has reported that saxagliptin- and alogliptin-containing drugs may increase the risk of heart failure, especially in patients who already have cardiovascular <u>or</u> renal disease. Drugs in this risk group include Nesina (alogliptin) and Onglyza (saxagliptin)

▷ *alogliptin* (B) take twice daily with meals; max 25 mg/day
Pediatric: <18 years: not recommended
> **Nesina** *Tab:* 6.25, 12.5, 25 mg
▷ *linagliptin* (B) 5 mg once daily
Pediatric: <18 years: not recommended
> **Tradjenta** *Tab:* 5 mg
▷ *saxagliptin* (B) 2.5-5 mg once daily
Pediatric: <18 years: not recommended
> **Onglyza** *Tab:* 2.5, 5 mg
▷ *sitagliptin* (B) as monotherapy <u>or</u> as combination therapy with metfor- min <u>or</u> a TZD
Pediatric: <18 years: not recommended
> **Januvia** 25-100 mg once daily
> *Tab:* 25, 50, 100 mg

DIPEPTIDYL PEPTIDASE-4 (DPP-4) INHIBITOR/BIGUANIDE COMBINATIONS

Comment: DPP-4 inhibitor/*metformin* combinations are contraindicated with renal impairment (men: SCr ≥1.5 mg/dL; women: SCr ≥1.4 mg/dL) <u>or</u> abnormal CrCl, metabolic acidosis, ketoacidosis, or history of angioedema. Temporarily suspend for surgery or IV administered iodinated contrast agents. Avoid in the elderly, malnourished, dehydrated, or with clinical or lab evidence of hepatic disease. For other DPP-4 and/or *metformin* precautions, see mfr pkg insert. The FDA has reported that *saxagliptin*- and *alogliptin*-containing drugs may increase the risk of heart failure, especially in patients who already have cardiovascular or renal disease. These drugs include: Onglyza (*saxagliptin*), Kombiglyze XR (*saxagliptin/metformin*), Nesina (*alogliptin*), Kazano (*alogliptin/metformin*), and Oseni (*alogliptin/pioglitazone*).

▶ *alogliptin/metformin* (B) take twice daily with meals; max *algogliptin* 25 mg/day, max *metformin* 2000 mg/day

    Pediatric: <18 years: not recommended

       Kazano

         Tab: Kazano 12.5/500: *algo* 12.5 mg/*met* 500 mg

             Kazano 2.5/1000: *algo* 12.5 mg/*met* 1000 mg

▶ *linagliptin/metformin* (B) take twice daily with meals; max *linagliptin* 5 mg/day, max *metformin* 2000 mg/day

    Pediatric: <18 years: not recommended

       Jentadueto

         Tab: Jentadueto 2.5/500: *lina* 2.5 mg/*met* 500 mg

              Jentadueto 2.5/850: *lina* 2.5 mg/*met* 850 mg

              Jentadueto 2.5/1000: *lina* 2.5 mg/*met* 1000 mg

▶ *saxagliptin/metformin* (B) take once daily with meals; max *saxagliptin* 5 mg/day, max *metformin* 2000 mg/day

    Pediatric: <18 years: not recommended

       Kombiglyze XR

         Tab: Kombiglyze XR 5/500: *saxa* 5 mg/*met* 500 mg

              Kombiglyze XR 2.5/1000: *saxa* 2.5 mg/*met* 1000 mg

              Kombiglyze XR 5/1000: *saxa* 5 mg/*met* 1000 mg

Comment: The FDA has reported that *saxagliptin*-containing drugs may increase the risk of heart failure, especially in patients who already have cardiovascular or renal disease. The drug Kombiglyze XR (*saxagliptin/metformin*) is in this risk group. *metformin* is contraindicated with renal impairment, metabolic acidosis, ketoacidosis. Suspend *metformin*, prior to, and for 48 hours after, surgery or receiving IV iodinated contrast agents.

▶ *sitagliptin/metformin* (B) take twice daily with meals; max *sitagliptin* 100 mg/day, max *metformin* 2000 mg/day

    Pediatric: <18 years: not recommended

       Janumet

         Tab: Janumet 50/500: *sita* 50 mg/*met* 500 mg

              Janumet 50/1000: *sita* 50 mg/*met* 1000 mg

       Janumet XR

         Tab: Janumet XR 50/500: *sita* 50 mg/*met* 500 mg ext-rel

              Janumet XR 50/1000: *sita* 50 mg/*met* 1000 mg ext-rel

              Janumet XR 100/1000: *sita* 100 mg/*met* 1000 mg ext-rel

Comment: *metformin* is contraindicated with renal impairment, metabolic acidosis, ketoacidosis. Suspend *metformin*, prior to, and for 48 hours after, surgery or receiving IV iodinated contrast agents.

MEGLITINIDE/BIGUANIDE COMBINATION

▶ *repaglinide/metformin* (C)(G) take in 2-3 divided doses within 30 minutes before food; max 4/1000 per meal and 10/2000 per day

Pediatric: not recommended
> **Prandimet**
> *Tab:* **Prandimet 1/500:** *repa* 1 mg/*met* 500 mg
> **Prandimet 2/500:** *repa* 2 mg/*met* 500 mg

Comment: *metformin* is contraindicated with renal impairment, metabolic acidosis, ketoacidosis. Suspend *metformin*, prior to, and for 48 hours after, surgery or receiving IV iodinated contrast agents.

DIPEPTIDYL PEPTIDASE-4 (DPP-4) INHIBITOR/HMG-COA REDUCTASE INHIBITOR COMBINATION

▷ *sitagliptin/simvastatin* (B) take once daily in the PM; swallow whole; adjust dose if needed after 4 weeks; *Concomitant verapamil* or *diltiazem:* max 100/10 once daily; *Concomitant amiodarone, amlodipine,* or *ranolazine:* max 100/20 once daily; *Homogenous familial hypercholesterolemia:* max 100/40 once daily; *Chinese patients taking lipid-modifying doses (>1 g/day niacin) of niacin-containing products:* caution with 100/40 dose; increase risk of myopathy
Pediatric: <18 years: not recommended
> **Juvisync**
> *Tab:* **Juvisync 100/10:** *sita* 100 mg/*simva* 10 mg
> **Juvisync 100/20:** *sita* 100 mg/*simva* 20 mg
> **Juvisync 100/40:** *sita* 100 mg/*simva* 40 mg

DOPAMINE RECEPTOR AGONIST

▷ *bromocriptine mesylate* (B) take with food in the morning within 2 hours of waking; initially 0.8 mg once daily; may increase by 0.8 mg/ week; max 4.8 mg/week; *Severe psychotic disorders:* not recommended
Pediatric: not recommended
> **Cycloset** *Tab:* 0.8 mg
> **Comment:** **Cycloset** is an adjunct to diet and exercise to improve glycemic control. Contraindicated with syncopal migraines, nursing mothers, and other ergot-related drugs.

Bile Acid Sequestrant

▷ *colesevelam* (B) *Monotherapy:* 3 tabs bid or 6 tabs once daily or one **1.875 g pkt bid** or one 3.75 g pkt once daily
Pediatric: not recommended
> **WelChol** *Tab:* 625 mg; *Pwdr for oral susp:* 1.875 g pwdr pkts (60/carton); 3.75 g pwdr pkts (30/carton) (citrus; phenylalanine)
> **Comment:** *colesevelam* (WelChol) is indicated as an adjunctive therapy to improve glycemic control in adults with type 2 diabetes. It can be added to *metformin*, sulfonylureas, or *insulin* alone or in combination with other antidiabetic agents

 TYPHOID FEVER (SALMONELLA TYPHI)

PRE-EXPOSURE PROPHYLAXIS

▷ *typhoid* vaccine, oral, live, attenuated strain

Vivotif Berna 1 cap every other day, 1 hour before a meal, with a lukewarm (not > body temperature) <u>or</u> cold drink for a total of 4 doses; do not crush <u>or</u> chew; complete therapy at least 1 week prior to expected exposure; re-immunization recommended every 5 years if repeated exposure

> *Pediatric:* <6 years: not recommended; ≥6 years: same as adult
> *Cap:* ent-coat

▷ *typhoid Vi polysaccharide* vaccine (C)

Typhim Vi 0.5 ml IM in deltoid; re-immunization recommended every 2 years if repeated exposure

> *Pediatric:* <2 years: not recommended; ≥2 years: same as adult
> *Vial:* 20, 50 dose; *Prefilled syringe:* 0.5 ml

Comment: Febrile illness may require delaying administration of the vaccine; have *epinephrine* 1:1000 readily available.

TREATMENT

▷ *azithromycin* (B) 8-10 mg/kg/day; *Mild Illness:* treat x 7 days; *Severe Illness:* treat x 14 days

Pediatric: 8-10 mg/kg/day; max 500 mg/day; *Mild Illness:* treat x 7 days; *Severe Illness:* treat x 14 days; *see page 548 for dose by weight*

> **Zithromax** *Tab:* 250, 500, 600 mg; *Oral susp:* 100 mg/5 ml (15 ml); 200 mg/5 ml (15, 22.5, 30 ml) (cherry); *Pkt:* 1 g for reconstitution (cherry-banana)
> **Zithromax Tri-pak** *Tab:* 3 x 500 mg tabs/pck
> **Zithromax Z-pak** *Tab:* 6 x 250 mg tabs/pck
> **Zmax** *Oral susp:* 2 g ext-rel for reconstitution (cherry-banana) (148 mg Na+)

▷ *cefixime* (B) *Mild Illness:* 15-20 mg/kg/day x 7-14 days; *Severe Illness:* 20 mg/kg/day x 10-14 days

Pediatric: <6 months: not recommended; 6 months-12 years, <50 kg: *Mild Illness:* 15-20 mg/kg/day x 7-14 days; *Severe Illness:* 20 mg/kg/day x 10-14 >50 kg: same as adult; *see page 552 for dose by weight*

> **Suprax** *Tab:* 400 mg; *Cap:* 400 mg; *Oral susp:* 100, 200 mg/5 ml (50, 75, 100 ml) (strawberry)

▷ *ciprofloxacin* (C) 15 mg/kg/day; *Mild Illness:* treat x 5-7 days; *Severe Illness:* treat x 10-14 days

Pediatric: <18 years: not recommended

> **Cipro (G)** *Tab:* 250, 500, 750 mg; *Oral susp:* 250, 500 mg/5 ml (100 ml) (strawberry)
> **Cipro XR** *Tab:* 500, 1000 mg ext-rel
> **ProQuin XR** *Tab:* 500 mg ext-rel

Comment: *ciprofl oxacin* is contraindicated <18 years-of-age, and during pregnancy and lactation. Risk of tendonitis or tendon rupture, especially 60 years-of-age and older.

▷ *ofloxacin* (C) 15 mg/kg/day; *Mild Illness:* treat x 5-7 days; *Severe Illness:* treat x 10-14 days

Pediatric: <18 years: not recommended

> *Pediatric:* <18 years: not recommended
> **Floxin** *Tab:* 200, 300, 400 mg

Comment: *ofloxacin* is contraindicated <18 years-of-age, and during pregnancy and lactation. Risk of tendonitis or tendon rupture, especially 60 years-of-age and older.

▷ *cefotaxime* 80 mg/kg/day IM/IV x 10-14 days; max 2 g/day
  Pediatrics: 80 mg/kg/day IM/IV x 10-14 days; max 2 g/day
    Claforan *Vial:* 500 mg; 1, 2 g
▷ *ceftriaxone* (B)(G) 75 mg/kg/day IM/IV x 10-14 days; max 2 g/day
  Pediatrics: 75 mg/kg/day IM/IV x 10-14 days; max 2 g/day
    Rocephin *Vial:* 250, 500 mg; 1, 2 g
▷ *trimethoprim/sulfamethoxazole* (D)(G) 8-40 mg/kg/day x 14 days
  Pediatric: <2 months: not recommended; ≥2 months: 8-40 mg/kg/day of
  sulfamethoxazole in 2 divided doses bid x 10 days; *see page 576 for dose by weight*
    Bactrim, Septra 2 tabs bid x 10 days
      Tab: trim 80 mg/*sulfa* 400 mg*
    Bactrim DS, Septra DS 1 tab bid x 10 days
      Tab: trim 160 mg/*sulfa* 800 mg*
    Bactrim Pediatric Suspension, Septra Pediatric Suspension 20 ml bid x 10
    days
      Oral susp: trim 40 mg/*sulfa* 200 mg per 5 ml (100 ml) (cherry) (alcohol 0.3%)
  Comment: *trimethoprim/sulfamethoxazole* is not recommended in pregnancy
  <u>or</u> lactation. *CrCl 15-30 mL/min:* reduce dose by 1/2; *CrCl <15 mL/min:* not
  recommended

ULCER: DIABETIC, NEUROPATHIC (LOWER EXTREMITY) ULCER: VENOUS INSUFFICIENCY (LOWER EXTREMITY)

NUTRITIONAL SUPPLEMENT

▷ *L-methylfolate calcium (as metafolin)/pyridoxyl 5-phosphate/methylcobalamin* (NR)
take 1 cap daily
Pediatric: not recommended
  Metanx *Cap:* metafo 3 mg/*pyrid* 35 mg/*methyl* 2 mg (gluten-free, yeast-free,
  lactose-free)
  Comment: **Metanx** is indicated as adjunct treatment of endothelial dysfunction <u>and/or</u> hyperhomocysteinemia in patients who have lower extremity
  ulceration.

DEBRIDING/CAPILLARY STIMULANT AGENT

▷ *trypsin/balsam peru/castor oil* (NR) apply at least twice daily; may cover with a wet
bandage
  Granulex *Aerosol liq:* tryp 0.12 mg/*bal peru* 87 mg/*cast* 788 mg per 0.82 ml

GROWTH FACTOR

▷ *becaplermin* (C) apply once daily with a cotton swab <u>or</u> tongue depressor; then cover
with saline moistened gauze dressing; rinse after 12 hours; then re-cover with a clean
saline dressing
  Regranex *Gel:* 0.01% (2, 7.5, 15 g) (parabens)
  Comment: Store in refrigerator; do not freeze. Not for use in wounds that close by
  primary intention.

ULCER: PRESSURE/DECUBITUS

DEBRIDING/CAPILLARY STIMULANT AGENT

Granulex (*trypsin* 0.1 mg/*balsam peru* 72.5 mg/castor oil 650 mg per 0.82 ml)
apply at least twice daily; may cover with a wet bandage
> *Aerosol liq:* (2, 4 oz)

GROWTH FACTOR

➤ *becaplermin* (C) apply once daily with a cotton swab <u>or</u> tongue depressor; then cover
with saline moistened gauze dressing; rinse after 12 hours; then recover with a clean
saline dressing
> **Regranex** *Gel:* 0.01% (2, 7.5, 15 g) (parabens)

Comment: Store in refrigerator; do not freeze. Not for use in wounds that close by
primary intention.

ULCERATIVE COLITIS

Comment: Standard treatment regimen is anti-infective, anti-spasmodic, and bowel
rest; progressing to clear liquids; then to high fiber.

Parenteral Corticosteroids *see page* 499
Oral Corticosteroids *see page* 497

➤ *budesonide micronized* (C) take 9 mg once daily in the AM for up to 8 weeks; may repeat an 8-week course; *Maintenance of remission:* 6 mg once daily for up yo 3 months;
taper other systemic steroids when transferring to *bunesonide*
Pediatric: not recommended
> **Entocort EC** *Cap:* 3 mg ent-coat granules
> **Uceris** *Tab:* 9 mg ext-rel

RECTAL GLUCOCORTICOSTEROIDS

➤ *hydrocortisone* rectal (C)
Pediatric: not recommended
> **Anusol-HC Suppositories** 1 supp rectally 3 times daily <u>or</u> 2 supp rectally twice
> daily for 2 weeks; max 8 weeks
>> *Rectal supp:* 25 mg (12, 24/pck)
> **Cortenema** 1 enema q HS x 21 days <u>or</u> until symptoms controlled
>> *Enema:* 100 mg/60 ml (1, 7/pck)
> **Cortifoam** 1 applicator full once daily-bid x 2-3 weeks and every 2nd day there-
> after until symptoms are controlled
>> *Aerosol:* 80 mg/applicator (14 application/container)
> **Proctocort** 1 supp rectally in AM and PM x 2 weeks; for more severe cases, may
> increase to 1 supp rectally 3 times daily <u>or</u> 2 supp rectally twice daily; max 4-8
> weeks
>> *Rectal supp:* 30 mg (12, 24/pck)

Comment: Use *hydrocortisone* foam as adjunctive therapy in the distal portion of
the rectum when *hydrocortisone* enemas cannot be retained.

RECTAL CORTICOSTEROID/ANESTHETIC

Hydrocortisone/Pramoxine

> **Proctofoam HC** apply to anal/rectal area 3-4 times daily; max 4-8 weeks
> *Rectal foam: hydrocort 1%/ pram 1% (10 g w. applicator)*

SALICYLATES

▷ *balsalazide disodium* (B)

> **Colazal** 2.25 g 3 times daily x 8 weeks; max 12 weeks; swallow whole or sprinkle contents into apple sauce
> *Pediatric:* <5 years: not recommended; ≥5 years: 2.25 g 3 times daily or 750 mg once daily x 8 weeks; swallow whole or sprinkle contents into apple sauce
> *Cap:* 750 mg

Comment: *balsalazide* 6.75 g provides 2.4 g of *mesalazine* to the colon.

> **Giazo** take 3 tabs bid; max 8 weeks
> *Tab:* 1.1 g (sodium 126 mg/tab) film-coat

▷ *mesalamine* (B)

> *Pediatric:* not recommended
> **Apriso** take 1.5 g once daily in the AM for maintenance of remission
> *Cap:* 0.375 g ext-rel (phenylalanine 0.56 mg/cap)
> **Asacol HD** 1600 mg tid x 6 weeks; maintenance 1.6 g/day in divided doses; swallow whole; do not crush or chew
> *Tab:* 800 mg delayed-rel
> **Canasa** 1 g qid for up to 8 weeks
> *Rectal supp:* 1 g del-rel (30, 42/pck)
> **Delzicol** 800 mg tid x 6 weeks; maintenance once daily for up to 8 weeks; *Maintenance:* 1.6 g/day in 2-4 divided doses once daily; swallow whole; do not crush or chew
> *Cap:* 400 mg del-rel
> **Lialda** 2.4-4.8 g once daily for up to 8 weeks; maintenance 2.4 g once daily; swallow whole; do not crush or chew
> *Tab:* 1.2 g del-rel
> **Pentasa** 1 g qid for up to 8 weeks
> *Cap:* 250, 500 mg cont-rel
> **Rowasa Suppository** 1 supp rectally bid x 3-6 weeks; retain for 1-3 hours or longer
> *Rectal supp:* 500 mg (12, 24/pck)
> **Sulfite-Free Rowasa Rectal Suspension** 4 g rectally by enema q HS; retain for 8 hours x 3-6 weeks
> *Enema:* 4 g/60 ml (7, 14, 28/pck; kit, 7, 14, 28/pck w. wipes)

▷ *olsalazine* (C) 1 g/day in 2 divided doses

> **Dipentum** *Cap:* 250 mg

▷ *sulfasalazine* (B; D in 2nd, 3rd)(G)

> *Pediatric:* <2 years: not recommended; 2-16 years: initially 40-60 mg/kg/day in 3 to 6 divided doses; max 30 mg/kg/day in 4 divided doses; max 2 g/day; >16 years: same as adult
> **Azulfidine** initially 1-2 g/day; increase to 3-4 g/day in divided doses pc until clinical symptoms controlled; maintenance 2 g/day; max 4 g/day
> *Tab:* 500*mg

Azulfidine EN-Tabs initially 500 mg in the PM x 7 days; then 500 mg bid x 7 days; then 500 mg in the AM and 1 g in the PM x 7 days; then 1 g bid; max 4 g/day
   Tab: 500 mg ent-coat

TUMOR NECROSIS FACTOR (TNF) BLOCKER

▷ *adalimumab* (B) initially 180 mg SC (as 4 injections in 1 day <u>or</u> divided over 2 days) on week 0; then 80 mg at week 2; start 40 mg every other week maintenance at week 4; only continue if evidence of clinical remission by 8 weeks; administer in abdomen <u>or</u> thigh; rotate sites
Pediatric: <18 years not recommended
   Humira *Prefilled syringe:* 20 mg/0.4 ml; 40 mg/0.8 ml single-dose (2/pck; 2, 6/ starter pck) (preservative-free)
▷ *infliximab* (B) administer by IV infusion over 2 hours; 5 mg/kg weeks 0, 2, 6; then once every 8 weeks
Pediatric: <6 years: not recommended; ≥6 years: same as adult
   Vial: 100 mg pwdr for reconstitution for IV infusion (preservative-free)
▷ *vedolizumab* (B) administer by IV infusion over 30 minutes; 300 mg at weeks 0, 2, 6; then once every 8 weeks
Pediatric: not established
   Entyvio
      Vial: 300 mg (20 ml) single dose, pwdr for IV infusion after reconstitution (preservative-free)

ANTI-DIARRHEAL AGENTS

▷ *difenoxin/atropine* (C) 2 tabs; then 1 tab after each loose stool <u>or</u> 1 tab q 3-4 hours; max 8 tabs/day x 2 days
   Motofen *Tab:* dif 1 mg/*atro* 0.025 mg
▷ *diphenoxylate/atropine* (C)(G) 2 tabs <u>or</u> 10 ml qid
   Lomotil *Tab:* diphen 2.5 mg/*atro* 0.025 mg; *Liq:* diphen 2.5 mg/*atro* 0.025 mg/5 ml (2 oz w. dropper)
▷ *loperamide* (B)(G)
   Imodium (OTC) 4 mg initially; then 2 mg after each loose stool; max 16 mg/day
      Cap: 2 mg
   Imodium A-D (OTC) 4 mg initially; then 2 mg after each loose stool; usual max 8 mg/day x 2 days
      Cplt: 2 mg; *Liq:* 1 mg/5 ml (2, 4 oz)
   Imodium Advanced (OTC) 2 tabs chewed after first loose stool; then 1 after the next loose stool; max 4 tabs/day
      Chew tab: loperamide 2 mg/simethicone 125 mg

◯ URETHRITIS: NONGONOCOCCAL (NGU)

Comment: The following treatment regimens for NGU are published in the **2015 CDC Sexually Transmitted Diseases Treatment Guidelines**. Treatment regimens are for adults only; consult a specialist for treatment of patients less than 18 years-of-age. Treatment regimens are presented by generic drug name first, followed by information about brands and dose forms. All persons who have confirmed <u>or</u> suspected urethritis should be tested for gonorrhea and chlamydia. Men treated for NGU should be instructed to abstain from sexual intercourse for 7 days after a single-dose regimen or until completion of a 7-day regimen.

RECOMMENDED REGIMEN: UNCOMPLICATED NGU

▷ *azithromycin* 1 g in a single dose or 100 mg orally bid x 7 days
   plus
▷ *doxycycline* 100 mg bid x 7 days

PERSISTENT/RECURRENT NGU

Men Initially Treated With Azithromycin+Doxycycline

▷ *azithromycin* 1 g PO in a single dose

Men Who Fail a Regimen of Azithromycin

▷ *moxifloxacin* 400 mg PO once daily x 7 days

Heterosexual Men Who Live in Areas Where *T. Vaginalis* is Highly Prevalent

▷ *metronidazole* 2 g PO in a single dose
   or
▷ *tinidazole* 2 g PO in a single dose

ALTERNATIVE REGIMENS

▷ *erythromycin base* 500 mg PO qid x 7 days

   or

▷ *erythromycin ethylsuccinate* 800 mg PO qid x 7 days

   or

▷ *levofloxacin* 500 mg once daily x 7 days

   or

▷ *ofloxacin* 300 mg PO bid x 7 days

DRUG BRANDS AND DOSE FORMS

▷ *azithromycin* (B)
   Zithromax *Tab:* 250, 500, 600 mg; *Oral susp:* 100 mg/5 ml (15 ml); 200 mg/5 ml (15, 22.5, 30 ml) (cherry); *Pkt:* 1 g for reconstitution (cherry-banana)
   Zithromax Tri-pak *Tab:* 3 x 500 mg tabs/pck
   Zithromax Z-pak *Tab:* 6 x 250 mg tabs/pck
   Zmax *Oral susp:* 2 g ext-rel for reconstitution (cherry-banana) (148 mg Na⁺)
▷ *doxycycline* (D)(G)
   Adoxa *Tab:* 50, 75, 100, 150 mg ent-coat
   Doryx *Tab:* 75, 100, 150 mg del-rel
   Monodox *Cap:* 50, 75, 100 mg
   Oracea *Cap:* 40 mg del-rel
   Vibramycin *Cap:* 50, 100 mg; *Syr:* 50 mg/5 ml (raspberry; sulf-ites); *Oral susp:* 25 mg/5 ml (raspberry-apple)
   Vibra-Tab *Tab:* 100 mg film-coat

Comment: *doxycycline* is contraindicated <8 years-of-age, in pregnancy, and lactation (discolors developing tooth enamel). A side effect may be photo-sensitivity (photophobia). Do not give with antacids, calcium supplements, milk or other dairy, or within two hours of taking another drug.

▷ *erythromycin base* (B)
　　Ery-Tab *Tab:* 250, 333, 500 mg ent-coat
　　PCE *Tab:* 333, 500 mg

Comment: *erythromycin* may increase INR with concomitant *warfarin*, as well as increase serum level of *digoxin*, benzodiazepines and statins.

▷ *erythromycin ethylsuccinate* (B)(G)
　　EryPed *Oral susp:* 200 mg/5 ml (100, 200 ml) (fruit); 400 mg/5 ml (60, 100, 200 ml) (banana); *Oral drops:* 200, 400 mg/5 ml (50 ml) (fruit); *Chew tab:* 200 mg wafer (fruit)
　　E.E.S. *Oral susp:* 200, 400 mg/5 ml (100 ml) (fruit)
　　E.E.S. Granules *Oral susp:* 200 mg/5 ml (100, 200 ml) (cherry)
　　E.E.S. 400 Tablets *Tab:* 400 mg

Comment: *erythromycin* may increase INR with concomitant *warfarin*, as well as increase serum level of *digoxin*, benzodiazepines and statins.

▷ *levofloxacin* (C)
　　Levaquin *Tab:* 250, 500, 750 mg; *Oral soln:* 25 mg/ml (480 ml) (benzyl alcohol); *Inj conc:* 25 mg/ml for IV infusion after dilution (20, 30 ml single-use vial) (preservative-free); *Premix soln:* 5 mg/ml for IV infusion (50, 100, 150 ml) (preservative-free)

Comment: *levofloxacin* is contraindicated <18 years-of-age, and during pregnancy and lactation. Risk of tendonitis or tendon rupture, especially 60 years-of-age and older.

▷ *metronidazole* (not for use in 1st; B in 2nd, 3rd)(G)
　　Flagyl *Tab:* 250*, 500*mg
　　Flagyl 375 *Cap:* 375 mg
　　Flagyl ER *Tab:* 750 mg ext-rel

Comment: Alcohol is contraindicated during treatment with oral *metronidazole* and for 72 hours after therapy due to a possible *disulfiram*-like reaction (nausea, vomiting, flushing, headache).

▷ *moxifloxacin* (C)(G)
　　Avelox Tab: 400 mg

Comment: *moxifloxacin* is contraindicated <18 years-of-age, and during pregnancy and lactation. Risk of tendonitis or tendon rupture, especially 60 years-of-age and older.

▷ *ofloxacin* (C)(G)
　　Floxin *Tab:* 200, 300, 400 mg

Comment: *ofloxacin* is contraindicated <18 years-of-age, and during pregnancy and lactation. Risk of tendonitis or tendon rupture, especially 60 years-of-age and older.

▷ *tinidazole* (not for use in 1st; B in 2nd, 3rd)
　　Tindamax *Tab:* 250*, 500*mg

Comment: Alcohol is contraindicated during treatment with oral *tinidazole* and for 72 hours after therapy due to a possible *disulfiram*-like reaction (nausea, vomiting, flushing, headache).

◯ URINARY RETENTION: UNOBSTRUCTIVE

▷ *bethanechol* (C) 10-30 mg tid
     Urecholine *Tab:* 5, 10, 25, 50 mg
     Comment: Contraindicated in presence of urinary obstruction. *atropine* 0.4 mg
     administered SC reverses *bethanechol* toxicity.

◯ URINARY TRACT INFECTION (UTI, CYSTITIS: ACUTE)

URINARY TRACT ANALGESIA

▷ *phenazopyridine* (B)(G) 95-200 mg q 6 hours prn; max 2 days
     Pediatric: not recommended
     AZO Standard, Prodium, Uristat (OTC) *Tab:* 95 mg
     AZO Standard Maximum Strength (OTC) *Tab:* 97.5 mg
     Pyridium, Urogesic *Tab:* 100, 200 mg

ANTI-INFECTIVES: THERAPY IN ADULT FEMALE WITH UNCOMPLICATED UTI

▷ *amoxicillin/clavulanate* (B)(G) 500 mg tid or 875 mg bid x 10 days
     Augmentin *Tab:* 250, 500, 875 mg; *Chew tab:* 125, 250 mg (lemon-lime); 200,
     400 mg (cherry-banana) (phenylalanine); *Oral susp:* 125 mg/5 ml (banana), 250
     mg/5 ml (75, 100, 150 ml) (orange); 200, 400 mg/5 ml (50, 75, 100 ml) (orange)
     (phenylalanine)
          Pediatric: 40-45 mg/kg/day divided tid x 10 days or 90 mg/kg/day divided
          bid x 10 days *see pages 545-546 for dose by weight*
     Augmentin ES-600 *Oral susp:* 600 mg/5 ml (50, 75, 100, 125, 150, 200 ml)
     (strawberry cream) (phenylalanine) every 12 hours
          Pediatric: <3 months: not recommended; ≥3 months, <40 kg: 90 mg/kg/day
          in 2 divided doses; ≥40 kg: not recommended
     Augmentin XR 2 tabs q 12 hours x 7-10 days
          Pediatric: <16 years: use other forms; ≥16 years: same as adult
          Tab: 1000*mg ext-rel
▷ *ciprofloxacin* (C)
     Pediatric: <18 years: not recommended
     Cipro (G) *Tab:* 250, 500, 750 mg; *Oral susp:* 250, 500 mg/5 ml (100 ml)
     (strawberry)
     Cipro XR *Tab:* 500, 1000 mg ext-rel
     ProQuin XR *Tab:* 500 mg ext-rel
     Comment: *ciprofloxacin* is contraindicated <18 years-of-age, and during pregnancy
     and lactation. Risk of tendonitis or tendon rupture, especially 60 years-of-age and
     older.
▷ *fosfomycin* (B) 1 pkt in 3-4 oz cold water x 1 dose
     Monurol *Single-dose pkts:* 1-3 g (mandarin orange; sucrose)
▷ *levofloxacin* (C) 250 mg once daily x 3 days
     Pediatric: <18 years: not recommended

Levaquin *Tab:* 250, 500, 750 mg; *Oral soln:* 25 mg/ml (480 ml) (benzyl alcohol); *Inj conc:* 25 mg/ml for IV infusion after dilution (20, 30 ml single-use vial) (preservative-free); *Premix soln:* 5 mg/ml for IV infusion (50, 100, 150 ml) (preservative-free)

Comment: *levofloxacin* is contraindicated <18 years-of-age, and during pregnancy and lactation. Risk of tendonitis or tendon rupture, especially 60 years-of-age and older.

➤ *norfloxacin* (C) 400 mg once daily x 3 days
Pediatric: <18 years: not recommended
   Noroxin *Tab:* 400 mg
Comment: *norfloxacin* is contraindicated <18 years-of-age, and during pregnancy and lactation. Risk of tendonitis or tendon rupture, especially 60 years-of-age and older.

➤ *ofloxacin* (C)(G) 200 mg q 12 hours x 3 days
Pediatric: <18 years: not recommended
   Floxin *Tab:* 200, 300, 400 mg
   Floxin UroPak *Tab:* 200 mg (6/pck)
Comment: *ofloxacin* is contraindicated <18 years-of-age, and during pregnancy and lactation. Risk of tendonitis or tendon rupture, especially 60 years-of-age and older.

➤ *trimethoprim* (C)(G)
   Primsol 100 mg q 12 hours or 200 mg once daily x 10 days
      Pediatric: <6 months: not recommended; ≥6 months: 10 mg/kg/day in 2 divided doses x 10 days
      Oral soln: 50 mg/5 ml (bubble gum; dye-free, alcohol-free)
   Proloprim 100 mg q 12 hours or 200 mg once daily x 10 days
      Pediatric: not recommended
      Tab: 100, 200 mg
   Trimpex 100 mg q 12 hours or 200 mg once daily x 10 days
      Pediatric: not recommended
      Tab: 100 mg

➤ *trimethoprim/sulfamethoxazole* (D)(G)
Pediatric: <2 months: not recommended; >2 months: 40 mg/kg/day of *sulfamethoxazole* in 2 divided doses bid x 10 days; *see page 576 for dose by weight*
   Bactrim, Septra 2 tabs bid x 10 days
      Tab: trim 80 mg/*sulfa* 400 mg*
   Bactrim DS, Septra DS 1 tab bid x 10 days
      Tab: trim 160 mg/*sulfa* 800 mg*
   Bactrim Pediatric Suspension, Septra Pediatric Suspension
      Oral susp: trim 40 mg/*sulfa* 200 mg per 5 ml (100 ml) (cherry) (alcohol 0.3%)
Comment: *trimethoprim/sulfamethoxazole* is not recommended in pregnancy or lactation. *CrCl 15-30 mL/min:* reduce dose by 1/2; *CrCl <15 mL/min:* not recommended

ANTI-INFECTIVES: STANDARD REGIMEN FOR UTI

➤ *acetyl sulfisoxazole* (C)(G)
   Gantrisin initially 2-4 g in a single or divided doses; then 4-8 g/day in 4-6 divided doses x 7 days
      Tab: 500 mg
   Gantrisin

Pediatric: <2 months: not recommended; ≥2 months: initial dose 75 mg/kg/day; then 150 mg/kg/day in 4-6 divided doses x 7 days; max 6 g/day
Oral susp: 500 mg/5 ml (4, 16 oz); *Syr:* 500 mg/5 ml (16 oz)

▷ *amoxicillin* (B)(G) 500-875 mg bid or 250-500 mg tid x 7 days
Pediatric: <40 kg (88 lb): 20-40 mg/kg/day in 3 divided doses x 7 days or 25-45 mg/kg/day in 2 divided doses x 7 days; *see page 543 for dose by weight*
    Amoxil *Cap:* 250, 500 mg; *Tab:* 875*mg; *Chew tab:* 125, 200, 250, 400 mg (cherry-banana-peppermint) (phenylalanine); *Oral susp:* 125, 250 mg/5 ml (80, 100, 150 ml) (strawberry); 200, 400 mg/5 ml (50, 75, 100 ml) (bubble gum); *Oral drops:* 50 mg/ml (30 ml) (bubble gum)
    Moxatag *Tab:* 775 mg ext-rel
    Trimox *Tab:* 125, 250 mg; *Cap:* 250, 500 mg; *Oral susp:* 125, 250 mg/5 ml (80, 100, 150 ml) (raspberry-strawberry)

▷ *amoxicillin/clavulanate* (B)(G) 500 mg tid or 875 mg bid x 10 days
    Augmentin *Tab:* 250, 500, 875 mg; *Chew tab:* 125, 250 mg (lemon-lime); 200, 400 mg (cherry-banana) (phenylalanine); *Oral susp:* 125 mg/5 ml (banana), 250 mg/5 ml (75, 100, 150 ml) (orange); 200, 400 mg/5 ml (50, 75, 100 ml) (orange) (phenylalanine)
    Pediatric: 40-45 mg/kg/day divided tid x 10 days or 90 mg/kg/day divided bid x 10 days *see pages 545-546 for dose by weight*
    Augmentin ES-600 *Oral susp:* 600 mg/5 ml (50, 75, 100, 125, 150, 200 ml) (strawberry cream) (phenylalanine) every 12 hours
    Pediatric: <3 months: not recommended; ≥3 months, <40 kg: 90 mg/kg/day in 2 divided doses; ≥40 kg: not recommended
    Augmentin XR 2 tabs q 12 hours x 7-10 days
    Pediatric: <16 years: use other forms; ≥16 years: same as adult
    Tab: 1000*mg ext-rel

▷ *ampicillin* (B) 500 mg qid x 7-14 days
Pediatric: 50-100 mg/kg/day in 4 divided doses x 7-14 days; *see page 547 for dose by weight*
    Omnipen, Principen *Cap:* 250, 500 mg; *Oral susp:* 125, 250 mg/5 ml (100, 150, 200 ml) (fruit)

▷ *carbenicillin* (B) 1-2 tabs qid x 7-14 days
Pediatric: not recommended
    Geocillin *Tab:* 382 mg

▷ *cefaclor* (B)(G) 250-500 mg q 8 hours x 10 days; max 2 g/day
Pediatric: <1 month: not recommended; 20-40 mg/kg bid or q 12 hours x 10 days; max 1 g/ day; *see page 549 for dose by weight*
Tab: 500 mg; *Cap:* 250, 500 mg; *Susp:* 125 mg/5 ml (75, 150 ml) (strawberry); 187 mg/5 ml (50, 100 ml) (strawberry); 250 mg/5 ml (75, 150 ml) (strawberry); 375 mg/5 ml (50, 100 ml) (strawberry)
Pediatric: <16 years: ext-rel not recommended; ≥16 years: same as adult
    Cefaclor Extended Release *Tab:* 375, 500 mg ext-rel

▷ *cefadroxil* (B) 1-2 g in a single or 2 divided doses x 10 days
Pediatric: 30 mg/kg/day in 2 divided doses x 10 days; *see page 550 for dose by weight*
    Duricef *Cap:* 500 mg; *Tab:* 1 g; *Oral susp:* 250 mg/5 ml (100 ml); 500 mg/5 ml (75, 100 ml) (orange-pineapple)

▷ *cefixime* (B) 400 mg once daily x 10 days
Pediatric: <6 months: not recommended; 6 months-12 years, <50 kg: 8 mg/kg/day in a single or 2 divided doses x 10 days; >12 years, >50 kg: same as adult; *see page 552 for dose by weight*

Suprax *Tab:* 400 mg; *Cap:* 400 mg; *Oral susp:* 100, 200 mg/5 ml (50, 75, 100 ml) (strawberry)

▶ *cefpodoxime proxetil* (B) 100 mg bid x 7 days
Pediatric: <2 months: not recommended; 2 months-12 years: 10 mg/kg/day (max 400 mg/dose) *or* 5 mg/kg/day bid (max 200 mg/dose) x 7 days; >12 years: same as adult; *see page 553 for dose by weight*
Vantin *Tab:* 100, 200 mg; *Oral susp:* 50, 100 mg/5 ml (50, 75, 100 mg) (lemon creme)

▶ *cefuroxime axetil* (B)(G) 125-250 mg bid x 7-10 days
Pediatric: <3 months: not recommended; 3 months-12 years: 20-30 mg/kg/day in 2 divided doses x 7-10 days; >12 years: same as adult; *see page 556 for dose by weight*
Ceftin *Tab:* 250, 500 mg; *Oral susp:* 125, 250 mg/5 ml (50, 100 ml) (tutti-frutti)

▶ *cephalexin* (B)(G) 500 mg bid x 7-10 days
Pediatric: 25-50 mg/kg/day in 4 divided doses x 7-10 days; *see page 557 for dose by weight*
Keflex *Cap:* 250, 333, 500, 750 mg; *Oral susp:* 125, 250 mg/5 ml (100, 200 ml) (strawberry)

▶ *ciprofloxacin* (C) 500 mg bid *or* 1000 mg XR once daily x 3-14 days
Pediatric: <18 years: not recommended
Cipro (G) *Tab:* 250, 500, 750 mg; *Oral susp:* 250, 500 mg/5 ml (100 ml) (strawberry)
Cipro XR *Tab:* 500, 1000 mg ext-rel
ProQuin XR *Tab:* 500 mg ext-rel
Comment: *ciprofloxacin* is contraindicated <18 years-of-age, and during pregnancy and lactation. Risk of tendonitis or tendon rupture, especially 60 years-of-age and older.

▶ *doxycycline* (D)(G) 100 mg bid x 7-10 days
Pediatric: <8 years: not recommended; ≥8 years, <100 lb: 2 mg/lb on first day in 2 divided doses, followed by 1 mg/lb/day in a single *or* 2 divided doses x 7-10 days; ≥8 years, >100 lb: same as adult
Adoxa *Tab:* 50, 75, 100, 150 mg ent-coat
Doryx *Tab:* 75, 100, 150 mg del-rel
Monodox *Cap:* 50, 75, 100 mg
Oracea *Cap:* 40 mg del-rel
Vibramycin *Cap:* 50, 100 mg; *Syr:* 50 mg/5 ml (raspberry; sulfites); *Oral susp:* 25 mg/5 ml (raspberry-apple)
Vibra-Tab *Tab:* 100 mg film-coat
Comment: *doxycycline* is contraindicated <8 years-of-age, in pregnancy, and lactation (discolors developing tooth enamel). A side effect may be photo-sensitivity (photophobia). Do not give with antacids, calcium supplements, milk or other dairy, or within two hours of taking another drug.

▶ *enoxacin* (C) 200 mg q 12 hours x 7 days
Pediatric: <18 years: not recommended
Penetrex *Tab:* 200, 400 mg
Comment: *enoxacin* is contraindicated <18 years-of-age, and during pregnancy and lactation. Risk of tendonitis or tendon rupture, especially 60 years-of-age and older.

▷ *levofloxacin* (C) 250 mg once daily x 7-10 days
　　Pediatric: <18 years not recommended
　　　　Levaquin *Tab:* 250, 500, 750 mg; *Oral soln:* 25 mg/ml (480 ml) (benzyl alcohol);
　　　　Inj conc: 25 mg/ml for IV infusion after dilution (20, 30 ml single-use vial)
　　　　(preservative-free); *Premix soln:* 5 mg/ml for IV infusion (50, 100, 150 ml)
　　　　(preservative-free)
　　Comment: *levofloxacin* is contraindicated <18 years-of-age, and during pregnancy
　　and lactation. Risk of tendonitis or tendon rupture, especially 60 years-of-age and
　　older.
▷ *lomefloxacin* (C) 400 mg once daily x 10 days
　　Pediatric: <18 years: not recommended
　　　　Maxaquin *Tab:* 400 mg
Comment: *lomefloxacin* is contraindicated <18 years-of-age, and during pregnancy
and lactation. Risk of tendonitis or tendon rupture, especially 60 years-of-age and
older.
▷ *minocycline* (D)(G) 100 mg q 12 hours x 10 days
　　Pediatric: <8 years: not recommended; ≥8 years, <100 lb: 2 mg/lb on first day in 2 divided
　　doses, followed by 1 mg/lb q 12 hours x 9 more days; ≥8 years, >100 lb: same as adult
　　　　Dynacin *Cap:* 50, 100 mg
　　　　Minocin *Cap:* 50, 75, 100 mg; *Oral susp:* 50 mg/5 ml (60 ml) (custard) (sulfites,
　　　　alcohol 5%)
　　Comment: *minocycline* is contraindicated <8 years-of-age, in pregnancy, and
　　lactation (discolors developing tooth enamel). A side effect may be photo-
　　sensitivity (photophobia). Do not give with antacids, calcium supplements, milk or
　　other dairy, or within two hours of taking another drug.
▷ *nalidixic acid* (B) 1 g qid x 7-14 days
　　Pediatric: <3 months: not recommended; >3 months: 25 mg/lb/day in 4 divided
　　doses x 7-14 days
　　　　NegGram *Tab:* 250, 500 mg; 1 g; *Cap:* 250, 500 mg; *Oral susp:* 250 mg/5 ml
▷ *nitrofurantoin* (B)(G)
　　　　Furadantin 50-100 mg qid x 7-10 days
　　　　　　Pediatric: <1 month: not recommended; ≥1 month: 5-7 mg/kg/day in 4 divid-
　　　　　　ed doses x 7-10 days; *see page 571 for dose by weight*
　　　　　　Oral susp: 25 mg/5 ml (60 ml)
　　　　Macrobid 100 mg q 12 hours x 7-10 days
　　　　　　Pediatric: <12 years: not recommended; ≥12 years: same as adult
　　　　　　Cap: 100 mg
　　　　Macrodantin 50-100 mg qid x 5-7 days; long-term use 50-100 mg q HS
　　　　　　Cap: 25, 50, 100 mg
▷ *norfloxacin* (C) 400 mg x 7-10 days
　　Pediatric: <18 years: not recommended
　　　　Noroxin *Tab:* 400 mg
　　Comment: *norfloxacin* is contraindicated <18 years-of-age, and during pregnancy
　　and lactation. Risk of tendonitis or tendon rupture, especially 60 years-of-age and
　　older.
▷ *ofloxacin* (C)(G) 200 mg q 12 hours x 7-10 days
　　Pediatric: <18 years: not recommended
　　　　Floxin *Tab:* 200, 300, 400 mg

Comment: *ofloxacin* is contraindicated <18 years-of-age, and during pregnancy and lactation. Risk of tendonitis or tendon rupture, especially 60 years-of-age and older.

▷ *trimethoprim* (C)(G)

    Primsol 100 mg q 12 hours <u>or</u> 200 mg once daily x 10 days
        Pediatric: <6 months: not recommended; ≥6 months: 10 mg/kg/day in 2 divided doses divided q 12 hours x 10 days
        Oral soln: 50 mg/5 ml (bubble gum; dye-free, alcohol-free)
    Proloprim 100 mg q 12 hours <u>or</u> 200 mg once daily x 10 days
        Pediatric: not recommended
        Tab: 100, 200 mg
    Trimpex 100 mg q 12 hours <u>or</u> 200 mg once daily x 10 days
        Pediatric: not recommended
        Tab: 100 mg

▷ *trimethoprim/sulfamethoxazole* (D)(G)

    Pediatric: <2 months: not recommended; ≥2 months: 40 mg/kg/day of *sulfamethoxazole* in 2 divided doses bid x 10 days; *see page 576 for dose by weight*
    Bactrim, Septra 2 tabs bid x 10 days
        Tab: trim 80 mg/*sulfa* 400 mg*
    Bactrim DS, Septra DS 1 tab bid x 10 days
        Tab: trim 160 mg/*sulfa* 800 mg*
    Bactrim Pediatric Suspension, Septra Pediatric Suspension
        Oral susp: trim 40 mg/*sulfa* 200 mg per 5 ml (100 ml) (cherry) (alcohol 0.3%)
    Comment: *trimethoprim/sulfamethoxazole* is not recommended in pregnancy <u>or</u> lactation. *CrCl 15-30 mL/min:* reduce dose by 1/2; *CrCl <15 mL/min:* not recommended

PARENTERAL THERAPY

▷ *ertapenem* (B) 1 g once daily; *CrCl <30 mL/min:* 500 mg once daily; treat x 10-14 days; may switch to an oral antibiotic after 3 days if warranted; *IV infusion:* administer over 30 minutes; *IM injection:* reconstitute with lidocaine only
    Pediatric: <18 years: not recommended
    Ivanz *Vial:* 1 g pwdr for reconstitution

LONG-TERM PROPHYLACTIC/SUPPRESSION THERAPY

▷ *methenamine hippurate* (C) 1 tab bid
    Pediatric: <6 years: not recommended; ≥6-12 years: 1/2 tab bid
    Hiprex, Urex *Tab:* 1 g

URINARY TRACT ANALGESIC/ANTISPASMODICS

▷ *hyoscyamine* (C)(G)

    Anaspaz 1-2 tabs q 4 hours prn; max 12 tabs/day
        Pediatric: <2 years: not recommended; ≥2-12 years: 0.0625-0.125 mg q 4 hours prn; max 0.75 mg/day; >12 years: same as adult
        Tab: 0.125*mg
    Levbid 1-2 tabs q 12 hours prn; max 4 tabs/day
        Pediatric: <12 years: not recommended; ≥12 years: same as adult
        Tab: 0.375*mg ext-rel
    Levsin 1-2 tabs q 4 hours prn; max 12 tabs/day

Pediatric: <6 years: not recommended; 6-12 years: 1 tab q 4 hours prn; ≥12 years: same as adult
Tab: 0.125*mg

Levsin Drops 1-2 ml q 4 hours prn; max 60 ml/day
Pediatric: 3.4 kg: 4 drops q 4 hours prn; max 24 drops/day; 5 kg: 5 drops q 4 hours prn; max 30 drops/day; 7 kg: 6 drops q 4 hours prn; max 36 drops/day; 10 kg: 8 drops q 4 hours prn; max 40 drops/day
Oral drops: 0.125 mg/ml (15 ml) (orange) (alcohol 5%)

Levsin Elixir 5-10 ml q 4 hours prn
Pediatric: <10 kg: use drops; 10-19 kg: 1.25 ml q 4 hours prn; 20-39 kg: 2.5 ml q 4 hours prn; 40-49 kg: 3.75 ml q 4 hours prn; >50 kg: 5 ml q 4 hours prn
Elix: 0.125 mg/5 ml (16 oz) (orange) (alcohol 20%)

Levsinex SL 1-2 tabs q 4 hours SL <u>or</u> po; max 12 tabs/day
Pediatric: 2-12 years: 1 tab q 4 hours; max 6 tabs/day; >12 years: same as adult
Tab: 0.125 mg sublingual

Levsinex Timecaps 1-2 caps q 12 hours; may adjust to 1 cap q 8 hours
Pediatric: 2-12 years: 1 cap q 12 hours; max 2 caps/day; >12 years: same as adult
Cap: 0.375 mg time-rel

NuLev dissolve 1-2 tabs on tongue, with <u>or</u> without water, q 4 hours prn; max 12 tabs/day
Pediatric: <2 years: not recommended; 2-12 years: dissolve 1 tab on tongue, with <u>or</u> without water, q 4 hours prn; max 6 tabs/day
ODT: 0.125 mg (mint) (phenylalanine)

▷ *methenamine/phenyl salicylate/methylene blue/benzoic acid/atropine sulfate/hyoscyamine* (C)(G) 2 tabs qid prn
Pediatric: <6 years: not recommended
    Urised *Tab:* meth 40.8 mg/*phenyl salic* 18.1 mg/*meth blue* 5.4 mg/*benz acid* 4.5 mg/*atro sulf* 0.03 mg/*hyoscy* 0.03 mg
    Comment: Urised imparts a blue-green color to urine which may stain fabrics.

▷ *methenamine/phenyl salicylate/methylene blue/na phosphate onobasic/hyoscyamine* (C) 1 cap qid prn
Pediatric: <6 years: not recommended; ≥6 years: same as adult
    Uribel *Cap:* meth 118 mg/*phenyl salic* 36 mg/*meth blue* 10 mg/*naphos mono* 40.8 mg/*hyoscy* 0.12 mg

▷ *methenamine/phenyl salicylate/methylene blue/na biphosphate/hyoscyamine* (C) 1 tab qid prn
Pediatric: <6 years: not recommended; ≥6 years: same as adult
    Urelle *Cap:* meth 81 mg/*phenyl salic* 32.4 mg/*meth blue* 10.8 mg/*na biphos* 40.8 mg/ *hyoscy* 0.12 mg

▷ *phenazopyridine* (B)(G) 95-200 mg q 6 hours prn; max 2 days
Pediatric: not recommended
    AZO Standard, Prodium, Uristat (OTC) *Tab:* 95 mg
    AZO Standard Maximum Strength (OTC) *Tab:* 97.5 mg
    Pyridium, Urogesic *Tab:* 100, 200 mg
    Comment: *phenazopyridine* imparts an orange-red color to urine which may stain fabrics.

PROPHYLACTIC/SUPPRESSION THERAPY

▷ *methenamine hippurate* (C) 1 g bid

Pediatric: <6 years: 0.25 g/30 lb qid; 6-12 years: 25-50 mg/kg/day in 2 divided doses <u>or</u> 0.5-1 g bid; >12 years: same as adult
> **Hiprex** *Tab:* 1 g; *Oral susp:* 500 mg/5 ml (480 ml)

⦾ UROLITHIASIS (RENAL CALCULI, KIDNEY STONES)

Acetaminophen for IV Infusion *see Pain page 296*
Oral Prescription NSAIDs *see page 489*
Other Oral Analgesics *see Pain page 298*
Opioids and Other Analgesics *see page 298*

ANTISPASMOTIC

▷ *flavoxate* (B)(G)
> **Urispaz** 100-200 mg tid-qid

PARENTERAL NARCOTICS

Aid to Stone Passage: Alpha-1A Blockers

▷ *alfuzosin* (B)(G) 10 mg once daily taken immediately after the same meal each day
> **UroXatral** *Tab:* 10 mg ext-rel
▷ *tamsulosin* (B)(G) initially 0.4 mg once daily; may increase to 0.8 mg once daily after 2-4 weeks if needed
> **Flomax** *Cap:* 0.4 mg
> Comment: May take **Flomax** 0.4 mg with **Avodart** 0.5 mg once daily as combination therapy.
▷ *buprenorphine* (C) 0.3 mg IM q 6 hours prn
> **Buprenex** *Amp:* 0.3 mg/ml (1 ml)
▷ *meperidine* (B; D in 2nd, 3rd)(II)(G) 50-100 mg IM q 3-4 hours prn
> **Demerol** *Tubex:* 25, 50, 75, 100 mg/ml (2 ml); *Vial:* 25 mg/ml (1 ml); 50 mg/ml (1, 30 ml); 75 mg/ml; (1 ml); 100 mg/ml (1, 20 ml)
> *Amp:* 25, 50, 75, 100 mg/ml (1 ml)
▷ *morphine sulfate* (C)(II)(G) 10-15 mg q 3-4 hours prn
> *Vial:* 1 mg/ml (1, 60 ml); 5 mg/ml (1 ml); 8 mg/ml (1 ml); 10 mg/ml (1, 2, 10 ml); 15 mg (1, 20 ml); *Amp:* 8 mg/ml (1 ml); 10 mg/ml (1 ml); 15 mg/ml (1 ml)

PREVENTION OF CALCIUM STONES

▷ *chlorothiazide* (B)(G) 50 mg bid
> **Diuril** *Tab:* 250*, 500*mg; *Oral susp:* 250 mg/5 ml (237 ml)
▷ *hydrochlorothiazide* (B)(G) 50 mg bid
> **Esidrix** *Tab:* 25, 50mg
> **Microzide** *Cap:* 12.5 mg

PREVENTION OF CYSTINE STONES

▷ *penicillamine* (D) 1-4 g/day
> *Pediatric:* not recommended

Cuprimine *Cap:* 125, 250 mg
Depen *Titratable tab:* 250 mg
▷ *potassium citrate* (C) 30 mEq qid
Urocit-K *Tab:* 5, 10, 15 mEq ext-rel
Comment: *potassium citrate* is contraindicated in hyperkalemia.

PREVENTION OF URIC ACID STONES

▷ *allopurinol* (C)(G) 200-300 mg in 1-3 doses; max 800 mg/day
Zyloprim *Tab:* 100*, 300*mg
▷ *potassium citrate* (C)
Urocit-K *Tab:* 5, 10, 15 mEq ext-rel
Comment: *potassium citrate* is contraindicated in hyperkalemia. Encourage
patients to limit salt intake and maintain liberal hydration (urine volume should be
at least 2 liters/day). Target urine pH is 6.0-7.0 and urine citrate at least 320 mg/day
and close to the normal mean of 640 mg/day. Take with food.

⬤ URTICARIA: CHRONIC IDIOPATHIC (CIU)

▷ *hydroxyzine* (C)(G) 25 mg tid prn; max 600 mg/day
Pediatric: <6 years: 50 mg/day divided qid prn; ≥6 years: 50-100 mg/day divided qid
prn; max 600 mg/day
AtaraxR *Tab:* 10, 25, 50, 100 mg; *Syr:* 10 mg/5 ml (alcohol 0.5%)
VistarilR *Cap:* 25, 50, 100 mg; *Oral susp:* 25 mg/5 ml (4 oz) (lemon)
Oral Drugs for Allergy, Cough, and Cold Symptoms *see page* 524

⬤ URTICARIA: ACUTE (HIVES)

MILD/MODERATE URTICARIA

Oral Drugs for Allergy, Cough, and Cold *see page* 524
Topical Corticosteroids *see page* 494
Oral Corticosteroids *see page* 497

SEVERE URTICARIA

Parenteral Antihistamines

▷ *diphenhydramine* (C)(G) 25-50 mg IM immediately; then q 6 hours
Pediatric: 1.25 mg/kg up to 25 mg IM x 1 dose; then q 6 hours
Benadryl Injectable *Vial:* 50 mg/ml (1 ml single-use); 50 mg/ml (10 ml multi-
dose); *Amp:* 10 mg/ml (1 ml); *Prefilled syringe:* 50 mg/ml (1 ml)

Parenteral Corticosteroids *see page* 499

▷ *epinephrine* (C) 1:1000 0.01 ml/kg SC; max 0.3 ml
Pediatric: 0.01 mg/kg SC

⬤ VAGINAL IRRITATION: EXTERNAL

▷ Replens Vaginal Moisturizer (NR)(OTC) apply as needed; for external use only
Bottle: 2 oz

▷ **Vagisil Intimate Moisturizer (NR)(OTC)** apply as needed; for external use only
Bottle: 2 oz

Comment: **Vagisil** has no effect on condom integrity.

VERTIGO

▷ *meclizine* **(B)(G)** 25-100 mg/day in divided doses
Pediatric: not recommended
    Antivert *Tab:* 12.5, 25, 50*mg
    Bonine (OTC) *Cap:* 15, 25, 30 mg; *Tab:* 12.5, 25, 50 mg; *Chew tab/Film-coat tab:* 25 mg
    Dramamine II (OTC) *Tab:* 25*mg
    Zentrip *Strip:* 25 mg orally-disint

VITILIGO

REPIGMENTATION ENHANCEMENT

▷ *methoxsalen* **(C)** Apply to well-defined area of vitiligo; then expose area to source of UVA (ultraviolet A) <u>or</u> sunlight; initial exposure no more than 1/2 predicted minimal erythemal dose; repeat weekly
Pediatric: <12 years: not recommended
    Oxsoralen *Lotn:* 1% (30 ml)

Comment: *methoxsalen* may only be applied by a health care provider. Do not dispense to patient.

▷ *trioxsalen* **(C)** 10 mg daily, taken 2-4 hours before ultraviolet light exposure; max 14 days and 28 tabs
Pediatric: <12 years: not recommended
    Trisoralen *Tab:* 5 mg

Depigmenting Agents *see Hyperpigmentation page* 198

WART: COMMON (VERRUCA VULGARIS)

▷ *salicylic acid* **(NR)(G)**
    Duo Film (OTC) apply daily-bid; max 12 weeks; *Liq:* 17% (1/2 oz w. applicator)
    Duo Film Patch for Kids (OTC) apply 1 patch q 48 hours; max 12 weeks
        Patch: 40% (18/pck)
    Occlusal HP (OTC) apply daily-bid; max 12 weeks
        Liq: 17% (10 ml w. applicator)
    Wart-Off (OTC) apply one drop at a time to sufficiently cover wart, let dry; repeat 1-2 times daily; max 12 weeks
        Liq: 17% (0.45 oz)

WART: PLANTAR (VERRUCA PLANTARIS)

▷ *salicylic acid* **(NR)(G)**
    Duo Plant Gel (OTC) apply daily bid; max 12 weeks

Gel: 17% (1/2 oz)
Mediplast cut to size of wart and apply; remove q 1-2 days, peel keratin, and reapply; repeat as long as needed
Occlusal-HP (OTC) apply once daily-bid; max 12 weeks
   Liq: 17% (10 ml w. applicator)
Wart-Off (OTC) apply one drop at a time to sufficiently cover wart, let dry; repeat 1-2 times daily; max 12 weeks
   Liq: 17% (0.45 oz)
▷ *trichloroacetic acid* (NR) apply after wart is pared and repeat weekly

 WART: VENEREAL HUMAN PAPILLOMA VIRUS (HPV), CONDYLOMA ACUMINATA

Comment: This section contains treatment regimens for genital warts published in the **2015 CDC Sexually Transmitted Diseases Treatment Guidelines** as well as other treatment options. Due to the increased risk of cervical cancer with HPV, Pap smears should be done q 3 months during active disease and then q 3-6 months for the next 2 years.

PATIENT-APPLIED AGENTS

Regimen 1

▷ *imiquimod* (C)
   Pediatric: not recommended
     Aldara (G) rub into lesions before bedtime and remove with soap and water 6-10 hours later; treat 3 times per week; max 16 weeks
       Crm: 5% (12 single-use pkts/carton)
     Zyclara rub into lesions before bedtime and remove with soap and water 8 hours later; treat 3 times per week; max 1 packet per treatment; max 8 weeks
       Crm: 3.75% (28 single-use pkts/carton) (parabens)

Regimen 2

▷ *podofilox 0.5% cream* (C) apply bid (q 12 hours) x 3 days; then discontinue for 4 days; may repeat if needed; max 4 treatment cycles
   Condylox *Soln:* 0.5% (3.5 ml); *Gel:* 0.5% (3.5 g)

Regimen 3

▷ *sinecatechins 15% ointment* (C) apply to each lesion tid for up to 16 weeks
   Veregen *Oint:* 15% (15, 30 g)

PROVIDER-ADMINISTERED AGENTS

Regimen 1

▷ Cryotherapy with liquid nitrogen <u>or</u> cryoprobe; repeat applications every 1-2 weeks as needed

Regimen 2

▷ **trichloroacetic acid (TCA) 80-90%** (C) apply to warts; repeat weekly if needed
Comment: TCA is the preferred treatment during pregnancy. Immediate application of sodium bicarbonate paste following treatment decreases pain.

Regimen 3

▷ **podofilox 0.5% cream** (C) apply bid (q 12 hours) x 3 days; then discontinue for 4 days; may repeat if needed; max 4 treatment cycles
      Condylox *Soln:* 0.5% (3.5 ml); *Gel:* 0.5% (3.5 g)

Regimen 4

▷ **interferon alfa-n3** (C) 0.05 ml injected into base of wart twice weekly for up to 8 weeks; max 0.5 ml/session (20 warts/session)
      Alferon N Vial: 5 million units/ml (1 ml)

Regimen 5

▷ **interferon alfa-2b** (C) 0.1 ml injected into base of wart three times weekly for up to 3 weeks; max 0.5 ml/session (5 warts/session)
      Intron A Vial: 1 million units/0.1 ml (0.5, 1 ml)

Regimen 6

▷ Surgical removal either by tangential scissor excision, tangential shave excision, curettage, or electrosurgery

◯ WHIPWORM (TRICHURIASIS)

ANTIHELMINTICS

▷ **albendazole** (C) 400 mg as a single dose; may repeat in 3 weeks; take after a meal
   Pediatric: <2 years: 200 mg daily x 3 days; may repeat in 3 weeks; 2-12 years: 400 mg daily x 3 days; may repeat in 3 weeks; >12 years: same as adult
      Albenza *Tab:* 200 mg
▷ **mebendazole** (C)(G) 100 mg bid x 3 days; may repeat in 2-3 weeks if needed; take after a meal
   Pediatric: same as adult (chew or crush and mix with food)
      Vermox *Chew tab:* 100 mg
▷ **pyrantel pamoate** (C) 11 mg/kg x 1 dose; max 1 g/dose; take after a meal
   Pediatric: 25-37 lb: 1/2 tsp x 1 dose; 38-62 lb: 1 tsp x 1 dose; 63-87 lb: 1 tsp x 1 dose; 88-112 lb: 2 tsp x 1 dose; 113-137 lb: 2 tsp x 1 dose; 138-162 lb: 3 tsp x 1 dose; 163-187 lb: 3 tsp x 1 dose; >187 lb: 4 tsp x 1 dose
      Antiminth (OTC) *Cap:* 180 mg; *Liq:* 50 mg/ml (30 ml); 144 mg/ml (30 ml); *Oral susp:* 50 mg/ml (60 ml)
      Pin-X (OTC) *Cap:* 180 mg; *Liq:* 50 mg/ml (30 ml); 144 mg/ml (30 ml); *Oral susp:* 50 mg/ml (30 ml)
▷ **thiabendazole** (C) 25 mg/kg bid x 7 days; max 1.5 g/dose; take after a meal
   Pediatric: same as adult; <30 lb: consult mfr literature; >30 lb: 2 doses/day with meals; 30-50 lb: 250 mg bid with meals; >50 lb: 10 mg/lb/dose bid with meals; max 3g/day

Mintezol *Chew tab:* 500*mg (orange); *Oral susp:* 500 mg/5 ml (120 ml) (orange)
Comment: *thiabendazole* is not for prophylaxis. May impair mental alertness.

⬤ WOUND: INFECTED, NONSURGICAL, MINOR

TETANUS PROPHYLAXIS

Previously Immunized (within previous 5 years)

▷ *tetanus toxoid* vaccine **(C)** 0.5 ml IM x 1 dose
    Vial: 5 Lf units/0.5 ml (0.5, 5 ml); *Prefilled syringe:* 5 Lf units/0.5 ml (0.5 ml)

Not Previously Immunized

see Tetanus *page* 398

TOPICAL ANTI-INFECTIVES

▷ *mupirocin* **(B)(G)** apply to lesions bid
    Pediatric: same as adult
        Bactroban *Oint:* 2% (22 g); *Crm:* 2% (15, 30 g)
        Centany *Oint:* 2% (15, 30 g)

ORAL ANTI-INFECTIVES

▷ *azithromycin* **(B)** 500 mg x 1 dose on day 1, then 250 mg daily on days 2-5 or 500 mg daily x 3 days or Zmax 2 g in a single dose
    Pediatric: 10 mg/kg x 1 dose on day 1, then 5 mg/kg/day on days 2-5; max 500 mg/day; *see page 548 for dose by weight*
        Zithromax *Tab:* 250, 500, 600 mg; *Oral susp:* 100 mg/5 ml (15 ml); 200 mg/5 ml (15, 22.5, 30 ml) (cherry); *Pkt:* 1 g for reconstitution (cherry-banana)
        Zithromax Tri-pak *Tab:* 3 x 500 mg tabs/pck
        Zithromax Z-pak *Tab:* 6 x 250 mg tabs/pck
        Zmax *Oral susp:* 2 g ext-rel for reconstitution (cherry-banana) (148 mg Na⁺)
▷ *amoxicillin/clavulanate* **(B)(G)** 500 mg tid or 875 mg bid x 10 days
        Augmentin *Tab:* 250, 500, 875 mg; *Chew tab:* 125, 250 mg (lemon-lime); 200, 400 mg (cherry-banana) (phenylalanine); *Oral susp:* 125 mg/5 ml (banana), 250 mg/5 ml (75, 100, 150 ml) (orange); 200, 400 mg/5 ml (50, 75, 100 ml) (orange) (phenylalanine)
        Pediatric: 40-45 mg/kg/day divided tid x 10 days or 90 mg/kg/day divided bid x 10 days; *see pages 545-546 for dose by weight*
        Augmentin ES-600 *Oral susp:* 600 mg/5 ml (50, 75, 100, 125, 150, 200 ml) (strawberry cream) (phenylalanine) every 12 hours
        Pediatric: <3 months: not recommended; ≥3 months, <40 kg: 90 mg/kg/day in 2 divided doses; ≥40 kg: not recommended
        Augmentin XR 2 tabs q 12 hours x 7-10 days
        Pediatric: <16 years: use other forms; ≥16 years: same as adult
        Tab: 1000*mg ext-rel
▷ *cefaclor* **(B)(G)** 250-500 mg q 8 hours x 10 days; max 2 g/day
    Pediatric: <1 month: not recommended; 20-40 mg/kg bid or q 12 hours x 10 days; max 1 g/ day; *see page 549 for dose by weight*

Tab: 500 mg; *Cap:* 250, 500 mg; *Susp:* 125 mg/5 ml (75, 150 ml) (strawberry); 187 mg/5 ml (50, 100 ml) (strawberry); 250 mg/5 ml (75, 150 ml) (strawberry); 375 mg/5 ml (50, 100 ml) (strawberry)
Pediatric: <16 years: ext-rel not recommended
   Cefaclor Extended Release *Tab:* 375, 500 mg ext-rel
▶ *cefadroxil* 1 g/day in 1-2 divided doses x 10 days
Pediatric: 15-30 mg/kg/day in 2 divided doses x 10 days; *see page 550 for dose by weight*
   Duricef *Cap:* 500 mg; *Tab:* 1 g; *Oral susp:* 250 mg/5 ml (100 ml); 500 mg/5 ml (75, 100 ml) (orange-pineapple)
▶ *cefdinir* (B) 300 mg bid or 600 mg daily x 10 days
Pediatric: <6 months: not recommended; 6 months-12 years: 14 mg/kg/day in 1-2 divided doses x 10 days; *see page 551 for dose by weight*
   Omnicef *Cap:* 300 mg; *Oral susp:* 125 mg/5 ml (60, 100 ml) (strawberry)
▶ *cefpodoxime proxetil* (B) 400 mg bid x 7-14 days
Pediatric: <2 months: not recommended; 2 months-12 years: 10 mg/kg/day (max 400 mg/ dose) or 5 mg/kg/day bid (max 200 mg/dose) x 7-14 days; *see page 553 for dose by weight*
   Vantin *Tab:* 100, 200 mg; *Oral susp:* 50, 100 mg/5 ml (50, 75, 100 mg; lemon cream)
      Pediatric: see page 553 for dose by weight
▶ *cefprozil* (B) 250-500 mg q 12 hours or 500 mg daily x 10 days
Pediatric: <2 years: not recommended; 2-12 years: 7.5 mg/kg-15 mg/kg q 12 hours x 10 days; >12 years: same as adult; *see page 554 for dose by weight*
   Cefzil *Tab:* 250, 500 mg; *Oral susp:* 125, 250 mg/5 ml (50, 75, 100 ml) (bubble gum, phenylalanine)
▶ *cephalexin* (B)(G) 2 g 1 hour before procedure
Pediatric: 50 mg/kg/day in 4 divided doses x 10 days; *see page 557 for dose by weight*
   Keflex *Cap:* 250, 333, 500, 750 mg; *Oral susp:* 125, 250 mg/5 ml (100, 200 ml) (strawberry)
      Pediatric: see page 557 for dose by weight
▶ *clarithromycin* (C)(G) 500 mg or 500 mg ext-rel for 7-10 days
Pediatric: see page 558 for dose by weight
   Biaxin *Tab:* 250, 500 mg
   Biaxin Oral Suspension *Oral susp:* 125, 250 mg/5 ml (50, 100 ml) (fruit-punch)
   Biaxin XL *Tab:* 500 mg ext-rel
▶ *dirithromycin* (C)(G) 500 mg daily x 7 days
Pediatric: <12 years: not recommended
   Dynabac *Tab:* 250 mg
▶ *erythromycin base* (B)(G) 500 mg qid x 14 days
Pediatric: 30-50 mg/kg/day in 2-4 divided doses x 10 days
   Ery-Tab *Tab:* 250, 333, 500 mg ent-coat
   PCE *Tab:* 333, 500 mg
Comment: *erythromycin* may increase INR with concomitant *warfarin*, as well as increase serum level of *digoxin*, benzodiazepines and statins.
▶ *erythromycin ethylsuccinate* (B)(G) 400 mg qid x 7 days
Pediatric: 30-50 mg/kg/day in 4 divided doses x 7 days; may double dose with severe infection; max 100 mg/kg/day; *see page 563 for dose by weight*
   EryPed *Oral susp:* 200 mg/5 ml (100, 200 ml) (fruit); 400 mg/5 ml (60, 100, 200 ml) (banana); *Oral drops:* 200, 400 mg/5 ml (50 ml) (fruit); *Chew tab:* 200 mg wafer (fruit)

E.E.S. *Oral susp:* 200, 400 mg/5 ml (100 ml) (fruit)
E.E.S. **Granules** *Oral susp:* 200 mg/5 ml (100, 200 ml) (cherry)
E.E.S. **400 Tablets** *Tab:* 400 mg
Comment: *erythromycin* may increase INR with concomitant **warfarin**, as well as increase serum level of **digoxin**, benzodiazepines and statins.

▷ *gemifloxacin* (C) 320 mg daily x 5-7 days
Pediatric: <18 years: not recommended
Factive *Tab:* 320*mg
Comment: *gemifloxacin* is contraindicated <18 years-of-age, and during pregnancy and lactation. Risk of tendonitis or tendon rupture, especially 60 years-of-age and older.

▷ *levofloxacin* (C) *Uncomplicated:* 500 mg daily x 7 days; *Complicated:* 750 mg daily x 7 days
Pediatric: <18 years: not recommended
Levaquin *Tab:* 250, 500, 750 mg
Comment: *levofloxacin* is contraindicated <18 years-of-age, and during pregnancy and lactation. Risk of tendonitis or tendon rupture, especially 60 years-of-age and older.

▷ *loracarbef* (B) 200-400 mg bid x 7 days
Pediatric: 15 mg/kg/day in 2 divided doses x 7 days; *see page 570 for dose by weight*
Lorabid *Pulvule:* 200, 400 mg; *Oral susp:* 100 mg/5 ml (50, 100 ml); 200 mg/
5 ml (50, 75, 100 ml) (strawberry bubble gum)

▷ *ofloxacin* (C)(G) 400 mg bid x 10 days
Pediatric: <18 years: not recommended
Floxin *Tab:* 200, 300, 400 mg
Comment: *ofloxacin* is contraindicated <18 years-of-age, and during pregnancy and lactation. Risk of tendonitis or tendon rupture, especially 60 years-of-age and older.

◯ WRINKLES: FACIAL (CROW'S FEET, FROWN LINES, SMILE LINES)

TOPICAL RETINOIDS

Comment: Wash the affected area with a soap-free cleanser; pat dry and wait 20 to 30 minutes; then apply topical retinoid sparingly to affected area. Use only once daily in the PM. Avoid eyes, ears, nostrils, and mouth.

▷ *adapalene* (C)
Pediatric: <12 years: not recommended
Differin *Crm:* 0.1% (15, 45 g); *Gel:* 0.1% (15, 45 g); *Pad:* 0.1% (30/pk; alcohol 30%)
Differin Solution *Soln:* 0.1% (30 ml; alcohol 30%)

▷ *tazarotene* (X) apply daily at HS
Pediatric: not recommended
Avage Cream *Crm:* 0.1% (5, 30 g)
Tazorac Cream *Crm:* 0.05, 0.1% (15, 30, 60 g)
Tazorac Gel *Gel:* 0.05, 0.1% (30, 100 g)

▷ *tretinoin* (C) apply daily at HS
Pediatric: <12 years: not recommended

Atralin Gel *Gel:* 0.05% (45 g)
Avita *Crm:* 0.025% (20, 45 g); *Gel:* 0.025% (20, 45 g) **Renova** *Crm:* 0.02% (40 g); 0.05% (40, 60 g)
Retin-A Cream *Crm:* 0.025, 0.05, 0.1% (20, 45 g)
Retin-A Gel *Gel:* 0.01, 0.025% (15, 45 g; alcohol 90%)
Retin-A Liquid *Soln:* 0.05% (alcohol 55%)
Retin-A Micro Gel *Gel:* 0.04, 0.08, 0.1% (20, 45 g)
Tretin-X Cream *Crm:* 0.075% (35 g) (parabens-free, alcohol-free, propylene glycol-free)
Retin-A Micro *Microspheres:* 0.04, 0.1% (20, 45 g)

Comment: Effective for mitigation of fine wrinkles, mottled hyperpigmentation, and tactile roughness of skin. No mitigating effect on deep wrinkles, skin yellowing, lentigines, telangiectasia, skin laxity, keratinocytic atypia, melanocytic atypia, or dermal elastosis. Avoid sun exposure. Cautious use of concomitant astringents, alcohol-based products, sulfur-containing products, salicylic acid-containing products, soap, and other topical agents.

XEROSIS

MOISTURIZING AGENTS

Aquaphor Healing Ointment (OTC) *Oint:* 1.75, 3.5, 14 oz (alcohol)
Eucerin Daily Sun Defense (OTC) *Lotn:* 6 oz (fragrance-free)
  Comment: Eucerin Daily Sun Defense is a moisturizer with SPF 15 sunscreen.
Eucerin Facial Lotion (OTC) *Lotn:* 4 oz
Eucerin Light Lotion (OTC) *Lotn:* 8 oz
Eucerin Lotion (OTC) *Lotn:* 8, 16 oz
Eucerin Original Creme (OTC) *Crm:* 2, 4, 16 oz (alcohol)
Eucerin Plus Creme (OTC) *Crm:* 4 oz
Eucerin Plus Lotion (OTC) *Lotn:* 6, 12 oz
Eucerin Protective Lotion (OTC) *Lotn:* 4 oz (alcohol)
  Comment: Eucerin Protective is a moisturizer with SPF 25 sunscreen.
Lac-Hydrin Cream (OTC) *Crm:* 280, 385 g
Lac-Hydrin Lotion (OTC) *Lotn:* 225, 400 g
Lubriderm Dry Skin Scented (OTC) *Lotn:* 6, 10, 16, 32 oz
Lubriderm Dry Skin Unscented (OTC) *Lotn:* 3.3, 6, 10, 16 oz (fragrance-free)
Lubriderm Sensitive Skin Lotion (OTC) *Lotn:* 3.3, 6, 10, 16 oz (lanolin-free)
Lubriderm Dry Skin (OTC) *Lotn:* 2.5, 6, 10, 16 oz (scented); 1, 2.5, 6, 10, 16 oz (fragrance-free)
Lubriderm Bath & Shower Oil (OTC) 1-2 capfuls in bath or rub onto wet skin as needed, then rinse
  Oil: 8 oz
Moisturel apply as needed
  Crm: 4, 16 oz; *Lotn:* 8, 12 oz; *Clnsr:* 8.75 oz

Topical Oil

 fluocinolone acetamide 0.01% topical oil **(C)**
  Pediatric: <6 years: not recommended; ≥6 years: apply sparingly bid for up to 4 weeks

Derma-Smoothe/FS Topical Oil apply sparingly tid
Topical oil: 0.01% (4 oz; peanut oil)

⬤ ZOLLINGER-ELLISON SYNDROME

PROTON PUMP INHIBITORS

Comment: If hepatic impairment, <u>or</u> if patient is Asian, consider reducing the PPI dose.

▷ *dexlansoprazole* (B) 30-60 mg daily for up to 4 weeks
Pediatric: <18 years: not recommended
   Dexilant *Cap:* 30, 60 mg ent-rel granules; may open and sprinkle on applesauce; do not crush <u>or</u> chew granules

▷ *esomeprazole* (B)(OTC)(G) 20-40 mg daily; max 8 weeks; take 1 hour before food; swallow whole <u>or</u> mix granules with food <u>or</u> juice and take immediately; do not crush <u>or</u> chew granules
Pediatric: <1 year: not recommended; 1-11 years, <20 kg: 10 mg; >20 kg: 10-20 mg once daily; 12-17 years: 20-40 mg once daily; max 8 weeks
   Nexium *Cap:* 20, 40 mg ent-coat del-rel pellets
   Nexium for Oral Suspension *Oral susp:* 10, 20, 40 mg ent-coat del-rel granules/pkt; mix in 2 tblsp water and drink immediately; 30 pkt/carton

▷ *lansoprazole* (B)(OTC)(G) 15-30 mg daily for up to 8 weeks; may repeat course; take before eating
Pediatric: <1 year: not recommended; 1-11 years, <30 kg: 15 mg once daily; >11 years: same as adult
   Prevacid *Cap:* 15, 30 mg ent-coat del-rel granules; swallow whole <u>or</u> mix granules with food <u>or</u> juice and take immediately; do not crush <u>or</u> chew granules; follow with water
   Prevacid for Oral Suspension *Oral susp:* 15, 30 mg ent-coat del- rel granules/pkt; mix in 2 tblsp water and drink immediately; 30 pkt/carton (strawberry)
   Prevacid SoluTab *ODT:* 15, 30 mg (strawberry; phenylalanine)
   Prevacid 24HR *Oral granules:* 15 mg ent-coat del-rel granules; swallow whole <u>or</u> mix granules with food <u>or</u> juice and take immediately; do not crush <u>or</u> chew granules; follow with water

▷ *omeprazole* (C)(OTC)(G) 20-40 mg daily; take before eating; swallow whole <u>or</u> mix granules with applesauce and take immediately; do not crush <u>or</u> chew; follow with water
Pediatric: <1 year: not recommended; 5-<10 kg: 5 mg daily; 10-<20 kg: 10 mg daily; ≥20 kg: same as adult
   Prilosec *Cap:* 10, 20, 40 mg ent-coat del-rel granules
      Pediatric: <18 years: not recommended
   Prilosec *Tab:* 20 mg del-rel (regular, wild berry)

▷ *pantoprazole* (B) initially 40 mg bid
Pediatric: not recommended
   Protonix (G) *Tab:* 40 mg ent-coat del-rel
   Protonix for Oral Suspension *Oral susp:* 40 mg ent-coat del-rel granules/pkt; mix in 1 tsp apple juice for 5 seconds <u>or</u> sprinkle on 1 tsp apple sauce, and swallow immediately; do not mix in water <u>or</u> any other liquid <u>or</u> food; take ap-

proximately 30 minutes prior to a meal; 30 pkt/carton any other liquid or food; take approximately 30 minutes prior to a meal; 30 pkt/carton

▷ *rabeprazole* (B)(OTC)(G) initially 20 mg daily; then titrate; may take 100 mg daily in divided doses or 60 mg bid

Pediatric: <12 years: not recommended; ≥12 years: 20 mg once daily; max 8 weeks

AcipHex *Tab:* 20 mg ent-coat del-rel

SECTION II

APPENDICES

APPENDIX A: FDA PREGNANCY CATEGORIES

Category	Description
A	Controlled studies in women have failed to demonstrate risk to the fetus in the first trimester of pregnancy and there is no evidence of risk in later trimesters.
B	Animal reproduction studies have not demonstrated risk to the fetus, but there are no controlled studies in pregnant women, or animal studies have demonstrated an adverse effect, but controlled studies in pregnant women have not documented risk to the fetus in the first trimester of pregnancy and there is no evidence of risk in later trimesters.
C	Risk to the fetus cannot be ruled out. Animal reproduction studies have demonstrated adverse effects on the fetus (i.e., teratogenic or embryocidal effects or other) but there are no controlled studies in pregnant women or controlled studies in women and animals are not available.
D	There is positive evidence of human fetal risk, but benefits from use by pregnant women may be acceptable despite the potential risk (e.g., if the drug is needed in a life-threatening situation or for a serious disease for which safer drugs cannot be used or are ineffective.
X	Studies in animals or humans have demonstrated fetal abnormalities or there is evidence of fetal risk based on human experience, or both, and the risk of using the drug in pregnant women clearly outweighs any possible benefit. The drug is contraindicated in women who are pregnant or who may become pregnant.

APPENDIX B: U.S. SCHEDULE OF CONTROLLED SUBSTANCES

Schedule	Description
I	High potential for abuse and of no currently accepted medical use. Not obtainable by prescription, but may be legally procured for research, study, or instructional use. (Examples: *heroin, LSD, marijuana, mescaline, peyote*)
II	High abuse potential and high liability for severe psychological or physical dependence potential. Prescription required and cannot be refilled. Prescription must be written in ink or typed and signed. A verbal prescription may be allowed in an emergency by the dispensing pharmacist, but must be followed by a written prescription within 72 hours. Includes opium derivatives, other opioids, and short-acting barbiturates.

(continued)

(continued)

Schedule	Description
III	Potential for abuse is less than that for drugs in schedules I and II. Moderate to low physical dependence and high psychological dependence potential. Prescription required. May be refilled up to 5 times in 6 months. Prescription may be verbal (telephone) <u>or</u> written. Includes certain stimulants and depressants not included in the above schedules, and prepararations containing limited quantities of certain opioids.
IV	Lower potential for abuse than Schedule III drugs. Prescription required. May be refilled up to 5 times in 6 months. Prescription may be verbal (telephone) <u>or</u> written.
V	Abuse potential less than that for Schedule IV drugs. Preparations contain limited quantities of certain narcotic drugs. Generally intended for antitussive and anti-diarrheal purposes and may be distributed without a prescription provided that • such distribution is made only by a pharmacist; • not more than 240 ml <u>or</u> not more than 48 solid dosage units of any substance containing opium, nor more than 120 ml <u>or</u> not more than 24 solid dosage units of any other controlled substance may be distributed at retail to the same purchaser in any given 48-hour period without a valid prescription order; • the purchaser is at least 18 years old; • the pharmacist knows the purchaser <u>or</u> requests suitable identification; • the pharmacist keeps an official written record of: name and address of purchaser, name, and quantity of controlled substance purchased, date of sale, initials of dispensing pharmacist. This record is to be made available for inspection and copying by the U.S. officers authorized by the Attorney General; • other federal, state, <u>or</u> local law does not reuire a prescription order. Under jurisdiction of the Federal Controlled Substances Act. Refillable up to 5 times within 6 months.

APPENDIX C: JNC-8* AND ASH** HYPERTENSION EVALUATION AND TREATMENT RECOMMENDATIONS¶

APPENDIX C.1: BLOOD PRESSURE CLASSIFICATION

Classification	SBP mmHg		DBP mmHg
Normal	<120	<u>and</u>	<80
Prehypertension	120-139	<u>or</u>	80-89

(continued)

(*continued*)

Classification	SBP mmHg		DBP mmHg
Hypertension, Stage 1	140-159	or	90-99
Hypertension, Stage 2	≥160	or	≥100

¶Adapted from: PL Detail-Document, Treatment of Hypertension: JNC 8 and More. *Pharmacist's Letter/ Prescriber's Letter*, February 2014.

APPENDIX C.2: BLOOD PRESSURE RCOMMENDATIONS

Classification	SBP mmHg	DBP mmHg
Optimal	<120	<80
Normal	<130	<85
High normal	130-139	85-89

APPENDIX C.3: IDENTIFIABLE CAUSES OF HYPERTENSION (JNC-8)

- Obstructive sleep apnea
- Chronic kidney disease
- Primary aldosteronism
- Renovascular disease
- Excess sodium ingestion
- Herbal supplements
- Coarctation of the aorta
- Pheochromocytoma
- Thyroid disease
- Parathyroid disease
- Cushing's syndrome

- *Prescription Drugs:* oral contraceptives, sympathomimetics, venlafaxine, bupropion, clozapine, buspirone, bromocriptine, carbamazepine, metoclopramide
- *Illicit, Over-the-Counter Drugs, and Herbal Products:* excess alcohol consumption, alcohol withdrawal, anabolic steroids, cocaine, cocaine withdrawal, phenylpropanolamine analogs, ephedra alkalois, ergotcontaining herbal products, St. John's wart, nicotine withdrawal

APPENDIX C.4: CVD RISK FACTORS (JNC-8)

- Hypertension
- Obesity (BMI ≥30 kg/m²)
- Dyslipidemia
- Diabetes mellitus
- Cigarette smoking
- Physical inactivity

- Microalbuminuria, eGFR <60 mL/min
- Age (men >55 yrs, women >65 yrs)
- Family History of premature CVD (men <55 yrs, women <65 yrs)

APPENDIX C.5: DIAGNOSTIC WORKUP OF HYPERTENSION (JNC-8)

- Assess risk factors and comorbidities
- Reveal identifiable causes of hypertension
- Assess for presence of target organ damage
- History and physical examination

(*continued*)

(*continued*)

> - Urinalysis, blood glucose, hematocrit, lipid panel, potassium, creatinine, calcium, (*optional* urine albumin/Cr ratio), EKG

APPENDIX C.6: BLOOD PRESSURE MEASUREMENT RECOMMENDATIONS (JNC-8)

> - Blood pressure should be measured after the patient has emptied their bladder and has been seated for 5 minutes with back supported and legs resting on the ground (not crossed)
> - Arm used for measurement should rest on a table, at heart level.
> - Use a sphygmomanometer/stethoscope or automated electronic device (preferred) with the correct size arm cuff
> - Take two readings one to two minutes apart, and average the readings (preferred)
> - Measure blood pressure in both arms at initial valuation; use the higher reading for measurements thereafter
> - Confirm the diagnosis of HTN at a subsequent visit one to four weeks after the first
> - If blood pressure is very high (e.g., systolic 180 mmHg or higher), or timely follow-up unrealistic, treatment can be started after just one set of measurements

APPENDIX C.7: PATIENT-SPECIFIC FACTORS TO CONSIDER WHEN SELECTING DRUG THERAPY(IES) (JNC-8* AND ASH**)

> JNC-8:
> - Nonblack, including those with diabetes: thiazide, CCB, ACEI, or ARB
> - African American, including those with diabetes: thiazide or CCB
> - CKD; regimen should include an ACEI or ARB (including African Americans)
> - Can initiate with two agents, especially if systolic >20 mmHg above goal or diastolic >10 mmHg above goal
> - If goal not reached: stress adherence to medication and lifestyle, increase dose or add a second or third agent from one of the recommended classes
> - Choose a drug outside of the classes recommended above only if these options have been exhausted. Consider specialist referral
>
> ASH:
> - **Nonblack <60 years of age:** *First-line:* ACEI or ARB; *Second-line (add-on):* CCB or thiazide; *Third-line:* CCB plus ACEI or ARB plus thiazide
> - **Nonblack 60 years of age and older:** *First-line:* CCB or thiazide preferred, ACEI, or ARB; *Second-line (add-on):* CCB, thiazide, ACEI, or ARB (don't use ACEI plus ARB); *Third-line:* CCB plus ACEI or ARB plus thiazide
> - **African American:** *First-line:* CCB or thiazide; *Second-line (add-on):* ACEI or ARB. *Third-line:* CCB plus ACEI or ARB plus thiazide

(*continued*)

(continued)

Comorbidities (ASH):
- **Diabetes:** *First-line:* ACEI or ARB (can start with CCB or thiazide in African Americans); *Second-line:* add CCB or thiazide (can add ACEI or ARB in African Americans); *Third-line:* CCB plus ACEI or ARB plus thiazide
- **CKD:** *First-line:* ARB or ACEI (ACEI for African Americans) *Second-line (add-on):* CCB or thiazide; *Third-line:* CCB plus ACEI or ARB plus thiazide
- **CAD:** *First-line:* BB plus ARB or ACEI; *Second-line (add-on):* CCB or thiazide; *Third-line:* BB plus ARB or ACEI plus CCB plus thiazide
- **Stroke history:** *First-line:* ACEI or ARB; *Second-line:* add CCB or thiazide; *Third-line:* CCB plus ACEI or ARB plus thiazide
- **Heart failure:** ACEI or ARB plus BB plus diuretic plus aldosterone antagonist. Amlodipine can be added for additional BP control (Start with ACEI, BB, diuretic. Can add BB even before ACE-I optimized. Use diuretic to manage fluid.)
- In patients 60 years of age or older who do not have diabetes or chronic kidney disease, the goal blood pressure level is now <150/90 mmHg
- In patients 18 to 59 years of age without major comorbidities, and in patients 60 years of age or older who have diabetes, chronic kidney disease, or both conditions, the new goal blood pressure level is <140/90 mmHg

APPENDIX C.8: BLOOD PRESSURE MANAGEMENT CHANGES FROM JNC VII TO JNC-8¶

- First-line and later-line treatments should now be limited to 4 classes of medications: thiazide-type diuretics, calcium channel blockers (CCBs), ACEIs, and ARBs
- Second- and third-line alternatives included higher doses or combinations of ACEIs, ARBs, thiazide type diuretics, and CCBs
- Several medications are now designated as later-line alternatives, including the following:
  - Beta-blockers
  - Alpha-blockers
  - Alpha$_1$/beta-blockers (e.g., carvedilol)
  - Vasodilating beta-blockers (e.g., nebivolol)
  - Central alpha$_2$-adrenergic agonists (e.g, clonidine)
  - Direct vasodilators (e.g., hydralazine)
  - Loop diuretics (e.g., furosemide)
  - Aldosterone antagonists (e.g., spironolactone)
  - Peripherally acting adrenergic antagonists (e.g., reserpine)
- When initiating therapy, patients of African descent without chronic kidney disease should use CCBs and thiazides instead of ACEIs.
- Use of ACEIs and ARBs is recommended in all patients with chronic kidney disease regardless of ethnic background, either as first-line therapy or in addition to first-line therapy.

(continued)

(*continued*)

> - ACEIs and ARBs should not be used in the same patient simultaneously.
> - CCBs and thiazide-type diuretics should be used instead of ACEIs and ARBs in patients over the age of 75 with impaired kidney function due to the risk of hyperkalemia, increased creatinine, and further renal impairment.

¶Adapted from: PL Detail-Document, Treatment of Hypertension: JNC 8 and More. *Pharmacist's Letter/ Prescriber's Letter*, February 2014.

APPENDIX D: ATP-IV TARGET LIPID RECOMMENDATIONS¶

APPENDIX D.1: TARGET TC, TG, HDL-C, NON-HDL-C

Total cholesterol	<200 mg/dL
Triglyceride	<150 mg/dL
High-density lipoprotein (HDL)	>40 mg/dL (male) >50 mg/dL (female)
Non-high-density lipoprotein (Non-HDL-C)	<130 mg/dL; 30 mg/dL above the LDL-C treatment target

¶Adapted from the National Cholesterol Education Program Expert Panel on Detection, Evaluation, and Treatment of High Blood Cholesterol in Adults (Adult Treatment Panel IV, 2012)

APPENDIX D.2: TARGET LDL-C†

Risk Assessment††	LDL Target	Initiate TLC†††	Initiate Drug Therapy
0-1	<160 mg/dL	≥160 mg/dL	≥190 mg/dL (optional at 160-189 mg/dL)
2 <u>or</u> more plus 10-year risk <10%	<130 mg/dL	≥130 mg/dL	≥160 mg/dL
2 <u>or</u> more plus 10-year risk <20%	<130 mg/dL <100 mg/dL optional	≥130 mg/dL	≥130 mg/dL
CHD <u>or</u> CHD risk equivalents 10-year risk >20%	<100 mg/dL <70 mg/dL optional	≥100 mg/dL	≥100 mg/dL

†Treatment decisions based on LDL cholesterol.

††Risk factors include age (men ≥45 years and women ≥55 years).

†††Therapeutic lifestyle changes (e.g., exercise, weight loss, low fat diet).

APPENDIX D.3: NON-HDL-C[1]

		Non-HDL-C is calculated as total cholesterol minus HDL-C. The addition of non-HDL-C to the Lipid Panel reflects the recognition of this calculated value as a predictive factor in cardiovascular disease based on the National Cholesterol Education III studies. The reference ranges for non-HDL-C are based on National Cholesterol Education III guidelines: Non-HDL-C is thought to be a better predictor of CVD than LDL-C; treatment goal for non-HDL-C is usually 30 mg/dL above the LDL-C treatment target. For example, if the LDL-C treatment goal is <70 mg/dL, the non-HDL-C treatment target would be <100 mg/dL.
Desirable	<130 mg/dL	
Borderline high	139-159 mg/dL	
High	160-189 mg/dL	
Very high	≥190 mg/dL	

[1]Adapted from the National Cholesterol Education Program Expert Panel on Detection, Evaluation, and Treatment of High Blood Cholesterol in Adults (Adult Treatment Panel IV, 2012).

APPENDIX E: EFFECTS OF SELECTED DRUGS ON INSULIN ACTIVITY

Hyper- and Hypo-glycemic Drug Effects	
Drugs That May Cause Hyperglycemia	Drugs That May Cause Hypoglycemia
Calcium channel blockers	Alcohol
Thiazide diuretics	Beta-blockers
Corticosteroids	MAO inhibitors
Nicotinic acid	Salicylates
Oral contraceptives	NSAIDs
Phenytoin	Warfarin
Sympathomimetics diazoxide	Phenylbutazone

APPENDIX F: GLYCOSYLATED HEMOGLOBIN (HBA1C) AND AVERAGE BLOOD GLUCOSE EQUIVALENT

HbA1c and Average Blood Glucose Equivalent			
HbA1c	GLU	HbA1c	GLU
4%	60 mg/dL	14%	360 mg/dL
5%	90 mg/dL	15%	390 mg/dL
6%	120 mg/dL	16%	420 mg/dL
7%	150 mg/dL	17%	450 mg/dL
8%	180 mg/dL	18%	480 mg/dL
9%	210 mg/dL	19%	510 mg/dL
10%	240 mg/dL	20%	540 mg/dL
11%	270 mg/dL	21%	570 mg/dL
12%	300 mg/dL	22%	600 mg/dL
13%	330 mg/dL	23%	630 mg/dL

APPENDIX G: ROUTINE IMMUNIZATION RECOMMENDATIONS[¶]

- Prior to 1 year-of-age, administer IM vaccinations in the vastus lateralis muscle
- After 1 year-of-age, administer vaccinations in the posterolateral upper arm
- Influenza vaccine should be administered annually for all ages ≥6 months of age
- Inactivated vaccines (e.g., pneumococcal, meningococcal, and inactivated influenza vaccines), are generally acceptable and live vaccines are generally avoided, in persons with immune deficiencies or immuneocompromising conditions
- Additional information about routine vaccinations, unknown vaccination status, travel vaccinations, vaccinations in pregnancy, and other vaccines, is available at:
  www.cdc.gov/vaccines/hcp/acip-recs/index.html
  www.cdc.gov/mmwr/preview/mmwrhtml rr6002a1/htm
  wwwnc.cdc.gov/travel/destinations/list
  www.cdc.gov/vaccines/adult/rec-vac/pregnant.html
  www.cdc.gov/flu/protect/vaccine/vaccines/htm
- DTaP (diphtheria-tetanus-toxoid, acellular pertussis); minimum age 6 wks
- DTaP should not be administered at or after the 7th birthday
- The 4th dose of DTaP vaccine can be administered as early as age 12 months, provided that the interval between doses 3 and 4 is at least 6 months
- DTaP and IPV should be administered at or before school entry
- HAV (hepatitis A vaccine) is recommended for all children at 1 year (12-23 months) of age

(continued)

(*continued*)

- **HAV** 2-dose series should be administered at least 6 months apart
- **HBV** (*hepatitis B vaccine*) is a 3-dose series initiated at birth; administer 2nd dose at 1-2 months; administer the 3rd dose at age 6 months (<u>not</u> before ≥24 weeks)
- **HBV** should be offered to all children who have <u>not</u> received the full series
- Infants born to HVsAG-positive mothers should be tested for HBsAG and antibody to HBsAg after completion of the **HBV** series (at age 9-18 months)
- **Hib** (*hemophilus influenzae* type b conjugate vaccine) minimum age 6 months
- **Hib** is <u>not</u> recommended if age >5 years
- **HPV** (*human papillovirus vaccine*) vaccine should be administered anytime between 11 and 12 years-of-age
- **HPV** is a 3-series vaccine administered months 0, 1, 6; females may recive HPV/4 or HPV/2; males should receive HPV/2
- **HPV** if <u>not</u> previously received at 11 <u>or</u> 12 years-of-age, may be iniitiated at any time between 13 and 26 years-of-age
- **IIV** (*inactivated influenza vaccine*) can be administered >6 months (use age-appropriate formulation), pregnant women, and persons with hives-only allergy to eggs
- **IHD** (*influenza high dose*) (**Fluzone High Dose**) may be recommended to persons ≥65 years of age
- **IPV** (*inactivated poliovirus vaccine*) minimum age 4 weeks
- An all-**IPV** schedule is recommended to eliminate the risk of vaccine-associated paralytic polio (VAPP) associated with **OPV** (*oral poliovirus vaccine*)
- **LAIV** (*live attenuated influenza vaccine*) may be administered intranasally (**FluMist**)
- **Men** (*meningococcal vaccine*) should be administered to all children at the 11-12 year old visit as well as to unvaccinated adolescents 15 years-of-age (usually at high school entry)
- **Men** should be administered to all college freshmen living in dormitories\
- Use MPSV4 for children aged 2-10 years and MCV4 for older children, although MPSV4 is an acceptable alternative for prophylaxis in men
- **MMR** (*mumps-measles-rubella*) should be administered at age 12 months in high-risk areas; if indicated, tuberculin testing can be done at the same visit
- **MMR** should be administered at age 11-12 years unless 2 doses were given after the first birthday; the interval between doses should be at least 4 weeks
- **MMR** adults born <1957 are generally considered immune to measles and mumps; all adults born ≥1957 should have documentation of at least I dose of MMR vaccine unless there is a medical contraindication <u>or</u> laboratory evidence of immunity to each of the 3 disease components; documentation of provider-diagnosed disease is <u>not</u> acceptable evidence of immunity to any of the 3 disease components
- **PCV-13** (*pneumococcal vaccine*) does <u>not</u> replace 23-valent pneumococcal polysaccharide in children age ≥24 months
- **PCV-13** when PCV-13 and PCV-23 are indicated, administer PCV-13 first; do <u>not</u> administer PCV-13 and PCV-23 in the same visit
- **PCV-13** adults ≥65 years-of-age, who have <u>not</u> received PCV-13 <u>or</u> PCV-23, should receive PCV-13 followed by PCV-23 6-12 months later
- **PCV-23** (*pneumococcal vaccine 23 trivalent*) minimum age 6 weeks
- **PCV-23** adults ≥65 years of age, who have received **PCV-23**, but <u>not</u> received PCV-13, should receive. **PCV-13** at least I year later; adults ≥65 years of age, who have <u>not</u> received **PCV-23**, should receive

(*continued*)

(*continued*)

- **PCV-13** followed by **PCV-23** 6-12 months later
- **RIV** (*recombinant influenza vaccine*; **FluBlok**) may be administered to any adult >18 years-of-age, including pregnant women
- **RIV** does <u>not</u> contain any egg protein; can be administered to anyone with egg allergy at any severity
- Older infants and children previously vaccinated with **PCV** should receive 3 doses (if age 7-11 months), 2 doses (if age 12-23 months) <u>or</u> 1 dose (if age >24 months)
- **Rot** (*rotavirus vaccine*) is a live attenuated oral vaccine for infants age >6 weeks <u>or</u> <32 weeks *only*; administer the 1st dose at 6-12 weeks-of-age; administer 2nd and 3rd doses at 4-10-week intervals for a total of 3 doses
- **Rot** If an incomplete dose is administered, *do <u>not</u>* administer a replacement dose, but continue with the remaining doses in the recommended series
- **Td** (*tetanus-diphtheria vaccine*) should be repeated every 10 years throughout life (<u>or</u> if at-risk injury ≥5 years after previous dose)
- **Td** should <u>not</u> be administered until minimum age ≥7 years
- **TdaP** (*tetanus-diphtheria-acellular pertussis*) administer 1 dose to pregnant women during each pregnancy, preferably during 27-36 weeks gestation, regardless of interval since prior Td <u>or</u> TdaP
- **TdaP** persons ≥11 years of age who have <u>not</u> received **Tdap** vaccine <u>or</u> for whom vaccine status is unknown, should receive 1 dose of **TdaP** followed by a **Td** booster every 10 years
- **Var** should be administered to children at age 11-12 years who have <u>not</u> had chicken-pox <u>or</u> who report having had chickenpox but do <u>not</u> have laboratory documentation of immunity
- **Var** If <u>not</u> received between age 11 and 12 years, administer 2 doses at least 4 weeks apart anytime after 12 years-of-age <u>or</u> a 2nd dose if previously only received 1 dose
- **VarZ** (*herpes zoster vaccine*) should be administered in a single dose once at ≥60 years-of-age, whether <u>or</u> <u>not</u> the person reports a prior episode of active herpes zoster infection
- **VarZ** is contraindicated in pregnancy and immune deficiency
- DTaP and IPV can be initiated as early as 4 weeks in areas of high endemicity <u>or</u> outbreak.

¶Adapted from DHHS CDC 2015.

APPENDIX G.1: CONTRAINDICATIONS TO VACCINES¶

All vaccines	Previous anaphylactic reaction to the vaccine Moderate <u>or</u> severe illness with <u>or</u> without fever
TDaP/DTaP, Td	Encephalopathy within 7 days of administration of previous dose
Hib	Previous anaphylactic reaction to the vaccine Moderate <u>or</u> severe illness with <u>or</u> without fever
HBV	Anaphylactic reaction to baker's yeast

(*continued*)

(continued)

HAV	Previous anaphylactic reaction to the vaccine Moderate <u>or</u> severe illness with <u>or</u> without fever
Influenza	Allergy to eggs (*except* **FluBlok** which does <u>not</u> contain any egg protein)
IPV	Anaphylactic reaction to neomycin <u>or</u> streptomycin
Pneumococcal	Hypersensitivity to diphtheria toxoid
MMR	Pregnancy, immunodeficiency, anaphylactic reaction to eggs <u>or</u> neomycin
Meningococcal	Encephalopathy within 7 days of administration of previous dose
Rotavirus	<6 months <u>or</u> >32 months
HPV	Pregnancy; pregnancy testing is <u>not</u> required; however, if administered, defer the remaining dose(s) until completion <u>or</u> termination of pregnancy
Varicella	Pregnancy
Herpes zoster	Pregnancy

¶ Adapted from DHHS CDC 2015.

APPENDIX G.2: ROUTE OF ADMINISTRATION AND DOSE OF VACCINES¶

Vaccine	Route	Dose
Single Vaccines		
Diphtheria-Tetanus-Pertussis (DTaP, Dtap, DT)	IM	0.5 ml
Haemophilus influenza type b (Hib)	IM	0.5 ml
Hepatitis A vaccine (HAV)	IM	0.5 ml: age <18 yrs 1.0 ml: age ≥19 yrs
Hepatitis B vaccine (HBV)	IM	0.5 ml: age <18 yrs 1.0 ml: age ≥19 yrs
Human Papillomavirus (HPV)	IM	0.5 ml
Influenza (**Fluzone Intradermal**)	ID	0.5 ml
Influenza, inactivated (IIV), recombinant (RIV)	IM	0.25 ml: age 6-35 months 0.5 ml: age ≥3 yrs
Influenza, live attenuated (LAIV)	NS	0.2 ml; 0.1 ml in each nostril
Meningococcal conjugate	IM	0.5 ml

(continued)

(*continued*)

Vaccine	Route	Dose
Meningococcal polysaccharide (MPSV)	SC	0.5 ml
Meningococcal sero group B (Men B)	IM	0.5 ml
Mumps-Measles-Rubella (MMR)	SC	0.5 ml
Pneumococcal conjugate (PCV)	IM	0.5 ml
Pneumococcal polysaccharide (PPSV)	IM/SC	0.5 ml
Polio, Inactivated (IPV)	IM/SC	0.5 ml
Rotavirus (**Rotarix**)	PO	1 ml
Rotavirus (**Rotateq**)	PO	2 ml
Tetanus (Td)	IM	0.5 ml
Varicella	SC	0.5 ml
Herpes Zoster	SC	0.65 ml: age ≥60 yrs
Combination Vaccines		
MMR-Var (**ProQuad**)	SC	0.5 ml: age ≤12 yrs
HBV-HAV (**Twinrix**)	IM	1 ml: >18 yrs
DTaP-HBV-IPV (**Pediarix**)	IM	0.5 ml
DTaP-IPV-Hib (**Pentacel**)	IM	0.5 ml
DTaP-IPV (**Kinrix, Quadracel**)	IM	0.5 ml
Hib-HBV (**Comvax**)	IM	0.5 ml
Hib-MenCY (**MenHibrix**)	IM	0.5 ml

¶ Adapted from DHHS CDC 2015.

APPENDIX G.3: ADVERSE REACTIONS TO VACCINES¶

Vaccine	Signs and Symptoms	Treatment
Inactivated antigens: DTP, Dtap, DTaP, Td, IPV, influenza inactiveted (IIV) recombinant (RIV) Live attenuated viruses: MMR, Meningococcal, rotavirus, varicella, herpes zoster	Local tenderness Erythema Swelling Low-grade fever Drowsiness Fretfulness Decreased appetite Prolonged crying Unusual cry	*acetaminophen* or *ibuprofen* for age and/or weight; *aspirin* and *aspirin*-containing products are contraindicated

¶ Adapted from DHHS CDC 2015.

APPENDIX G.4: MINIMUM INTERVALS BETWEEN VACCINE DOSES[1]

Type	#1 to #2	#2 to #3	#3 to #4	#4 to #5
HBV	4 weeks	5 months		
HAV	6 months			
DTaP	4 weeks	4 weeks	6 months	6 months
IPV	4 weeks	4 weeks	4 weeks	
MMR	4 weeks			
Var	4 weeks			
Rotavirus	4 weeks	4 weeks; do not administer >32 weeks of age		
PCV-13	4 weeks (if #1 at age <12 months and current age <24 months); 8 weeks (as last dose if #1 at age >12 months or current age 24-59 months); No more doses needed if healthy and #1 at age ≥24 months	4 weeks if age <12 months; 8 weeks (as last dose if age ≥12 months); No more doses needed if healthy and previous dose at age ≥24 months	8 weeks (as last dose; only necessary for age 12 months to 5 years who received 3 doses before age 12 months)	
Hib	4 weeks (if #1 at age <12 months); 8 weeks (as last dose if #1 at age 12-14 months); No more doses needed if healthy and #1 at age ≥15 months	4 weeks if age 12 months; 8 weeks (as last dose if age ≥12 months); No more doses needed if previous dose at age ≥15 months	8 weeks (as last dose; only necessary for age 12 months to 2 years who received 3 doses before age 12 months)	
HPV	4 weeks	20 weeks (24 weeks after #1		

[1] Adapted from DHHS CDC 2015.

APPENDIX G.5: RECOMMENDED CHILDHOOD IMMUNIZATION SCHEDULE[1]

Type	Birth	1 month	2 months	4 months	6 months	6-18 months	12-15 months	15-18 months	4-6 years	11-12 years
HBV	•	•			•					
DTaP			•	•	•				•	
IPV			•	•		•			•	
Hib			•	•	•		•			
Rotavirus			•	•	•					
MMR							•		•	
TDaP										•
Varicella			•	•	•		•		•	
PVC-13			•	•	•		•			
HAV								•		
Meningitis										•
HPV•										•••

[1]Adapted from DHHS CDC 2015.

•=immunization due.

Shaded box=immunization due.

•••HPV 3-dose series, months 0, 1, 6.

APPENDIX G.6: RECOMMENDEND CHILDHOOD IMMUNIZATION CATCH-UP SCHEDULE[1]

Vaccine	Minimum Interval Between Doses			
	#1 to #2	#2 to #3	#3 to #4	#4 to #5
HBV	4 weeks	8 weeks (16 weeks after #1)		
DTaP	4 weeks	4 weeks	6 months	6 months
IPV	4 weeks	4 weeks	4 weeks	
MMR	4 weeks			
Var	4 weeks			
Rotavirus	4 weeks	4 weeks; do not administer >32 weeks of age		
PCV	2 months	2 months	2 months	6-15 months
HPV	4 weeks	20 weeks (24 weeks after #1		

[1]Adapted from DHHS CDC 2015.

APPENDIX G.7: RECOMMENDED ADULT IMMUNIZATION SCHEDULE[1]

Type	19-21 yrs	22-26 yrs	27-49 yrs	50-59 yrs	60-65 yrs	≥65 yrs
Influenza	1 dose annually					
HBV	3 dose series: months 0, 1, 6					
Td/TdaP	Substitute Tdap for Td one time; then continue Td once every 10 years					
MMR*	Born >1957: 2 doses					
Varicella*	Without evidence of immunity: 2 doses, 4 weeks apart					
Herpes zoster*					1 time dose	
PVC-13/ PVC-23					1 time dose	
HAV	Single Antigen, 2 doses: months 0, 6-12 (Havrix); 0, 6-18 (Vaqta)					
Meningitis	1 or more doses					

(continued)

(*continued*)

Type	19-21 yrs	22-26 yrs	27-49 yrs	50-59 yrs	60-65 yrs	≥65 yrs
HPV (female)*β	3 doses; months 0, 1, 6					
HPV (male)β	3 doses; months 0, 1, 6					

¶Adapted from DHHS CDC 2015.
*Contraindicated in pregnancy.
βOnly if <u>not</u> previously vaccinated between 11-12 years-of-age.

APPENDIX H: CONTRACEPTIVES: CONTRAINDICATIONS AND RECOMMENDATIONS

- All contraceptives are pregnancy category X
- No non-barrier contraceptives protect against STDs
- **Absolute Contraindication:**
  - HTN >35 years-of-age
  - DM >35 years-of-age
  - LDL-C >160 <u>or</u> TG >250
  - Known <u>or</u> suspected pregnancy
  - Known <u>or</u> suspected carcinoma of the breast
  - Known <u>or</u> suspected carcinoma of the endometrium
  - Known <u>or</u> suspected estrogen-dependent neoplasia
  - Undiagnosed abnormal genital bleeding
  - Cerebral vascular <u>or</u> coronary artery disease
  - Cholestatic jaundice of pregnancy <u>or</u> jaundice with prior use
  - Hepatic adenoma <u>or</u> carcinoma <u>or</u> benign liver tumor
  - Active <u>or</u> past history of thrombophlebitis <u>or</u> thromboembolic disorder
- **Relative Contraindications**
  - Lactation
  - Asthma
  - Ulcerative colitis
  - Migraine <u>or</u> vascular headache
  - Cardiac <u>or</u> renal dysfunction
  - Gestational diabetes, prediabetes, diabetes mellitus
  - Diastolic BP 90 mmHg <u>or</u> greater <u>or</u> hypertension by any other criteria
  - Psychic depression
  - Varicose veins
  - Smoker >35 years-of-age
  - Sickle-cell <u>or</u> sickle-hemoglobin C disease
  - Cholestatic jaundice during pregnancy, active gallbladder disease
  - Hepatitis <u>or</u> mononucleosis during the preceding year

(*continued*)

(*continued*)
- First-order family history of fatal or nonfatal rheumatic CVD or diabetes prior to age 50 years
- Drug(s) with known interaction(s)
- Elective surgery or immobilization within 4 weeks
- Age >50 years
- **Recommendations**
  - Start the first pill on the first Sunday after menses begins. Thereafter, each new pill pack will be started on a Sunday.
  - Take each daily pill in the same 3-hour window (e.g., 9A-12N, 12N-3P; a 4-hour window prior to bedtime is not recommended).
  - If 1 pill is missed, take it as soon as possible and the next pill at the regular time.
  - If 2 pills are missed, take both pills as soon as possible and then two pills the following day. A barrier method should be used for the remainder of the pill pack.
  - If 3 pills are missed before 10th cycle day, resume taking OCs on a regular schedule and take precautions.
  - If 3 pills are missed after the 10th cycle day, discard the current pill pack and begin a new one 7 days after the last pill was taken.
  - If very low-dose OCs are used or if combination OCs are begun after the th day of the menstrual cycle, an additional method of birth control should be used for the first 7 days of OC use.
  - If nausea occurs as a side effect, select an OC with *lower **estrogen*** content.
  - If breakthrough bleeding occurs during the first half of the cycle, select an OC with *higher **progesterone*** content.
  - Symptoms of a serious nature include loss of vision, diplopia, unilateral numbness, weakness, or tingling, severe chest pain, severe pain in left arm or neck, severe leg pain, slurring of speech, and abdominal tenderness or mass.

APPENDIX H.1: 28-DAY ORAL CONTRACEPTIVES

Comment: **Beyaz**, **Loryna**, **Syeda**, **Safyral**, **Yasmin**, and **Yaz** are contraindicated with renal and adrenal insufficiency. Monitor k^+ level during the first cycle if the patient is at risk for hyperkalemia for any reason. If the patient is taking drugs that increase potassium (e.g., ACEIs, ARBS, NSAIDs, K^+ sparing diuretics), the patient is at risk for hyperkalemia.

Combined Oral Contraceptive	Estrogen (mcg)	Progesterone (mg)
Alesse-21, Alesse-28 (X)(G) *ethinyl estradiol/levonorgestrel*	20	0.1
Altavera (X) *ethinyl estradiol/levonorgestrel*	30	0.15
Apri (X)(G) *ethinyl estradiol/desogestrel*	30	0.15
Aranelle (X)(G) *ethinyl estradiol/norethindrone*	35	0.5 1 0.5

(*continued*)

(*continued*)

Combined Oral Contraceptive	Estrogen (mcg)	Progesterone (mg)
Aviane (X)(G) *ethinyl estradiol/levonorgestrel*	20	0.1
Balziva (X)(G) *ethinyl estradiol/norethindrone*	35	0.4
Beyaz (X)(G) *ethinyl estradiol/drospirenone* plus levomefolate calcium 0.451 mcg (28 tabs)	20	3
Blisovi 24Fe (X)(G) *ethinyl estradiol/norethindrone* plus *ferrous fumarate* 75 mg (4 tabs)	20	1
Brevicon-21, Brevicon-28 (X)(G) *ethinyl estradiol/norethindrone*	35	0.5
Camrese (X) *ethinyl estradiol/levonorgestrel*	30 10	0.15
Camrese Lo (X) *ethinyl estradiol/levonorgestrel*	20 10	0.1
Cesia (X)(G) *ethinyl estradiol/desogestrel*	25 25 25	0.1 0.125 0.15
Cryselle (X)(G) *ethinyl estradiol/norgestrel*	30	0.3
Cyclessa (X)(G) *ethinyl estradiol/desogestrel*	25 25 25	0.1 0.125 0.15
Demulen 1/35-21, Demulen 1/35-28 (X) **(G)** *ethinyl estradiol/ethynodiol diacetate*	35	1
Demulen 1/50-21, Demulen 1/50-28 (X) **(G)** *ethinyl estradiol/ethynodiol diacetate*	50	1
Desogen (X)(G) *ethinyl estradiol/desogestrel diacetate*	30	0.15
Enpresse (X)(G) *ethinyl estradiol/levonorgestrel*	30 40 30	0.05 0.075 0.125

(*continued*)

(*continued*)

Combined Oral Contraceptive	Estrogen (mcg)	Progesterone (mg)
Estrostep Fe (X) *ethinyl estradiol/norethindrone* plus *ferrous fumarate* 75 mg	20 30 35	1 1 1
Femcon Fe (X)(G) *ethinyl estradiol/norethindrone* plus *ferrous fumarate* 75 mg	35	0.4
Generess Fe Chew tab (X)(G) *ethinyl estradiol/norethindrone* plus *ferrous fumarate* 75 mg	25	0.8
Genora (X)(G) *ethinyl estradiol/norethindrone*	35 35 35	0.5 1 0.5
Gianvi (X)(G) *ethinyl estradiol/drospirenone*	20	3
Gildess 1.5/30 (X)(G) *ethinyl estradiol/norethindrone*	30	1.5
Introvale (X) *ethinyl estradiol/levonorgestrel*	30	0.15
Jenest-28 (X) *ethinyl estradiol/norethindrone*	35 35	0.5 1
Jolessa (X)(G) *ethinyl estradiol/levonorgestrel*	30	0.15
Junel 1/20 (X)(G) *ethinyl estradiol/norethindrone*	20	1
Junel 1.5/30 (X)(G) *ethinyl estradiol/norethindrone*	30	1.5
Junel Fe 1/20 (X)(G) *ethinyl estradiol/norethindrone* plus *ferrous fumarate* 75 mg	20	1
Junel Fe 1.5/30 (X)(G) *ethinyl estradiol/norethindrone* plus *ferrous fumarate* 75 mg	30	1.5
Kaitlib Fe Chew Tab (X)(G) *ethinyl estradiol/norethindrone* plus *ferrous fumarate* 75 mg	25	0.8

(*continued*)

(*continued*)

Combined Oral Contraceptive	Estrogen (mcg)	Progesterone (mg)
Kariva (X)(G) *ethinyl estradiol/desogestrel*	20 10	0.15 0.15
Kelnor 1/35 (X)(G) *ethinyl estradiol/ethynodiol diacetate*	35	1
Leena (X) *ethinyl estradiol/norethindrone*	35 35 35	0.5 1 0.5
Lessina 28 (X)(G) *ethinyl estradiol/levonorgestrel*	20	0.1
Levlen 21, Levlen 28 (X)(G) *ethinyl estradiol/levonorgestrel*	30	0.15
Levlite 28 (X)(G) *ethinyl estradiol/levonorgestrel*	20	0.1
Levora-21, Levora-28 (X)(G) *ethinyl estradiol/levonorgestrel*	30	0.15
Loestrin 21 1/20 (X)(G) *ethinyl estradiol/norethindrone*	20	1
Loestrin 21 1.5/30 (X)(G) *ethinyl estradiol/norethindrone*	30	1.5
Loestrin Fe 1/20 (X)(G) *ethinyl estradiol/norethindrone* plus *ferrous fumarate* 75 mg	20	1
Loestrin Fe 1.5/30 (X)(G) *ethinyl estradiol/norethindrone* plus *ferrous fumarate* 75 mg (4 tabs)	30	1.5
Loestrin 24 Fe (X)(G) *ethinyl estradiol/norethindrone* plus *ferrous fumarate* 75 mg (4 tabs)	20	1
Lo Loestrin Fe (X) *ethinyl estradiol/norethindrone* plus *ferrous fumarate* 75 mg (2 tabs)	10	1
Lomedia 24 Fe (X)(G) *ethinyl estradiol/norethindrone* plus *ferrous fumarate* 75 mg	20	1

(*continued*)

(*continued*)

Combined Oral Contraceptive	Estrogen (mcg)	Progesterone (mg)
Lo/Ovral-21, Lo/Ovral-28 (X)(G) *ethinyl estradiol/norgestrel*	30	0.3
Loryna (X) *ethinyl estradiol/drospirenone*	20	3
Low-Ogestrel-21, **Low-Ogestrel-28 (X)(G)** *ethinyl estradiol/norgestrel*	30	0.3
Lutera (X)(G) *ethinyl estradiol/levonorgestrel*	20	0.1
Lybrel (X) *ethinyl estradiol/levonorgestrel*	20	0.09
Mircette (X)(G) *ethinyl estradiol/desogestrel diacetate*	20 10	0.15
Microgestin 1/20 (X)(G) *ethinyl estradiol/norethindrone*	20	1
Microgestin Fe 1/20 (X)(G) *ethinyl estradiol/norethindrone* plus *ferrous fumarate* 75 mg	20	1
Microgestin 1.5/30 (X)(G) *ethinyl estradiol/norethindrone*	30	1.5
Microgestin Fe 1.5/30 (X)(G) *ethinyl estradiol/norethindrone* plus *ferrous fumarate* 75 mg	30	1.5
Minastrin24FE (X) *ethinyl estradiol/norethindrone* plus *ferrous fumarate* 75 mg	20	1
Modicon 0.5/35-28 (X)(G) *ethinyl estradiol/norethindrone*	35	0.5
MonoNessa (X)(G) *ethinyl estradiol/norgestimate*	35	0.25
Natazia (X) *estradiol valerate/dienogest*	30 20 20 10	— 2 3 —

(*continued*)

(*continued*)

Combined Oral Contraceptive	Estrogen (mcg)	Progesterone (mg)
Necon 0.5/35-21, Necon 0.5/35-28 (X)(G) *ethinyl estradiol/norethindrone*	35	0.5
Necon 1/35-21, Necon 1/35-28 (X)(G) *ethinyl estradiol/norethindrone*	35	0.5
Necon 10/11-21, Necon 10/11-28 (X)(G) *ethinyl estradiol/norethindrone*	35 35	0.5 1
Necon 1/50-21, Necon 1/50-28 (X)(G) *mestranol/norethindrone*	50	1
Nelova 0.5/35-21, Nelova 0.5/35-28 (X)(G) *ethinyl estradiol/norethindrone*	35	0.5
Nelova 1/35-21, Nelova 1/35-28 (X)(G) *ethinyl estradiol/norethindrone*	35	1
Nelova 10/11-21, Nelova 10/11-28 (X)(G) *ethinyl estradiol/norethindrone*	35 35	0.5 1
Nelova 1/50-21, Nelova 1/50-28 (X)(G) *mestranol/norethindrone*	50	1
Neocon 7/7/7 (X)(G) *ethinyl estradiol/norethindrone*	35 35 35	0.5 0.75 1
Nordette-21, Nordette-28 (X)(G) *ethinyl estradiol/levonorgestrel*	30	0.15
Norinyl 1+35-21, Norinyl 1+35-28 (X)(G) *ethinyl estradiol/norethindrone*	35	1
Norinyl 1+50-21, Norinyl 1+50-28 (X)(G) *mestranol/norethindrone*	50	1
Nortrel 0.5/35 (X)(G) *ethinyl estradiol/norethindrone*	35	0.5
Nortrel 1/35-21, Nortrel 1/35-28 (X)(G) *ethinyl estradiol/norethindrone*	35	1
Nortrel 7/7/7-28 (X)(G) *ethinyl estradiol/norethindrone*	35 35 35	0.5 0.75 1
Ocella (X)(G) *ethinyl estradiol/drospirenone*	30	3

(*continued*)

(*continued*)

Combined Oral Contraceptive	Estrogen (mcg)	Progesterone (mg)
Ortho-Cept 28 (X)(G) *ethinyl estradiol/desogestrel*	30	0.15
Ortho-Cyclen 28 (X)(G) *ethinyl estradiol/norgestimate*	35	0.25
Ortho-Novum 1/35-21, Ortho-Novum 1/35-28 (X)(G) *ethinyl estradiol/norethindrone*	35	1
Ortho-Novum 1/50-21, Ortho-Novum 1/50-28 (X)(G) *mestranol/norethindrone*	50	1
Ortho-Novum 7/7/7-28 (X)(G) *ethinyl estradiol/norethindrone*	35 35 35	0.5 0.75 1
Ortho-Novum 10/11-28 (X) *ethinyl estradiol/norethindrone*	35 35	0.5 1
Ortho Tri-Cyclen 21, Ortho Tri-Cyclen 28 (X)(G) *ethinyl estradiol/norgestimate*	35 35 35	0.18 0.215 0.25
Ortho Tri-Cyclen Lo (X)(G) *ethinyl estradiol/norgestimate*	25 25 25	0.18 0.215 0.25
Ovcon 35 Fe (X)(G) *ethinyl estradiol/norethindrone* plus *ferrous fumarate* 75 mg (4 tabs)	35	0.4
Ovcon 50-28, Ovcon 50-28 (X) *ethinyl estradiol/norethindrone*	50	1
Ovral-21, Ovral-28 (X)(G) *ethinyl estradiol/norgestrel*	50	0.5
Portia (X)(G) *ethinyl estradiol/levonorgestrel*	30	0.15
Previfem (X) *ethinyl estradiol/norgestimate*	35	0.25
Quasense (X) *ethinyl estradiol/levonorgestrel*	30	0.15

(*continued*)

(*continued*)

Combined Oral Contraceptive	Estrogen (mcg)	Progesterone (mg)
Reclipsen (X)(G) *ethinyl estradiol/desogestrel* plus *ferrous fumarate* 75 mg (4 tabs)	30	0.15
Safyral (X) *ethinyl estradiol/drospirenone* plus *levomefolate calcium* 0.451 mg	30	3
Sprintec 28 (X)(G) *ethinyl estradiol/norgestimate*	35	0.25
Syeda (X) *ethinyl estradiol/drospirenone*	30	3
Tarina Fe 1/20 (X)(G) *ethinyl estradiol/norethindrone* plus *ferrous fumarate* 75 mg (7 tabs)	20	1
Tilia Fe (X)(G) *ethinyl estradiol/norethindrone* plus *ferrous fumarate* 75 mg (7 tabs)	20 30 35	1 1 1
Tri-Legest 21 (X)(G) *ethinyl estradiol/norethindrone*	20 30 35	1 1 1
TriLegest Fe (X)(G) *ethinyl estradiol/norethindrone* plus *ferrous fumarate* 75 mg (7 tabs)	20 30 35	1 1 1
Tri-Levlen 21, Tri-Levlen 28 (X)(G) *ethinyl estradiol/levonorgestrel*	30 40 30	0.05 0.075 0.125
Tri-Lo-Estarylla (X)(G) *ethinyl estradiol/norgestimate*	25 25 25	0.18 0.215 0.25
Tri-Lo-Sprintec (X)(G) *ethinyl estradiol/norgestimate*	25 25 25	0.18 0.215 0.25
TriNessa (X)(G) *ethinyl estradiol/norgestimate*	35 35 35	0.18 0.215 0.25

(*continued*)

(continued)

Combined Oral Contraceptive	Estrogen (mcg)	Progesterone (mg)
Tri-Norinyl 21, Tri-Norinyl 28 (X)(G) *ethinyl estradiol/norethindrone*	35 35 35	0.5 1 0.5
Triphasil-21, Triphasil-28 (X)(G) *ethinyl estradiol/levonorgestrel*	30 40 30	0.050 0.075 0.125
Tri-Previfem (X)(G) *ethinyl estradiol/norgestimate*	35 35 35	0.18 0.215 0.25
Tri-Sprintec (X)(G) *ethinyl estradiol/norgestimate*	35 35 35	0.18 0.215 0.25
Trivora (X)(G) *ethinyl estradiol/levonorgestrel*	30 40 30	0.05 0.075 0.125
Velivet (X)(G) *ethinyl estradiol/desogestrel*	25 25 25	0.1 0.125 0.15
Yasmin (X)(G) *ethinyl estradiol/drospirenone*	30	3
Yaz (X)(G) *ethinyl estradiol/drospirenone*	20	3
Zovia 1/35E-28 (X)(G) *ethinyl estradiol/ethynodiol diacetate*	35	1
Zovia 1/50E-28 (X)(G) *ethinyl estradiol/ethynodiol diacetate*	50	1

APPENDIX H.2: EXTENDED-CYCLE ORAL CONTRACEPTIVES

91 Day
➤ *ethinyl estradiol/levonorgestrel* (X) 1 tab daily x 91 days; repeat (no tablet-free days)
    Ashlyna (G) *Tab: levnorgest* 15 mcg/*eth est* 30 mcg (84) + *eth est* 10 mcg (7)
    (91 tabs/pck)
    Jolessa (G) *Tab: levonorgest* 15 mcg/*eth est* 30 mcg (84) + inert tabs (7m91 tabs/pck)
    LoSeasonique *Tab: levnorgest* 0.1 mcg/*eth est* 20 mcg (84) + *eth est* 10 mcg (7)
    (91 tabs/pck)

(continued)

(continued)

Quartette *Tab: levonorgest* 15 mcg/*eth est* 30 mcg (84) + *eth est* 10 mcg (7) (91 tabs/pck)

Quasense (G) *Tab: levonorgest* 15 mcg/*eth est* 30 mcg (84) + inert tabs (7) (91 tabs/pck)

Seasonale (G) *Tab: levonorgest* 15 mcg/*eth est* 30 mcg (84) + inert tabs (7) (91 tabs/pck)

Seasonique (G) *Tab: levnorgest* 15 mcg/*eth est* 30 mcg (84) + *eth est* 10 mcg (7) (91 tabs/pck)

365 Day

▶ *ethinyl estradiol/levonorgestrel* (X) 1 tab daily x 28 days; repeat (no tablet-free days)
Lybrel *Tab: levnorgest* 0.09 mcg/*eth est* 20 mcg (28 tabs/pck)

APPENDIX H.3: PROGESTERONE-ONLY ORAL CONTRACEPTIVES ("MINI-PILL")

Brand	Progesterone	Mcg
Comment: Take progestin-only pills at the same time each day (within a 3-hour time window). If a pill is missed, another method of contraception should be used for the remainder of the pill pack.		
Camila	*norethindrone* (X)(G)	35
Errin	*norethindrone* (X)(G)	35
Jolivette	*norethindrone* (X)(G)	35
Micronor	*norethindrone* (X)(G)	35
Nora-BE	*norethindrone* (X)(G)	35
Nor-QD	*norethindrone* (X)(G)	35
Ovrette	*norgestrel* (X)	7.5

APPENDIX H.4: INJECTABLE CONTRACEPTIVES

H.4.1: Injectable Progesterone

90 Days
Comment: Administer first dose within 5 days of onset of normal menses, within 5 days postpartum if not breastfeeding, <u>or</u> at 6 weeks postpartum if breastfeeding exclusively. Do not use for >2 years unless other methods are inadequate.

▶ *medroxyprogesterone* (X)(G)
Depo-Provera 150 mg deep IM q 3 months
Vial: 150 mg/ml (1 ml); *Prefilled syringe:* 150 mg/ml
Depo-SubQ 104 mg SC q 3 months
Prefilled syringe: 104 mg/ml (0.65 ml) (parabens)

APPENDIX H.5: TRANSDERMAL CONTRACEPTIVE

Ethinyl Estradiol/ Norelgestromin
Comment: Apply the transdermal patch to the abdomen, buttock, upper-outer arm, or upper torso. *Do* not apply the transdermal patch to the breast. Rotate the site (however, may use the same anatomical area).

▷ *ethinyl estradio/norelgestromin* (X) apply one patch once weekly x 3 weeks; then 1 patch-free week; then repeat sequence
norelgestromin/ethinyl estradiol (X)
   Ortho Evra
      Transdermal patch: eth est 20 mcg/norel 150 mcg per day (1, 3/pck)

APPENDIX H.6: CONTRACEPTIVE VAGINAL RINGS

Ethinyl Estradiol/ Etonogestrel
Comment: The vaginal ring should be inserted prior to, or on 5th day, of the menstrual cycle. Use of a backup method is recommended during the first week. When switching from oral contraceptives, the vaginal ring should be inserted anytime within 7 days after the last active tablet and no later than the day a new pill pack would have been started (no back up method is needed). If the ring is accidently expelled for less than 3 hours, it should be rinsed with cool to lukewarm water and reinserted promptly. If ring removal lasts for more than 3 hours, an additional contraceptive method should be used. If the ring is lost, a new ring should be inserted and the regimen continued without alteration.

▷ *etonogestrel/ethinyl estradiol* (X) insert 1 ring vaginally and leave in place for 3 weeks; then remove for 1 ring-free week; then repeat
   NuvaRing
      Vag ring: eth est 15 mcg/eton 120 mcg per day (1, 3/pck)

APPENDIX H.7: SUBDERMAL CONTRACEPTIVES

Comment: Implants must be inserted within 7 days of the onset of menses. A complete physical examination is required annually. Remove if pregnancy, thromboembolic disorder including thrombophlebitis, jaundice, visual disturbances. Not for use by patients with hypertension, diabetes, hyperlipidemia, impaired liver function, epilepsy, asthma, migraine, depression, cardiac or renal insufficiency, thromboembolic disorder including thrombophlebitis, pro-longed immobilization, or who are smokers.

▷ *etonogestrel* (X) implant rod subdermally in the upper inner non-dominant arm; remove and replace at the end of 3 years
   Implanon, Nexplanon
      Implantable rod: 68 mg implant for subdermal insertion (w. insertion device; latex-free)

(continued)

(continued)

> *levonorgestrel* (X) implant rods subdermally in the upper inner nondominant arm; remove and replace at the end of 5 years
>   **Norplant**
>   *Implantable rods:* 6-36 mg implants (total 216 mg) for subdermal insertion (1 kit w. sterile supplies)

APPENDIX H.8: INTRAUTERINE CONTRACEPTIVES

Comment: Indicated in women who have had at least one child and who are in a stable, mutually monogamous relationship. Reexamine after menses within 3 months to check placement.

> *levonorgestrel* (X)
>   **Liletta** *IUD:* 52 mg (replace at least every 3 years)
>   **Mirena** *IUD:* 52 mg (replace at least every 5 years)
>   **Skyla** *IUD:* 13.5 mg (replace at least every 3 years)

APPENDIX H.9: EMERGENCY CONTRACEPTION

Comment: Emergency contraception must be started within 72 hours after unprotected intercourse following a negative urine hCG pregnancy test. If vomiting occurs within 1 hour of taking a dose, repeat the dose.

> *ethinyl estradiol/levonorgestrel* (X) 2 tabs as soon as possible after unprotected intercourse <u>or</u> contraceptive failure, then 2 more 12 hours after first dose
> *Pediatric:* premenarchal: not applicable
>   **Preven**
>   *Tab: eth est* 50 mcg/*lev* 250 mcg (4/pck) + *Pregnancy test:* 1 hCG home pregnancy test
>   **Yuzpe Regimen**
>   *Tab: eth est* 50 mcg/*lev* 250 mcg (4/pck)

> *levonorgestrel* (X)(OTC)(G)
>   Comment: <17 years of age (prescription required; ≥17 years of age (OTC)
>   *Pediatric:* premenarchal: not applicable
>   **My Way** take 1 tab as soon as possible, within 72 hours, after unprotected sex <u>or</u> suspected contraceptive failure
>   *Tab:* 1.5 mg
>   **Plan B One Step** take 1 tab as soon as possible, within 72 hours, after unprotected sex <u>or</u> suspectedcontraceptive failure
>   *Tab:* 1.5 mg
>   **EContra EZ** take 1 tab within 72 hours after unprotected sex <u>or</u> suspected contraceptive failure
>   *Tab:* 1.5 mg

(continued)

(continued)

▷ **ulipristal (X)**
  Pediatric: premenarchal: not applicable
    ella 1 tab as soon as possible within 120 hours (5 days) after unprotected
    intercourse *or* contraceptive failure; may repeat dose if vomiting occurs
    within 3 hours
      Tab: 30 mg

 **APPENDIX I: ANESTHETIC AGENTS
FOR LOCAL INFILTRATION AND
DERMAL/MUCOSAL MEMBRANE APPLICATION**

Agents and Indications	
Brand/*generic*	**Indication(s)**
AnaMantle HC *lidocaine 3%/hydrocortisone 0.5%*	Local anesthetic/steroid; for hemorrhoids, pruritus ani, anal fissure
Decadron Phosphate with Xylocaine *dexamethasone 4 mg/lidocaine 10 mg/ ml (5 ml)*	Local anesthetic/steroid; infiltration by injection
Dyclone *dyclonine 0.5%, 0.1%*	Local anesthetic; infiltration by injection
Duranest (B) *etidocaine 1%* (30 ml) **Duranest (B) w. Epinephrine** *Inj: etido 1.5%/epi 1:200,000 (30 ml)* *Dental Cartridge: etido 1.5%/epi 1:200,000 (1.8 ml)*	Nerve block and local anesthetic; mouth, pharynx, larynx, trachea, esophagus, anogenital area, urethra Local anesthetic: dental procedures
Ela-Max 4% Cream (B) *lidocaine 4%* **Ela-Max 5% Cream (B)** *lidocaine 5%*	Local dermal anesthetic and for anorectal irritation and pain
Emla Cream (B) (5, 30 g) **Emla Anesthetic Disc (B)** (2 discs/box) *lidocaine 2.5%/prilocaine 2.5%*	Local dermal anesthetic; preparation for phlebotomy, PIV starts, injections
Flector Patch (C/D) (30/box) *diclofenac epolamine 180 mg*	Local dermal NSAID analgesic
Exparel (B) *Vial:* 13.3 mg/ml (20 ml) *bupivacaine liposome 1.3% susp for inj*	Surgical site injection for postop pain management

(continued)

(continued)

Agents and Indications	
Brand/*generic*	**Indication(s)**
LidaMantle (B) cream (1, 2 oz) **LidaMantle (B)** lotion (177 ml) **Lidoderm** cream **(B)** (85 g) *lidocaine 3%* **Lidoderm (B)(G)** adhesive patch (10 cm x14 cm; 30/box) *lidocaine 5%*	Local dermal anesthetic lotion, cream, and adhesive patch
Ophthaine (B) (15 ml) *proparacaine 0.5% ophthalmic solution*	Ophthalmic anesthetic for examination/removal of foreign body (eye)
Pliaglis Cream (B) (30 g) *lidocaine 7%/tetracaine 7%*	Local dermal anesthetic for superficial dermatological procedures
Qutenza (B) (1, 2 patches, each *with 50 g tube of cleansing gel)* *capsaicin 8% patch*	Local dermal NSAID analgesic for postherpetic neuralgia
Synera Topical Patch (B) (2, 10/pck) *lidocaine 70 mg/tetracaine 70 mg*	Local dermal anesthetic for venous access or skin lesion removal
Tetracaine Ophthalmic Solution (B) (15 ml) *proparacaine 0.5% ophthalmic solution*	Ophthalmic anesthetic for examination/removal of foreign body (eye)
Xylocaine Jelly (B) (5, 10, 20, 30 ml) *lidocaine 2% aqueous*	For procedures of the urethra, painful urethritis, and endotracheal intubation
Xylocaine Ointment (B) (3.5, 35 g) *lidocaine 5% water miscible*	For procedures of the urethra, painful urethritis, and endotracheal intubation
Xylocaine Topical Solution (B) (100 ml) *lidocaine 2% solution* **Xylocaine Viscous (B)** (50 ml) *lidocaine 2% viscous solution*	Anesthetic for the nasal and oropharyngeal mucosa and the proximal portions of the GI tract
Zingo *lidocaine monohydrate 0.5 mg*	Hand-held, needle-free device, helium-powered delivery system that numbs site in 1-3 minutes delivers 0.5 mg sterile lidocaine HCL monohydrate sterile lidocaine HCL pwdr for intradermal injection for the management of venous access pain

(continued)

(continued)

Agents and Indications	
Brand/*generic*	Indication(s)
Zostrix (B) (0.7, 1.5, 3 oz) *capsaicin 0.025% cream* **Zostrix HP (B)** (1, 2 oz) *capsaicin 0.075% emollient cream*	Local dermal NSAID analgesic

APPENDIX J: ORAL PRESCRIPTION NSAIDs

Comment: NSAIDs should be taken with food to decrease gastric upset. Dosing of NSAIDs should be scheduled rather than PRN for maximal benefit. NSAIDs are contraindicated with sulfonamide or *aspirin* allergy, 3rd trimester pregnancy (causes premature closure of the ductus arteriosus), and coronary artery bypass graft (CABG) surgery. Concomitant use of *misoprostol* (**Cytotec**) with NSAIDs reduces gastric upset and potential for ulceration; however, *misoprostol* is pregnancy category X. Administration of *misoprostol* in pregnancy can cause spontaneous abortion, premature birth, birth defects, and uterine rupture (beyond the 8th week of pregnancy). NSAIDs and *warfarin* (**Coumadin**) are synergistic. With all patients, use the lowest effective dose for the shortest time necessary. NSAIDs should be taken with food to reduce the risk of gastrointestinal adverse side effects (GIASE).

GI ADVERSE SIDE EFFECTS:
(+) MILD; (++) FREQUENT; (+++) MORE FREQUENT/SEVERE

▷ *celecoxib* (C/D)(G)(+) 100 mg twice daily or 200 mg once daily or 200 mg twice daily or 400 mg once daily; <50 kg, start at lowest dose
Pediatric: <2 years: not recommended; ≥2 years, >10<25 kg: 50 mg twice daily; ≥25 kg: 100 mg once daily
Celebrex
Cap: 50, 100, 200, 400 mg

▷ *diclofenac sodium* (D)(+++)
Pediatric: not recommended
Dyloject administer 37.5 mg IV bolus over 15 seconds q 6 hours; max 150 mg/day
Vial: 37.5 mg/ml (25/box)
Pennsaid 1% in 10 drop increments, dispense and rub into front, side, and back of knee: usually 40 drops (40 mg) qid
Topical soln: 1.5% (150 ml)

(continued)

(*continued*)

Pennsaid 2% apply 2 pump actuations (40 mg) and rub into front, side, and back of knee bid
  Topical soln: 2% (20 mg/pump actuation; 112 g)
Solaraze Gel apply to affected areas bid
  Gel: 3% (30 mg (100 g))
Voltaren 50 mg bid <u>or</u> qid <u>or</u> 75 mg bid <u>or</u> 25 mg qid with an additional 25 mg at HS if necessary
  Tab: 25, 50, 75 mg ent-coat
Voltaren XR 100 mg once daily; rarely, 100 mg bid may be used
  Tab: 100 mg ext-rel
Zorvolex 35 mg tid
  Gelcap: 18, 35 mg ext-rel

▷ *diclofenac potassium* (C/D)(G)(+++) 50 mg tid <u>or</u> qid <u>or</u> 25 mg tid <u>or</u> qid and may add 25 mg at HS
Pediatric: not recommended
    Cataflam
      Tab: 50 mg
    Zipsor
      Gel cap: 25 mg

▷ *diclofenac sodium* plus *misoprostol* (X)(++)
Pediatric: not recommended
    Arthrotec
      Tab: 50, 75 mg

▷ *diflunisal* (C/D)(G)(+++) initially 1 g as a single dose followed by 500 mg q 8-12 hours <u>or</u> 500 mg as a single dose followed by 250 mg q 8-12 hours
Pediatric: <12 years: not recommended
    Dolobid
      Tab: 500*mg

▷ *etodolac* (C/D)(G)(+)
Pediatric: not recommended
    Lodine initially 600 mg to 1 g/day in 2-3 divided doses; usual max 1 g/day in divided doses; may increase to 1.2 g/day when needed
      Tab: 400, 500 mg; *Cap:* 200, 300 mg
    Lodine XL 400 mg to 1 g once daily; max 1.2 g/day
      Tab: 400, 500, 600 mg ext-rel

▷ *fenoprofen* (B/D)(++) 300-600 mg tid-qid; max 3.2 g/day
Pediatric: not recommended
    Nalfon
      Tab: 200 mg

▷ *flurbiprofen* (B/D)(G)(++) 200-300 mg/day in 2-4 divided doses; max single dose 100 mg; reduce dosage for renal impairment
Pediatric: not recommended
    Ansaid
      Tab: 50, 100 mg

(continued)

▷ ***ibuprofen/famotidine*** (B/D)(++) 1 tab 3 times daily; swallow whole; use lowest effective dose for the shortest duration
Pediatric: not recommended
> **Duexis**
>> *Tab:* ibu 800 mg/*fam* 26.6 mg

▷ ***indomethecin*** (B/D)(G)(+++) 75-100 mg daily in 3-4 divided doses; max 200 mg/day
Pediatric: <14 years: not recommended
> **Indocin**
>> *Cap:* 25, 50 mg; *Rectal supp:* 50 mg; *Oral susp:* 25 mg/5 ml; *Vial:* 1 mg pwdr for reconstitution and IV infusion
> **Indocin SR**
>> *Cap:* 75 mg ext-rel
> **Tivorbex**
>> *Cap:* 20, 40 mg

▷ ***ketoprofen*** (C/D)(G)(++) 75 mg tid <u>or</u> 50 mg qid; max 300 mg/day
Pediatric: <18 years: not recommended
> **Orudis**
>> *Cap:* 50, 75 mg
> **Oruvail**
>> *Cap:* 100, 150, 200 mg ext-rel

▷ ***ketorolac tromethamine*** (C/D)(G)(+++)
Pediatric: <17 years: not recommended
> **Sprix** *17-64 years:* 1 spray each nostril (total dose 31,5 mg) every 6-8 hours prn; max 4 doses/24 hours (total daily dose 126 mg); ≥*65 years, renal impairment* <u>or</u> <*50 kg:* 1 spray in one nostril (total dose 15.75 mg) every 6-8 hours; max 4 doses/24 hours (63 mg); discard used bottle after 24 hours
>> *Nasal spray:* 15.75 mg/100 mcl nasal spray (8 sprays, 1.7 g)
> **Toradol** 60 mg as a single IM dose; max 30 mg as a single IV dose; may administer 30 mg IV and 30 mg IM as a single dose; oral dosing is indicated <u>*only*</u> as continuation therapy to IM <u>or</u> IV dosing; oral formulation should <u>*never*</u> be administered as an initial dose; initiate oral dosing at 20 mg followed by 10 mg q 4-6 hours prn; max oral dosing 40 mg/day; >65 years, initiate oral dosing at 10 mg followed by 10 mg q 4-6 hours prn; max 40 mg/day; the combined duration of IV/IM/PO dosing is not to exceed 5 days
>> *Tab:* 10 mg; *Inj* 15, 30, 60 mg/ml

▷ ***magnesium chol salicylate*** (C/D)(G)(+)
Pediatric:
> **Trilisate**
>> *Tab:* 10 mg

▷ ***meclofenamate sodium*** (B/D)(G)(++) 50-100 mg q 4-6 hours <u>or</u> 300-400 mg/day in 3-4 equal doses; max 400 mg/day
Pediatric: <14 years: not recommended
> **Meclofen**
>> *Cap:* 50, 100 mg

(continued)

(*continued*)

▶ ***mefenamic acid*** (C)(G)(++) 500 mg once; then, 250 mg q 6 hours
Pediatric: <14 years: not recommended
Ponstel
Cap: 250 mg

▶ ***meloxicam*** (C/D)(G)(+) 7.5 mg once daily; max 15 mg/day; hemodialysis max 7.5 mg/day
Pediatric: <2 years: not recommended; ≥2 years: 0.125 mg/kg; max 7.5 mg once daily
Mobic
Tab: 7.5, 15 mg; *Oral susp:* 7.5 mg/5 ml (100 ml) (raspberry)
Relafen
Tab: 500, 750 mg

▶ ***nabumetone*** (C/D)(G)(+) 1-2 g/day in a single dose <u>or</u> 2 divided doses; max 2 g/day; <50 kg, max 1 g/day
Pediatric: not recommended

▶ ***naproxen*** (B)(G)(++) 275-550 mg twice daily <u>or</u> 275 mg every 6-8 hours; max 1.375 g first day; then, max 1.1 g/day; acute gout: 825 mg once, then 275 mg every 8 hours
Pediatric: <2 years: not recommended; ≥2 years: 5 mg/kg bid; max 15 mg/kg/day has been used; use suspension
Naprosyn
Tab: 250, 375, 500 mg
Naprosyn Suspension
Oral susp: 125 mg/5 ml

▶ ***naproxen/esomeprazole (as magnesium trihydrate)*** (C/D)(++) one 375/20 <u>or</u> one 500/20 tab twice daily; take at least 30 minutes before meals; take lowest effective dose
Pediatric: <18 years: not recommended
Vimovo 375/20
Tab: nap 375 mg/*eso* 20 mg
Vimovo 500/20
Tab: nap 500 mg/*eso* 20 mg

▶ ***oxaprozin*** (C/D)(++) 1.2 g once daily; max 1.8 g <u>or</u> 26 mg/kg daily, whichever is less, in divided doses; low body weight, milder disease, <u>or</u> on dialysis: initially 600 mg once daily; max 1.2 g daily
Pediatric: <6 years: not recommended; 6-16 years, 21-31 kg: 600 mg once daily; 32-54 kg: 900 mg once daily; ≥55 kg: 1.2 g once daily
Daypro *Tab:* 600*

▶ ***piroxicam*** (C/D)(G)(+++) 20 mg once daily
Pediatric: not recommended
Feldene
Cap: 10, 20 mg
Comment: Because of the long half-life, steady state blood levels of ***piroxicam*** are not reached for 7-12 days. Therefore, there is a progressive response over several weeks.

(*continued*)

(continued)

> **salsalate (C/D)(G)(+)** 1.5 g bid <u>or</u> 1 g tid
> *Pediatric:* not recommended
> > **Disalcid**
> > *Tab:* 500*, 750*mg; *Cap:* 500 mg

> **sulindac (B/D)(G)(+++)** 150-200 mg bid; max 400 mg/day; usually x 7-14 days
> *Pediatric:* not recommended
> > **Clinoril**
> > *Tab:* 150*, 200*mg
> > **Tolectin DS**
> > *Cap:* 400 mg
> > **Tolectin 600**
> > *Tab:* 600 mg film-coat

> **tolmetin (C/D)(G)(+++)** initially 400 mg tid; usual range 600 mg to 1.8 g/day in divided doses; max 1,800 mg/day
> *Pediatric:* <2 years: not recommended; ≥2 years: 20 mg/kg divided tid to qid; usual range 15-30 mg/kg/day divided tid to qud: max 30 mg/kg/day
> > **Tolectin** *Tab:* 200*mg

> **nabumetone (C/D)(G)(+)** 1-2 g/day in a single dose <u>or</u> 2 divided doses; max 2 g/day; <50 kg, max 1 g/day
> *Pediatric:* not recommended

> **naproxen (B)(G)(++)** 275-550 mg bid <u>or</u> 275 mg q 6-8 hours; max 1.375 g first day, then, max 1.1 g/day; *Acute gout attack:* 825 mg once, then 275 mg every 8 hours
> *Pediatric:* <2 years: not recommended; ≥2 years: 5 mg/kg bid; max 15 mg/kg/day has been used; use suspension
> > **Naprosyn**
> > *Tab:* 250, 375, 500 mg
> > **Naprosyn Suspension**
> > *Oral susp:* 125 mg/5 ml

> **naproxen/esomeprazole (as magnesium trihydrate) (C/D)(++)** 1 x 375/20 <u>or</u> 1 x 500/20 tab bid; take at least 30 minutes before meals; take lowest effective dose
> *Pediatric:* <18 years: not recommended
> > **Vimovo 375/20**
> > *Tab: nap* 375 mg/*eso* 20 mg
> > **Vimovo 500/20**
> > *Tab: nap* 500 mg/*eso* 20 mg

> **oxaprozin (C/D)(++)** 1.2 g once daily; max 1.8 g <u>or</u> 26 mg/kg daily, whichever is less, in divided doses; *Low body weight, milder disease,* <u>or</u> *on dialysis:* initially 600 mg once daily; max 1.2 g daily
> *Pediatric:* <6 years: not recommended; 6-16 years, 21-31 kg: 600 mg once daily; 32-54 kg: 900 mg once daily; ≥55 kg: 1.2 g once daily
> > **Daypro**
> > *Tab:* 600*

(*continued*)

▷ *piroxicam* (C/D)(G)(+++) 20 mg once daily
    Pediatric: not recommended
        Feldene
            Cap: 10, 20 mg

Comment: Because of the long half-life, steady state blood levels of *piroxicam* are not reached for 7-12 days. Therefore, there is a progressive response over several weeks.

▷ *salsalate* (C/D)(G)(+) 1.5 g bid <u>or</u> 1 g tid
    Pediatric: not recommended
        Disalcid
            Tab: 500*, 750*mg; *Cap:* 500 mg
        Tolectin 600
            Tab: 600 mg film-coat

APPENDIX K: TOPICAL CORTICOSTEROIDS BY POTENCY

Comment: All topical, oral, and parenteral corticosteroids are pregnancy category C. Use with caution in infants and children. Steroids should be applied sparingly and for the shortest time necessary. Do not use in the diaper area. Do not use an occlusive dressing. Systemic absorption of topical corticosteroids can induce reversible hypothalamic-pituitary-adrenal (HPA) axis suppression with the potential for clinical glucocorticoid insufficiency.

Potency guide:
- Face: Low potency
- Ears/scalp margin: Intermediate potency
- Eyelids: Hydrocortisone in ophthalmic ointment base 1%
- Chest/back: Intermediate potency
- Skin folds: Low potency

Generic	Brand/Formulation/Frequency	Strength/Volume
Low Potency		
alclometasone dipropionate (C)	**Aclovate** Crm bid-tid	0.05% (15,45, 60 g)
	Aclovate Oint bid-tid	0.05% (15,45, 60 g)
fluocinolone acetonide (C)	**Synalar** Crm bid-qid	0.025% (15, 60 g)
hydrocortisone base <u>or</u> *acetate* (C)(G)	**Anusol-HC** Crm bid-qid	2.5% (30 g)
	Hytone Crm bid-qid	1% (1, 2 oz)
	Hytone Oint bid-qid	1% (1 oz)
	Hytone Lotn bid-qid	1% (2 oz)

(*continued*)

(*continued*)

Generic	Brand/Formulation/Frequency	Strength/Volume
	Hytone Crm bid-qid	2.5% (1, 2 oz)
	Hytone Oint bid-qid	2.5% (1 oz)
	Hytone Lotn bid-qid	2.5% (1 oz)
	U-cort Crm bid-qid	1% (7, 28, 35 g)
triamcinolone acetonide (C)(G)	**Kenalog** Crm bid-qid	0.025% (15, 80 g)
	Kenalog Lotn bid-qid	0.025% (60 ml)
	Kenalog Oint bid-qid	0.025% (15, 60, 80 g)
Intermediate Potency		
betamethasone valerate (C)(G)	**Luxiq** Foam bid	0.12% (100 g)
clocortolone pivalate (C)	**Cloderm** Crm bid	
desonide (C)(G)	**Desonate** Gel/Formulation bid-tid	0.05% (15, 60 g)
	DesOwen Crm bid-tid	0.05% (15, 60 g)
	DesOwen Lotn bid-tid	0.05% (2, 4 fl oz)
	DesOwen Oint bid-tid	0.05% (15, 60 g)
	Tridesilon Crm bid-qid	0.05% (15, 60 g)
	Tridesilon Oint bid-qid	0.05% (15, 60 g)
	Verdeso Foam	
desoximetasone (C)(G)	**Topicort-LP** Emol Crm bid	0.05% (15, 60 g, 4 oz)
fluocinolone acetonide (C)(G)	**Capex** Shampoo	0.01% (4 oz)
	Derma-Smoothe/FS Oil tid	0.01% (4 oz)
	Derma-Smoothe/FS Shampoo	0.01% (4 oz)
	Synalar Crm bid-qid	0.025% (15, 30, 60 g)
	Synalar Oint bid-qid	0.025% (15, 60 g)
flurandrenolide (C)	**Cordran-SP** Crm bid to tid	0.025% (30, 60 g)
	Cordran Oint bid-tid	0.025% (30, 60 g)
	Cordran-SP Crm bid-tid	0.05% (15, 30, 60 g)
	Cordran Lotn bid-tid	0.05% (15, 60 ml)
	Cordran Oint bid-tid	0.05% (15, 30, 60 g)
fluticasone propionate (C)(G)	**Cutivate** Oint bid	0.005% (15, 30, 60 g)
	Cutivate Crm qd-bid	0.05% (15, 30, 60 g)
	Cutivate Lotn qd-bid	0.05%

(*continued*)

(*continued*)

Generic	Brand/Formulation/ Frequency	Strength/Volume
hydrocortisone probutate (C)	**Pandel** Crm qd-bid	0.1% (15, 45 g)
hydrocortisone butyrate (C)(G)	**Locoid** Crm bid-tid **Locoid** Oint bid-tid **Locoid** Soln bid-tid	0.1% (15, 45 g) 0.1% (15, 45 g) 0.1% (30, 60 ml)
hydrocortisone valerate (C)(G)	**Westcort** Crm bid-tid **Westcort** Oint bid-tid	0.2% (15, 45, 60, 120 g) 0.2% (15, 45, 60 g)
mometasone furoate (C)	**Elocon** Crm qd **Elocon** Lotn qd **Elocon** Oint qd	0.1% (15, 45 g) 0.1% (30, 60 ml) 0.1% (15, 45 g)
prednicarbate	**Dermatop** Emol Crm bid **Dermatop** Oint bid	0.1% (15, 60 g)
triamcinolone acetonide (C)(G)	**Kenalog** Crm bid-tid **Kenalog** Lotn bid-tid **Kenalog** Emul Spray bid-tid	0.1% (15, 60, 80 g) 0.1% (60 ml) 0.2% (63, 100 g)
High Potency		
amcinonide (C)(G)	Crm bid-tid Lotn bid Oint bid	0.1% (15, 30, 60 g) 0.1% (20, 60 ml) 0.1% (15, 30, 60 g)
Betamethasone dipropionate (C)	**Sernivo Spray** Emul Spray bid	0.05% (60, 120 ml)
betamethasone dipropionate, augmented (C)	**Diprolene AF** Emol Crm qd-bid **Diprolene** Lotn qd-bid	0.05% (15, 50 g) 0.05% (30, 60 ml)
desoximetasone (C)(G)	**Topicort** Gel bid **Topicort** Emol Crm bid **Topicort** Oint bid	0.05% (15, 60 g) 0.25% (15, 60 g) 0.25% (15, 60 g)
diflorasone diacetate (C)	**Psorcon e** Emol Crm bid **Psorcon e** Emol Oint qd-tid	0.05% (15, 30, 60 g) 0.05% (15, 30, 60 g)
fluocinonide (C)	**Lidex** Crm bid-qid **Lidex** Gel bid-qid **Lidex** Oint bid-qid **Lidex** Soln bid-qid **Lidex-E** Emol Crm bid-qid	0.05% (15, 30, 60, 120 g) 0.05% (15, 30, 60 g) 0.05% (15, 30, 60, 120 g) 0.05% (20, 60 ml) 0.05% (15, 30, 60 g)

(*continued*)

(*continued*)

Generic	Brand/Formulation/Frequency	Strength/Volume
Flurandrenolide (C)	**Cordan** Oint bid-tid **Cordan** Crm bid-tid	0.05% (15, 30, 60 g) 0.025% (30, 60, 120 g) 0.05% (15, 30, 60, 120 g)
halcinonide (C)	**Halog** Crm bid-tid **Halog** Oint bid-tid **Halog** Soln bid-tid **Halog-E** Emol Crm qd-tid	0.1% (15, 30, 60, 240 g) 0.1% (15, 30, 60, 120 g) 0.1% (20, 60 ml) 0.1% (15, 30, 60 g)
triamcinolone acetonide (C)(G)	**Kenalog** Crm bid-tid	0.5% (20 g)
Super High Potency		
betamethasone dipropionate, augmented (C)	**Diprolene** Oint qd-bid **Diprolene** Gel qd-bid	0.05% (15, 50 g) 0.05% (15, 50 g)
clobetasol propionate (C)(G)	**Clobex** Shampoo daily **Clobex** Spray bid **Cormax** Oint bid **Cormax** Scalp App **Olux** Foam **Olux E** Foam **Temovate** Crm bid **Temovate** Gel bid **Temovate** Oint bid **Temovate** Scalp App bid **Temovate-E** Emol Crm bid	0.05% (4 oz) 0.05% (2, 4.5 oz) 0.05% (15, 45 g) 0.05% (15, 45 g) 0.05% (50, 100 g) 0.05% (50, 100 g) 0.05% (15, 30, 45, 60 g) 0.05% (15, 30, 60 g) 0.05% (15, 30, 45, 60 g) 0.05% (25, 50 ml) 0.05% (15, 30, 60 g)
fluocinonide (C)	**Vanos** Oint qd-tid	0.1% (30, 60, 120 g)
flurandrenolide (C)	**Cordran** Tape q 12 hours	4 mcg/sq cm (roll of 3"x 80")
halobetasol propionate (C)	**Ultravate** Crm qd-bid **Ultravate** Oint qd to bid	0.05% (15, 45 g) 0.05% (15, 45 g)

 APPENDIX L: ORAL CORTICOSTEROIDS

Comment: Systemic corticosteroids increase glucose intolerance, reduce the action of insulin and oral hypoglycemic agents, reduce adrenal cortex activity, decrease immunity, mask signs of infection, impair wound healing, suppress growth in

(*continued*)

(*continued*)

children, and promote osteoporosis, fluid retention, and weight gain. Use systemic
steroids with caution, using the lowest possible dose to affect clinical response, and
withdraw (wean) gradually in tapering doses to avoid adrenal insufficiency. The
American Academy of Rheumatology (AAR) recommends the following daily doses
for anyone on a chronic systemic corticosteroid regimen: Calcium 1,200-1,500 mg/
day and vitamin D 800-1,000 IU/day.

▷ *betamethasone* (C)(G) initially 0.6-7.2 mg daily
  Pediatric: same as adult
    Celestone *Tab:* 0.6 mg; *Syr:* 0.6 mg/5 ml (120 ml)

▷ *cortisone* (D)(G) initially 25-300 mg daily <u>or</u> every other day
  Pediatric: not recommended
    Cortone Acetate *Tab:* 25 mg

▷ *xamethasone* (C)(G) initially 0.75-9 mg/day
  Pediatric: same as adult
    Decadron *Tab:* 0.5*, 0.75*, 4*mg; *Syr:* 0.5 mg/5 ml (100 ml)
    Decadron 5-12 Pak *Tabs:* 0.75*mg (12/pck)

▷ *hydrocortisone* (C)(G) 20-240 mg daily
  Pediatric: 2-8 mg/day
    Cortef *Tab:* 5, 10, 20 mg; *Oral susp:* 10 mg/5 ml
    Hydrocortone *Tab:* 10 mg

▷ *methylprednisolone* (C)(G) 4-48 mg/day
  Pediatric: same as adult
    Medrol *Tab:* 2*, 4*, 8*, 16*, 24*, 32*mg
    Medrol Dosepak *Dosepak:* 4*mg tabs (21/pck)

▷ *prednisolone* (C)(G) initially 5-60 mg/day in 1-2 doses x 3-5 days
  Pediatric: 0.14-2 mg/kg/day in 3-4 doses x 3-5 days
    Flo-Pred *Susp:* 5, 15 mg/5 ml
    Orapred *Soln:* 15 mg/5 ml (grape) (dye-free, alcohol 2%)
    Orapred ODT *Tab:* 10, 15, 30 mg orally disintegrating (grape)
    Pediapred *Soln:* 5 mg/5 ml (raspberry, sugar-, alcohol-, dye-free)
    Prelone *Syr:* 15 mg/5 ml
    Comment: **Flo-Pred** does not require refrigeration <u>or</u> shaking prior to use.

▷ *prednisone* (C)(G) initially 5-60 mg/day in 1-2 doses x 3-5 days
  Pediatric: 0.14-2 mg/kg/day in 3-4 doses x 3-5 days
    Deltasone *Tab:* 2.5*, 5*, 10*, 20*, 50*mg

▷ *prednisone* (*delayed release*) (C) initially 5-60 mg/day in 1-2 doses x 3-5 days
  Pediatric: 0.14-**2 mg**/kg/day in 3-4 doses x 3-5 days
    RAYOS *Tab:* 1, 2, 5 mg del-rel

▷ *triamcinolone* (C)(G) initially 4-48 mg/day in 1-2 doses x 3-5 days
  Pediatric: 0.14-2 mg/kg/day in 3-4 doses x 3-5 days
    Aristocort *Tab:* 4*mg
    Aristocort Forte *Susp:* 40 mg/ml (benzoyl alcohol)
    Aristocort Aristopak *Tab:* 4*mg (16/pck)

● APPENDIX M: PARENTERAL CORTICOSTEROID THERAPY

Comment: Systemic glucocorticosteroids increase glucose intolerance, reduce the action of insulin and oral hypoglycemic agents, reduce adrenal cortex activity, decrease immunity, mask signs of infection, impair wound healing, suppress growth in children, and promote osteoporosis, fluid retention, and weight gain. Use systemic steroids with caution, using the lowest possible dose to affect clinical response, and withdraw (wean) gradually in tapering doses to avoid adrenal insufficiency. The American Academy of Rheumatology (AAR) recommends the following daily doses for anyone on a chronic systemic corticosteroid regimen: Calcium 1,200-1,500 mg/day and vitamin D 800-1,000 IU/day.

▷ *betamethasone* (C)(G)
> **Celestone** 0.5-9 mg IM/IV x 1 dose
> *Vial:* 3 mg/ml (10 ml)
> **Celestone Soluspan** 0.5-9 mg IM/IV x 1 dose; usual IM dose 6 mg
> *Vial:* 6 mg/ml (10 ml)

▷ *cortisone* (D)(G) 20-300 mg IM
> *Pediatric:* not recommended
> **Cortone Acetate** *Vial:* 50 mg/ml (10 ml)

▷ *dexamethasone* (C)(G) initially 0.5-9 mg IM/IV daily
> **Dalalone D.P.** *Vial:* 16 mg/ml (1, 5 ml)
> **Decadron** *Vial:* 4, 24 mg/ml for IM use (5 ml, sulfites)
> **Decadron-LA** *Vial:* 8 mg/ml (1, 5 ml)

▷ *hydrocortisone* (C)(G) initially 100-500 mg IM/IV daily
> *Pediatric:* 2-8 mg/kg loading dose (max 250 mg); then 8 mg/kg/day
> **Hydrocortone** *Vial:* 50 mg/ml (5 ml)
> **Solu-Cortef** *Vial:* 100 mg (2 ml); 250 mg (2 ml); 500 mg (4 ml); 1 g (8 ml)

▷ *hydrocortisone phosphate* (C)(G) for IM, IV, and SC injection
> **Hydrocortone** *Vial:* 50 mg/ml (2 ml)

▷ *methylprednisolone* (C)(G) 40-120 mg IM/week for 1-4 weeks
> **Depo-Medrol** *Vial:* 20 mg/ml (5 ml); 40 mg/ml (5, 10 ml); 80 mg/ml (5 ml)

▷ *methylprednisolone sodium succinate* (C)(G) 10-40 mg IV initially; then, IM <u>or</u> IV
> *Pediatric:* 1-2 mg/kg loading dose; then 1.6 mg/kg/day in divided doses at least 6 hours apart
> **Solu-Medrol** *Vial:* 40 mg (1 ml); 125 mg (2 ml); 500 mg (4 ml); 1 g (8 ml); 2 g (8 ml)

▷ *triamcinolone* (C)(G) 40 mg IM/week
> **Aristocort** *Vial:* 25 mg/ml (5 ml)
> **Aristocort Forte** *Vial:* 40 mg/ml (1, 5 ml) *(do not administer IV)*
> **Aristospan** *Vial:* 5 mg/ml (5 ml); 20 mg/ml (1, 5 ml)
> **TAC-3** *Vial:* 3 mg/ml (5 ml) for intralesional and intradermal use

Injectable Corticosteroid/Anesthetic

▷ *dexamethasone/lidocaine* (C) 0.1-0.75 ml into painful area
> **Decadron Phosphate with Xylocaine** *Vial: dexa* 4 mg/*lido* 10 mg per ml (5 ml)

APPENDIX N: INHALATIONAL CORTICOSTEROID THERAPY

Comment: Inhaled glucocorticosteroids are indicated for the long-term control of asthma. Inhaled corticosteroids are not indicated for exercise induced asthma <u>or</u> for relief of acute symptoms (i.e., "rescue"). Low doses are indicated for mild persistent asthma, medium doses are indicated for moderate persistent asthma, and high doses are reserved for severe cases. Titrate to lowest effective dose. To reduce the potential for adverse effects with inhalers, the patient should use a spacer <u>or</u> holding chamber and rinse the mouth and spit after every inhalation treatment. Linear growth should be monitored in children. When inhaled doses exceed 1000 mcg/day, consider supplements of calcium (1-1.5 g/day), vitamin D (400 IU/day), and *estrogen* replacement therapy for postmenopausal women.

▷ *beclomethasone* (C)
   Beclovent 2 inhalations tid-qid <u>or</u> 4 inhalations bid; max 20 inhalations/day
      Pediatric: <6 years: not recommended; 6-12 years: 1-2 inhalations tid-qid <u>or</u> 4 inhalations bid; max 10 inhalations/day
      Inhaler: 42 mcg/actuation (6.7 g, 80 inh); 16.8 g (200 inh)
   Qvar *Previously using only bronchodilators:* initiate 40-80 mcg bid; max 320 mcg/day; *Previously using an inhaled corticosteroid:* initiate 40-160 mcg bid; max 320 mcg/day; *Previously taking a systemic corticosteroid:* attempt to wean off the systemic drug after approximately 1 week after initiating Qvar
      Pediatric: not recommended
      Inhaler: 40, 80 mcg/actuation metered-dose aerosol w. dose counter (8.7 g, 120 inh) (CFC-free)
   Vanceril 2 inhalations tid to qid <u>or</u> 4 inhalations bid
      Pediatric: <6 years: not recommended; 6-12 years: 1-2 inhalations tid to qid
      Inhaler: 42 mcg/actuation (16.8 g, 200 inh)
   Vanceril Double Strength 2 inhalations bid
      Pediatric: <6 years: not recommended; 6-12 years: 1-2 inhalations bid; >12 years: same as adult
      Inhaler: 84 mcg/actuation (12.2 g, 120 inh)

▷ *budesonide* (B)(G)
   Pulmicort Respules use turbuhaler
      Pediatric: <12 months: not recommended; ≥12 months to 8 years: *Previously using only bronchodilators:* initiate 0.5 mg/day once daily <u>or</u> in 2 divided doses; may start at 0.25 mg/day; *Previously using inhaled orticosteroids:* initiate 0.5 mg/day daily <u>or</u> in 2 divided doses; max 1 mg/day; *Previously using oral orticosteroids:* initiate 1 mg/day daily <u>or</u> in 2 divided doses
      Inhal susp: 0.25 mg/2 ml (30/box)
   Pulmicort Turbuhaler 1-2 inhalations bid; *Previously on oral corticosteroids:* 2-4 inhalations bid
      Pediatric: <6 years: not recommended; ≥6 years: 1-2 inhalations bid
      Turbuhaler: 200 mcg/actuation (200 inh)

(continued)

(*continued*)

➤ *flunisolide* (C)(G)
    AeroBid, AeroBid M initially 2 inhalations bid; max 8 inhalations/day
      Pediatric: <6 years: not recommended; 6-15 years: 2 inhalations bid; ≥16
      years: same as adult
      Inhaler: 250 mcg/actuation (7 g, 100 inh)

➤ *fluticasone* (C)(G)
    Flovent HFA initially 88 mcg bid; if previously using an inhaled corticoste-
    roid, initially 88-220 mcg bid; if previously taking an oral corticosteroid,
    initially 880 mcg/day
      Pediatric: use **Rotadisk:** initially 50-88 mcg inh bid; <4 years: not recom-
      mended; 4-11 years: initially 50-88 mcg bid; >11 years: initially 100 mcg
      bid; if previously using an inhaled corticosteroid, initially 100-200 mcg
      bid; *Previously taking an oral corticosteroid;* initially 1000 mcg bid
      Inhaler: 44 mcg/actuation (7.9 g, 60 inh; 13 g, 120 inh); 110 mcg/actuation
      (13 g, 120 inh); 220 mcg/ actuation (13 g, 120 inh)
    Rotadisk 50 mcg/actuation (60 blisters/disk); 100 mcg/actuation (60 blisters/
    disk); 250 mcg/actuation (60 blisters/disk)

➤ *mometasone furoate* (C) *Previously using a bronchodilator* <u>or</u> *inhaled corticoste-*
roid: 220 mcg q PM <u>or</u> bid; max 440 mcg q PM <u>or</u> 220 mcg bid; *Previously using an*
oral corticosteroid: 440 mcg bid; max 880 mcg/day
    Pediatric: <12 years: not recommended
    Asmanex Twisthaler
      Inhaler: 220 mcg/actuation (6.7 g, 80 inh); 16.8 g (200 inh)

⭕ APPENDIX O: ORAL ANTIARRHYTHMIA DRUGS

Antiarrhythmics by Classification With Dose Forms		
Brand/*generic* **Pregnancy Category**	**Class/Indication(s)**	**Dose** **Form(s)**
Betapace *sotalol* (B)	*Class:* Class II and III Antiarrhythmic *Indications:* Documented life-threatening ventricular arrhythmias	*Tab:* 80*, 120*, 160*, 240*mg
Betapace AF *sotalol* (B)	*Class:* Class II and III Antiarrhythmic *Indications:* Maintenance of normal sinus rhythm in patients with highly symptomatic atrial fibrillation <u>or</u> atrial flutter who are currently in sinus rhythm	*Tab:* 80*, 120*, 160*mg
Calan *verapamil* (C)(G)	*Class:* Calcium Channel Blocker *Indications:* Control (with *digitalis*) of ventricular rate in patients with chronic atrial fibrillation <u>or</u> atrial flutter; prophylaxis of repetitive paroxysmal supraventricular tachycardia	*Tab:* 40, 80*, 120*mg

(*continued*)

(*continued*)

Antiarrhythmics by Classification With Dose Forms		
Brand/*generic* **Pregnancy Category**	**Class/Indication(s)**	**Dose Form(s)**
Cordarone *amiodarone* (D)(G)	*Class:* Class III Antiarrhythmic *Indications:* Documented life threatening recurrent refractory ventricular fibrillation <u>or</u> hemodynamically unstable ventricular tachycardia	*Tab:* 200*mg
Quinidex *quinidine sulfate* (C) (G)	*Class:* Class I Antiarrhythmic *Indications:* Atrial and ventricular arrhythmias	*Tab:* 300 mg ext-rel
Inderal *propranolol* (C)(G) **Inderal XL** *propranolol* ext-rel (C)(G) **InnoPran XL** *Propranolol* ext-rel (C)	*Class:* Beta-Blocker *Indications:* Atrial and ventricular arrhythmias; tachyarrhythmias due to *digitalis* intoxication; reduce mortality and risk of reinfarction in stabilized patients after myocardial infarction	*Tab:* 10*, 20*, 40*, 60*, 80*mg *Cap:* 60, 80, 120, 160 mg sust-rel *Cap:* 80, 120 mg ext-rel
Mexitil *mexiletine* (C)	*Class:* Class IB Antiarrhythmic *Indications:* Documented life-threatening ventricular arrhythmias	*Cap:* 150, 200, 250 mg
Multaq *dronedarone* (C)	*Class:* IB Antiarrhythmic *Indications:* Paroxysmal <u>or</u> persistent atrial fibrillation <u>or</u> atrial flutter	*Tab:* 400 mg
Norpace *disopyramide* (C)	*Class:* Class I Antiarrhythmic *Indications:* Documented life threatening ventricular arrhythmias	*Cap:* 100, 150 mg
Procanbid *procainamide* (C)(G)	*Class:* Class IA Antiarrhythmic *Indications:* Life threatening ventricular arrhythmias	*Tab:* 500, 1000 mg ext-rel
Quinaglute *quinidine gluconate* (C)(G)	*Class:* Class I Antiarrhythmic *Indications:* Atrial and ventricular arrhythmias	*Tab:* 324 mg ext-rel

(*continued*)

(*continued*)

Antiarrhythmics by Classification With Dose Forms		
Brand/*generic* Pregnancy Category	Class/Indication(s)	Dose Form(s)
Rythmol *propafenone* (C)(G)	*Class:* Class IC Antiarrhythmic *Indications:* Documented lifethreatening ventricular arrhythmias; prolonged recurrence of paroxysmal atrial fibrillation and/or atrial flutter or paroxysmal supraventricular tachycardia associated with disabling symptoms in patients without structural heart disease	*Tab:* 150*, 225*, 300*mg
Sectral *acebutolol* (B)(G)	*Class:* Beta-Blocker *Indications:* Ventricular arrhythmias	*Cap:* 200, 400 mg
Sotylize *sotalol* (B)	*Class:* Class II and III Antiarrhythmic *Indications:* Documented life threatening ventricular arrhythmias, and highly symptomatic AF/AF	*Oral soln:* 5 mg/ml
Tambocor *flecainide acetate* (C)(G)	*Class:* Class IC Antiarrhythmic *Indications:* Documented life threatening ventricular arrhythmias; paroxysmal atrial fibrillation and/or atrial flutter or paroxysmal supraventricular tachycardia in patients without structural heart disease	*Tab:* 50, 100*, 150* mg
Tenormin *atenolol* (C)(G)	*Class:* Beta-Blocker *Indications:* Reduce mortality and in stabilized patients after myocardial infarction	*Tab:* 25, 50, 100 mg *Inj:* 5 mg/ml (10 ml) for IV administration
timolol maleate (C) (G)	*Class:* Beta-Blocker *Indications:* Reduce mortality and in stabilized patients after myocardial infarction	*Tab:* 5, 10*, 20*mg

(*continued*)

(*continued*)

Antiarrhythmics by Classification With Dose Forms		
Brand/*generic* Pregnancy Category	Class/Indication(s)	Dose Form(s)
Tikosyn *dofetilide* (C)	*Class:* Class III Antiarrhythmic *Indications:* Maintenance of normal sinus rhythm in patients with atrial fibrillation or atrial flutter of >1 week duration who were converted to normal sinus rhythm (only for highly symptommatic patients); conversion to normal sinus rhythm	*Cap:* 125, 250, 500 mcg
Tonocard *tocainide* (C)(G)	*Class:* Class I Antiarrhythmic *Indications:* Documented lifethreatening ventricular arrhythmias	*Tab:* 400*, 600*mg
Toprol XL *metoprolol* (C)(G)	*Class:* Beta-Blocker *Indications:* Ischemic, hypertensive, or cardiomyopathic heart failure	*Tab:* 25*, 50*, 100*, 200*mg

◯ APPENDIX P: ORAL ANTINEOPLASIA DRUGS

Antineoplastics With Classification With Dose Forms		
Brand/*generic* Pregnancy Category	Class/Indications	Dose Forms
Alkeran *melphalan* (D)	Alkylating Agent	*Tab:* 2*mg
Arimidex *anastrozole* (D)	Aromatase Inhibitor	*Tab:* 1 mg
Aromasin *exemestane* (D)	Aromatase Inactivator	*Tab:* 25 mg
Arranon *nelarabine* (D)	Nucleoside Analog	*Vial:* 250 mg for IV infusion
Casodex *Bicalutamide* (X)	Antiandrogen	*Tab:* 50 mg
Cytoxan *Cyclophosphamide* (D)	Alkylating Agent	*Tab:* 25, 50 mg

(*continued*)

(*continued*)

Antineoplastics With Classification With Dose Forms		
Brand/*generic* Pregnancy Category	**Class/Indications**	**Dose Forms**
Eligard *leuprolide acetate* (**X**)	GnRH Analogue	*Inj:* 7.5 mg ext-rel per monthly SC injection
Eulexin *flutamide* (**D**)	Antiandrogen	*Cap:* 125 mg
Faslodex *fulvestrant* (**D**)(**G**)	Estrogen Receptor Antagonist	*Prefilled syringe for IM inj:* 50 mg/ml (2.5, 5 ml/syringe)
Femara *letrozole* (**D**)	Aromatase Inhibitor	*Tab:* 2.5 mg
Gleevec *imatinib mesylate* (**D**)	Signal Transduction Inhibitor	*Cap:* 100 mg
Hydrea *hydroxyurea* (**D**)(**G**)	Substituted Urea	*Cap:* 500 mg
Iressa *gefitinib* (**D**)	Epidermal Growth Factor receptor tyrosine kinase inhibitor	*Tab:* 250 mg
Leukeran *chlorambucil* (**D**)(**G**)	Alkylating Agent	*Tab:* 2 mg
Leupron *leuprolide* (**X**)	GnRH Analogue	*Susp for IM inj:* 1 mg (daily); 7.5 mg depot (monthly); 22.5 mg depot (every 3 months); 30 mg depot (every 4 months)
Megace, Megace Oral Suspension, Megace ES, *megestrol acetate* (**D**) (**G**)	Progestin	*Tab:* 20*, 40*mg; *Susp:* 40 mg/ml; ES concentrate: 125 mg/ml, 625 mg/5 ml
Nexavar *sorafenib* (**D**)	Multikinase Inhibitor	*Tab:* 200 mg
Nolvadex *tamoxifen citrate* (**D**) (**G**)	Antiestrogen	*Tab:* 10, 20 mg

(*continued*)

(continued)

Antineoplastics With Classification With Dose Forms		
Brand/*generic* Pregnancy Category	**Class/Indications**	**Dose Forms**
Tarceva *erlotinib* (D)	Kinase Inhibitor	*Tab:* 25, 100, 150 mg
Velcade *bortezomib* (D)	Proteasome Inhibitor	*Vial:* 3.5 mg (pwdr for IV injection after reconstitution)
Viadur *leuprolide acetate* (X)	GnRH Analogue	*SC implant:* 65 mg depot (replace every 12 months)
Xeloda *capecitabine* (D)	Fluoropyrimidine (prodrug of *5-fluorouracil*)	*Tab:* 150, 500 mg
Zoladex *goserelin acetate* (D)	GnRH Analogue	*SC implant:* 3.6 mg depot (28 days), 10.8 mg depot (3-month)
Zometa *zoledronic acid* (D)	Bisphosphonate	*Vial:* 4 mg pwdr for reconstitution for IV infusion, single dose

APPENDIX Q: ORAL AND DEPOT ANTIPSYCHOSIS DRUGS

ANTIPSYCHOSIS DRUGS WITH DOSE FORMS

Comment: Patients receiving an antipsychosis agent should be monitored closely for the following adverse side effects: neuroleptic malignant syndrome, extrapyramidal reactions, tardive dyskinesia, blood dyscrasias, anticholinergic effects, drowsiness, hypotension, photosensitivity, retinopathy, and lowered seizure threshold. Use lower doses for elderly or debilitated patients. Prescriptions should be written for the smallest practical amount. Foods and beverages containing alcohol are contraindicated for patients receiving psychotropic drug therapy.

➤ *aripiprazole* (C)(G)
  Abilify *Tab:* 2, 5, 10, 15, 20, 30 mg; *Oral soln:* 1 mg/ml (150 ml; orange crèam; parabens)
  Abilify Discmelt *Tab:* 15 mg orally disintegrating (vanilla) (phenylalanine)
  Abilify Maintena *Vial:* 300, 400 mg ext-rel pwdr for IM injection after reconstitution; 300, 400 mg single dose prefilled dual chamber syringes w. supplies

(continued)

(*continued*)

> *asenapine* (C)
>> **Saphris** *SL tab:* 2.5, 5, 10 mg

> *brexpizole* (C)
>> **Rexulti** *Tab:* 0.25, 0.5, 1, 2, 3, 4 mg

> *bupropion* (C)
>> **Forfivo XL** *Tab:* 450 mg ext-rel

> *cariprazine* (NR)
>> **Vraylar** *Cap:* 1.5, 3, 4.5, 6 mg

> *chlorpromazine* (C)(G)
>> **Thorazine** *Tab:* 10, 25, 50, 100, 200 mg; *Cap:* 30, 75, 150 mg sust-rel; *Syr:* 10 mg/5 ml (4 oz, orange-custard); *Vial/Amp:* 25 mg/ml (1, 2 ml) (sulfites)

> *clozapine* (B)(G)
>> **Clozapine ODT** (G) *ODT:* 150, 200 mg
>> **Clozaril** (G) *Tab:* 25*, 100* mg; *ODT:* 150, 200 mg
>> **FazaClo ODT** (G) *ODT:* 12.5, 25, 100, 150, 200 mg (phenylalanine)
>> **Versacloz** *Oral susp:* 50 mg/ml (100 ml)

> *fluphenazine* (C)(G)
>> **Prolixin** *Tab:* 1, 2.5, 5*, 10 mg (tartrazine); *Conc:* 5 mg/ml (4 oz w. calib dropper) (alcohol 14%); *Elix:* 5 mg/ml (2 oz w. calib dropper) (alcohol 14%); *Vial:* 25 mg/ml (10 ml)

> *fluphenazine decanoate* (C)(G)
>> **Prolixin Decanoate** *Vial:* 25 mg/ml (5 ml) (benzyl alcohol)

> *fluphenazine* (C)(G)
>> **Prolixin Ethanate** *Vial:* 25 mg (5 ml) (benzyl alcohol)

> *fluphenazine decanoate* (C)(G)
>> **Prolixin Decanoate** *Vial:* 25 mg/ml (5 ml) (benzyl alcohol)

> *haloperidol* (B)(G)
>> **Haldol** *Tab:* 0.5*, 1*, 2*, 5*, 10*, 20 mg

> *iloperidone* (C)
>> **Fanapt** *Tab:* 1, 2, 4, 6, 8, 10, 12 mg

> *loxapine* (C)
>> **Adasuve** *Oral inhal pwdr:* 10 mg single-use disposable inhaler (5/box)

> *lurasidone* (B)
>> **Latuda** *Tab:* 20, 40, 80 mg

> *olanzapine fumarate* (C)(G)
>> **Zyprexa** *Tab:* 2.5, 5, 7.5, 10, 15, 20 mg
>> **Zyprexa Zydis** *ODT:* 5, 10, 15, 20 mg (phenylalanine)

(*continued*)

(*continued*)

> *paliperidone* (C)(G)
>> **Invega** *Tab:* 3, 6, 9 mg ext-rel
>> **Invega** Sustenna *Prefilled syringe:* 39, 78, 117, 156, 234 mg ext-rel suspension w. needle
>> **Invega** Trinza *Prefilled syringe:* 273, 410, 546, 819 mg ext-rel suspension

> *prochlorperazine* (C)(G)
>> **Compazine** *Tab:* 5, 10 mg; *Cap:* 10, 15 mg susrel; *Syr:* 5 mg/5 ml (4 oz; fruit); *Supp:* 2.5, 5, 25 mg

> *quetiapine* (C)(G)
>> **Seroquel** *Tab:* 25, 100, 200, 300 mg
>> **Seroquel** XR *Tab:* 50, 150, 200, 300, 400 mg ext-rel

> *risperidone* (C)(G)
>> **Risperdal** *Tab:* 0.25, 0.5, 1, 2, 3, 4 mg; *Soln:* 1 mg/ml (30 ml w. pipette); *Consta (Inj):* 25, 37.5, 50 mg
>> **Risperdal** M-Tabs *M-tab:* 0.5, 1, 2, 3, 4 mg orally-disint (phenylalanine)

> *thioridazine* (C)(G) *Tab:* 10, 25, 50, 100 mg

> *trifluoperazine* (C)(G)
>> **Stelazine** *Tab:* 1, 2, 5, 10 mg; *Conc:* 10 mg/ml; (2 oz w. calib dropper (banana-vanilla) (sulfites); *Vial:* 2 mg/ml (10 ml)

> *ziprasidone* (C)(G)
>> **Geodon** *Cap:* 20, 40, 60, 80 mg

APPENDIX R: ORAL ANTICONVULSANT DRUGS

ANTICONVULSANT DRUGS WITH DOSE FORMS

> *carbarbamazepine* (D)(G)
>> **Carbatrol** *Cap:* 200, 300 mg ext-rel
>> **Equetro** *Cap:* 100, 200, 300 mg ext-rel
>> **Tegretol** *Tab:* 100*, 200*mg; *Chew tab:* 100*mg
>> **Tegretol** Suspension *Oral susp:* 100 mg/5 ml (450 ml)(citrus vanilla; sorbitol)
>> **Tegretol-XR** *Tab:* 100, 200, 400 mg ext-rel

> *clobazam* (C)(IV)
>> **Onfi** *Tab:* 10*, 20*mg;
>> **Onfi** Oral Suspension *Oral susp:* 2.5 mg/ml (120 ml w. 2 dosing syringes) (berry)

> *clonazepam* (D)(IV)(G)
>> **Clonazepam ODT** *ODT:* 0.125, 0.25, 0.5, 1, 2, oral-dis
>> **Klonopin** *Tab:* 0.5*, 1, 2 mg

(*continued*)

(*continued*)

▷ *diazepam* (D)(IV)(G)
> **Diastat** *Rectal gel delivery system:* 2.5 mg
> **Diastat AcuDial** *Rectal gel delivery system:* 10, 20 mg
> **Valium** *Tab:* 2*, 5*, 10*mg
> **Valium Injectable** *Vial:* 5 mg/ml (10 ml); *Amp:* 5 mg/ml (2 ml); *Prefilled syringe:* 5 mg/ml (5 ml)
> **Valium Intensol** *Conc oral soln:* 5 mg/ml (30 ml w. dropper) (alcohol 19%)
> **Valium Oral Solution** *Oral soln:* 5 mg/5 ml (500 ml) (winter green-spice)

▷ *divalproex sodium* (D)(G)
> **Depakene** *Cap:* 250 mg; *Syr:* 250 mg/5 ml (16 oz)
> **Depakote** *Tab:* 125, 250, 500 mg
> **Depakote ER** *Tab:* 250, 500 mg ext-rel
> **Depakote Sprinkle** *Cap:* 125 mg

▷ *eslicarbazepine* (C)
> **Aptiom** *Tab:* 200*, 400, 600*, 800* mg

▷ *ezogabine* (C)
> **Potiga** *Tab:* 50, 200, 300, 400 mg

▷ *felbamate* (C)(G)
> **Felbatol** *Tab:* 400*, 600*mg
> **Felbatol Oral Suspension** *Oral susp:* 600 mg/5 ml (4, 8, 32 oz)
> **Peganone** *Tab:* 250, 500 mg

▷ *bapentin* (C)
> **Horizant** *Tab:* 300, 600 ext-rel
> **Neurontin** (G) *Cap:* 100, 300, 400 mg; *Tab:* 600*, 800*mg
> **Neurontin Oral Solution** *Oral soln:* 250 mg/5 ml (480 ml) (strawberry-anise)

▷ *lacosamide* (C)(V)
> **Vimpat** *Tab:* 50, 100, 150, 200 mg; *Oral soln:* 10 mg/ml (200, 465 ml); *Vial:* 10 mg/ml soln for IV infusion, single-use (20 ml)

▷ *lamotrigine* (C)(G)
> **Lamictal** *Tab:* 25*, 100*, 150*, 200*mg
> **Lamictal Chewable Dispersible Tab** *Chew tab:* 2, 5, 25, 50 mg (black current)
> **Lamictal ODT** *ODT:* 25, 50, 100, 200 mg oral-dis
> **Lamictal XR** *Tab:* 25, 50, 100, 200, 250, 300 mg ext-rel

▷ *levetiracetam* (C)
> **Elepsia** *Tab:* 1000, 1500 mg ext-rel
> **Keppra** *Tab:* 250*, 500*, 750*, 1000*mg
> **Keppra Oral Solution** *Oral soln:* 100 mg/ml (16 oz) (grape) (dye-free)
> **Keppra XR** *Tab:* 500, 750 mg ext-rel
> **Levitiracetam IV** (G) *Premixed:* 500, 1,000, 1,500 mg for IV infusion (100 ml)

▷ *mephobarbital* (D)(II)
> **Mebaral** *Tab:* 32, 50, 100 mg

(*continued*)

(*continued*)

> *methsuximide* (C)
>   **Celontin Kapseals** *Cap:* 150, 300 mg
> *oxcarbazepine* (C)(G)
>   **Trileptal** *Tab:* 150, 300, 600 mg; *Oral susp:* 300 mg/5 ml (lemon) (alcohol)
>   **Oxtella XR** *Tab:* 150, 300, 600 mg ext-rel
> *perampanel* (C)(III)
>   **Fycompa** *Tab:* 2, 4, 6, 8, 10, 12 mg
> *phenytoin* (D)(G), *primidone* (D)(G)
>   **Dilantin** *Cap:* 30, 100 mg extre
>   **Dilantin Infatabs** *Chew tab:* 50 mg
>   **Dilantin Oral Suspension** *Oral susp:* 125 mg/5 ml (237 ml) (alcohol 6%)
>   **Phenytek** *Cap:* 200, 300 mg ext-rel
> *pregabalin* (C)(V)
>   **Lyrica** *Cap:* 25, 50, 75, 100, 200, 225, 300 mg
>   **Lyrica Oral Solution** *Oral soln:* 20 mg/ml
> *primidone* (C)
>   **Mysoline** *Tab:* 50*, 250* mg
>   **Mysoline Oral Solution** *Oral susp:* 250 mg/5 ml (8 oz)
> *rufinamide* (C)
>   **Banzel** *Tab:* 200*, 400* mg
>   **Banzel Oral Solution** *Susp:* 40 mg/ ml (orange) (lactose-free, gluten-free, dye-free)
> *tiagabine* (C)(G)
>   **Gabitril** *Tab:* 2, 4, 12, 16 mg
> *topiramate* (D)(G)
>   **Topamax** *Tab:* 25, 50, 100, 200 mg
>   **Topamax Sprinkle Caps** *Cap:* 15, 25, 50 mg
>   **Trokendi XR** *Cap:* 100, 200 mg ext-rel
>   **Qudexy** *Tab:* 25, 50, 100, 150, 200 mg ext-rel
>   **Qudexy XR** *Cap:* 25, 50, 100, 150, 200 mg ext-rel
> *vigabatrin* (C)
>   **Sabril** *Tab:* 500 mg
>   **Sabril for Oral Solution** 500 mg/pkt pwdr for reconstitution
> *zonisamide* (C)
>   **Zonegran** *Cap:* 25, 50, 100 mg

APPENDIX S: ORAL ANTI-HIV DRUGS WITH DOSE FORMS

Agenerase

prenavir (C)
Cap: 50 mg (plus Vit E 36 IU/cap), 150 mg (plus Vit E 109 IU/cap); *Oral soln:* 15 mg/ml (*plus* Vit E 46 IU/ml) (240 ml) (grape, bubble gum) (peppermint) (propylene glycol)

(*continued*)

(*continued*)

Aptivus

tipranavir (C)
Gel cap: 250 mg (alcohol); *Oral soln:* 100 mg/ml (95 ml w. dosing syringe) (Vit E 116 IU/ml) (buttermint-butter, toffee)

Comment: *valganciclovir* is indicated for the treatment of AIDS-related cytomegalovirus (CMV) retinitis.

Atripla

efavirenz/emtricitabine/tenofovir disoproxil (D)
Tab: efa 600 mg/*emtri* 200 mg/*teno diso* 300 mg

Combivir

abacavir/amivudine/zidovudine (C)(G)
Tab: aba/lami 150/*zido* 300 mg

Complera

emtricitabine/tenofovir disoproxil fumarate/rilpivirine (B)
Tab: emtri 200 mg/*teno diso* 300 mg/*rilpiv* 25 mg

Crixivan

indinavir sulfate (C)
Cap: 100, 200, 333, 400 mg

Cytovene

ganciclovir (C)(G)
Cap: 250, 500 mg; *Vial:* 50 mg/ml single-dose (500 mg, 10 ml)

Descovy

emtricitabine/tenofovir alafenamide/rilpivirine (NR)
Tab: emtri 200 mg/*teno ala* 25 mg

Edurant

rilpivirine (B)
Tab: 25 mg

Emtriva

emtricitabine (B)
Cap: 200 mg; *Oral soln:* 10 mg/ml (170 ml) (cotton candy)

Epivir

lamivudine (C)
Tab: 150*, 300*mg; *Oral soln:* 10 mg/ml (240 ml) (strawberry-banana) (sucrose 3 g/15 ml)

(*continued*)

Epzicom

abacavir sulfate/lamivudine (B)
Tab: aba 600 mg/*lami* 300 mg

Evotaz

atazanavir/cobicistat (B)
Tab: ataz 300/*cobi* 150 mg

Fortovase

aquinavir (B)
Soft gel cap: 200 mg

Fuzeon

enfuvirtide (B)
Vial: 90 mg/ml pwdr for SC inj after reconstitution (1 ml, 60 vials/kit) (preservative-free)

Genvoya

elvitegravir/cobicistat/emtricitabine/tenofovir alafenamide (TAF) (B)
Tab: elv 150 mg/*cob* 150 mg/*emtri* 200 mg/*teno alafen* 10 mg

Hivid

zalcitabine (C)
Tab: 0.375, 0.75 mg

Isentress

raltegravir (C)
Tab: 400 mg film-coat; *Chew tab:* 25, 100*mg (orange-banana) (phenylalanine);
Oral susp: 100 mg/pct pwdr for oral susp (banana)

Intelence

etravirine (C)
Tab: 25*, 100, 200 mg

Invirase

saquinavir mesylate (B)
Hard gel cap: 200 mg

Kaletra

lopinavir plus ritonavir (C)
Cap: lopin 133.3 mg/*riton* 33.3 mg; *Oral soln: lopin* 80 mg/*riton* 20 mg per ml
(160 ml w. dose cup) (cotton candy) (alcohol 42%)
Hard gel cap: 200 mg

Lexiva

fosamprenavir (C)
Tab: 700 mg; *Oral soln:* 50 mg/ml (grape, bubble gum) (peppermint)

(*continued*)

(*continued*)

Norvir

ritonavir (B)
Soft gel cap: 100 mg (alcohol); *Oral soln:* 80 mg/ml (8 oz) (peppermint-caramel) (alcohol)

Odefsey

emtricitabine/rilivirine/tenofovir alafenamide (NR)
Tab: emtri 200 mg/rilpiv 25 mg/tenof alafen 25 mg

Prexcobix

dirunavir/cobicistat (C)
Tab: diru 800 mg/cobi 150 mg/teno DF 300 mg

Prezcobix

darunavir/cobicistat (B)
Tab: daru 800/cobi 150 mg

Prezista

darunavir (C)
Tab: 75, 150, 600, 800 mg; *Oral susp:* 100 mg/ml (200 ml) (strawberry cream)

Rescriptor

delavirdine mesylate (C)
Tab: 100, 200 mg

Retrovir

zidovudine (C)
Tab: 300 mg; *Cap:* 100 mg; *Syr:* 50 mg/5 ml (240 ml) (strawberry); *Vial:* 10 mg/ml (20 ml vial for IV infusion) (peservative-free)

Reyataz

atazanavir (B)
Cap: 100, 150, 200, 300 mg

Selzentry

maraviroc (B)
Tab: 150, 300 mg

Stribild

elvitegravir/cobicistat/emtricitabine/tenofovir disoproxil fumarate (B)
Tab: elv 150 mg/cob 150 mg/emtri 200 mg/teno diso fumar 300 mg

Sustiva

efavirenz (C)
Tab: 75, 150, 600, 800 mg; *Cap:* 50, 200 mg

(*continued*)

Tivicay

dolutegavir (B)
Tab: 50 mg

Triumeq

abacavir sulfate/dilutegravir/lamivudine (C)
Tab: aba 600 mg/*dilu* 50 mg/*lami* 300 mg

Trizivir

abacavir sulfate/lamivudine/zidovudine (C)(G)
Tab: aba 300 mg/*lami* 150 mg/*zido* 300 mg

Truvada

emtricitabine/tenofovir disoproxil fumarate (B)
Cap: 200, 300 mg

Valcyte

valganciclovir (C)(G)
Tab: 450 mg

Videx EC

didanosine (C)
Cap: 125, 200, 250, 400 mg ent-coat del-rel; *Chew tab:* 25, 50, 100, 150, 200 mg (mandarin orange) (buffered with calcium carbonate and magnesium hydroxide, phenylalanine); *Pwdr for oral soln:* 2, 4 g (120, 240 ml)

Viracept

nelfinavir mesylate (B)
Tab: 250, 625 mg; *Pwdr for oral soln:* 50 mg/g (144 g) (phenylalanine)

Viramune

nevirapine (C)(G)
Tab: 200*mg; *Oral susp:* 50 mg/5 ml (240 ml)

Viramune XR

nevirapine (C)
Tab: 400 mg ext-rel

Viread

tenofovir disoproxil fumarate (C)
Tab: 150, 200, 250, 300 mg; *Oral pwdr:* 40 mg/1 g pwdr

Vistide

cidofovir (C)
Inj: 75 mg/ml (5 ml vials for IV infusion) (preservative free)

(*continued*)

(continued)

> Comment: *cidofovir* is indicated for the treatment of AIDS-related cytomegalovirus (CMV) retinitis.

Zerit

> *stavudine* (C)
> *Cap:* 15, 20, 30, 40 mg; *Oral soln:* 1 mg/ml pwdr for reconstitution (200 ml) (fruit) (dye-free)

Ziagen

> *abacavir sulfate* (C)
> *Tab:* 300*mg; *Oral soln:* 20 mg/ml (240 ml) (strawberry-banana) (parabens, propylene glycol)

◉ APPENDIX T: COUMADIN (WARFARIN)

T.1: COUMADIN TITRATION AND DOSE FORMS

> ▷ *warfarin* (X)(G) dosage initially 2-5 mg/day; usual maintenance 2-10 mg/day; adjust dosage to maintain INR in therapeutic range:
> *Venous thrombosis:* 2.0-3.0
> *Atrial fibrillation:* 2.0-3.0
> *Post MI:* 2.5-3.5
> *Mechanical and bioprosthetic heart valves:* 2.0-3.0 for 12 weeks after valve insertion, then 2.5-3.5 long-term
> *Pediatric:* not recommended <18 years
> **Coumadin** *Tab:* 1*, 2*, 2.5*, 3*, 4*, 5*, 6*, 7.5*, 10* mg
> **Coumadin for Injection** *Vial:* 2 mg/ml (2.5 ml)
> Comment: **Coumadin for Injection** is for peripheral IV administration only.

T.2: COUMADIN OVER-ANTICOAGULATION REVERSAL

> ▷ *phytonadione (vitamin K)* (G) 2.5-10 mg PO or IM; max 25 mg
> **AquaMEPHYTON**
> *Vial:* 1 mg/0.5 ml (0.5 ml); 10 mg/ml (1, 2.5, 5 ml)
> **Mephyton**
> *Tab:* 5 mg

T.3: AGENTS THAT INHIBIT COUMADIN'S ANTICOAGULATION EFFECTS

Increase Metabolism	Decrease Absorption	Other Mechanism(s)
azathioprine	azathioprine	coenzyme Q10
carbamazepine	cholestyramine	estrogen
dicloxacillin	colestipol	griseofulvin
ethanol	sucralfate	oral contraceptives
griseofulvin		

(continued)

(*continued*)

Increase Metabolism	Decrease Absorption	Other Mechanism(s)
nafcillin		ritonavir
pentobarbital		spironolactone
phenobarbital		trazodone
phenytoin		vitamin C (high
primidone		dose)
rifabutin		vitamin K
rifampin		

APPENDIX U: LOW MOLECULAR WEIGHT HEPARINS

Comment: Administer by subcutaneous injection *only*, in the abdomen, and rotate sites. Avoid concomitant drugs that affect hemostasis (e.g., oral anticoagulants and platelet aggregation inhibitors, including *aspirin*, NSAIDs, *dipyridamole*, *sulfinpyrazone*, *ticlopidine*). Pediatrics not recommended.

▷ *ardeparin* (C)
   Normiflo *Soln for inj:* 5,000 anti-Factor Xa U/0.5 ml; 10,000 anti-Factor Xa U/0.5 ml (sulfites, parabens)

▷ *dalteparin* (B)
   Fragmin *Prefilled syringe:* 2500 IU/0.2 ml, 5000 IU/0.2 ml (10/box) (preservative-free); *Multi-dose*
      vial: 1,000 IU/ml (95,000 IU, 9.5 ml) (benzyl alcohol)

▷ *danaparoid* (B)
   Orgaran *Amp:* 750 anti-Xa units/0.6 ml (0.6 ml, 10/box); *Prefilled syringe:* 750 anti-Xa units/ 0.6 ml (0.6 ml, 10/box) (sulfites)

▷ *enoxaparin* (B)(G)
   Lovenox *Prefilled syringe:* 30 mg/0.3 ml, 40 mg/0.4 ml, 60 mg/0.6 ml, 80 mg/0.8 ml (100 mg/ml)
      (preservative-free); *Vial:* 100 mg/ml (3 ml)

▷ *tinzaparin* (B)
   Innohep *Vial:* 20,000 *anti-Factor Xa* IU/ml (2 ml) (sulfites, benzyl alcohol)

APPENDIX V: FACTOR XA INHIBITOR THERAPY

FACTOR XA INHIBITOR THERAPY

▷ *apixaban* (C) 5 mg bid; reduce to 2.5 mg bid if any two of the following: ≥80 years, ≤60 kg, serum Cr ≥1.5

(*continued*)

(continued)

Pediatric: not recommended
Eliquis *Tab:* 2.5, 5 mg
Comment: **Eloquis** is indicated to reduce the risk of stroke and systemic embolism in patients with nonvalvular atrial fibrillation (NVAF).

▷ *edoxaban* (C) transition to and from **Savaysa**; assess CrCl prior to initiation:
NVAF CrCl >50 mL/min: 60 mg once daily; *CrCl 15-50 mL/min:* 30 mg once daily
DVT/PE CrCl >50 mL/min: 60 mg once daily following initial parental anticoagulant; *CrCl 15-50 mL/min, <60 kg, or concomitant Pgp inhibitors:* 30 mg once daily
Pediatric: not established
Savaysa *Tab:* 15, 30, 60 mg
Comment: **Savaysa** is indicated to reduce the risk of stroke and systemic embolism in patients with nonvalvular atrial fibrillation (NVAF), treatment of DVT and pulmonary embolism (PE) following 5-10 days of initial therapy with with parenteral anticoagulant. Not for use in persons with NVAF with CrCl >95 mL/min.

▷ *fondaparinux* (B) Administer SC; administer first dose no earlier than 6-8 hours after hemostasis is achieved, start warfarin usually within 72 hours of last dose of *fondaparinux*
Post-op: 2.5 mg once daily x 5-9 days
Hip/Knee Replacement: once daily x 11 days
Hip Fracture: once daily x 32 days
Abdominal Surgery: once daily x 10 days
Prophylaxis: do not use <50 kg
Treatment: once daily for at least 5 days until INR=2-3 (usually 5-9 days); max 26 days; <50 kg: 5 mg; 50-100 kg: 7.5 mg; >100 kg: 10 mg
Pediatric: not established
Arixtra *Soln for SC inj:* 2.5 mg/0.5 ml, 5 mg/0.4 ml, 7.5 mg/0.6 ml, 10 mg/0.8 ml *prefilled syringe* (10/box) (preservative-free)

▷ *prasugrel* (B) *Loading dose:* 60 mg once in a single-dose; *Maintenance:* 10 mg once daily; *<60 kg:* consider 5 mg once daily; take with aspirin 75-325 mg once daily
Pediatric: not recommended
Effient *Tab:* 5, 10 mg
Comment: *Effient* is indicated to reduce the risk of thrombotic cardiovascular events in persons with acute coronary syndrome (ACS) who aret to be managed with percutaneous coronary intervention (PCI) including unstable angina, non-ST elevation myocardial infarction (NSTEMI) and STEMI. Do not start if active pathological bleeding (e.g., peptic ulcer, intracranial hemorrhage), prior TIA or stroke, or if patient likely to undergo urgent CABG. Discontinue 7 days before surgery and if TIA or stroke occurs.

▷ *rivaroxaban* (C) take with food
Treatment of DVT or PE: 15 mg twice daily for the first 21 days; then 20 mg once daily

(continued)

(continued)

> *Reduction in risk of DVT or PE recurrence:* 20 mg once daily with the evening meal; *CrCl <30 mL/min:* avoid
> *Prophylaxis of DVT:* take 6-10 hours after surgery when hemostasis established, then 20 mg once daily with the evening meal; *CrCl 30-50 mL/min:* 10 mg; *CrCl <30 mL/min:* avoid; discontinue if acute renal failure develops; monitor closely for
> blood loss
> *Hip:* treat for 35 days; *Knee:* treat for 12 days
> *Nonvalvular AF:* take once daily with the evening meal; *CrCl >50 mL/min:* 20 mg; *CrCl 15-50 mL/min:* 15 mg; *CrCl >15 mL/min:* avoid
> *Pediatric:* not recommended
> > **Xarelto** *Cap:* 10, 15, 20 mg
> > **Comment:** **Xarelto** is indicated to reduce the risk of stroke and systemic embolism in nonvalvular atrial fibrillation (AF), to treat deep vein thrombosis (DVT) and pulmonary embolism (PE), to reduce the risk of recurrence of DVT and/or PE following 6 months treatment for DVT and/or PE, and prophylaxis of DVT which may lead to PE in patients undergoing knee or hip replacement surgery. **Xarelto** eliminates the need for bridging with heparin or lmwh; no need for routine monitoring of INR or other coagulation parameters; no need for dose adjustments for age, weight, or gender; no known dietary restrictions. Switching from *warfarin* or other anticoagulant, see mfr literature.

APPENDIX W: DIRECT THROMBIN INHIBITOR THERAPY

> ⊳ *aspirin* (D) single dose once daily
> *Pediatric:* not established
> > **Durlaza** *Cap:* 162.5 mg 24-hr ext-rel (30, 90/bottle)
> > **Comment:** Presently there is only one reversal agent for this drug class. *idarucizumab* (**Praxbind**) is a specific reversal agent for dabigatran (**Pradaxa**). It is a humanized monoclonal antibody fragment (Fab) that binds to dabigatran and its acylglucuronide metabolites with higher affinity than the binding affinity of dabigatran to thrombin, neutralizing its anticoagulant effects.

IDARUCIZUMAB REVERSAL AGENT: HUMANIZED MONOCLONAL ANTIBODY FRAGMENT (FAB)

> ⊳ *idarucizumab* (NR) administer 5 g (2 vials) IV drip or push; administer within 1 hour of removal from vial
> *Pediatric:* not established
> > **Praxbind** *Vial:* 2.5 g/50 ml, single-use (preservative-free)
> > **Comment:** Presently, there is inadequate human and animal data to assess risk of *idarucizumab* (**Praxbind**) use in pregnancy. Risk/benefit should be considered prior to use.

(continued)

(continued)

> ***dabigatran etexilate mesylate*** **(C)** swallow whole; *CrCl >30 mL/min:* 150 mg bid; *CrCl 15-30 mL/min:* 75 mg twice daily; *CrCl <15 mL/min:* not recommended
> *Pediatric:* not recommended
> > **Pradaxa** *Cap:* 75, 150 mg
> > Comment: **Pradaxa** is indicated to reduce the risk of stroke and systemic embolism in nonvalvular AF, DVT prophylaxis, PE prophylaxis in patients who have undergone hip replacement surgery, treatment of DVT and PE in patients who have been treated with a parenteral anticoagulant for 5-10 days, and to reduce the risk of recurrent DVT and PE in patients who have been previously treated. **Pradaxa** is contraindicated in patients with a mechanical prosthetic heart valve.

> ***desirudin (recombinant hirudin)*** **(C)** 15 mg SC every 12 hours, preferably in the abdomen <u>or</u> thigh, starting up to 5-15 minutes before surgery (after induction of regional block anesthesia, if used); may continue for 9-12 days post-op; *CrCl <60 mL/min:* reduce dose (see mfr literature)
> *Pediatric:* not recommended
> > **Iprivask** *Pwdr for SC inj after reconstitution:* 15mg/single-usevial (10/box) (preservative-free, diluent contains mannitol)
> > Comment: **Iprivask** is indicated for DVT prophylaxis in patients undergoing hip replacement surgery. It is not interchangeable with other hirudins.

APPENDIX X: PLATELET AGGREGATION INHIBITOR THERAPY

> ***cilostazol*** **(B)** 100 mg bid
> *Pediatric:* not recommended
> > **Pletal** *Tab:* 50, 100 mg
> > Comment: **Pletal** is an (antiplatelet/vasodilator [PDE III inhibitor])

> ***clopidogrel*** **(B)** 75 mg once daily
> *Pediatric:* not recommended
> > **Plavix** *Tab:* 75, 300 mg
> > Comment: **Plavix** is indicated for the reduction of atherosclerotic events in recent MI <u>or</u> stroke, established PAD, non-ST-segment elevation acute coronary syndrome (unstable angina/non-STEMI), <u>or</u> STEMI.

> ***dipyridamole*** **(B)(G)** 75-100 mg qid
> *Pediatric:* not recommended
> > **Persantine** *Tab:* 25, 50, 75 mg
> > Comment: *dipyridamole* is indicated as an adjunct to oral anticoagulants after cardiac valve replacement surgery to prevent thromboembolism.

> ***dipyridamole/aspirin*** **(B)(G)** swallow whole; one cap bid
> *Pediatric:* not recommended
> > **Aggrenox** *Cap:* dipyr 200 mg/*asa* 25 mg

(continued)

(*continued*)

▷ *pentoxifylline* (C) [hemorrheologic (xanthine)]
  Pediatric: not recommended
    Trental *Tab:* 400 mg sust-rel

▷ *prasugrel* (C)
  Pediatric: not recommended
    Effient *Tab:* 5, 10 mg
    Comment: Effient is indicated to reduce the risk of cardiovascular events in patients with acute coronary syndrome (ACS) who are to be managed with percutaneous coronary intervention (unstable angina or non-STEMI), and STEMI when managed with either primary or delayed PCI.

▷ *ticagrelor* (C) initiate 180 mg loading dose once in a single dose with aspirin 325 mg loading dose in a single dose; maintenance 90 mg twice daily with aspirin 75-100 mg once daily; ACS patients may start *ticagrelor* after a loading dose of *clopidogrel*
    Brilinta *Tab:* 90 mg
  Comment: Effient is indicated to reduce the risk of cardiovascular events in patients with acute coronary syndrome (ACS) (unstable angina, Non-ST elevation (NSTEMI), myocardial infarction, or STEMI).

▷ *ticlopidine* (B) 250 mg bid
  Pediatric: not recommended
    Ticlid *Tab:* 250 mg
    Comment: Ticlid is indicated to reduce the risk of thrombotic stroke in selected patients intolerant of aspirin.

APPENDIX Y: PROTEASE-ACTIVATED RECEPTOR-1 (PAR-1) INHIBITOR THERAPY

▷ *vorapaxar* (B) administer 2.08 mg once daily; use with *aspirin* or *clopidogrel*
  Pediatric: not established
    Zontivity *Tab:* 2.08 mg (equivalent to 2.5 mg vorapaxar sulfate)
    Comment: Zontivity is indicated to reduce thrombotic cardiovascular events in patients with a history of myocardial infarction or with peripheral arterial disease (PAD). Contraindicated with active pathological bleeding (e.g., peptic ulcer, intra-cranial hemorrhage), prior TIA or stroke. Not recommended with severe hepatic impairment.

APPENDIX Z: PRESCRIPTION PRENATAL VITAMINS

Comment: It is recommended that prenatal vitamins be started at least 3 months prior to conception to improve preconception nutritional status, and continued

(*continued*)

(continued)

throughout pregnancy and the postnatal period, in lactating and nonlactating women, and throughout the childbearing years.

▷ **CitraNatal 90 DHA** take 1 tab* and 1 DHA cap daily
Tab: thiamine 3 mg, riboflavin 3.4 mg, niacinamide 20 mg, pyridoxine HCL 20 mg, folic acid 1 mg, Vit C 120 mg, Vit D₃ 400 IU, Vit E 30 IU, calcium (as citrate) 160 mg, copper (as oxide) 2 mg, iodine (as potassium iodide) 150 mcg, iron (as carbonyl) 90 mg, zinc (as oxide) 25 mg, docusate sodium 50 mg
Cap: docosahexaenoic acid (DHA) 300 mg

▷ **CitraNatal Assure** take 1 tab and 1 DHA cap daily
Tab: thiamine 3 mg, riboflavin 3.4 mg, niacinamide 20 mg, pyridoxine HCL 25 mg, folic acid 1 mg, Vit C 120 mg, Vit D₃ 400 IU, Vit E 30 IU, calcium (as citrate) 125 mg, copper (as oxide) 2 mg, iodine (as potassium oxide) 150 mcg, iron (as carbonyl and ferrous gluconate) 35 mg, zinc (as oxide) 25 mg, docusate sodium 50 mg
Cap: docosahexaenoic acid (DHA) 300 mg

▷ **CitraNatal B-Calm** take 1 tab every 8 hours; begin with tab #1.
Tab: pyridoxine HCL 25 mg, folic acid 1 mg, Vit C 120 mg, Vit D₃ 400 IU, calcium (as citrate) 120 mg, iron (as carbonyl) 20 mg
Tab: pyridoxine 25 mg
Comment: CitraNatal B-Calm may be used as an adjunct treatment to help minimize pregnancy-related nausea and vomiting.

▷ **CitraNatal DHA** take 1 tab and 1 DHA cap daily
Tab: thiamine 3 mg, riboflavin 3.4 mg, niacinamide 20 mg, pyridoxine HCL 20 mg, folic acid 1 mg, Vit C 120 mg, Vit D₃ 400 IU, Vit E 30 IU, calcium (as citrate) 125 mg, copper (as oxide) 2 mg, iodine (as potassium oxide) 150 mcg, iron (as carbonyl and gluconate) 27 mg, zinc (as oxide) 25 mg, docusate sodium 50 mg
Cap: docosahexaenoic acid (DHA) 250 mg

▷ **CitraNatal Harmony** take 1 gelcap daily
Gelcap: pyridoxine HCL 25 mg, folic acid 1 mg, Vit D₃ 400 IU, Vit E 30 IU, calcium (as citrate) 104 mg, iron (as carbonyl and ferrous fumarate) 27 mg, docusate sodium 50 mg, docosahexaenoic acid (DHA) 260 mg

▷ **CitraNatal Rx** take 1 tab* and 1 DHA cap daily
Tab: thiamine 3 mg, riboflavin 3.4 mg, niacinamide 20 mg, pyridoxine HCL 20 mg, folic acid 1 mg, Vit C 120 mg, Vit D₃ 400 IU, Vit E 30 IU, calcium (as citrate) 125 mg, copper (as oxide) 2 mg, iodine (as potassium iodide) 150 mcg, iron (as carbonyl and gluconate) 27 mg, zinc (as oxide) 25 mg, docusate sodium 50 mg

▷ **Duet DHA Balanced** take 1 tab and 1 gelcap daily
Tab: Vit A (as beta carotene) 2800 IU, thiamine 1.5 mg, riboflavin 2 mg, niacinamide 20 mg, pyridoxine HCL 50 mg, Vit B₁₂ 12 mcg, folic acid 1 mg, Vit C 120 mg, Vit D₃ 640 IU, Vit E 15 IU, calcium (as carbonate) 215 mg, iron (as polysaccharide iron complex and sodium iron EDTA, Ferrazone) 25 mg, copper (as oxide) 1.8 mg, magnesium (as oxide) 25 mg, zinc (as oxide) 25 mg, iodine (as potassium iodide) 210 mcg, selenium 65 mcg, choline (as bartrate) 55 mg

(continued)

(continued)

> *Gelcap:* omega 3 fatty acids 267 mg (includes docosahexaenoic acid [DHA], eicosapentaenoic acid [EPA], alpha-linolenic acid [ALA], docasapentaeoic acid [DPA]) (gelatin, gluten-free)

▷ **Duet DHA Complete** take 1 tab and 1 gelcap daily
Tab: Vit A (as beta carotene) 3000 IU, thiamine 1.8 mg, riboflavin 4 mg, niacinamide 20 mg, pyridoxine HCL 50 mg, Vit B_{12} 12 mcg, folic acid 1 mg, Vit C 120 mg, Vit D_3 800 IU, Vit E 3 mg, calcium (as carbonate) 230 mg, iron (as polysaccharide iron complex and sodium iron EDTA, ferrazone) 27 mg, copper (as oxide) 2 mg, magnesium (as oxide) 25 mg, zinc (as oxide) 25 mg, iodine 220 mcg
Gelcap: omega 3 fatty acids ≥430 mg (as docosahexaenoic acid (DHA) ≥295 mg, as other omega-3 fatty acids ≥135 mg (eicosapentaenoic acid (EPA), docasapentaenoic acid (DHA) (gluten-free)

▷ **Natachew** take 1 chew tab daily
Chew tab: Vit A 1000 IU (as beta carotene), thiamine 2 mg, riboflavin 3 mg, niacinamide 20 mg, pyridoxine HCL 10 mg, B12 12 mcg, folic acid 1 mg, Vit C 120 mg, Vit D3 400 IU, Vit E 11 IU, iron (as ferrous fumarate) 29 mg (wildberry)

▷ **Natafort** take 1 tab daily
Tab: Vit A 1000 IU (as acetate and beta carotene), thiamine 2 mg, riboflavin 3 mg, niacinamide 20 mg, pyridoxine HCL 10 mg, B12 12 mcg, folic acid 1 mg, Vit C 120 mg, Vit D3 400 IU, Vit E 11 IU, iron (as carbonyl and sulfate) 60 mg

▷ **Neevo DHA** take 1 cap daily
Cap: l-methylfolate (as Metafolin) 1.3 mg, thiamin1.4 mg, riboflavin 1.4 mg, niacinamide 18 mg, pyridoxine HCL 25 mg, B12 1 mg, Vit D3, 5 mcg, Vit E 15 IU, calcium (as carbonate) 110 mg, iron (ferrous fumarate) 27 mg, iodine (as potassium iodide) 220 mcg, magnesium (as oxide) 60 mg, docosahexaenoic acid (DHA, vegetarian source (algal oil) 581.92 mg (soy, gelatin, sorbitol, glycerin)
Comment: **Neevo DHA** is indicated as a nutritional supplement during pregnancy, and the prenatal and postnatal periods, in women with dietary needs for the biologically active form of folate, who are at risk for hyperhomocysteinemia, impaired folic acid absorption, <u>and/or</u> impaired folic acid metabolism due to 667C >T mutations in the MTHFR gene.

▷ **Nexa Plus** take 1 cap daily
Cap: pyridoxine HCL 25 mg, folic acid 1.25 mg, Vit C 28 mg, Vit D3 800 IU, Vit E 30 IU, biotin 250 mcg, calcium (as carbonate [158 mg] + docusate calcium [2 mg] 160 mg, iron (as ferrous fumarate) 29 mg, docosahexaenoic acid (DHA, plant-based source [algal oil]) 350 mg (soy)

▷ **Nexa Select** take 1 softgel cap daily
Softgel cap: pyridoxine HCL 25 mg, folic acid 1.25 mg, Vit C 28 mg, Vit D3 800 IU, Vit E 30 IU, calcium (as phosphate) 160 mg, iron (as ferrous fumarate) 29 mg, docosahexaenoic acid (DHA) plant-based source (algal oil) 325 mg, docusate sodium 55 mg (soy)

▷ **Prenate AM** take 1 tab daily
Tab: pyridoxine HCL 75 mg, folate (as folic acid 400 mcg + Quatrefolic 1.1 mg [equivalent to 600 mcg folic acid]) 1 mg, Vit B12 12 mcg, calcium (as carbonate) 200 mg, ginger extract 500 mg, lingon-berry 25 mg

(continued)

(continued)

> **Prenate Chewable** take 1 chew tab daily
> *Chew tab:* pyridoxine HCL 10 mg, Vit B12 125 mcg, calcium (as carbonate) 500 mg, Vit D3 300 IU, biotin 280 mcg, boron amino acid chelate 250 mcg, folate (as Quatrefolic) 1 mg, magnesium (as oxide) 50 mg, blueberry extract 25 mg (Dutch chocolate)

> **Prenate DHA** take 1 gel cap daily
> *Gelcap:* pyridoxine HCL 26 mg, folate (as folic acid) 400 mcg + Quatrafolic 1.1 mg [equivalent to 600 mcg folic acid]) 1 mg, Vit B12 13 mcg, Vit C 90 mg, Vit D3 220 IU, Vit E 10 IU, calcium (as carbonate) 145 mg, iron (as ferrous fumarate) 28 mg, magnesium (as oxide) 50 mg, docosahexaenoic acid (DHA) 300 mg (fish oil, soy, gelatin)

> **Prenate Elite** take 1 gel cap daily
> *Gelcap:* Vit A (as beta-carotene) 2600 IU, thiamine 3 mg, riboflavin 3.5 mg, pyridoxine HCl 21 mg, niacinamide 21 mg, pantothenic acid 6 mg, folate (as folic acid 400 mcg + Quatrefolic 1.1 mg [equivalent to 600 mcg folic acid]) 1 mg, Vit B12 13 mcg, Vit C 75 mg, Vit D3 450 IU, Vit E 10 IU, biotin 330 mcg, calcium (as carbonate) 100 mg, iron (as ferrous fumarate) 27 mg, magnesium (as oxide) 25 mg, copper (as oxide) 1.5 mg, iodine 150 mcg, iron (as ferrous fumarate) 26 mg, zinc (as oxide) 15 mg

> **Prenate Enhance** take 1 gel cap daily
> *Gelcap:* pyridoxine HCL 25 mg, folate (as folic acid 400 mcg + Quatrefolic 1.1 mg [equivalent to 600 mcg folic acid]) 1 mg, Vit B12 12 mcg, Vit C 85 mg, Vit D3 1000 IU, Vit E 10 IU, biotin 500 mcg, calcium (as carbonate + Formical) 155 mg, iodine (as potassium) 150 mcg, iron (as ferrous fumarate) 28 mg, magnesium (as oxide) 50 mg, docosahexaenoicacid (DHA) 400 mg (soy, gelatin)

> **Prenate Essential** take 1 gel cap daily
> *Gelcap:* pyridoxine HCL 26 mg, folate (as folic acid 400 mcg + Quatrefolic 1.1 mg [equivalent to 600 mcg folic acid]) 1 mg, Vit B12 13 mcg, Vit C 90 mg, Vit D3 220 IU, Vit E 10 IU, biotin 280 mcg, calcium (as carbonate) 145 mg, iodine (as potassium iodide) 150 mcg, iron (as ferrous fumarate) 29 mg, magnesium (as oxide) 50 mg, docosahexaenoic acid (DHA) 300 mg, eicosapentaenoic acid (EPA) 40 mg (fish oil, soy, gelatin)

> **Prenate Mini** take 1 gel cap daily
> *Gelcap:* pyridoxine HCL 26 mg, folate (as folic acid) 400 mcg + Quatrefolic 1.1 mg [equivalent to 600 mcg folic acid]) 1 mg, Vit B12 13 mcg, Vit C 60 mg, Vit D3 220 IU, Vit E 10 IU, calcium (as carbonate) 100 mg, iron (as carbonyl iron) 29 mg, iodine (as potassium iodide) 150 mcg, biotin 280 mcg, magnesium (as oxide) 25 mg, docosahexaenoic acid (DHA) 300 mg, blueberry extract 25 mg (fish oil, soy, gelatin)

> **Prenate Restore** take 1 gel cap daily
> *Gelcap:* pyridoxine HCL 25 mg, folate (as folic acid 400 mcg + Quatrefolic 1.1 mg [equivalent to 600 mcg folic acid]) 1 mg, Vit B12 12 mcg, Vit C 85 mg, Vit D3 1000 IU, Vit E 10 IU, biotin 500 mcg, calcium (as carbonate + Formical) 155 mg, iron (as ferrous fumarate) 27 mg, magnesium (as oxide) 45 mg, docosahexaenoic

(continued)

(continued)

> acid (DHA) 400 mg, *Bacillus coagulans* 150 million CFU (as lactospore) 10 mg
> (soy, gelatin)
>
> ▷ **Prenexa** take 1 gel cap daily
> *Gelcap:* pyridoxine HCL 25 mg, folic acid 1.25 mg, Vit C 28 mg, Vit D3 400 IU,
> Vit E 30 IU, calcium (as phosphate) 160 mg, iron (as ferrous fumarate) 27 mg,
> docosahexaenoic acid (DHA) plant-based source (algal oil) 300 mg, docusate
> sodium 55 mg (soy)

APPENDIX AA: ORAL PRESCRIPTION DRUGS FOR THE MANAGEMENT OF ALLERGY, COUGH, AND COLD SYMPTOMS

Oral prescription drugs for the management of allergy symptoms, cough, and symptoms of the common cold are listed in alphabetical order by brand name.

Legend:	acriv	acrivastine
	benzo	benzonatate
	brom	brompheniramine
	carb	carbinoxamine
	carbeta	carbetapentane
	chlor	chlorpheniramine
	cod	codeine
	cypro	cyproheptadine
	deslorat	desloratadine
	dexchlo	dexchlorphenirimine
	dextro	dextromethorphan
	diphen	diphenhydramine
	hydrox	hydroxyzine
	guaiac	potassium guaiacosulfonate
	guaif	guaifenesin
	homat	homatropine
	hydro	hydrocodone

(continued)

(*continued*)

hydrox	hydroxyzine
levocetir	levocetirizine
meth	methscopolamine
phenyle	phenylephrine
prometh	promethazine
pseud	pseudoephedrine
pyril	pyrilamine tannate

▷ **Allerex (C)** 1 AM tab in the morning and 1 PM tab in the evening prn
Pediatric: not recommended
AM tab: meth 2.5 mg/*pseud* 120 mg ext-rel; *PM tab: meth* 2.5 mg/*chlor* 8 mg/*phenyle* 10 mg* ext-rel (*Dose Pack 20:* 10 AM tabs+10 PM tabs; *Dose Pack 60:* 30 AM tabs+30 PM tabs)

▷ **Allures-D (C)** 1 tab q 12 hours prn
Pediatric: not recommended
Tab: meth 2.5 mg/*pseud* 120 mg ext-rel

▷ **Allerex DF (C)** 1 AM tab in the morning and 1 PM tab in the evening prn
Pediatric: not recommended
AM tab: meth 2.5 mg/*chlor* 4 mg/*PM tab: meth* 2.5 mg/*chlor* 8 mg* (*Dose Pack 20:* 10 AM tabs+10 PM tabs; *Dose Pack 60:* 30 AM tabs+30 PM tabs)

▷ **Allerex PE (C)** 1 AM tab in the morning and 1 PM tab in the evening prn
Pediatric: not recommended
AM tab: meth 2.5 mg/*phenyle* 40 mg/*PM tab: meth* 8 mg/*phenyle* 10 mg* (*Dose Pack 20:* 10 AM tabs+10 PM tabs; *Dose Pack 60:* 30 AM tabs+30 PM tabs)

▷ **Allerex Suspension (C)** 15 ml q 12 hours prn
Pediatric: <6 years: not recommended
6-12 years: 2.5-5 ml q 12 hours prn
Susp: chlor 3 mg/*phenyle* 7.5 mg ext-rel (raspberry)

▷ **Atarax (B)(G)** 25 mg tid <u>or</u> qid prn
Pediatric: <2 years: not recommended
2-6 years: 6.25 mg q 4-6 hours prn
6-12 years: 12.5-25 mg q 4-6 hours prn
Tab: hydrox 10, 25, 50, 100 mg; *Syr:* 10 mg/5 ml (alcohol 0.5%)

▷ **Bromfed DM (C)(G)** 2 tsp q 4 hours prn: max 6 doses/day
Pediatric: <2 years: not recommended
2-6 years: 1/2 tsp q 4 hours prn
6-12 years: 1 tsp q 4 hours prn
Max 6 doses/day
Tannate susp: brom 2 mg/*pseudo* 30 mg/*dextro* 10 mg per 5 ml (butterscotch; alcohol 0.95%)

▷ **Clarinex (C)** 1 tab daily prn
Pediatric: <6 years: not recommended
>6 years: ½-1 tab once daily
Tab: deslorat 5 mg

(*continued*)

(*continued*)

▷ **Clarinex RediTabs (C)** 5 mg daily prn
  Pediatric: <6 years: not recommended
  6-12 years: 2.5 mg once daily
  ODT: deslorat 2.5, 5 mg (tutti-frutti; phenylalanine)
▷ **Clarinex Syrup (C)** 1 tab daily prn
  Pediatric: <6 months: not recommended
  6-11 months: 1 mg (2 ml) daily prn
  1-5 years: 1.25 mg (2.5 ml) daily prn
  6-11 years: 2.5 mg (5 ml) daily prn
  >12 years: 5 mg (10 ml) daily prn
  Tab: deslorat 0.5 mg per ml (4 oz)(tutti-frutti; phenylalanine)
▷ **Duratuss AC 12 (C)** 1-2 tsp q 12 hours prn
  Pediatric: <2 years: not recommended
  2-6 years: 1/2 tsp q 12 hrs prn
  >6 years: 1 tsp q 12 hours prn *Susp:diphen* 12.5 mg/*dextro* 15 mg/*phenyle* 15 mg per 5 ml (strawberry banana; sugar-free, alcohol-free, phenylalanine)
▷ **Duratuss DM (C)** 1 tsp q 4 hours prn
  Pediatric: <2 years: not recommended
  2-6 years: 1/4 tsp q 4 hrs prn
  >6 years: ½ tsp q 4 hours prn *Susp: dextro* 25 mg/*guaif* 225 mg per 5 ml (grape) (sugar-free, alcohol-free)
▷ **Duratuss DM 12 (C)** 1-2 tsp q 12 hours prn; max 6 tabs/day
  Pediatric: <2 years: not recommended
  2-6 years: 1/2 tsp q 12 hrs prn
  >6 years: ½-1 tsp q 12 hours prn *Susp: dextro* 15 mg/*guaif* 225 mg per 5 ml (grape; sugar-free, alcohol-free)
▷ **Flowtuss Oral Solution (C)(II)(G)** 1-2 tsp q 4-6 hours prn; max 6 tsp/24 hours
  Pediatric: <6 years: not recommended
  6-12 years: 1/2 tsp q 4-6 hours prn; max 15 ml/day
  >12 years: same as adult
  Oral soln: hydro 2.5 mg/*guaif* 200 mg per 5 ml (black raspberry)
Comment: *hydrocodone* is known to be excreted in human milk.
▷ **Hycodan (C)(III)** 1 tab q 4-6 hours prn; max 6 tabs/day
  Pediatric: <6 years: not recommended
  6-12 years: 1/2 tab q 4-6 hours prn; max 3 tabs/day
  Tab: hydro 5 mg/*homat* 1.5 mg
Comment: *hydrocodone* is known to be excreted in human milk.
▷ **Hycodan Syrup (C)(II)(G)** 1 tsp q 4-6 hours prn
  Pediatric: <6 years: not recommended
  6-12 years: 1/2 tsp q 4-6 hours prn; max 15 ml/day
  >12 years: same as adult
  Syr: hydro 5 mg/*homat* 1.5 mg per 5 ml
Comment: *hydrocodone* is known to be excreted in human milk.
▷ **Hycofenix Oral Solution (C)(II)** 1 tsp q 4-6 hours prn
  Pediatric: <6 years: not recommended
  6-12 years: 1/2 tsp q 4-6 hours prn; max 15 ml/day
  >12 years: same as adult

(*continued*)

(continued)

    Oral soln: hydro 2.5 mg/pseudoephedrine 30 mg /quafenesin 200 mg per 5 ml
    (black raspberry)

Comment: ***hydrocodone*** is known to be excreted in human milk.

▷ **Palgic (C)** 4 mg daily prn; max 24 mg/day in divided doses 6-8 hours apart
    Pediatric: <2 year: not recommended
    2-3 years: 2 mg tid <u>or</u> qid prn <u>or</u> 0.2-0.4 mg/kg/day divided tid <u>or</u> qid
    3-6 years: 2-4 mg daily prn <u>or</u> 0.2-0.4 mg/kg/day divided tid <u>or</u> qid
    >6 years: same as adult
    Tab: carb 4*mg; *Syr: carb* 4 mg per 5 ml (bubble gum)

▷ **Periactin (B)(G)** initially 4 mg tid prn, then adjust as needed; usual range 12-16
    mg/day; max 32 mg/day
    Pediatric: < 2 years: not recommended
    2-6 years: 2 mg 2-3 times/day: max 12 mg daily
    7-14 years: 4 mg 2-3 times/day: max 16 mg daily
    >14 years: same as adult
    Tab: cypro 4*mg; *Syr: cypro* 2 mg per 5 ml

▷ **Prolex-DH (C)(III)** 1-1½ tsp qid prn
    Pediatric: <3 years: not recommended
    3-6 years: 1/4-1/2 tsp qid prn
    6-12 years: 1/2-1 tsp qid prn
    Liq: hydro 4.5 mg/*pot guaiac* 300 mg per 5 ml (tropical fruit punch; alcohol-free,
    sugar-free)

▷ **Phenergan (C)(G)** 25 mg po <u>or</u> rectally tid ac and HS prn
    Pediatric: <2 years: not recommended
    >2 years: 0.5 mg/lb <u>or</u> 6.25-25 mg po <u>or</u> rectally tid
    Tab: 12.5*, 25*, 50 mg; *Syr: prom* 6.25 mg per 5 ml; *Syr fortis: prom* 25 mg per 5 ml;
    Rectal supp: prom 12.5, 25, 50 mg

▷ **Promethazine DM (C)(V)(G)** 1 tsp q 4-6 hours prn
    Pediatric: <6 years: not recommended
    6-12 years: ½-1 tsp q 4-6 hours prn
    Syr: prometh 6.25 mg/*dex* 15 mg per 5 ml (alcohol 7%)

Comment: Contraindicated with asthma.

▷ **Promethazine VC (C)(V)(G)** 1 tsp q 4-6 hours prn; max 30 ml/day
    Pediatric: 2-6 years: 1.25 ml q 4-6 hours prn; max 7.5 ml/day
    6-12 years: 2.5 ml q 4-6 hours prn; max 15 ml/day
    >12 years: same as adult
    Syr: prometh 6.25 mg/*phenyle* 5 mg per 5 ml (alcohol 7%)

Comment: Contraindicated with asthma.

▷ **Promethazine VC w. Codeine (C)(V)(G)** 1 tsp q 4-6 hours prn; max 30 ml/day
    Pediatric: <6 years: not recommended
    6-12 years: ½-1 tsp q 4-6 hours prn; max 30 ml/day
    >12 years: same as adult
    Syr: prometh 6.25 mg/*phenyle* 5 mg/cod 10 mg per 5 ml (alcohol 7%)

Comment: Contraindicated with asthma.

▷ **Promethazine w. Codeine (C)(V)(G)** 1 tsp q 4-6 hours prn
    Pediatric: <6 years: not recommended
    6-12 years: ½-1 tsp q 4-6 hours prn

(continued)

(continued)

 Liq: prometh 6.25 mg/*cod* 10 mg per 5 ml (alcohol 7%)
Comment: Contraindicated with asthma.
▷ **Rynatan (C)** 1-2 tabs q 12 hours prn
 Pediatric: not recommended
 Tab: chlor 9 mg/*phenyle* 25 mg
▷ **Rynatan Pediatric Suspension (C)**
 Pediatric: <2 years: not recommended
 2-6 years: ½-1 tsp q 12 hours prn
 >6-12 years: 1-2 tsp q 12 hours prn
 Susp: chlor 4.5 mg/*phenyle* 5 mg
▷ **Ryneze (C)** 1 tab q 12 hours prn
 Pediatric: <6 years: not recommended
 6-12 years: 1/2 tab q 12 hours prn
 Tab: chlor 8 mg/*meth* 2.5 mg
▷ **Robitussin AC (C)(III)(G)** 2 tsp q 4 hours prn; max 60 ml/day
 Pediatric: <2 years: not recommended
 2-6 years: 1/4-1/2 tsp q 4 hours prn
 6-12 years: 1 tsp q 4 hours prn
 Liq: cod 10 mg/*guaif* 100 mg per 5 ml
▷ **Rondec Syrup (C)(G)** 1 tsp qid prn; max 30 ml/day
 Pediatric: <2 years: not recommended
 2-5 years: 1/4 tsp q 4-6 hours prn; max 7.5 ml/day
 6-11 years: 1/2 tsp q 4-6 hours prn; max 15 ml/day
 >11 years: same as adult
 Syr: phenyle 12.5 mg/*chlor* 4 mg per 5 ml (bubblegum; sugar-free, alcohol-free)
▷ **Semprex-D (B)** 1 cap q 4-6 hours prn; max 4 doses/day
 Pediatric: not recommended
 Cap: acriv 8 mg/*pseud* 60 mg
▷ **Tanafed DMX (C)(G)** 2-4 tsp q 12 hours prn
 Pediatric: <2 years: not recommended
 2-6 years: ½-1 tsp q 12 hours prn
 6-12 years: 1-2 tsp q 12 hours prn
 Susp: dexchlor 2.5 mg/*pseud* 75 mg/*dextro* 25 mg per 5 ml (cotton candy, alcohol-free)
▷ **Tessalon Caps (C)** 100-200 mg tid prn; max 600 mg/day
 Pediatric: <10 years: not recommended
 >10 years: same as adult
 Cap: benzo 200 mg
Comment: Swallow whole. Do not suck or chew.
▷ **Tessalon Perles (C)** 100-200 mg tid prn; max 600 mg/day
 Pediatric: <10 years: not recommended
 >10 years: same as adult
 Perles: benzo 100 mg
Comment: Swallow whole. Do not suck or chew.
▷ **Tussi-12 D Tablets (C)** 1-2 tabs q 12 hours prn
 Pediatric: <6 years: use susp
 6-11 years: ½-1 tab q 12 hours prn
 Tab: carbeta 60 mg/*pyril* 40 mg/*phenyle* 10*mg

(continued)

(*continued*)

▶ **Tussi-12 D S (C)** 1-2 tsp q 12 hours prn
  Pediatric: <2 years: individualize
  2-6 years: ½-1 tsp q 12 hours prn
  6-12 years: 1-2 tsp q 12 hours prn
  Liq: carbeta 30 mg/*pyril* 30 mg/*phenyle* 5 mg per 5 ml (strawberry-currant; tartrazine)
▶ **TussiCaps 5 mg/4 mg (C)(III)** 2 caps q 12 hours prn; max 4 caps/day
  Pediatric: <6 years: not recommended
  6-11 years: 1 cap q 12 hours prn; max 2 caps/day
  >11 years: same as adult
  Cap: hydro 5 mg/*chlor* 4 mg ext-rel (alcohol)
▶ **TussiCaps 10 mg/8 mg (C)(III)** 1 cap q 12 hours prn; max 2 caps/day
  Pediatric: not recommended
  Cap: hydro 10 mg/*chlor* 8 mg ext-rel (alcohol)
▶ **Tussionex (C)(III)** 1 tsp q 12 hours prn
  Pediatric: <6 years: not recommended
  6-12 years: ½ tsp q 12 hours prn
  S*usp: hydro* 10 mg/*chlor* 8 mg per 5 ml ext-rel
▶ **Tussi-Organidin DM NR Liquid (C)(III)** 5 ml q 4 hours prn; max 40 ml/day
  Pediatric: <6 months: not recommended
  6-23 months: 0.6 ml q 4 hours prn; max 3.7 ml/day
  2-5 years: 1.25 ml q 4 hours prn; max 7.5 ml/day
  6-11 years: 2.5 ml q 4 hours prn; max 15 ml/day
  Liq: dextro 10 mg/*guaif* 300 mg per 5 ml (grape; sugar-free, alcohol-free)
▶ **Tussi-Organidin NR (C)(V)** 1 tsp q 4 hours prn; max 40 ml/day
  Pediatric: <2 years: not recommended
  2 years: 1.5 ml q 4-6 hours prn; max 6 ml/day
  3 years: 1.75 ml q 4-6 hours prn; max 7 ml/day
  4 years: 2 ml q 4-6 hours prn; max 8 ml/day
  5 years: 2.25 ml q 4-6 hours prn; max 9 ml/day
  6-11 years: 2.5 ml q 4 hours prn; max 20 ml/day
  Liq: cod 10 mg/*guaif* 300 mg per 5 ml (grape; sugar-free, alcohol-free)
▶ **Tuzistra XR (C)(III)** 1-2 tsp q 12 hours prn; max 20 ml/day
  Pediatric: <18 years: not recommended
  Liq: cod 14.7 *mg/chlor* 2.8 mg per 5 ml (cherry)
▶ **Vistaril (C)(G)** 25 mg tid or qid prn
  Pediatric: <6 years: 50 mg/day prn
  6-12 years: 50-100 mg daily prn
  Cap: hydrox 25, 50, 100 mg; *Susp: hydrox* 25 mg/5 ml (lemon)
▶ **Xyzal, Xyzal Oral Solution (B)** 2.5-5 mg in the evening prn
  CrCl 30-50 mL/min: 2.5 mg every other day
  CrCl 10-30 mL/min: 2.5 mg twice weekly
  CrCl <10 mL/min or hemodialysis: contraindicated
  Pediatric: <6 months: not recommended
  6 months to 5 years: max 1.25 mg once daily in the PM prn
  6-11 years: max 2.5 mg once daily in the PM prn
  Tab: levocetir 5*mg film-coat; *Oral soln: levocetir* 0.5 mg/ml (150 ml)

(*continued*)

APPENDIX BB: SYSTEMIC ANTI-INFECTIVE DRUGS

Comment:
- Adverse effects of aminoglycosides include nephrotoxicity and ototoxicity.
- Use cephalosporins with caution in persons with penicillin allergy due to potential cross allergy.
- Sulfonamides are contraindicated with sulfa allergy and G6PD deficiency. A high fluid intake is indicated during sulfonamide therapy.
- Tetracyclines should be taken on an empty stomach to facilitate absorption. Tetracyclines should not be taken with milk.
- Tetracyclines are contraindicated during pregnancy and breastfeeding, and in children <8 years of age, due to the risk of developing tooth enamel discoloration.
- Systemic quinolones and fluoroquinolones are contraindicated in pregnancy and children <18 years of age due to the risk of joint dysplasia.

Anti-infectives by Class With Dose Forms		
Generic Name	Brand Name	Dose Form/Volume
Amebicide		
chloroquine phosphate (C)	**Aralen**	*Tab:* 500 mg; *Inj:* 50 mg/ml (5 ml)
iodoquinol (C)	**Yodoxin**	*Tab:* 210, 650 mg
metronidazole (**not for use in 1st; B in 2nd, 3rd**)(G)	**Flagyl**	*Tab:* 250*, 500* mg
	Flagyl 375	*Cap:* 375 mg
	Flagyl ER	*Tab:* 750 mg ext-rel
tinidazole (C)	**Tindamax**	*Tab:* 250*, 500* mg
Antihelmintic		
albendazole (C)(G)	**Albenza**	*Tab:* 200 mg
mebendazole (C)(G)	**Emverm, Vermox**	*Chew tab:* 100 mg
	Pin-X	*Cap:* 180 mg; *Liq:* 50 mg/ml (30 ml); 144 mg/ml (30 ml); *Oral susp:* 50 mg/ml (30 ml)
thiabendazole(C)	**Mintezol**	*Chew tab:* 500*mg (orange); *Oral susp:* 500 mg/5 ml (120 ml) (orange)
Antifungal		
atovaquone (C)	**Mepron**	*Susp:* 750 mg/5ml (210 ml)
clotrimazole (B)(G)	**Mycelex Troche**	10 mg (70, 40/bottle)

(*continued*)

(*continued*)

Anti-infectives by Class With Dose Forms		
Generic Name	**Brand Name**	**Dose Form/Volume**
fluconazole (C)(G)	Diflucan	*Tab:* 50, 100, 150, 200 mg; *Oral susp:* 10, 40 mg/ml (35 ml) (orange)
griseofulvin, microsize (C)	Grifulvin V	*Tab:* 250, 500 mg; *Oral susp:* 125 mg/5 ml (120 ml) (alcohol 0.02%)
	Gris-PEG	*Tab:* 125, 250 mg
itraconazole (C)	Sporanox	*Cap:* 100 mg; *Soln:* 10 mg/ml (150 ml); *Pulse Pack:* 100 mg caps (7/pck)
ketoconazole (C)(G)	Nizoral	*Tab:* 200 mg
nystatin (C)(G)	Mycostatin	*Pastille:* 200,000 units/pastille (30 pastilles/ pck); *Oral susp:* 100,000 units/ml (60 ml w. dropper)
terbinafine (B)(G)	Lamisil	*Tab:* 250 mg
vorconazole (D)	Vfend	*Tab:* 50, 200 mg
Antimalarial		
atovaquone/ proguanil (C)	Malarone	*Tab: atov* 250 mg/*proq* 100 mg
	Malarone Pediatric	*Tab: atov* 62.5 mg/*proq* 25 mg
chloroquine (C)(G)	Aralen	*Tab:* 500 mg; *Amp:* 50 mg/ml (5 ml)
doxycycline (D)(G)	Actilate	*Tab:* 75, 150**mg
	Adoxa	*Tab:* 50, 100 mg enteric-coated
	Doryx	*Cap:* 100 mg
	Monodox	*Cap:* 50, 100 mg
	Oracea	*Cap:* 40 mg
	Vibramycin	*Cap:* 50, 100 mg; *Syr:* 50 mg/5 ml (raspberry-apple) (sulfites); *Oral susp:* 25 mg/5 ml (raspberry-apple)
	Vibra-Tab	*Tab:* 100 mg film-coat
hydroxychloroquine (C)(G)	Plaquenil	*Tab:* 200 mg
mefloquine (C)	Lariam	*Tab:* 250 mg

(*continued*)

(*continued*)

Anti-infectives by Class With Dose Forms		
Generic Name	Brand Name	Dose Form/Volume
Antiprotozoal/Antibacterial		
metronidazole (not for use in 1st; B in 2nd, 3rd)(G)	Flagyl, Protostat	*Tab:* 250*, 500* mg
	Flagyl 375	*Cap:* 375 mg
	Flagyl ER	*Tab:* 750 mg ext-rel
tinidazole (C)	Tindamax	*Tab:* 250*, 500*mg
Antiviral (for HIV-specific antiviral drugs see page 510)		
acyclovir (C)(G)	Zovirax	*Cap:* 200 mg; *Tab:* 400, 800 mg; *Oral susp:* 200 mg/5 ml (banana)
amantadine (C)(G)	Symmetrel	*Tab:* 100 mg; *Syr:* 50 mg/5ml (16 oz) (raspberry)
famciclovir (B)	Famvir	*Tab:* 125, 250, 500 mg
lamivudine (C)	Epivir-HBV	*Tab:* 100 mg; *Oral soln:* 5 mg/ml (240 ml) (strawberry-banana)
oseltamivir (C)	Tamiflu	*Cap:* 75 mg
rimantadine (C)	Flumadine	*Tab:* 100 mg
valacyclovir (B)	Valtrex	*Tab:* 500 mg; 1 g
zanamivir	Relenza	*Tab: lami* 150/*zido* 300 mg
Antitubercular		
ethambutol (EMB) (B)(G)	Myambutol	*Tab:* 100, 400*mg
isoniazid (INH) (C)(G)	generic only	*Tab:* 100, 300*mg; *Syr:* 50 mg/5 ml; *Inj:* 100 mg/ml
pyrazinamide (PZA) (C)	generic only	*Tab:* 500*mg
rifampin (C)(G)	Priftin	*Tab:* 150 mg
	Rifadin	*Cap:* 150, 300 mg
rifampin/isoniazid (C)	Rifamate	*Cap: rif* 300 mg/*iso* 150 mg
rifampin/isoniazid/ pyrazinamide (C)	Rifater	*Tab: rif* 120 mg/*iso* 50 mg/*pyr* 300 mg

(*continued*)

(*continued*)

Anti-infectives by Class With Dose Forms		
Generic Name	Brand Name	Dose Form/Volume
Aminoglycoside		
amikacin (C)	Amikin	*Vial:* 500 mg, 1 g (2 ml)
gentamicin (C)(G)	Garamycin	*Vial:* 20, 80 mg/2 ml
streptomycin (D)(G)	Streptomycin	*Amp:* 1 g/2.5 ml <u>or</u> 400 mg/ml (2.5 ml)
Cephalosporin		
First Generation Cephalosporin		
cefadroxil (B)	Duricef	*Cap:* 500 mg; *Tab:* 1 g; *Oral susp:*250 mg/5 ml (100 ml); 500 mg/5 ml (75, 100 ml) (orange-pineapple)
cefazolin (B)	Ancef, Zolicef	*Vial:* 500 mg; 1, 10 g
cephalexin (B)	Keflex	*Cap:* 250, 333, 500, 750 mg; *Oral susp:*125, 250 mg/5 ml (100, 200 ml)
Second Generation Cephalosporin		
cefaclor (B)(G)	*generic only*	*Tab:* 500 mg; *Cap:* 250, 500 mg; *Susp:* 125 mg/5 ml (75, 150 ml) (strawberry); 187 mg/5 ml (50, 100 ml) (strawberry); 250 mg/5 ml (75, 150 ml) (strawberry); 375 mg/5 ml (50, 100 ml) (strawberry)
	Cefaclor Extended Release	*Tab:* 375, 500 mg ext-rel
cefamandole (B)	Mandol	*Vial:* 1, 2 g
cefotetan (B)	Cefotan	*Vial:* 1, 2 g
cefoxitin (B)	Mefoxin	*Vial:* 1, 2 g
cefprozil (B)	Cefzil	*Tab:* 250, 500 mg; *Oral susp:* 125, 250 mg/5 ml (50, 75, 100 ml) (bubble gum) (phenylalanine)
ceftaroline (B)	Teflaro	*Vial:* 400, 600 mg
cefuroxime axetil (B)	Ceftin	*Tab:* 250, 500 mg; *Oral susp:* 125, 250 mg/5 ml (50, 100 ml) (tutti-frutti)

(*continued*)

(*continued*)

Anti-infectives by Class With Dose Forms		
Generic Name	**Brand Name**	**Dose Form/Volume**
cefuroxime sodium (B)(G)	Zinacef	*Vial:* 750 mg; 1.5 g
loracarbef (B)	Lorabid	*Pulvule:* 200, 400 mg; *Oral susp:* 100 mg/5 ml (50, 100 ml); 200 mg/5 ml (50, 75, 100 ml) (strawberry bubble gum)
Third Generation Cephalosporin		
cefoperazone (B)	Cefobid	*Vial:* 1, 2 g pwdr for reconstitution
cefotaxime (B)	Claforan	*Vial:* 500 mg; 1, 2 g pwdr for reconstitution
cefpodoxime (B)	Vantin	*Tab:* 100, 200 mg; *Oral susp:* 50, 100 mg/5 ml (50, 75, 100 ml) (lemon creme)
ceftazidime (B)	Ceptaz	*Vial:* 1, 2 g pwdr for reconstitution
	Fortaz	*Vial:* 500 mg; 1, 2 g pwdr for reconstitution
	Tazicef	*Vial:* 1, 2 g pwdr for reconstitution
	Tazidime	*Vial:* 1, 2 g pwdr for reconstitution
ceftazidime/ avibactam (B)	Avycaz	*Vial:* 2.5 g pwdr for reconstitution
ceftibuten (B)	Cedax	*Cap:* 400 mg; *Oral susp:* 90 mg/5 ml (30, 60, 90, 120 ml); 180 mg/5 ml (30, 60, 120 ml) (cherry)
Third/Fourth Generation Cephalosporin		
cefdinir (B)	Omnicef	*Cap:* 300 mg; *Oral susp:* 125 mg/5 ml (60, 100 ml) (strawberry)
cefditoren pivoxil (C)	Spectracef	*Tab:* 200 mg
cefepime (B)	Maxipime	*Vial:* 1 g pwdr for reconstitution
cefixime (B)	Suprax	*Tab/Cap:* 400 mg; *Oral Susp:* 100 mg/ 5 ml (50, 75, 100 ml)(strawberry)

(*continued*)

(continued)

Anti-infectives by Class With Dose Forms		
Generic Name	Brand Name	Dose Form/Volume
ceftaroline (B)	Teflaro	*Vial:* 400, 600 mg
ceftriaxone (B)(G)	Rocephin	*Vial:* 250, 500 mg; 1, 2 g
cytolozane/ tazobactam (B)	Zerbaxa	*Vial:* 1.5 g pwdr for reconstitution
Fluoroquinolone and Quinolone		
First-Generation Quinolone		
enoxacin (C)	Penetrex	*Tab:* 200, 400 mg
Second-Generation Fluoroquinolone		
ciprofloxacin (C) (G)	Cipro	*Tab:* 250, 500, 750 mg; *Oral susp:* 250, 500 mg/5 ml (100 ml) (strawberry) *IV conc:* 10 mg/ml after dilution (20, 40 ml); *IV premix:* 2 mg/ml (100, 200 ml)
	Cipro XR	*Tab:* 500, 1000 mg ext-rel
	ProQuin XR	*Tab:* 500 mg ext-rel
lomefloxacin (C)	Maxaquin	*Tab:* 400 mg
norfloxacin (C)(G)	Noroxin	*Tab:* 400 mg
ofloxacin (C)(G)	Floxin	*Tab:* 200, 300, 400 mg
Third-Generation Fluoroquinolone		
levofloxacin (C)(G)	Levaquin	*Tab:* 250, 500, 750 mg
Fourth-Generation Fluoroquinolone		
gemifloxacin (C)(G)	Factive	*Tab:* 320*mg
moxifloxacin (C) (G)	Avelox	*Tab:* 400 mg
Ketolide		
telithromycin (C)	Ketek	*Tab:* 300, 400 mg
Macrolide		

(continued)

(*continued*)

Anti-infectives by Class With Dose Forms		
Generic Name	Brand Name	Dose Form/Volume
azithromycin (B)	Zithromax	*Tab:* 250, 500, 600 mg; *Pkt:* 1 g for reconstitution (cherry-banana)
	ZithPed Syr	*Oral susp:* 100 mg/5 ml, (15 ml); 200 mg/5 ml (15, 22.5, 30 ml) (cherry)
	Zithromax Tri-Pak	*Tab:* 3 x 500 mg tabs/pck
	Zithromax Z-Pak	*Tab:* 6 x 250 mg tabs/pck
	Zmax	Pkt: 2 g for reconstitution (cherry-banana)
clarithromycin (C)(G)	Biaxin	*Tab:* 250, 500 mg; *Oral susp:* 125, 250 mg/5 ml (50, 100 ml)(fruit punch)
	Biaxin XL	*Tab:* 500 mg ext-rel
dirithromycin (C)(G)	*generic only*	*Tab:* 250 mg
erythromycin base (B)(G)	Ery-Tab	*Tab:* 250, 333, 500 mg ent-coat
	PCE	*Tab:* 333, 500 mg
erythromycin estolate (B)(G)	Ilosone	*Pulvule:* 250 mg; *Tab:* 500 mg; *Liq:* 125, 250 mg/5 ml (100 ml)
erythromycin ethylsuccinate (B)(G)	E.E.S.	*Tab:* 400 mg; *Oral susp:* 200 mg/5 ml (100, 200 ml) (cherry); 200, 400 mg/5 ml (100 ml)(fruit)
	EryPed	*Oral susp:* 200 mg/5 ml (100, 200 ml) (fruit); 400 mg/5 ml (60, 100, 200 ml) (banana); *Oral drops:* 200, 400 mg/5 ml (50 ml) (fruit); *Chew tab:* 200 mg wafer (fruit)
erythromycin stearate (B)(G)	Erythrocin	*Film tab:* 250, 500 mg
Penicillin		
amoxicillin (B)(G)	Amoxil	*Cap:* 250, 500 mg; *Tab:* 500, 875* mg; *Chew tab:* 125, 200, 250, 400 mg (cherry-banana-peppermint) (phenylalanine); *Oral susp:*125, 250 mg/ml (80, 100, 150 ml) (bubble gum); 200, 400 mg/5ml (50, 75, 100 ml) (bubble gum); *Oral drops:* 50 mg/ml (30 ml) (bubble gum)

(*continued*)

(continued)

Anti-infectives by Class With Dose Forms		
Generic Name	Brand Name	Dose Form/Volume
	Moxatag	*Tab:* 775 mg ext-rel
	Trimox	*Cap:* 250, 500 mg; *Oral susp:* 125, 250 mg/5ml (80, 100, 150 ml) (raspberry-strawberry)
amoxicillin/ clavulanate (B)(G)	Augmentin	*Tab:* 250, 500, 875 mg; *Chew tab:* 125, 250 mg (lemon lime); 200, 400 mg (cherry-banana; phenylalanine); *Oral susp:* 125 mg/5 ml (banana), 250 mg/5 ml (orange) (75, 100, 150 ml); 200, 400 mg/5ml (50, 75, 100 ml) (orange)
	Augmentin ES-600	*Oral susp:* 600 mg/5 ml (50, 75, 100, 125, 150, 200 ml) (strawberry cream) (phenylalanine)
	Augmentin XR	*Tab:* 1000*mg ext-rel
ampicillin (B)(G)	Omnipen	*Cap:* 250, 500 mg; *Oral susp:* 125, 250 mg/ml (100, 150, 200 ml)
	Principen	*Cap:* 250, 500 mg; *Syr:* 125, 250 mg/5 ml
ampicillin/ sulbactam (B)(G)	Unasyn	*Vial:* 1.5, 3 g
carbenicillin (B)	Geocillin	*Tab:* 382 mg film-coat
dicloxacillin (B)(G)	Dynapen	*Cap:* 125, 250, 500 mg; *Oral susp:* 62.5 mg/5 ml (80, 100, 200 ml)
ertapenem (B)	Ivanz	*Vial:* 1 g pwdr for reconstitution
meropenem (B)(G)	Merrem	*Vial:* 500 mg; 1 g pwdr for reconstitution (sodium 3.92 mEq/g)
penicillin G benzathine (B)(G)	Bicillin LA, Bicillin C-R	*Cartridge-needle unit:* 600,000 million units (1 ml); 1.2 million units (2 ml); 2.4 million units (4 ml)
	Permapen	*Prefilled syringe:* 1.2 million units
penicillin G procaine (B)(G)	*generic only*	*Prefilled syringe:* 1.2 million units

(continued)

(continued)

Anti-infectives by Class With Dose Forms		
Generic Name	Brand Name	Dose Form/Volume
penicillin v potassium (B)(G)	Pen-Vee K	Tab: 250, 500 mg; Oral soln: 125 mg/5 ml (100, 200 ml); 250 mg/5 ml (100, 150, 200 ml)
piperacillin/ tazobactam (B)(G)	Zosyn	Vial: 2, 3, 4 g pwdr for reconstitution
Sulfonamide		
sulfamethoxazole (B/D)(G)	Gantrisin Pediatric	Oral susp: 500 mg/5 ml; Syr: 500 mg/5 ml
trimethoprim (C) (G)	Primsol	Oral soln: 50 mg/5 ml (bubble gum) (dye-free, alcohol-free)
	Trimpex	Tab: 100 mg
	Proloprim	Tab: 100, 200 mg
trimethoprim/ sulfamethoxazole (C)(G)	Bactrim, Septra	Tab: trim 80 mg/sulfa 400 mg*
	Bactrim DS, Septra DS	Tab: trim 160 mg/sulfa 800 mg*; Oral susp: trim 40 mg/sulfa 200 mg per 5 ml (100 ml) (cherry) (alcohol 0.3%)
Tetracycline		
demeclocycline (D)	Declomycin	Tab: 300 mg
doxycycline (D)(G)	Adoxa	Tab: 50, 100 mg ent-coat
	Doryx	Cap: 100 mg
	Monodox	Cap: 50, 100 mg
doxycycline (D)(G)	Vibramycin	Cap: 50, 100 mg; Syr: 50 mg/5 ml; (raspberry) (sulfites); Oral susp: 25 mg/5 ml (raspberry-apple); IV conc: doxy 100 mg/asc acid 480 mg after dilution; doxy 200 mg/asc acid 960 mg after dilution
	Vibra-Tab	Tab: 100 mg film-coat
minocycline (D)(G)	Dynacin	Cap: 50, 100 mg
	Minocin	Cap: 50, 100 mg; Oral susp: 50 mg/5 ml (60 ml) (custard) (sulfites, alcohol 5%); Vial: 100 mg soln for inj:

(continued)

(*continued*)

Anti-infectives by Class With Dose Forms		
Generic Name	**Brand Name**	**Dose Form/Volume**
tetracycline (D)(G)	**Achromycin V**	*Cap:* 250, 500 mg
	Sumycin	*Tab:* 250, 500 mg; *Oral susp:* 125 mg/5 ml (fruit) (sulfites)
Macrolide/Sulfisoxazole		
erythromycin ethylsuccinate/ sulfisoxazole (C)(G)	**Pediazole**	*Oral susp:* eryth 200 mg/*sulf* 600 mg per 5 ml (100, 150, 200 ml) (strawberry-banana)
Miscellaneous		
aztreonam (B)	**Cayston**	*Vial:* 75 mg pwdr for reconstitution (preservative-free)
chloramphenicol (C)(G)	**Chloromycetin**	*Vial:* 1 g
clindamycin (B)(G)	**Cleocin**	*Cap:* 75 (tartrazine), 150 (tartrazine), 300 mg; *Oral susp:* 75 mg/5 ml (100 ml) (cherry); *Vial:* 150 mg/l (2, 4 ml) (benzyl alcohol)
dalbavancin (C)	**Dalvance**	*Vial:* 500 mg pwdr for IV infusion (preservative-free)
daptomycin (B)	**Cubicin**	*Vial:* 500 mg pwdr for reconstitution
doripenem (B)	**Doribax**	*Vial:* 500 mg pwdr for reconstitution
fosfomycin (B)	**Monurol**	*Sachet:* 3 g single-dose (mandarin orange; sucrose)
imipenem/cilastatin (C)(G)	**Primaxin**	*Vial:* imip 500 mg/*cila* 500 mg; imip 750 mg/*cila* 750 mg pwdr for reconstitution
lincomycin (B)(G)	**Lincocin**	*Vial:* 300 mg/ml (10 ml)
linezolid (C)(G)	**Zyvox**	*Tab:* 400, 600 mg; *Oral susp:* 100 mg/5 ml (orange) (phenylalanine); *IV:* 2 mg ml (100, 200, 300 ml)
meropenem (B)	**Merrem**	*Vial:* 500 mg; 1 g (sodium 3.92 mEq/g)

(*continued*)

(*continued*)

Anti-infectives by Class With Dose Forms		
Generic Name	Brand Name	Dose Form/Volume
nitrofurantoin (B) (G)	**Furadantin**	*Oral susp:* 25 mg/5 ml (60 ml)
	Macrobid	*Cap:* 100 mg
	Macrodantin	*Cap:* 25, 50, 100 mg
quinupristin/ dalfopristin (B)	**Synercid**	*Vial:* 150 mg/350 mg, 180 mg/420 mg
tygecycline (D)(G)	**Tygacil**	*Vial:* 50 mg pwdr for reconstitution
rifaximin (C)	**Xifaxan**	*Tab:* 200, 550 mg
telavancin (C)	**Vibativ**	*Vial:* 250, 750 mg pwdr for reconstitution for IV infusion (preservative-free)
vancomycin (C)(G)	**Vancocin**	*Cap:* 125, 250 mg; *Vial:* 500 mg, 1 g pwdr for reconstitution for IV infusion

APPENDIX CC.1: *ACYCLOVIR* (ZOVIRAX SUSPENSION)

Weight												
Pounds	15	20	25	30	35	40	45	50	55	60	65	70
Kilograms	6.8	9	11.4	13.6	15.9	18.2	20.5	22.7	25	27.3	29.5	31.8
Single Dose (ml)/Frequency/Strength/5-Day Volume (ml)												
20 mg/kg/d ml/dose qid	3.5	4.5	5.5	6.5	8	9	10	11.5	12.5	13.5	14.5	16
mg/5ml	200	200	200	200	200	200	200	200	200	200	200	200
Volume (ml)	70	90	110	130	160	180	200	230	250	270	290	320

Zovirax Oral Suspension <2 years: not recommended; >2 years, <40 kg: 20 mg/kg dosed qid x 5 days; ≥2 years, >40 kg: 800 mg dosed qid x 5 days; *Oral susp:* 200 mg/5 ml (banana).

542 ■ Appendix CC.2: *Amantadine* (Symmetrel Syrup)

APPENDIX CC.2: *AMANTADINE* (SYMMETREL SYRUP)

Weight												
Pounds	15	20	25	30	35	40	45	50	55	60	65	70
Kilograms	6.8	9	11.4	13.6	15.9	18.2	20.5	22.7	25	27.3	29.5	31.8
Single Dose (ml)/Frequency/Strength/10-Day Volume (ml)												
4 mg/kg/d ml/dose bid	3	4	5	6	7	8	9	10	11	12	13	14
mg/5ml	50	50	50	50	50	50	50	50	50	50	50	50
Volume (ml)	30	40	50	60	70	80	90	100	110	120	130	140
8 mg/lb/d ml/dose bid	6	8	10	12								
mg/5ml	50	50	50	50								
Volume (ml)	60	80	100	60								

Symmetrel Suspension (C)(G) Symmetrel <1 year: not recommended; 1-8 years: max 150 mg/day; 9-12 years: 2 tsp bid; >12 years: 100 mg bid or 200 mg once daily; *Syr*: 50 mg/5 ml (raspberry).

APPENDIX CC.3: *AMOXICILLIN* (AMOXIL SUSPENSION, TRIMOX SUSPENSION)

Weight												
Pounds	15	20	25	30	35	40	45	50	55	60	65	70
Kilograms	6.8	9	11.4	13.6	15.9	18.2	20.5	22.7	25	27.3	29.5	31.8
Single Dose (ml)/Frequency/Strength/10-Day Volume (ml)												
20 mg/kg/d ml/dose tid	2	2.5	3	3.5	4	5	5.5	6	7	7.5	8	9
mg/5ml	125	125	125	125	125	125	125	125	125	125	125	125
Volume (ml)	60	75	90	105	120	150	165	180	210	225	240	270
30 mg/kg/d ml/dose tid	3	3.5	2.5	3	3	3.5	4	4.5	5	5.5	6	6.5
mg/5ml	125	125	250	250	250	250	250	250	250	250	250	250
Volume (ml)	90	105	75	90	90	105	120	135	150	165	180	195
40 mg/kg/d ml/dose bid	5	7	4.5	5	6	7	8	9	10	11	12	13
mg/5ml	125	125	250	250	250	250	250	250	250	250	250	250
Volume (ml)	100	140	90	100	120	140	160	180	200	220	240	250
45 mg/kg/d ml/dose bid	4	2.5	3	4	4.5	5	6	6.5	7	7.5	8.5	9

(continued)

APPENDIX CC.3: *AMOXICILLIN (AMOXIL SUSPENSION, TRIMOX SUSPENSION)* (*continued*)

mg/5ml	200	400	400	400	400	400	400	400	400	400	400	400
Volume (ml)	80	50	60	80	90	100	120	130	140	150	170	180
90 mg/kg/d ml/dose bid	8	5	6	7	9	10	12	13	14	15	17	18
mg/5ml	200	400	400	400	400	400	400	400	400	400	400	400
Volume (ml)	160	100	120	140	180	200	240	260	280	300	340	360

<40 kg (88 lb): 20-30 mg/kg/day in 3 divided doses or 40-90 mg/kg/day in 2 divided doses; >40 kg: same as adult.

Amoxil Suspension (B)(G) 125, 250 mg/5ml (80, 100, 150 ml) (strawberry); 200, 400 mg/5 ml (50, 75, 100 ml) (bubble gum).

Trimox Suspension (B)(G) 125, 250 mg/5 ml (80, 100, 150 ml) (raspberry-strawberry).

APPENDIX CC.4: *AMOXICILLIN/CLAVULANATE* (AUGMENTIN SUSPENSION)

Weight												
Pounds	15	20	25	30	35	40	45	50	55	60	65	70
Kilograms	6.8	9	11.4	13.6	15.9	18.2	20.5	22.7	25	27.3	29.5	31.8
Single Dose (ml)/Frequency/Strength/10-Day Volume (ml)												
40 mg/kg/d ml/dose bid	5.5	7	4.5	5.5	6.5	7	8	9	10	11	12	13
mg/5ml	125	125	250	250	250	250	250	250	250	250	250	250
Volume (ml)	110	140	90	110	130	140	160	180	200	220	240	260
45 mg/kg/d ml/dose bid	3	4	5	6	7	8	9	10	11.5	12.5	13.5	14.5
mg/5ml	250	250	250	250	250	250	250	250	250	250	250	250
Volume (ml)	60	80	100	120	140	160	180	200	230	250	270	290
45 mg/kg/d ml/dose bid	4	2.5	3	4	4.5	5	6	6.5	7	7.5	8.5	9
mg/5ml	200	400	400	400	400	400	400	400	400	400	400	400
Volume (ml)	80	50	60	80	90	100	120	130	140	150	170	180
90 mg/kg/d ml/dose bid	4	5	6.5	8	9	10	11.5	13	14	15.5	16.5	18
mg/5ml	400	400	400	400	400	400	400	400	400	400	400	400
Volume (ml)	80	100	130	160	180	200	240	260	280	300	340	360

Augmentin Suspension (B)(G) 40–45 mg/kg/day divided tid or 90 mg/kg/day divided bid: 125mg/5 ml (75, 100, 150 ml) (banana), 250 mg/5 ml (75, 100, 150 ml) (orange); 200, 400 mg/5 ml (50, 75, 100 ml) (orange-raspberry) (phenylalanine).

APPENDIX CC.5: *AMOXICILLIN/CLAVULANATE* (AUGMENTIN ES 600 SUSPENSION)

Weight

Pounds	15	20	25	30	35	40	45	50	55	60	65	70
Kilograms	6.8	9	11.4	13.6	15.9	18.2	20.5	22.7	25	27.3	29.5	31.8

Single Dose (ml)/Frequency/Strength/10-Day Volume (ml)

	15	20	25	30	35	40	45	50	55	60	65	70
40 mg/kg/d ml/dose bid	1	1.5	2	2	2.5	3	3.5	4	4	4.5	5	5
mg/5ml	600	600	600	600	600	600	600	600	600	600	600	600
Volume (ml)	30	40	40	40	50	60	70	80	80	90	100	100
45 mg/kg/d ml/dose bid	1.25	1.5	2	2.5	3	3.5	4	4.5	5	5	5.5	6
mg/5ml	600	600	600	600	600	600	600	600	600	600	600	600
Volume (ml)	25	30	40	50	60	70	80	90	100	100	110	120
90 mg/kg/d ml/dose bid	2.5	3.5	4	5	6	7	8	8.5	9.5	10	11	12
mg/5ml	600	600	600	600	600	600	600	600	600	600	600	600
Volume (ml)	50	70	80	100	120	140	160	170	190	200	220	240

Augmentin ES 600 Suspension (B) <3 months: not recommended; ≥3 months, <40 kg: 90 mg/kg/day in 2 divided doses; ≥40 kg: not recommended; 600 mg/5 ml (50, 75, 100, 125, 150, 200 ml) (strawberry cream) (phenylalanine).

APPENDIX CC.6: *AMPICILLIN* (OMNIPEN SUSPENSION, PRINCIPEN SUSPENSION)

Weight

Pounds	15	20	25	30	35	40	45	50	55	60	65	70
Kilograms	6.8	9	11.4	13.6	15.9	18.2	20.5	22.7	25	27.3	29.5	31.8

Single Dose (ml)/Frequency/Strength/10-Day Volume (ml)

50 mg/kg/d ml/dose q6h	3.5	4.5	3	3.5	4	4.5						
mg/5ml	125	125	250	250	250	250						
Volume (ml)	140	180	120	140	160	180						
100 mg/kg/d ml/dose q6h	3.5	4.5	6	7	8	9						
mg/5ml	250	250	250	250	250	250						
Volume (ml)	140	180	240	280	320	360						

Omnipen Suspension, Principen Suspension (B)(G) >20 kg: 250–500 mg q 6 h 125, 250 mg/5 ml (100, 150, 200 ml) (fruit).

APPENDIX CC.7: *AZITHROMYCIN* (ZITHROMAX SUSPENSION, ZMAX SUSPENSION)

Weight								
Pounds	11	22	33	44	55	66	77	88
Kilograms	5	10	15	20	25	30	35	40
Single Dose (ml)/Frequency/Strength/Volume (ml)								
3 Day Regimen								
10 mg/kg qd	2.5	5	7.5	5	6	7.5	9	10
mg/5ml	100	100	100	200	200	200	200	200
Volume (ml)	7.5	15	22.5	15	18	22.5	27	30
5 Day Regimen								
10 mg/kg qd								
Day 1	2.5	5	7.5	5	6	7.5	7.5	10
Days 2–5	1.25	2.5	4	2.5	3	4	4	5
mg/5ml	100	100	100	200	200	200	200	200
Volume (ml)	10	15	23.5	15	18	23.5	23.5	30

Zithromax ES 600 Suspension (B)(G) 100 mg/5 ml (15 ml), 200 mg/5 ml (15, 22.5, 30 ml) (cherry-vanilla-banana).

APPENDIX CC.8: *CEFACLOR* (CECLOR SUSPENSION)

Weight													
Pounds	15	20	25	30	35	40	45	50	55	60	65	70	
Kilograms	6.8	9	11.4	13.6	15.9	18.2	20.5	22.7	25	27.3	29.5	31.8	
Single Dose (ml)/Frequency/Strength/10-Day Volume (ml)													
20 mg/kg/d ml/dose tid	2	2.5	3	3.5	4	5	5.5	6	7	7.5	8	8.5	
mg/5ml	125	125	125	125	125	125	125	125	125	125	125	125	
Volume (ml)	60	75	90	105	120	150	165	180	210	225	240	255	
20 mg/kg/d ml/dose tid	1.5	1.5	2	2.5	3	3	4	4	4.5	5	5.5	6	
mg/5ml	187	187	187	187	187	187	187	187	187	187	187	187	
Volume (ml)	45	45	60	75	90	90	105	120	135	150	165	180	
40 mg/kg/d ml/dose tid	2	2.5	3	3.5	4	5	5.5	6	6.5	7	8	8.5	
mg/5ml	250	250	250	250	250	250	250	250	250	250	250	250	
Volume (ml)	60	75	90	105	120	150	165	180	195	210	240	255	
40 mg/kg/d ml/dose tid	1.5	1.5	2	2.5	3	3	3.5	4	4.5	5	5	5.5	
mg/5ml	375	375	375	375	375	375	375	375	375	375	375	375	
Volume (ml)	45	45	60	75	90	90	105	120	135	150	150	165	

Ceclor Suspension (B) <6 months: not recommended; 125, 250 mg/5 ml (75, 150 ml) (strawberry); 187, 375 mg/5ml (50, 100 ml) (strawberry).

APPENDIX CC.9: *CEFADROXIL* (DURICEF SUSPENSION)

Weight												
Pounds	15	20	25	30	35	40	45	50	55	60	65	70
Kilograms	6.8	9	11.4	13.6	15.9	18.2	20.5	22.7	25	27.3	29.5	31.8
Single Dose (ml)/Frequency/Strength/10-Day Volume (ml)												
30 mg/kg/d ml/dose bid	2	3	3.5	4	5	5.5	6	7	7.5	8	9	9.5
mg/5ml	250	250	250	250	250	250	250	250	250	250	250	250
Volume (ml)	40	60	75	80	100	110	120	140	150	160	180	190
30 mg/kg/d ml/dose qd	2	3	3.5	4	5	5.5	6	7	7.5	8	9	9.5
mg/5ml	500	500	500	500	500	500	500	500	500	500	500	500
Volume (ml)	20	30	35	40	50	55	60	70	75	80	90	95

Duricef Suspension (B) 250 mg/5 ml (100 ml) (orange-pineapple); 500 mg/5ml (75, 100 ml) (orange-pineapple).

APPENDIX CC.10: *CEFDINIR* (OMNICEF SUSPENSION)

Weight												
Pounds	15	20	25	30	35	40	45	50	55	60	65	70
Kilograms	6.8	9	11.4	13.6	15.9	18.2	20.5	22.7	25	27.3	29.5	31.8
Single Dose (ml)/Frequency/Strength/10-Day Volume (ml)												
7 mg/kg/d ml/dose bid	2	2.5	3	4	4.5	5	6	6.5	7	7.5	8	9
mg/5ml	125	125	125	125	125	125	125	125	125	125	125	125
Volume (ml)	40	50	60	80	90	100	120	130	140	150	160	180
14 mg/kg ml/dose bid	4	5	6	8	9	10	12	13	14	15	16	18
mg/5ml	125	125	125	125	125	125	125	125	125	125	125	125
Volume (ml)	40	50	60	80	90	100	120	130	140	150	160	180

Omnicef Suspension (B) <6 months: not recommended; 125 mg/5 ml (60, 100 ml) (strawberry).

◯ APPENDIX CC.11: *CEFIXIME* (SUPRAX ORAL SUSPENSION)

Weight												
Pounds	15	20	25	30	35	40	45	50	55	60	65	70
Kilograms	6.8	9	11.4	13.6	15.9	18.2	20.5	22.7	25	27.3	29.5	31.8
Single Dose (ml)/Frequency/Strength/10-Day Volume (ml)												
8 mg/kg/d ml/dose bid	1.3	1.8	2.2	2.5	3.1	3.5	4	4.5	5	5.5	6	6.5
mg/5ml	100	100	100	100	100	100	100	100	100	100	100	100
8 mg/kg/d ml/dose qd	2.7	3.6	4.5	5.5	6.3	7.2	8.2	9	10	11	12	13
mg/5ml	100	100	100	100	100	100	100	100	100	100	100	100
Volume (ml)	27	36	45	55	65	70	80	90	100	110	120	130

Supra Oral Suspension (B)(G) <6 months: not recommended; 100 mg/5 ml (50, 75, 100 ml) (strawberry).

APPENDIX CC.12: *CEFPODOXIME PROXETIL* (VANTIN SUSPENSION)

Weight												
Pounds	15	20	25	30	35	40	45	50	55	60	65	70
Kilograms	6.8	9	11.4	13.6	15.9	18.2	20.5	22.7	25	27.3	29.5	31.8
Single Dose (ml)/Frequency/Strength/10-Day Volume (ml)												
5 mg/kg/d ml/dose bid	3.5	4.5	5.5	7	8	9	10	11	12.5	13.5	15	16
mg/5ml	50	50	50	50	50	50	50	50	50	50	50	50
Volume (ml)	70	90	110	140	160	180	200	220	250	270	300	320
5 mg/kg/d ml/dose bid	2	2	3	3.5	4	4.5	5	5.5	6	7	7.5	8
mg/5ml	100	100	100	100	100	100	100	100	100	100	100	100
Volume (ml)	40	40	60	70	80	90	100	110	120	140	150	160

Vantin Suspension (B) <2 months: not recommended; 50, 100 mg/5 ml (50, 75, 100 ml) (lemon-crème).

APPENDIX CC.13: *CEFPROZIL* (CEFZIL SUSPENSION)

Weight

Pounds	15	20	25	30	35	40	45	50	55	60	65	70
Kilograms	6.8	9	11.4	13.6	15.9	18.2	20.5	22.7	25	27.3	29.5	31.8
Single Dose (ml)/Frequency/Strength/10-Day Volume (ml)												
7.5 mg/kg/d ml/dose bid	2	3	3.5	4	5	5.5	6	7	7.5	4	4.5	5
mg/5ml	125	125	125	125	125	125	125	125	125	250	250	250
Volume (ml)	40	60	70	80	100	110	120	140	150	80	90	100
15 mg/kg/d ml/dose bid	2	3	3.5	4	5	5	6	7	7.5	8	9	9.5
mg/5ml	250	250	250	250	250	250	250	250	250	250	250	250
Volume (ml)	40	60	70	80	100	100	120	140	150	160	180	190
20 mg/kg/d ml/dose qd	3	3.5	4.5	5.5	6.5	7	8	9	10	11	12	13
mg/5ml	250	250	250	250	250	250	250	250	250	250	250	250
Volume (ml)	60	70	90	110	130	140	160	180	200	220	240	260

Cefzil Suspension (B) ≤6 months: not recommended; 2–12 years: 7.5–20 mg/kg bid >12 years: same as adult, 250–500 mg once daily; 125, 250 mg/5 ml (50, 75, 100 ml) (bubble gum) (phenylalanine).

APPENDIX CC.14: *CEFTIBUTEN* (CEDAX SUSPENSION)

Weight												
Pounds	15	20	25	30	35	40	45	50	55	60	65	70
Kilograms	6.8	9	11.4	13.6	15.9	18.2	20.5	22.7	25	27.3	29.5	31.8
Single Dose (ml)/Frequency/Strength/10-Day Volume (ml)												
9 mg/kg/d ml/dose qd	3.5	4.5	6	7	8	9	10	11.5	12.5	13.5	15	16
90 mg/5ml	90	90	90	90	90	90	90	90	90	90	90	90
Volume (ml)	35	45	60	70	80	90	100	115	125	135	150	160
9 mg/kg/d ml/dose qd	1.75	2.3	3	3.5	4	4.5	5	5.4	6.2	6.6	7.5	8
180 mg/5ml	180	180	180	180	180	180	180	180	180	180	180	180
Volume (ml)	20	25	30	35	40	45	50	55	60	65	70	80

Cefzil Suspension (B) 90 mg/5 ml (30, 60, 90, 120 ml) (cherry); 180 mg/5ml (30, 60, 120 ml) (cherry).

APPENDIX CC.15: *CEFUROXIME AXETIL* (CEFTIN SUSPENSION)

Weight												
Pounds	15	20	25	30	35	40	45	50	55	60	65	70
Kilograms	6.8	9	11.4	13.6	15.9	18.2	20.5	22.7	25	27.3	29.5	31.8
Single Dose (ml)/Frequency/Strength/10-Day Volume (ml)												
20 mg/kg/d ml/dose bid	2.5	3.5	4.5	3	3	3.5	4	4.5	5	5.5	6	6.5
mg/5ml	125	125	125	250	250	250	250	250	250	250	250	250
Volume (ml)	50	70	90	60	60	70	80	90	100	110	120	130
30 mg/kg/d ml/dose bid	2	3	3.5	4	5	5.5	6	7	7.5	8	9	9.5
mg/5ml	250	250	250	250	250	250	250	250	250	250	250	250
Volume (ml)	40	60	70	80	100	110	120	140	150	160	180	190

Ceftin Suspension (B) 125, 250 mg/5 ml (50, 100 ml) (tutti-frutti).

APPENDIX CC.16: *CEPHALEXIN* (KEFLEX SUSPENSION)

Weight												
Pounds	15	20	25	30	35	40	45	50	55	60	65	70
Kilograms	6.8	9	11.4	13.6	15.9	18.2	20.5	22.7	25	27.3	29.5	31.8
Single Dose (ml)/Frequency/Strength/10-Day Volume (ml)												
25 mg/kg/d ml/dose tid	1	1.5	2	2	3	3	3.5	4	4	4.5	5	5
mg/5ml	125	125	125	125	125	125	125	125	125	125	125	125
Volume (ml)	30	45	60	60	90	90	105	120	120	135	150	150
25 mg/kg/d ml/dose qid	1	1	1.5	2	2	2.5	2.5	3	3	3.5	4	4
mg/5ml	250	250	250	250	250	250	250	250	250	250	250	250
Volume (ml)	40	40	60	80	80	100	100	120	120	140	160	160
50 mg/kg/d ml/dose tid	2	3	4	4.5	5	6	7	7.5	8	9	10	10.5
mg/5ml	250	250	250	250	250	250	250	250	250	250	250	250
Volume (ml)	60	90	120	135	150	180	210	225	240	270	300	315
50 mg/kg/d ml/dose qid	2	2	3	3.5	4	4.5	5	6	6	7	7.5	8
mg/5ml	250	250	250	250	250	250	250	250	250	250	250	250
Volume (ml)	80	80	120	140	160	180	200	240	240	280	300	320

Keflex Suspension (B)(G) <2 months: not recommended; 125, 250 mg/5 ml (100, 200 ml) (strawberry).

APPENDIX CC.17: *CLARITHROMYCIN* (BIAXIN SUSPENSION)

Weight												
Pounds	15	20	25	30	35	40	45	50	55	60	65	70
Kilograms	6.8	9	11.4	13.6	15.9	18.2	20.5	22.7	25	27.3	29.5	31.8
Single Dose (ml)/Frequency/Strength/10-Day Volume (ml)												
7.5 mg/kg/d ml/dose bid	2	3	3.5	4	5	5.5	6	7	7.5	8	9	10
mg/5ml	125	125	125	125	125	125	125	125	125	125	125	125
Volume (ml)	40	60	70	80	100	110	120	140	150	160	180	200
7.5 mg/kg/d ml/dose bid	1	1.5	2	2	2.5	3	3	3.5	4	4	4.5	5
mg/5ml	250	250	250	250	250	250	250	250	250	250	250	250
Volume (ml)	20	30	40	40	50	60	60	70	80	80	90	100

Biaxin Suspension (B) <6 months: not recommended; 125, 250 mg/5 ml (50, 100 ml) (fruit-punch).

APPENDIX CC.18: *CLINDAMYCIN* (CLEOCIN PEDIATRIC GRANULES)

Weight												
Pounds	15	20	25	30	35	40	45	50	55	60	65	70
Kilograms	6.8	9	11.4	13.6	15.9	18.2	20.5	22.7	25	27.3	29.5	31.8
Single Dose (ml)/Frequency/Strength/10-Day Volume (ml)												
8 mg/kg/d ml/dose tid	1	1.5	2	2.5	3	3	3.5	4	4.5	5	5	5.5
mg/5ml	75	75	75	75	75	75	75	75	75	75	75	75
Volume (ml)	30	45	60	75	90	90	105	120	135	150	150	165
16 mg/kg/d ml/dose tid	2.5	3	4	5	5.5	6.5	7	8	9	9.5	10.5	11
mg/5ml	75	75	75	75	75	75	75	75	75	75	75	75
Volume (ml)	75	90	120	150	165	105	210	240	270	285	315	330

Cleocin Pediatric Granules (B)(G) 75 mg/5 ml (100 ml) (cherry).

APPENDIX CC.19: *DICLOXACILLIN* (DYNAPEN SUSPENSION)

Weight												
Pounds	15	20	25	30	35	40	45	50	55	60	65	70
Kilograms	6.8	9	11.4	13.6	15.9	18.2	20.5	22.7	25	27.3	29.5	31.8
Single Dose (ml)/Frequency/Strength/10-Day Volume (ml)												
12.5 mg/kg/d ml/dose qid	2	2.5	3	3.5	4	4.5	5	6	6	7	7.5	8
mg/5ml	62.5	62.5	62.5	62.5	62.5	62.5	62.5	62.5	62.5	62.5	62.5	62.5
Volume (ml)	80	100	120	140	160	180	200	240	240	280	300	320
25 mg/kg/d ml/dose qid	3.5	4.5	6	7	8	9	10	11.5	12.5	13.5	15	16
mg/5ml	62.5	62.5	62.5	62.5	62.5	62.5	62.5	62.5	62.5	62.5	62.5	62.5
Volume (ml)	140	180	240	280	320	360	400	460	500	540	600	640

Dynapen Suspension (B)(G) 6.25 mg/5 ml (80, 100 ml) (raspberry-strawberry).

APPENDIX CC.20: *DOXYCYCLINE* (VIBRAMYCIN SYRUP/SUSPENSION)

Weight												
Pounds	15	20	25	30	35	40	45	50	55	60	65	70
Kilograms	6.8	9	11.4	13.6	15.9	18.2	20.5	22.7	25	27.3	29.5	31.8
Single Dose (ml)/Frequency/Strength/10-Day Volume (ml)												
1 mg/lb/d ml/dose qd	1.5	2	2.5	3	3.5	4	4.5	5	5.5	6	6.5	7
50 mg/5ml	50	50	50	50	50	50	50	50	50	50	50	50
Volume (ml)	15	20	25	30	35	40	45	50	55	60	65	70
1 mg/lb/d ml/dose qd	3	4	5	6	7	8	9	10	11	12	13	14
25 mg/5ml	25	25	25	25	25	25	25	25	25	25	25	25
Volume (ml)	30	40	50	60	70	80	90	100	110	120	130	140

Vibramycin Syrup (B)(G) <8 years: not recommended; double dose first day; 50 mg/5 ml (80, 100, ml) (raspberry-apple) (sulfites).

Vibramycin Suspension (B)(G) <8 years: not recommended; double dose first day; 25 mg/5 ml (80, 100, ml) (raspberry).

APPENDIX CC.21: *ERYTHROMYCIN ESTOLATE* (ILOSONE SUSPENSION)

Weight												
Pounds	15	20	25	30	35	40	45	50	55	60	65	70
Kilograms	6.8	9	11.4	13.6	15.9	18.2	20.5	22.7	25	27.3	29.5	31.8
Dose/Volume (10 days) in ml												
10 mg/kg/d ml/dose bid	3	3.5	4.5	5.5	6	7	8	9	10	5.5	6	6.5
mg/5ml	125	125	125	125	125	125	125	125	125	250	250	250
Volume (ml)	60	70	90	110	120	140	160	180	200	110	120	130
15 mg/kg/d ml/dose bid	4	5.5	7	8	9.5	5.5	6	7	7.5	8	9	9.5
mg/5ml	125	125	125	125	125	250	250	250	250	250	250	250
Volume (ml)	80	110	140	160	190	110	120	140	150	160	180	190
20 mg/kg/d ml/dose bid	3	3.5	4.5	5.5	6.5	7	8	9	10	11	12	13
mg/5ml	250	250	250	250	250	250	250	250	250	250	250	250
Volume (ml)	60	70	90	110	120	140	160	180	200	220	240	260
25 mg/kg/d ml/dose bid	3.5	4.5	5.5	7	8	9	10	11.5	12.5	13.5	15	16
mg/5ml	250	250	250	250	250	250	250	250	250	250	250	250
Volume (ml)	70	90	110	140	160	180	200	230	250	280	300	320

Ilosone Suspension (B)(G) 125, 250 mg/5 ml (100 ml).

APPENDIX CC.22: *ERYTHROMYCIN ETHYLSUCCINATE* (E.E.S. SUSPENSION, ERY-PED DROPS/SUSPENSION)

Weight												
Pounds	15	20	25	30	35	40	45	50	55	60	65	70
Kilograms	6.8	9	11.4	13.6	15.9	18.2	20.5	22.7	25	27.3	29.5	31.8
Single Dose (ml)/Frequency/Strength/10-Day Volume (ml)												
30 mg/kg/d ml/dose qid	1.5	2	2	2.5	3	3.5	4	4	4.5	5	5.5	6
mg/5ml	200	200	200	200	200	200	200	200	200	200	200	200
Volume (ml)	60	80	80	100	120	140	160	160	180	200	220	240
30 mg/kg/d ml/dose qid			1	1.5	1.5	2	2	2	2.5	2.5	3	3
mg/5ml			400	400	400	400	400	400	400	400	400	
Volume (ml)			60	60	80	80	80	100	100	120	120	
50 mg/kg/d ml/dose qid	2	3	3.5	4.5	5	5.5	6.5	7	8	8.5	9	10
mg/5ml	200	200	200	200	200	200	200	200	200	200	200	200

(continued)

APPENDIX CC.22: *ERYTHROMYCIN ETHYLSUCCINATE (E.E.S. SUSPENSION, ERY-PED DROPS/SUSPENSION) (continued)*

Volume (ml)	80	120	140	180	200	220	260	280	320	340	360	400
50mg/kg/d ml/dose qid	1	1.5	2	2	2.5	3	3	3.5	4	4.5	4.5	5
mg/5ml	400	400	400	400	400	400	400	400	400	400	400	400
Volume (ml)	40	60	80	80	100	120	140	140	160	180	180	200

Ery-Ped Drops/Suspension (B)(G) 200 mg/5 ml (100, 200 ml; fruit); 400 mg/5 ml (60, 100, 200 ml) (banana); Oral drops: 200, 400 mg/5 ml (50 ml) (fruit).

E.E.S. Suspension (B)(G) 200 mg/5 ml, 400 mg/5 ml (100 ml) (fruit).

E.E.S. Granules (B)(G) 200 mg/5 ml (100, 200 ml) (cherry).

APPENDIX CC.23: *ERYTHROMYCIN/SULFAMETHOXAZOLE* (ERYZOLE, PEDIAZOLE)

Weight												
Pounds	15	20	25	30	35	40	45	50	55	60	65	70
Kilograms	6.8	9	11.4	13.6	15.9	18.2	20.5	22.7	25	27.3	29.5	31.8
Single Dose (ml)/Frequency/Strength/10-Day Volume (ml)												
10 mg/kg/d ml/dose bid	3	4	5	6	6.5	7.5	8.5	9.5	10	11	12	13.5
mg/5ml	200	200	200	200	200	200	200	200	200	200	200	200
Volume (ml)	90	120	150	180	200	225	255	285	300	330	360	400

Eryzole (C)(G) <2 months: not recommended; *eryth* 200 mg/*sulf* 600 mg/5 ml (100, 150, 200, 250 ml).

Pediazole (C)(G) <2 months: not recommended; *eryth* 200 mg/*sulf* 600 mg/5 ml (100, 150, 200 ml) (strawberry-banana).

APPENDIX CC.24: *FLUCONAZOLE* (DIFLUCAN SUSPENSION)

Weight												
Pounds	15	20	25	30	35	40	45	50	55	60	65	70
Kilograms	6.8	9	11.4	13.6	15.9	18.2	20.5	22.7	25	27.3	29.5	31.8
Single Dose (ml)/Frequency/Strength/21-Day Volume (ml)												
3 mg/kg/d ml/dose qd	2	3	3.5	4	5	5.5	6	7	7.5	8	9	9.5
mg/ml	10	10	10	10	10	10	10	10	10	10	10	10
Volume (ml)	44	66	77	88	110	121	132	154	165	176	198	209
6 mg/kg/d ml/dose qd	4	5.5	2	2	2.5	3	3	3.5	4	4	4.5	5
mg/ml	10	10	40	40	40	40	40	40	40	40	40	40
Volume (ml)	88	121	44	44	55	66	66	77	88	88	99	110

Diflucan Suspension (B)(G) double-dose first day; 10, 40 mg/5 ml (35 ml) (orange).

APPENDIX CC.25: *FURAZOLIDONE* (FUROXONE LIQUID)

Weight												
Pounds	15	20	25	30	35	40	45	50	55	60	65	70
Kilograms	6.8	9	11.4	13.6	15.9	18.2	20.5	22.7	25	27.3	29.5	31.8
Single Dose (ml)/Frequency/Strength/7-Day Volume (ml)												
5 mg/kg/d ml/dose qid	2.5	3.5	4	5	6	7	8	8.5	9.5	10	11	12
mg/15 ml	50	50	50	50	50	50	50	50	50	50	50	50
Vol	100	140	160	200	240	280	320	340	380	400	440	480

Furoxone Liquid (C)(G) double-dose first day; 50 mg/15 ml (35 ml).

APPENDIX CC.26: *GRISEOFULVIN, MICROSIZE* (GRIFULVIN V SUSPENSION)

Weight												
Pounds	15	20	25	30	35	40	45	50	55	60	65	70
Kilograms	6.8	9	11.4	13.6	15.9	18.2	20.5	22.7	25	27.3	29.5	31.8
Single Dose (ml)/Frequency/Strength/30-Day Volume (ml)												
5 mg/lb/d ml/dose day	3	4	5	6	7	8	9	10	11	12	13	14
mg/5ml	125	125	125	125	125	125	125	125	125	125	125	125
Volume (ml)	90	120	150	180	210	240	270	300	330	360	390	420

Grifulvin V Suspension (C)(G) double-dose first day; 125 mg/5 ml (120 ml) (orange) (alcohol 0.02%).

APPENDIX CC.27: *ITRACONAZOLE* (SPORANOX SOLUTION)

Weight												
Pounds	15	20	25	30	35	40	45	50	55	60	65	70
Kilograms	6.8	9	11.4	13.6	15.9	18.2	20.5	22.7	25	27.3	29.5	31.8
Single Dose (ml)/Frequency/Strength/7-Day Volume (ml)												
5 mg/kg/d ml/dose qd	3.5	4.5	6	7	8	9	10	11.5	12.5	14	15	16
mg/ml	10	10	10	10	10	10	10	10	10	10	10	10
Volume (ml)	25	32	42	49	56	63	70	71	88	98	105	112

Sporanox V Solution (C)(G) double-dose first day; 10 mg/ml (150 ml) (cherry-caramel).

APPENDIX CC.28: *LORACARBEF* (LORABID SUSPENSION)

Weight

Pounds	15	20	25	30	35	40	45	50	55	60	65	70
Kilograms	6.8	9	11.4	13.6	15.9	18.2	20.5	22.7	25	27.3	29.5	31.8

Single Dose (ml)/Frequency/Strength/10-Day Volume (ml)

	15	20	25	30	35	40	45	50	55	60	65	70
15 mg/kg/d ml/dose bid	2.5	3.5	4	5	3	3.5	4	4	5	5	5.5	6
mg/5ml	100	100	100	100	200	200	200	200	200	200	200	200
Volume (ml)	50	70	80	100	60	70	80	80	100	100	110	120
30 mg/kg/d ml/dose bid	2.5	3.5	4	5	6	7	8	8.5	9.5	10	11	12
mg/5ml	200	200	200	200	200	200	200	200	200	200	200	200
Volume (ml)	50	70	80	100	120	140	160	170	190	200	220	240

Lorabid Suspension (B) 100 mg/5 ml (50, 100 ml) (strawberry bubble gum); 200 mg/5 ml (50, 75, 100 ml) (strawberry bubble gum).

APPENDIX CC.29: *NITROFURANTOIN* (FURADANTIN SUSPENSION)

Weight												
Pounds	15	20	25	30	35	40	45	50	55	60	65	70
Kilograms	6.8	9	11.4	13.6	15.9	18.2	20.5	22.7	25	27.3	29.5	31.8
Single Dose (ml)/Frequency/Strength/10-Day Volume (ml)												
5 mg/kg ml/dose qid	1.5	2.5	3	3.5	4	4.5	5	5.5	6	7	7.5	8
mg/5 ml	25	25	25	25	25	25	25	25	25	25	25	25
Volume (ml)	60	100	120	140	160	190	200	220	240	280	300	320

Furadantin Suspension (B)(G) 25 mg/5 ml (60 ml).

APPENDIX CC.30: *PENICILLIN V POTASSIUM* (PEN-VEE K SOLUTION, VEETIDS SOLUTION)

Weight												
Pounds	15	20	25	30	35	40	45	50	55	60	65	70
Kilograms	6.8	9	11.4	13.6	15.9	18.2	20.5	22.7	25	27.3	29.5	31.8
Single Dose (ml)/Frequency/Strength/10-Day Volume (ml)												
25 mg/kg/d ml/dose qid	2	2.5	3	3.5	4	4.5	5	5.5	6	7	7.5	8
mg/5ml	125	125	125	125	125	125	125	125	125	125	125	125
Volume (ml)	80	90	120	140	160	180	200	220	240	280	300	320
25 mg/kg/d ml/dose qid	1	1	1.5	2	2	2.5	2.5	3	3	3.5	4	4
mg/5ml	250	250	250	250	250	250	250	250	250	250	250	250
Volume (ml)	40	40	60	80	80	100	100	120	120	140	160	160
50 mg/kg/d ml/dose qid	2	2.5	3	3.5	4	4.5	5	6	6.5	7	7.5	8
mg/5ml	250	250	250	250	250	250	250	250	250	250	250	250
Volume (ml)	80	100	120	140	160	180	200	240	260	280	300	320

Pen-Vee K Solution (B)(G) 125 mg/5 ml (100, 200 ml), 250 mg/5 ml (100, 150, 200 ml).

Veetids Solution (B)(G) 125, 250 mg/5 ml (100, 200 ml).

APPENDIX CC.31: *RIMANTADINE* (FLUMADINE SYRUP)

Weight												
Pounds	15	20	25	30	35	40	45	50	55	60	65	70
Kilograms	6.8	9	11.4	13.6	15.9	18.2	20.5	22.7	25	27.3	29.5	31.8
Single Dose (ml)/Frequency/Strength/10-Day Volume (ml)												
5 mg/kg/d ml/dose qd	3.5	4.5	6	7	8	9	10	11.5	12.5	13.5	15	16
mg/5ml	50	50	50	50	50	50	50	50	50	50	50	50
Volume (ml)	35	45	60	70	80	90	100	115	125	135	150	160

Flumadine Syrup (B) >10 years: same as adult; 50 mg/5 ml (2, 8, 16 oz) (raspberry).

APPENDIX CC.32: TETRACYCLINE (SUMYCIN SUSPENSION)

Weight												
Pounds	15	20	25	30	35	40	45	50	55	60	65	70
Kilograms	6.8	9	11.4	13.6	15.9	18.2	20.5	22.7	25	27.3	29.5	31.8
Single Dose (ml)/Frequency/Strength/10-Day Volume (ml)												
25 mg/kg/d ml/dose qid	1.5	2.5	3	3.5	4	4.5	5	6	6.5	7	7.5	8
mg/5ml	125	125	125	125	125	125	125	125	125	125	125	125
Volume (ml)	60	100	120	140	160	180	200	240	260	280	300	320
50 mg/kg/d ml/dose qid	3.5	4.5	6	7	8	9	10	11.5	12.5	13.5	15	16
mg/5ml	125	125	125	125	125	125	125	125	125	125	125	125
Volume (ml)	140	180	240	280	320	360	400	460	500	540	600	640

Sumycin Suspension (D)(G) <8 years: not recommended; 125 mg/5 ml (100, 200 ml) (fruit) (sulfites).

APPENDIX CC.33: *TRIMETHOPRIM* (PRIMSOL SUSPENSION)

Weight												
Pounds	15	20	25	30	35	40	45	50	55	60	65	70
Kilograms	6.8	9	11.4	13.6	15.9	18.2	20.5	22.7	25	27.3	29.5	31.8
Single Dose (ml)/Frequency/Strength/10-Day Volume (ml)												
5 mg/kg/d ml/dose bid	3.5	4.5	6	7	8	9	10	11.5	12.5	13.5	15	16
mg/5ml	50	50	50	50	50	50	50	50	50	50	50	50
Volume (ml)	70	90	120	140	160	180	200	230	250	270	300	320

Primsol Suspension (C)(G) 50 mg/5 ml (50 mg/5 ml) (bubble gum) (dye-free, alcohol-free).

APPENDIX CC.34: *TRIMETHOPRIM/SULFAMETHOXAZOLE* (BACTRIM SUSPENSION, SEPTRA SUSPENSION)

Weight												
Pounds	15	20	25	30	35	40	45	50	55	60	65	70
Kilograms	6.8	9	11.4	13.6	15.9	18.2	20.5	22.7	25	27.3	29.5	31.8
Single Dose (ml)/Frequency/Strength/10-Day Volume (ml)												
10 mg/kg/d ml/dose bid	2	2	3	3.5	4	4.5	5	5.5	6	7	7.5	8
mg/5ml	200	200	200	200	200	200	200	200	200	200	200	200
Volume (ml)	40	40	60	70	80	90	100	110	120	140	150	160
20 mg/kg/d ml/dose bid	4	4	6	7	8	9	10	11	12	14	15	16
mg/5ml	200	200	200	200	200	200	200	200	200	200	200	200
Volume (ml)	80	80	120	140	160	180	200	220	240	280	300	320

Bactrim Pediatric Suspension, Septra Pediatric Suspension (C)(G) *trim* 40 mg/*sulfa* 200 mg/5 ml (100 ml) (cherry) (alcohol 0.3%).

APPENDIX CC.35: *VANCOMYCIN* (VANCOCIN SUSPENSION)

Weight												
Pounds	15	20	25	30	35	40	45	50	55	60	65	70
Kilograms	6.8	9	11.4	13.6	15.9	18.2	20.5	22.7	25	27.3	29.5	31.8
Single Dose (ml)/Frequency/Strength/10-Day Volume (ml)												
40 mg/kg/d ml/dose tid	2	2.5	3	3.5	4.5	5	5.5	6	7	7.5	8	8.5
mg/5ml	250	250	250	250	250	250	250	250	250	250	250	250
Volume (ml)	60	75	90	105	135	150	165	180	210	225	240	255
40 mg/kg/d ml/dose qid	1.5	2	2.5	3	3	3.5	4	4.5	5	5.5	6	6.5
mg/5ml	250	250	250	250	250	250	250	250	250	250	250	250
Volume (ml)	60	80	100	120	120	140	160	180	200	220	240	260
40 mg/kg/d ml/dose tid	1	1	1.5	2	2	2.5	3	3	3.5	3.5	4	4
mg/6ml	500	500	500	500	500	500	500	500	500	500	500	500
Volume (ml)	30	30	45	60	60	75	90	90	105	105	120	120
40 mg/kg/d ml/dose qid	1	1	1.5	1.5	1.5	2	2	2.5	2.5	3	3	3.5
mg/6ml	500	500	500	500	500	500	500	500	500	500	500	500
Volume (ml)	40	40	60	60	60	80	80	100	100	120	120	140

Vancomycin Suspension (C)(G).

RESOURCES

Information in the *The APRN's Complete Guide to Prescribing Drug Therapy 2017* is retrieved from professional juried nurse practitioner, medical, and pharmacy textbooks and professional publications, the Centers for Disease Control and Prevention, The National Institutes of Health, pharmaceutical company-created marketing materials, drug product package inserts, the Food and Drug Administration, and pharmaceutics websites as listed below:

Advance for Nurse Practitioners
http://nurse-practitioners.advanceweb.com

Advanced Practice Education Associates
www.apea.com

American Association of Nurse Practitioners
www.aanp.org

American Academy of Pediatrics (AAP)
http://aapexperience.org/

American College of Cardiology. Then and now: ATP III vs. IV: Comparison of ATP III and ACC/AHA guidelines.
http://www.acc.org/latest-in-cardiology/articles/2014/07/18/16/03/then-and-now-atp-iii-vs-iv

American Diabetes Association (ADA), Professional Diabetes Resources Online
http://professional.diabetes.org/content/clinical-practice-recommendations/?loc=rp-slabnav

American diabetes association standards of medical care. *Diabetes Care 2016, 38* (Suppl. 1).
http://care.diabetesjournals.org/content/38/Supplement_1

American Family Physician
http://www.aafp.org/online/en/home.html

American Geriatrics Society 2015 Beers Criteria Update Expert Panel. American geriatrics society 2015 updated Beers Criteria for potentially inappropriate medication use in older adults. *Journal of the American Geriatrics Society, 63*(11), 2227–2246.

American Headache Society
www.americanheadachesociety.org

American Pain Society
http://americanpainsociety.org/

CDC: Morbidity and Mortality Weekly Report (MMWR)
http://www.cdc.gov/mmwr/mmwr_wk.html

CDC 2015 Sexually Transmitted Diseases Treatment Guidelines
http://www.cdc.gov/std/tg2015/default.htm

Centers for Disease Control and Prevention
www.cdc.gov

Chow, A. W., Benninger, M. S., Brook, I., Brozek, J. L., Goldstein, E. J., Hicks, L. A., . . .
File, T. M., Jr., Infectious Disease Society of America. (2012). IDSA clinical practice
guideline for acute and bacterial rhinosinusitis in children and adults. *Clinical Infectious
Diseases, 54*(8), e72–e112.

Clinician Reviews
http://www.clinicianreviews.com/

Consultant 360
http://www.consultant360.com/home

Daily Med: NIH. US Library of Medicine
https://dailymed.nlm.nih.gov/dailymed/index.cfm

Domino, F. J., Baldor, R. A., Golding, J., & Stephens, M. B. *The 5-minute clinical consult
standard 2016.* Philadelphia, PA: Wolters Kluwer.

DRUGS.COM
www.drugs.com

DRUGS at FDA: FDA Approved Drug Products
http://www.accessdata.fda.gov/scripts/cder/drugsatfda/index.cfm

epocrates
https://online.epocrates.com/drugs

eMPR: Monthly Prescribing Reference (new FDA approved products, new generics,
new drug withdrawals, safety alerts)
http://www.empr.com/

FDA: Recalls, Market Withdrawals, and Safety alerts
http://www.fda.gov/Safety/Recalls/default.htm

Gilbert, D. N., Chambers, H. F., Eliopoulos, G. M., Saag, M. S., & Pavla, A. T. *The sanford
guide to antimicrobial therapy, 2016.* Sperryville, VA: Antimicrobial Therapy.

International Diabetes Federation (IDF) Clinical Practice Guidelines
http://www.idf.org/guidelines

James, P. A., Oparil, S., Carter, B. L., Cushman, W. C., Dennison-Himmelfarb, C., Handler, J., . . . Ortiz, E. (2014). 2014 evidence-based guidelines for the management of high blood pressure in adults: Report from the panel members appointed to the eighth joint national committee (JNC 8). *Journal of the American Medical Association, 311*(5), 507–520.

JNC 8 Guideline Summary. *Pharmacist's Letter/Prescriber's Letter*
https://www.scribd.com/doc/290772273/JNC-8-guideline-summary

Journal of the American Academy of Nurse Practitioners
https://www.aanp.org/publications/jaanp

Journal of the American Medical Association (JAMA) Internal Medicine
http://archinte.jamanetwork.com/journal.aspx

Journal of the American Geriatrics Society
http://onlinelibrary.wiley.com/journal/10.1111/(ISSN)1532-5415

Lieberthal, A. S., Carroll, A. E., Chonmaitree, T., Ganiats, T. G., Hoberman, A., Jackson, M. A., . . . Tunkel, D. E. (2013). The diagnosis and management of acute otitis media. *Pediatrics, 131*(3), e964–e999.

Mandell, L. A. Wunderink, R. G., Anzueto, A., Bartlett, J. G., Campbell, G. D., Dean, N. C., . . . Whitney, C. G. (2007). Infectious diseases society of America/American Thoracic Society consensus guidelines on the management of community-acquired pneumonia in adults. *Clinical Infectious Diseases, 44* (Suppl. 2), S27–S72.
https://enp-network.s3.amazonaws.com/NPA_Long_Island/pdf/Pneumonia.pdf

McMillan, J. A., Lee, C. K. K., Siberry, G. K., & Carroll, K. C. (2013). *The Harriet Lane handbook of pediatric antimicrobial therapy*. Philadelphia, PA: Elsevier Saunders.

MedlinePlus
https://www.nlm.nih.gov/medlineplus/ency/article/000165.htm

MedPage Today
http://www.medpagetoday.com/

Medscape
http://www.medscape.com/

National Academy of Medicine
http://nam.edu/

National Cholesterol Education Program Expert Panel on Detection, Evaluation, and Treatment of High Blood Cholesterol in Adults (Adult Treatment Panel IV, 2012).
http://circ.ahajournals.org/content/circulationaha/106/25/3143.full.pdf

National Heart Lung and Blood Institute (NHLBI)
  http://www.nhlbi.nih.gov/

New England Journal of Medicine (NEJM) Journal Watch General Medicine
  http://www.jwatch.org/general-medicine

Pharmacist's Letter
  www.pharmacistsletter.com

Physician's Desk Reference (PDR)
  http://www.pdr.net/

Prescriber's Letter
  http://prescribersletter.therapeuticresearch.com/pl/sample.aspx?cs=&s=PRL&
  AspxAutoDetectCookieSupport=1

Psychopharmacology
  http://link.springer.com/journal/213

Reference for Interpretation of Hepatitis C Virus (HCV) Test Results
  www.cdc.gov/hepatitis

RxLIST
  http://www.rxlist.com/script/main/hp.asp

RxLIST: Drugs A-Z
  http://www.rxlist.com/drugs/alpha_a.htm

Sanford Guide Web Edition
  https://webedition.sanfordguide.com

Solutions for Safer ER/LA Opioid Prescribing in a New Era of Health Care. American
Nurses Credentialing Center, Post Graduate Institute of Medicine
  www.cmeuniversity.com

The American Congress of Obstetrics and Gynecology (ACOG)
  http://www.acog.org/

The American Geriatric Society
  http://www.americangeriatrics.org

The Handbook of Antimicrobial Therapy (20th ed.). The Medical Letter

The Journal for Nurse Practitioners
  www.elsevier.com/locate/tjnp

The Medical Letter on Drugs and Therapeutics (subscription)
  http://secure.medicalletter.org/

The Nurse Practitioner Journal
   www.tnpj.com

Third Report of the National Cholesterol Education Program (NCEP) Expert Panel on Detection, Evaluation, and Treatment of High Blood Cholesterol in Adults (Adult Treatment Panel III) final report.
   http://www.ncbi.nlm.nih.gov/pubmed/12485966

Treatment Guidelines [Annual Volume]: The Medical Letter

Updated CDC guidance: Superbugs threaten hospital patients. *Medscape Education Clinical Briefs* (March 31, 2016).
   http://www.medscape.org/viewarticle/859361?nlid=105320_2713&src=wnl_cmemp_160523_mscpedu_nurs&impID=1106718&faf=1

U.S. Pharmacist Weekly Newsletter
   http://www.uspharmacist.com

Wald, E. R., Applegate, K. E., Bordley, C., Darrow, D. H., Glode, M. P., Marcy, S. M., . . . Weinberg, S. T., American Academy of Pediatrics. (2013). Clinical practice guidelines for the diagnosis and management of acute bacterial sinusitis in children 1 to 18 years. *Pediatrics, 132*(1), e262–280.
   http://www.ncbi.nlm.nih.gov/pubmed/23796742

WebMD: Drugs and Medications A to Z. Latest Drug News
   http://www.webmd.com/drugs/

See **Appendix A** for descriptions of FDA pregnancy categories
See **Appendix B** for descriptions of controlled drug categories
NR=not rated (not applicable *or* not yet assigned)

FDA Pregnancy Category	DEA Schedule	Drug	Page Numbers
C		*abacavir*, **Ziagen**	194, 515
C		**A/B Otic**, *antipyrine/benzocaine/glycerin*	289, 294
C		*abatacept*, **Orencia**	372
C		**Abilify**, *aripiprazole*	48, 52, 110, 506
NR		**Abreva**, *docosanol*	188
C		**Abstral**, *fentanyl citratesublingual tablet*	305
C		*acamprosate*, **Campral**	10
C		**Acanya**, *clindamycin/benzoyl peroxide gel*	5, 149
B		*acarbose*, **Precose**	423
B		**Accolate**, *zafirlukast*	28, 373
C		**Accuneb**, *albuterol*	31
D		**Accupril**, *quinapril*	175, 204
D		**Accuretic**, *quinapril/hydrochlorothiazide*	209
X		**Accutane**, *isotretinoin, retinoic acid*	7
B		*acebutolol*, **Sectral**	200, 503
D		**Aceon**, *perindopril*	204
B		**Acetadote**, *acetylcysteine*	3

FDA Pregnancy Category	DEA Schedule	Drug	Page Numbers
B		*acetaminophen*, **Feverall**, **Ofirmev**, **Panadol**, **Tempra**, **Tylenol**	143, 144, 296
C		*acetazolamide*, **Diamox**, **Diamox Sequels**	158
NR		*acetic acid*, **Domeboro Otic**	289
B		*acetylcysteine*, **Acetadote**	3
D		*acetylsalicylic acid*, *aspirin*, **Bayer**, **Easprin**, **Durlaza**, **Ecotrin**	144, 518
B		**AcipHex, Aciphex Sprinkle**, *rabeprazole*	154, 319, 455
X		*acitretin*, **Soriatane**	357
C		*aclidinium bromide*, **Tudorza Pressair**	64, 135
C		**Aclovate**, *alclometasone dipropionate*	494
C		**Actemra**, *tocilizumab*	371–372
D		**Acticlate**, *doxycycline*	4, 5, 21, 54, 55, 61, 72, 80, 82, 83, 139, 160, 165, 190, 246, 249, 316, 334, 351, 531
B		**Actigall**, *ursodiol*	46, 80
C		**Actimmune**, *interferon gamma-1b*	262
C	II	**Actiq**, *fentanyl citrate transmucosal unit*	305
X		**Activella**, *estradiol/ norethindrone*	256, 284
C		**Actoplus Met, Actoplus Met XR**, *pioglitazone/metformin*	425–426
C		**Actonel**, *risedronate (as sodium)*	286–287, 295

FDA Pregnancy Category	DEA Schedule	Drug	Page Numbers
B/D		**Azulfidine, Azulfidine EN-Tabs,** *sulfasalazine*	435–436
C		**Babylax,** *glycerin suppository*	137
NR		*bacillus athracis immune globulin intravenous (human),* **Anthrasil**	20
C		*bacitracin,* **Bacitracin Ophthalmic**	89
C		**Bacitracin Ophthalmic,** *bacitracin*	89
C		*baclofen,* **Lioresal**	262
C		**Bactrim, Bactrim DS,** *sulfamethoxazole/trimethoprim*	122, 165, 290, 293, 323, 329, 337, 338, 352, 353, 538
B		**Bactroban,** *mupirocin*	224, 387, 451
C	IV	**Balacet,** *propoxyphene napsilate/ acetaminophen*	304
B		*balsalazide,* **Colazal**	435
X		**Balziva,** *ethinyl estradiol/ norethindrone*	476
C		**Banzel,** *rufinamide*	510
C		**Baraclude,** *entecavir*	182
C		**Basaglar,** *insulin glargine (recombinant)*	419
D		**Bayer,** *aspirin*	144
C		*becaplermin,* **Regranex Gel**	433, 434
C		*beclomethasone dipropionate,* **Beconase AQ, QNASL, Qvar**	29, 373–374
C		**Beconase AQ,** *beclomethasone dipropionate*	373–374
B		*bedaquiline,* **Sirturo**	414
C	III	**Belbuca,** *buprenorphine*	279

FDA Pregnancy Category	DEA Schedule	Drug	Page Numbers
B		*budesonide*, Entocort EC, Pulmicort Respules, Pulmicort Flexhaler, Rhinocort, Rhinocort Aqua, Uceris	29, 101, 374, 434, 500
D		Bufferin, *aspirin/magnesium carbonate/magnesium oxide bumetanide*	145
C	III	Bunavail, *buprenorphine/ naloxone*	279–280
C		*bupivacaine liposome*, Exparel	487
C	III	Buprenex, *buprenorphine*	446
C	III	*buprenorphine*, Belbuca, Buprenex, Butrans, Subutex	279
C		*bupropion hydrobromide*, Aplenzin	109, 407
C		*bupropion hydrochloride*, Forfivo XL, Wellbutrin, Wellbutrin SR, Wellbutrin XL, Zyban	41, 109, 407, 507
B		BuSpar, *buspirone*	22, 310
B		*buspirone*, BuSpar	22, 310
B		*butenafine*, Mentax	67, 118, 400, 402, 404, 405
C		*butoconazole*, Femstat-3, Gynazole-1	70
C	IV	*butorphanol*, Stadol	173–174, 305
C		Butrans, *buprenorphine*	279, 304
C		Bydureon, *exenatide*	427
C		Byetta, *exenatide*	427
C		Bystolic, *nebivolol*	200
B		*cabergoline*, Dostinex	199
X		Cafergot, *ergotamine/caffeine*	167

FDA Pregnancy Category	DEA Schedule	Drug	Page Numbers
X		**Caduet,** *amlodipine/atorvastatin*	131, 215
C		**Calan, Calan SR,** *verapamil*	18, 170–171, 207, 501
C		*calcipotriene,* **Dovonex**	356
C		*calcitonin-salmon,* **Fortical, Miacalcin Injectable, Miacalcin Nasal Spray**	218, 284
C		*calcitriol,* **Rocaltrol, Vectical**	219, 221, 285, 356
C		*calcium acetate,* **PhosLo**	198
B		**Calcium Disodium Versenate,** *edetate calcium disodium (EDTA)*	244
C		*calcium polycarbophil,* **Fibercon, Konsyl**	95, 119
B/D		**Caldolor,** *ibuprofen*	296
X		**Camila,** *norethindrone*	484
C		**Campral,** *acamprosate*	10
X		**Camrese, Camrese Lo,** *ethinyl estradiol/levonorgestrel*	476
B		**Canasa,** *mesalamine*	100, 435
D		*candesartan,* **Atacand**	204
D		*capecitabine,* **Xeloda**	506
C		**Capex Shampoo,** *fluocinolone acetonide*	495
C		**Capitrol,** *chloroxine*	113
D		**Capoten,** *captopril*	174, 204
D		**Capozide,** *captopril/ hydrochlorothiazide*	209
B		*capsaicin,* **Capzasin-HP, Capzasin-P, Double Cap, Qutenza, Zostrix, Zostrix HP**	112, 115–116, 163, 241, 264, 265, 281–282, 297, 320, 340, 343, 354, 359, 368, 488

FDA Pregnancy Category	DEA Schedule	Drug	Page Numbers
C		**Celontin Kapseals,** *methsuximide*	510
X		**Cenestin,** *estrogens (conjugated)*	257
B		**Centany,** *mupirocin*	224, 387, 451
B		*cephalexin,* **Keflex**	42, 60, 74, 226, 248, 252, 292, 314, 325, 364, 381, 389, 410, 442, 452, 533, 557
B		*certolizumab,* **Cimzia**	102, 371
A		**Cerumenex,** *triethanolamine*	76
C		**Cesamet,** *nabilone*	269
C		**Cetamide,** *sulfacetamide*	57, 90, 394
B		*cetirizine,* **Zyrtec, Zyrtec Chewable Tablets**	87
C		*cevimeline,* **Evoxac**	386
C		**Chantix,** *varenicline*	407
C		**Chemet,** *succimer*	238, 244
B		**Children'sNasalCrom,** *cromolyn sodium*	375
D		*chlorambucil,* **Leukeran**	505
D	IV	*chlordiazepoxide,* **Librium**	9–10, 23, 311
B		*chlorhexidine gluconate,* **Peridex, PerioGard**	155
C		*chloroquine,* **Aralen**	251, 531
B		*chlorothiazide,* **Diuril**	131, 176, 202, 446
C		*chloroxine,* **Capitrol**	113
C		*chlorpromazine,* **Thorazine**	52–53, 190, 270, 507
C		*chlorpropamide,* **Diabinese**	422
B		*chlorthalidone,* **Thalitone**	132, 202

FDA Pregnancy Category	DEA Schedule	Drug	Page Numbers
C		Concerta, *methylphenidate*	39–40, 268
C		Condylox, *podofilox*	449, 450
B		Copaxone, *glatiramer acetate*	261
X		Copegus, *ribavirin*	183
C		Cordan, *flurandrenolide*	497
D		Cordarone, *amiodarone*	502
C		Cordran, Cordran SP, *flurandrenolide*	497
C		Coreg, *carvedilol*	175, 201
C		Corgard, *nadolol*	18, 170, 200
C		Cormax, *clobetasol propionate*	497
C		Cortaid, *hydrocortisone*	180, 434, 494
C		Cortane-B Otic, *hydrocortisone/ chloroxylenol/pramoxine*	288
C		Cortef, *hydrocortisone*	180, 434, 494
C		Cortenema, *hydrocortisone*	434
C		Cortifoam, *hydrocortisone*	180, 434, 494
C		Cortisporin Cream, Cortisporin Ophthalmic, Cortisporin Otic, *polymyxin B/neomycin/ hydrocortisone*	192, 289, 294
C		Cortisporin Ointment, *polymyxin B/bacitracin zinc/ neomycin/ hydrocortisone*	192
C		Corzide, *nadolol/ bendroflumethiazide*	211–212
C		Cosopt, *dorzolamide/timolol*	158
C		Cotazym, Cotazym S, *pancrelipase*	307
D		Coumadin, *warfarin*	322, 515–516

FDA Pregnancy Category	DEA Schedule	Drug	Page Numbers
X		Cytotec, *misoprostol*	319, 489
C		Cytovene, *ganciclovir*	511
D		Cytoxan, *cyclophosphamide*	504
C		*dabigatran etexilatemesylate*, Pradaxa	518, 519
X		*daclatasvir*, Daklinza	184
X		Daklinza, *daclatasvir*	184
C		*dalfampridine*, Ampyra	260
C		Daliresp, *roflumilast*	65
X	IV	Dalmane, *flurazepam*	147, 234
C		*dalteparin*, Fragmin	516
C		Dalvance, *dalbavancin*	74, 539
C		*dalbavancin*, Dalvance	74, 539
X		*danazol*, Danocrine	138, 146
X		Danocrine, *danazol*	138, 146
C		Dantrium, *dantrolene*	263
C		*dantrolene*, Dantrium	263
C		*dapagliflozin*, Farxiga	428
C		*dapsone*, Aczone	5, 149
B		*daptomycin*, Cubicin	539
C		*darbepoetin alpha*, Aranesp	15
C		*darifenacin*, Enablex	228
B		*darunavir*, Prezista	513
C	II	Daytrana, *methylphenidate*	40
C		Daypro, *oxaprozin*	492, 493
B		DDAVP Nasal Spray, *desmopressin*	138, 228
A		Debrox, *carbamide peroxide*	76

FDA Pregnancy Category	DEA Schedule	Drug	Page Numbers
C		*deferoxaminemesylate*, **Desferal**	244
C		*desipramine*, **Norpramin**	108, 117, 173, 342, 345, 413
C		*desirudin*, **Iprivask**	519
B		*desmopressin*, **DDAVP Nasal Spray, DDAVP Rhinal Tube Stimate**	138, 228
X		**Desogen-28**, *ethinyl estradiol/ desogestrel diacetate*	476
C		**Desonate**, *desonide*	111, 495
C		*desonide*, **Desonate, DesOwen, Tridesilon, Verdeso**	495
C		**DesOwen**, *desonide*	495
C		*desoximetasone*, **Topicort**	495, 496
C	II	**Desoxyn**, *methamphetamine*	39, 267, 273
C		**Desquam-X**, *benzoyl peroxide*	5
C		*desvenlafaxine*, **Pristiq**	107, 309, 347
C		**Detrol, Detrol LA**, *tolterodine*	228, 237
B		**Devrom**, *bismuth subgallate powder*	143
C		*dexamethasone*, **Decadron, Decadron LA, Maxidex**	85, 499
C	II	**Dexedrine**, *dextroamphetamine sulfate*	38, 267
B		**Dexilant**, *dexlansoprazole*	153, 318, 455
B		*dexlansoprazole*, **Dexilant**	153, 318, 455
C	II	*dexmethylphenidate*, **Focalin, Focalin XR**	39, 267
C	II	*dextroamphetamine sulfate*, **Dexedrine, Dextrostat**	38, 267

FDA Pregnancy Category	DEA Schedule	Drug	Page Numbers
B		**Double Cap,** *capsaicin*	112, 116, 163, 241, 264, 265, 282, 297, 320, 340, 343, 354, 359, 368
C		**Dovonex,** *calcipotriene*	356
C		*doxazosin,* **Cardura, Cardura XL**	45, 207, 230
C		*doxepin,* **Prudoxin, Silenor, Zonalon**	112, 343, 354
C		*doxercalciferol,* **Hectorol**	219, 221, 285
C		**Doxidan,** *docusate/ phenolphthalein*	97
D		*doxycycline,* **Acticlate, Adoxa, Doryx, Monodox, Oracea, Vibramycin, Vibra-Tab**	4, 5, 21, 54, 55, 61, 72, 80, 82, 83, 139, 160, 165, 190, 246, 249, 316, 334, 351, 377, 382–383, 389, 437, 442, 531, 538
B		**Dramamine,** *dimenhydrinate*	253, 259
B		**Dramamine II,** *meclizine*	243, 253, 259, 269, 448
C	III	*dronabinol,* **Marinol**	20, 269
C		*droxidopa,* **Northera**	223
C		**Dryvax,** *vaccina virus vaccine (dried calf lymph type)*	392
C		**Duac,** *clindamycin/benzoyl peroxide*	5, 149
X		**Duavee,** *conjugated estrogens/ bazedoxifene*	257, 284
A		**Duet DHA Balanced, Duet DHA Complete,** *prenatal vitamins*	521, 522
B/D		**Duexis,** *ibuprofen/famotidine*	491
C		*dulaglutide,* **Trulicity**	427

FDA Pregnancy Category	DEA Schedule	Drug	Page Numbers
D		**Efudex,** *fluorouracil, 5-fluorouracil, 5-FU*	9
C		**Elestat,** *epinastine*	87
C		*eletriptan,* **Relpax**	168
C		**Elidel,** *pimecrolimus*	112
X		**Eligard,** *leuprolide acetate*	505
B		**Elimite,** *permethrin*	380
C		**Eliquis,** *apixaban*	516–517
X		**ella,** *ulipristal*	487
B		**Elmiron,** *pentosan polysulfate sodium*	236
C		**Elocon,** *mometasone furoate*	496
B		*elvitegravir,* **Stribild**	513
C		**Emadine,** *emedastine difumarate*	86
C	II	**Embeda,** *morphine/naltrexone*	301
C		*emedastine difumarate,* **Emadine**	86
B		**Emend,** *aprepitant*	270
NR		**Emetrol,** *phosphorated carbohydrated solution*	269
C		*empagliflozen,* **Glyxambi**	429
C		**Emsam,** *selegiline*	109, 313, 349
B		*emtricitabine,* **Emtriva**	194, 511
B		**Emtriva,** *emtricitabine*	194, 511
B		**Emverm,** *mebendazole*	327, 530
C		**Enablex,** *darifenacin*	228
D		*enalapril,* **Epaned, Vasotec**	174, 204
B		**Enbrel,** *etanercept*	358, 361, 371
B		**Enduronyl, Enduronyl Forte,** *methyclothiazide/deserpidine*	133, 176, 202, 203

FDA Pregnancy Category	DEA Schedule	Drug	Page Numbers
B		*ethambutol,* Myambutol	414, 532
C		*ethotoin,* Peganone	509
C		*etodolac,* Lodine, Lodine XL	490
X		*etonogestrel,* Implanon, Nexplanon	485
C		Etrafon, *perphenazine/amitriptyline*	26
B		*etravirine,* Intelence	512
D		Eulexin, *flutamide*	505
C		Eurax, *crotamiton*	380
C	II	Evekeo, *amphetamine sulfate*	38, 266, 273
X		Evista, *raloxifene*	287
B		Evoclin Foam, *clindamycin*	5, 149
C		Evoxac, *cevimeline*	386
C	II	Exalgo, *hydromorphone*	300
D		Excedrin Migraine, *acetaminophen/aspirin/caffeine*	169
B		Excedrin PM, *acetaminophen/diphenhydramine*	235
C		Exelderm, *sulconazole nitrate*	401, 403, 404, 406
B		Exelon, *rivastigmine*	11
D		*exemestane,* Aromasin	504
C		*exenatide,* Bydureon, Byetta	427
D		Exforge, *amlodipine/valsartan*	214
D		Exforge HCT, *amlodipine/valsartan/hydrochlorothiazide*	214
B		Exjade, *deferasirox*	238
C		Exparel, *bupivacaine liposome*	487
C		Extavia, *interferon beta-1b*	262

FDA Pregnancy Category	DEA Schedule	Drug	Page Numbers
X		**Levlen-21, Levlen-28,** *ethinyl estradiol/levonorgestrel*	478
X		**Levlite-28,** *ethinyl estradiol/ levonorgestrel*	478
C		*levobunolol,* **Betagan**	157
C		*levocabastine,* **Livostin**	86
B		*levocetirizine,* **Xyzal**	529
C		*levodopa, l-dopa*	312
C		*levofloxacin,* **Levaquin**	61–62, 80, 140, 330, 335, 337, 365, 385–386, 390, 438–440, 443, 453, 535
C		*levofloxacin ophthalmic solution,* **Quixin**	90
C		*levomilnacipran,* **Fetzima**	106–107
X		*levonorgesterl,* **MyWay, Plan-B One Step**	486
X		**Levora-21, Levora-28,** *ethinyl estradiol/levonorgestrel*	478
A		*levothyroxine,* **Levoxyl, Synthroid, Unithroid**	223–224
C		**Levsin, Levsinex Timecaps,** *hyoscyamine*	83, 99, 228–229, 235–236, 240, 444–445
X		*levonorgestrel,* **EContra EZ**	487
X		*levonorgestrel IUD,* **Mirena, Skyla**	487
A		**Levoxyl,** *levothyroxine*	223
C		**Lexapro,** *escitalopram*	25, 106, 312
C		**Lexiva,** *fosamprenavir*	195, 512
B		**Lialda,** *mesalamine*	100, 435
D	IV	**Librium,** *chlordiazepoxide*	9–10, 23, 311

FDA Pregnancy Category	DEA Schedule	Drug	Page Numbers
B		*magnesium hydroxide*, **Milk of Magnesia**	96
C		**Malarone, Malarone Pediatric**, *atovaquone/proguanil*	250, 531
B		*maprotiline*, **Ludiomil**	110
B		*maraviroc*, **Selzentry**	513
C	III	**Marinol**, *dronabinol*	20, 269
C		**Marplan**, *isocarboxazid*	109
D		**Mavik**, *trandolapril*	175, 204
C		**Maxair, Maxair Autohaler**, *pirbuterol*	33
C		**Maxalt, Maxalt-MLT**, *rizatriptan*	168
C		**Maxaquin**, *lomefloxacin*	443, 535
C		**Maxidex Ophthalmic**, *dexamethasone*	85
C	II	**Maxidone**, *hydrocodone/ acetaminophen*	299
B		**Maxipime**, *cefepime*	534
C		**Maxitrol**, *neomycin/polymyxin B/ dexamethasone sodium phosphate*	91
C		**Maxzide**, *triamterene/ hydrochlorothiazide*	134, 177, 203
D	II	**Mebaral**, *mephobarbital*	509
C		*mebendazole*, **Emverm Vermox**	530
B		*mecasermin*, **Increlex**	166
B		*meclizine*, **Antivert, Bonine, Dramamine II, Zentrip**	243, 253, 259, 269, 448
B/D		*meclofenamate*	491
B		**Medihaler-ISO**, *isoproterenol*	32
C		**Medrol, Medrol Dosepak**, *methylprednisolone*	498

FDA Pregnancy Category	DEA Schedule	Drug	Page Numbers
C		Neosporin Ointment, Neosporin Ophthalmic Ointment, *neomycin/polymyxin B/bacitracin zinc*	394
C		*nepafenac*, Nevanac	88, 142, 297
C		Neptazane, *methazolamide*	158
C		Neupro Transdermal Patch, *rotigotine*	312, 367
C		Neurontin, *gabapentin*	116, 342, 366
C		Nevanac, *nepafenac*	88, 142, 297
C		*nevirapine*, Viramune	514
A		Neevo, Neevo DHA, *prenatal vitamins*	522
C		Nexiclon, Nexiclon XR, *clonidine*	208, 347
A		Nexa Plus, Nexa Select, *prenatal vitamins*	523
B		Nexium, *esomeprazole*	153, 318, 455
X		Nexplanon, *etonogestrel*	485
C		*niacin*, Niaspan, Slo-Niacin	129, 217
C		Niaspan, *niacin*	129, 217
C		*nicardipine*, Cardene, Cardene SR	17, 206
D		Nicoderm, Nicoderm CQ, *nicotine transdermal system*	407–408
X		Nicorette Gum, *nicotine polacrilex*	408
X		Nicorette Mini Lozenge, *nicotine polacrilex*	408
D		*nicotine nasal spray*, Nicotrol NS	408

FDA Pregnancy Category	DEA Schedule	Drug	Page Numbers
B		*penicillin v potassium*, **Pen-Vee K**	42, 55, 56, 75, 105, 141, 227, 326, 381, 411, 538, 572
NR		**Penlac Nail Laquer**, *ciclopirox topical solution*	227
C		**Pennsaid**, *diclofenac sodium*	297, 359, 489–490
C	IV	*pentazocine*, **Talwin**	303–305
D	II	*pentobarbital*, **Nembutal**	234
B		*pentosan polysulfate sodium*, **Elmiron**	236
C		*pentoxifylline*, **Trental**	322, 520
B		**Pen-Vee K**, *penicillin v potassium*	42, 55, 56, 75, 105, 141, 227, 326, 381, 411, 538, 572
B		**Pepcid, Pepcid AC, Pepcid RPD**, *famotidine*	152–153, 317
C		**Pepcid Complete**, *famotidine/CaCO2/Mg hydroxide*	153, 317
C/D		**Pepto-Bismol**, *bismuth subsalicylate*	119
C		*perampanel*, **Fycompa**	510
C	II	**Percocet**, *oxycodone/acetaminophen*	302–303
D	II	**Percodan, Percodan-Demi**, *oxycodone/oxycodone/terephthalate/aspirin*	303
C		**Peri-Colace**, *docusate/casanthranol*	97
B		**Peridex**, *chlorhexidine gluconate*	155
D		*perindopril*, **Aceon**	204
B		**PerioGard**, *chlorhexidine gluconate*	155

FDA Pregnancy Category	DEA Schedule	Drug	Page Numbers
C		**Stiolto Respimat,** *tiotropium/olodaterol*	64, 136
NR		**Strensiq,** *asfotase alfa*	222
D		*streptomycin*	328, 415, 533
X	III	**Striant,** *testosterone*	397
B		**Stribild,** *elvitegravir*	513
C	II	**Subsys,** *fentanyl citrate*	305
C	III	**Subutex,** *buprenorphine*	279
C		*succimer,* **Chemet**	238, 244
B		*sucralfate,* **Carafate**	142, 319
C		**Sular,** *nisoldipine*	206
C		*sulconazole,* **Exelderm, Extina**	401, 403, 404, 406
C		*sulfacetamide,* **Bleph-10, Cetamide, Isopto Cetamide, Klaron**	57, 90, 394
B/D		*sulfasalazine,* **Azulfidine, Azulfidine EN-Tabs**	435–436
C		*sulfinpyrazone,* **Anturane**	162
B/D		*sulfisoxazole,* **Gantrisin**	440–441, 538
C/D		*sulindac,* **Clinoril**	493
C		*sumatriptan,* **Alsuma Injectable, Imitrex, Imitrex Injectable, Imitrex Nasal Spray, Onzetra Xsail, Sumavel DosePro, Zecuity Transdermal, Zembrace SymTouch**	168
D		**Sumycin,** *tetracycline*	6, 27, 58, 62, 191, 247, 250, 339, 355, 377, 383, 391, 539, 574
B		**Suprax Oral Suspension,** *cefixime*	60, 292, 325, 382, 385, 410, 432, 441, 534, 552

FDA Pregnancy Category	DEA Schedule	Drug	Page Numbers
C		**Zembrace SymTouch,** *sumatriptan*	168
C		**Zemplar,** *paricalcitol*	198
C		**Zenpep,** *pancrelipase*	306–308
B		**Zentrip,** *meclizine*	243, 253, 259, 269, 447
B		**Zerbaxa,** *ceftolozane/tazobactam*	535
C		**Zerit,** *stavudine*	194, 515
C/D		**Zestoretic,** *lisinopril/ hydrochlorothiazide*	209
D		**Zestril,** *lisinopril*	175, 204
C		**Zetia,** *ezetimibe*	127
C		**Zetonna,** *ciclesonide*	374
C		**Ziac,** *bisoprolol/ hydrochlorothiazide*	211
C		**Ziagen,** *abacavir*	194, 515
C		**Ziana,** *tretinoin/clindamycin*	7
C		*ziconotide,* **Prialt**	306
C		*zidovudine, zdu,* **Retrovir**	194, 513
C		*zileuton,* **Zyflo, Zyflo CR**	28, 373
B		**Zinacef,** *cefuroxime*	534
C		**Zioptan,** *tafluprost*	158
C		*ziprasidone,* **Geodon**	50, 54, 508
C		**Zipsor,** *diclofenac potassium*	490
C		**Zirgan,** *ganciclovir*	242
B		**Zithromax, Zithromax Tri-Pak, Zmax,** *azithromycin*	42, 59, 71, 73, 76, 79–80, 82, 83, 93, 94, 160, 165, 225, 248, 249, 291, 322–324, 329–333, 336, 338, 380–383, 388, 409, 432, 437, 451, 536, 548